Oxford Medical Publications

A Life Course Approach to Women's Health

A Life Course Approach to Women's Health

Edited by

Diana Kuh

and

Rebecca Hardy

Medical Research Council National Survey of Health and
Development, Department of Epidemiology and Public Health
Royal Free and University College London Medical School

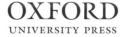

OXFORD
UNIVERSITY PRESS

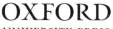

UNIVERSITY PRESS

Great Clarendon Street, Oxford OX2 6DP
Oxford University Press is a department of the University of Oxford.
It furthers the University's objective of excellence in research, scholarship,
and education by publishing worldwide in

Oxford New York
Auckland Bangkok Buenos Aires Cape Town Chennai
Dar es Salaam Delhi Hong Kong Istanbul Karachi Kolkata
Kuala Lumpur Madrid Melbourne Mexico City Mumbai Nairobi
São Paulo Shanghai Taipei Tokyo Toronto

Oxford is a registered trade mark of Oxford University Press
in the UK and in certain other countries

Published in the United States
by Oxford University Press, Inc., New York

A catalogue record for this title is available from the British Library.

Library of Congress Cataloging in Publication Data
A life course approach to women's health / edited by Diana Kuh and
Rebecca Hardy. (Life course approach to adult health; no. 1)

ISBN 0 19 263289 2 (Pbk.)

 1. Women–Health and hygiene.   2. Health promotion.
3. Epidemiology–Longitudinal studies.   4. Lifestyles–Health
aspects–Longitudinal studies.   5. Women–Health risk assessment.   I. Kuh,
Diana.   II. Hardy, Rebecca.   III. Series.

RA564.85 .L54 2002   613′.04244–dc21   2002075719

10 9 8 7 6 5 4 3 2 1

Typeset by Newgen Imaging Systems (P) Ltd., Chennai, India
Printed in Great Britain
on acid-free paper by
T. J. International Ltd, Padstow

*For our mothers and sisters, and
for Diana's daughter Ellie*

Foreword

The concept that early life experience determines health in later life is not new. After an investigation of the poor health of children in Aberdeen and Scotland, Leslie Mackenzie told the Royal Society of Edinburgh in 1905: "One truth we have already realized – if we would fit the man for his environment, we must begin with the child. 'The child is the father of the man.'" (see Harris, 2001).

In 1930 Andvord reported the outcome of tuberculosis in successive generations of Norwegians, the first quantitative medical study of the cohort effect. In 1934, Kermack, McKendrick, and McKinlay used data from England and Wales (1845–1925), Scotland (1860–1930), and Sweden (1755–1925) to show that birth cohorts with reduced mortality during childhood also experienced increased longevity throughout life (see Davey Smith, Kuh, 2001). Their analytic method was simple: Instead of reading cohort data in the conventional manner, down for each age group and across for each time period, Kermack's colleagues (Kermack himself was blind) drew freehand lines, one down for each age group and one across for each time period, an approach that (without computers or multivariate analysis) clearly showed a decline in death rates throughout the life course in successive generations. A generational approach to population data was rejected in the United Kingdom in 1949 because the effects of early life on adult health were largely attributed to the control of infectious diseases (see Kuh, Davey Smith, 1993).

A few papers examined the effects of early life on noncommunicable disease. In 1971, Abraham and colleagues reported that fat men whose school records showed that they were lean in childhood had more cardiovascular disease than those who had been fat all their lives. In 1984, Waaler reported that height (a surrogate for nutritional status in youth) was inversely associated with an excess risk of fatal cardiovascular disease and lung disease. Still, "With rather few exceptions, given such a dramatic illumination of a major biological and political issue, epidemiologists were slow to follow this lead." (Susser, 2001)

The life course theory of adult disease was rejuvenated by David Barker. Since 1986, Barker has built an impressive body of work showing that small babies or small/short children who become overweight adults are at an increased risk for cardiovascular disease, hypertension, diabetes, and other common chronic diseases (1986, 1992, 1998). Many papers by others followed, attempting either to discredit what is now called "the Barker hypothesis" or to debate the mechanism for a true association. Although the debate continues as to the mechanism(s) (social class, tobacco habit, fetal programming, stress, nutrition, thrifty phenotype, and so on), it is increasingly clear that many adult diseases are strongly influenced by fetal life or early childhood experiences. Childhood and adult health and longevity are also determined by the biologic consequences of the wealth of society and how it is distributed; how civil institutions buffer or exacerbate chronic stress and promote or undermine healthy living; and the nature of the family unit interaction (see Hertzman and Wiens, 1996). The complexity of these effects should keep those who are interested in the life course and the public health busy "sorting it out" for several more generations.

Although many questions remain, this thoughtful book that provides an excellent review of the evidence should persuade almost everyone that perinatal and childhood factors, some potentially modifiable, determine the risk of adult disease; the implications go beyond the study of risk factor-outcomes in individuals and point to community approaches (from whence the original observations came) to preventive medicine and social health solutions. The implications are particularly large for women, who as mothers provide multiple social, behavioral, and biological imprints, in utero and thereafter, that may determine the biological promise or vulnerability of children throughout life. The child is the mother of the woman and the man!

Elizabeth Barrett-Connor, M.D.
Division of Epidemiology
Department of Family and Preventive Medicine
University of California, San Diego
La Jolla, CA 92093-0607

References

Abraham S, Collins G, Nordsieck M. Relationship of childhood weight status to morbidity in adults. *HSMHA Health Rep* 1971;**86**:273–84.

Andvord KF. What can we learn from studying tuberculosis by generations? *Norsk Mag Loegevidensk* 1930;**91**:642–60.

Barker DJP, Osmond C. Infant mortality, childhood nutrition, and ischaemic heart disease in England and Wales. *Lancet* 1986;**1**:1077–81.

Barker DJP. *Mothers, Babies and Health in Later Life.* Edinburgh: Churchill Livingstone, 1998.

Davey Smith G, Kuh D. Commentary: William Ogilvy Kermack and the childhood origins of adult health and disease. *Int J Epidemiol* 2001;**30**:696–703.

Harris B. "The child is father of the man." The relationship between child health and adult mortality in the 19th and 20th centuries. *Int J Epidemiol* 2001;**30**:688–96.

Hertzman C, Wiens M. Child development and long-term outcomes: a population health perspective and summary of successful interventions. *Soc Sci Med* 1996;**43**:1083–95.

Kermack WO, McKendrick AG, McKinlay PL. Death rates in great Britain and Sweden: expression of specific mortality rates as products of two factors, and some consequences thereof. *J Hyg* 1934;**3334**:433–51.

Kermack WO, McKendrick AG, McKinlay PL. Death rates in great Britain and Sweden: some general regularities and their significance. *Lancet* 1934;**1**:698–70.

Kuh D, Davey Smith G. When is mortality risk determined? Historical insights into a current debate. *Soc Hist Med* 1993;**6**:101–23.

Susser M. Commentary: The longitudinal perspective and cohort analysis. *Int J Epidemiol* 2001;**30**:684–87.

Waaler HT. Height, weight and mortality. The Norwegian experience. *Acta Med Scand Suppl.* 1984;**679**:1–56.

Preface

In recent years women's health research has benefited enormously from the study of social and biological risk factors in integrated rather than competing aetiological models but the emphasis on adult factors remains. New epidemiological research shows the long-term importance of fetal and childhood experience in the development of common chronic diseases and disorders that pose the main threats to physical and mental health in midlife and beyond. It has been the catalyst for the development of a life course approach in epidemiology that studies the combined effects of both early and later life factors on adult health and disease risk. The aim of this book is to bring this research, scattered across the scientific literature, to the attention of those with an interest in women's health, and challenge the current emphasis on contemporary experience, particularly adult lifestyle. Contributors show how a life course approach can offer new insights into the causes of women's common health problems.

Our long-term interest in childhood influences on adult health comes from our work on the Medical Research Council National Survey of Health and Development. This is a prospective longitudinal study of over 5000 women and men who have been followed up since their birth in England, Scotland and Wales in March 1946. Our interest in women's health in midlife was stimulated by the information we collected from the women in this cohort about their health and social experiences during the menopause transition. We find that their midlife experiences relate in all kinds of expected and novel ways to their life history. Yet the literature on women's health and the literature on childhood origins of adult health rarely overlap. We decided to invite colleagues with expertise in a particular health problem to pull together these two strands of research. Authors of the chapters undertook a comprehensive review of the literature, interpreting the evidence and discussing the possible social and biological pathways through which experiences in earlier life might shape specific adult health outcomes. Other contributors provided commentaries on these chapters. In all, forty-eight researchers contributed to this book. Their interest and support for the project was terrific and this book would not have happened without them.

The range of health outcomes covered in this volume is wide and includes reproductive outcomes (menarche, pregnancy and menopause), breast cancer, cardiovascular disease, diabetes, musculoskeletal ageing, depression and psychological distress, body weight and body dissatisfaction. Even though each chapter reflects the views of individual authors, shared aims and a common life course framework provide a more consistent approach than is usual in such a broad collection of chapters. This conceptual framework is summarised in the introductory chapter. Key findings, common themes, and theoretical and methodological challenges are highlighted in the concluding chapter. It is not possible in one volume to cover all possible adult health outcomes where there is evidence of long-term early life influences. The life course framework is widely applicable and later books in the series will develop the ideas with respect to other topics such cognitive function, and other aspects of mental health.

As editors, this book has been an exciting and immense challenge. We have had thought provoking exchanges with contributors and forged new friendships and collaborations as a result. Most of the chapters were first presented at a one-day conference in Oxford, England in September 2001. It has been a privilege to edit this book and we have both gained an enormous amount from doing so. We thank all our contributors very much for their hard work. Special thanks are also extended to our families, friends, and colleagues who were so supportive of our involvement in this project. Jill Skehan's administrative help was invaluable at critical moments. Finally, we would like to give a special thanks to the women in the 1946 birth cohort study who have so kindly and willingly provided information about their lives.

London   D.K.
June 2002   R.H.

Acknowledgements

The authors would like to thank the following for permission to reproduce published material: Figure 2.1 reproduced from Ellison PT. Morbidity, mortality, and menarche. *Hum Biol* 1981;53:635–43 by permission of Wayne State University Press; Figure 3.1 reprinted from British Journal of Cancer Volume 83, De Stavola BL, Hardy R, Kuh D, dos Santos Silva I, Wadsworth M, Swerdlow AJ. Birthweight, childhood growth and risk of breast cancer in a British birth cohort, 964–8, 2000 by permission of the Nature Publishing Group; Figures 5.1 and 5.2 reproduced from Lawlor DA, Ebrahim S, Davey Smith G. Sex matters: secular and geographical trends in sex differences in ischaemic heart disease mortality. *Br Med J* 2001; 323:541–545 with permission of BMJ Publishing Group; Figure 10.10 reproduced from Chrousos GP. Integration of the immune and endocrine systems by interleukin-6, pp. 133–134. In: Papanicolaou DA. Moderator. The pathophysiologic roles of interleukin-6 in human disease. *Ann Intern Med* 1998;**128**:127–37 by permission of the American College of Physicians-American Society of Internal Medicine; Figure 10.11 reproduced from Yen SSC. Adrenal andropause and aging. *J Anti-Aging Med* 2000;**3**:315–28 by permission of Mary Ann Liebert, Inc., Publishers; Figures 16.1,16.2a and figure 16.2b reproduced from Kuh D and Davey Smith G, *When is mortality risk determined? Historical insights into a current debate*, Social History of Medicine 1993;6:101–23, by permission of Oxford University Press; figures 16.3a and 16.3b prepared by the Lung and Asthma Information Agency, St George's Hospital Medical School, London; figures 16.4a and 16.4b and figure 16.6 (updated) from Swerdlow A, Dos Santos Silva I and Doll R, *Cancer incidence and mortality in England and Wales: trends and risk factors* (2001), reproduced by permission of Oxford University Press; figure 16.5 reproduced from *Br J Cancer*, 73, Hermon C, Beral V. Breast cancer mortality rates are levelling off or beginning to decline in many western countries: an analysis of time trends, age-cohort and age-period models of breast cancer mortality in 20 countries, 955–60,1996, by permission of the publisher Churchill Livingstone; figure 16.7 reproduced from Kuh D.Power C, Rodgers B. Secular trends in social class and sex differences in height. *Int J Epidemiol* 1991;20:1001–9, by permission of Oxford University Press; Table 16.1 reproduced from Leon DA, Davey Smith G. Infant mortality, stomach cancer, stroke, and coronary heart disease: ecological analysis. *Br Med J* 2000;320:1705–6, by permission of BMJ Publishing Group.

Contents

Contributors

Dr Avan Aihie Sayer
MRC Clinical Scientist and Honorary Senior
Lecturer in Geriatric Medicine, MRC
Environmental Epidemiology Unit, University
of Southampton.

Kristy Ashleman
PhD student and Assistant Faculty Associate,
Human Development and Family Studies,
School of Human Ecology, University of
Wisconsin-Madison.

Professor Elizabeth Barrett-Connor
Professor and Chief, Division of Epidemiology,
Department of Family and Preventive Medicine,
School of Medicine, University of California,
San Diego.

Professor Mel Bartley
Professor in Medical Sociology, Department
of Epidemiology and Public Health, Royal Free
and University College London Medical School.

Dr Joan Bassey
Honorary Senior Research Fellow, School of
Biomedical Sciences, University of Nottingham.

Dr Yoav Ben-Shlomo
Senior Lecturer in Clinical Epidemiology,
Department of Social Medicine, University
of Bristol.

Professor Jane Cauley
Associate Professor, Department of
Epidemiology, University of Pittsburgh,
Pennsylvania.

Professor Nish Chaturvedi
Department of Epidemiology and Public
Health, Division of Primary Care & Population
Health Sciences, Imperial College School
of Medicine, London.

Professor Helen M Colhoun
Professor of Clinical Epidemiology, Eurodiab,
Department of Epidemiology and Public Health,
Royal Free & University College London Medical
School.

Professor Cyrus Cooper
Professor of Rheumatology, MRC
Environmental Epidemiology Unit,
University of Southampton.

Professor Sybil Crawford
Associate Professor, University of Massachusetts
School of Medicine, Worcester, Massachusetts.

Dr Bianca L De Stavola
Senior Lecturer in Medical Statistics, Medical
Statistics Unit, Department of Epidemiology
and Population Health, London School of
Hygiene and Tropical Medicine.

Dr William H Dietz
Director, Division of Nutrition and
Physical Activity, Centers for Disease
Control and Prevention, Atlanta, Georgia.

Professor George Davey Smith
Professor of Clinical Epidemiology, Department
of Social Medicine, University of Bristol.

Professor Shah Ebrahim
Professor of the Epidemiology of Ageing,
Department of Social Medicine,
University of Bristol.

Professor Rebecca Fuhrer
Department of Epidemiology and
Biostatistics and Occupational Health,
McGill University, Montreal.

Professor Hilary Graham
Professor of Social Policy, Department of
Applied Social Science, University of Lancaster.

Professor Ronald H Gray
John Hopkins University, School of Hygiene
and Public Health, Baltimore.

Professor Andrew J Hall
Professor of Infectious Disease Epidemiology,
Head of Unit of Infectious Disease
Epidemiology, London School of Hygiene and
Tropical Medicine.

Dr Rebecca Hardy
Medical Statistician, Medical Research Council
National Survey of Health and Development and
Honorary Senior Lecturer
Department of Epidemiology and Public Health,
Royal Free and University College London
Medical School.

Dr Kate Hunt
Senior Research Scientist, MRC Social and
Public health Sciences Unit, University
of Glasgow.

Dr Catherine Johannes
Epidemiologist, Ingenix Epidemiology,
Auburndale, WA.

Dr Quarraisha Karim
Southern African Fogarty AIDS training
Programme and Nelson R Mandela School
of Medicine, University of Natal, and Division
of Epidemiology, Columbia University.

Dr Diana Kuh
Senior Research Scientist, Medical Research
Council National Survey of Health and
Development and Professor of Life Course
Epidemiology, Department of Epidemiology
and Public Health, Royal Free &
University College London
Medical School.

Dr Catherine Law
Senior Lecturer, MRC Environmental
Epidemiology Unit, University of
Southampton.

Dr Debbie A Lawlor
MRC Research Fellow, Department of
Social Medicine, University of Bristol.

Professor David A Leon
Professor of Epidemiology, Department of
Epidemiology and Public Health, London
School of Hygiene and Tropical Medicine.

Professor Nadine F Marks
Associate Professor and Chair, Human
Development and Family Studies, School of
Human Ecology, University of
Wisconsin-Madison.

Dr Barbara Maughan
Reader, MRC Social, Genetic and Developmental
Psychiatry Research Centre, Institute of
Psychiatry, King's College, London.

Lindsay McLaren
PhD student, G.R.I.S., University of Montreal.

Dr Susan Morton,
PhD Student, Epidemiology Unit, Department
of Epidemiology and Population Health,
London School of Hygiene and Tropical
Medicine.

Dr Tessa Parsons
Lecturer, Centre for Paediatric Epidemiology
and Biostatistics, Institute of Child Health,
Royal Free & University College Medical
School, London.

Dr Nancy Potischman
Applied Research Program, Division
of Cancer Control and Population Sciences,
National Cancer Institute, Bethesda,
Maryland.

Professor Chris Power
Professor of Epidemiology & Public Health,
Centre for Paediatric Epidemiology and
Biostatistics, Institute of Child Health, Royal
Free & University College Medical School,
London.

Professor Janet Rich-Edwards
Assistant Professor, Department of Ambulatory
Care & Prevention, Harvard Medical School
and Harvard Pilgrim Health Care.

Dr Bryan Rodgers
Senior Fellow, Psychiatric Epidemiology
Research Centre, The Australian National
University, Canberra.

Dr Amanda Sacker
Senior Research Fellow, Department of
Epidemiology and Public Health, Royal
Free & University College London
Medical School.

Dr Isabel dos Santos Silva
Senior Lecturer in Epidemiology, Cancer
and Public Health Unit, Department of
Epidemiology and Population Health,
London School of Hygiene and Tropical
Medicine.

Dr Mary Schooling
Graduate of Department of Epidemiology and
Public Health, Royal Free & University College
London Medical School.

Dr Ingrid Schoon
Senior Lecturer in Psychology, City
University, London.

Professor David Serwadda
Institute of Public Health, Makerere University,
Kampala, Uganda.

Professor Stephen Stansfeld
Professor of Psychiatry, St Bartholomew's
and the Royal London School of Medicine
and Dentistry.

Professor Zena Stein
HIV Centre and New York State Psychiatric
Institute, Joseph L Mailman School of Public
Health, Columbia University, New York.

Professor Mervyn Susser
Emeritus Professor of Epidemiology
and Director of the Sergievsky Centre,
Columbia, New York.

Professor J Kevin Thompson
Professor of Psychology, University
of South Florida, Tampa, Florida.

Professor Carol M Worthman
Director of the Laboratory for Comparative
Human Biology, and Samuel Chandler Dobbs
Professor of Anthropology,
Emory University.

Professor Jane Wardle
Head of the Health Behaviour Unit,
Department of Epidemiology and
Public Health, Royal Free and University
College London Medical School.

Professor Maria J Wawer
Center for Population and Family
Health, New York.

Part I

Introduction

Chapter 1

A life course approach to women's health: does the past predict the present?

Diana Kuh and Rebecca Hardy

Chronic diseases become increasingly prevalent in midlife and present the main threat to women's health. The emphasis on adult lifestyle as the cause of these diseases is being increasingly challenged by research showing that the sources of risk may lie much earlier in life, or even in previous generations. A life course approach, introduced in this chapter and developed in the chapters that follow, assesses the biological and social factors at each stage of life that affect adult health outcomes. Particular attention is paid to the growing evidence for long-term effects of risk factors during childhood or fetal life on the more common chronic diseases and disorders in women. These are hypothesized to act through developmental processes. A life course approach also studies the biological, psychological, and social pathways that link early life experiences, reproductive events, conventional adult risk factors and health outcomes in later life. It asks whether the emerging life course models of health provide explanations for long-term disease trends, and whether they are relevant for understanding the future health of women now reaching middle-age in developed and less developed countries. This life course approach complements and extends recent research on women's health that has also emphasized the interactive nature of biological and social risk processes on disease risk but pays less attention to a temporal perspective. By bringing together these two strands of research this book makes a unique contribution to interdisciplinary research, offers important new insights into the causes of women's health and provides challenges for future life course research.

1.1 Introduction and overview

The central theme of this book is that the health of middle-aged and older women is shaped by biological, social, and psychosocial processes operating throughout life. The main causes of the burden of disease and disability in women aged 45–59 years living in established

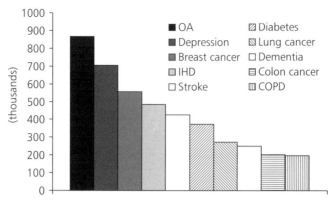

Fig. 1.1 Ten leading female DALYS (thousands) 45–59 years. Established market economies 1990.[1]

DALYS Disability Adjusted Life Years; OA Osteoarthritis; COPD Chronic Obstructive Pulmonary Disease.

market economies are cardiovascular diseases, cancers, osteoarthritis, depression, and diabetes[1] (Fig. 1.1). There is growing evidence that the sources of risk for these diseases occur across the life course, not just in adult life, and in some instances reach right back into fetal life, or the previous generation.[2–4] Contributors to this book use a life course approach[4,5] (Section 1.2) to review and examine the biological and social factors during gestation, childhood, adolescence, young adulthood, and later adult life that affect health outcomes in women. They bring together scientific evidence scattered across a number of disciplines to elucidate the pathways linking childhood experience to adult life.

Much of the evidence for the early origins of adult disease comes from cohort studies linking ischaemic heart disease, stroke, and diabetes in adulthood to body size at birth, in infancy or childhood. Many of the early studies, reviewed elsewhere,[6] had either few women or none at all (Section 1.4.1). This is now changing and it is time to review the findings for women, consider explanations for any gender differences, and set these findings alongside adolescent and adult sources of risk, including those that are unique to women such as reproductive factors. We thought it would be informative (and perhaps lead to a cross fertilization of ideas) to do the same for the literature on depression and psychological distress where there is a long tradition of research on their childhood origins. We also extend the life course approach to study other health outcomes of particular concern for women such as reproductive health, breast cancer, menopause and urogenital disorders, musculoskeletal disorders, and body image. These topics are all considered in Part II of this book.

The various biological and social pathways that link childhood to adult life are considered in Part III. This section begins with an up-to-date review of the development and ageing of the endocrine system, and the hormonal pathways across the life course that play a key role in the development of disease, the maintenance of health, and the rate of ageing of other body systems. Exposure to infectious diseases earlier in life can have long-term health consequences, and are particularly important in developing countries where these diseases are more prevalent. The impact of sexually transmitted diseases on the health of women and their offspring is the focus of the final chapter in Part III. Other chapters in Part III are concerned with the life course development of what are conventionally described as adult risk factors, such as health behaviours, body weight, social class, and social support. To the extent that these risk factors have their origins earlier in life they may help to explain the links between the childhood environment and adult health.

The research findings reviewed in this book come mainly from studies of women born in the first half of the twentieth century in the established market economies. In Part IV we first consider whether some of the early life risk factors that have been identified in these studies can also explain disease trends in these countries. The other chapter in Part IV examines cohort-related effects of extensive social and political change, and simultaneous change in the disease environment, on the life course and health experiences of Black women in South Africa. In Part V we conclude by drawing together our key findings and discussing their relevance for policy and for the future health of women born in the post-war period who are just reaching middle-age.

We hope that this book will stimulate others to apply a life course perspective to women's health. To further this goal, there are discussants for each of the chapters. Their role is to highlight the key points raised and gaps in current knowledge, and to assess the ways in which a life course approach could lead to new insights in their research field. Their commentaries are included at the end of each chapter. The following sections highlight the main themes of this book and link them to the chapters that follow.

1.2 An introduction to life course epidemiology

A life course approach offers an interdisciplinary framework or orientation for guiding and structuring research on health, human development, and ageing. Such an approach has been actively promoted for a long time in many scientific disciplines, including psychology, sociology, demography, anthropology, and biology.[7–10] Epidemiologists have been more recent converts.[5,11] As discussed elsewhere,[5] life course epidemiology has borrowed many of its concepts and ideas from these other scientific disciplines.[12–14]

Life course epidemiology starts from the premise that various biological and social factors throughout life, independently, cumulatively, and interactively, influence health and disease.[4,5] Investigation of this premise naturally starts at the beginning of life and assesses risk chronologically. Particular attention is paid to the long-term effects of risk factors acting in early life because of new and exciting research linking growth and development with adult chronic disease (Section 1.2.1) and to redress the balance on adult factors in most post war aetiological models of adult disease.

A life course approach to adult disease does not deny the importance of adult risk factors, such as smoking and obesity, that were so successfully identified by the early post war adult cohort studies. The purpose is to study the contribution of early life factors jointly with these later life risk factors to identify risk and protective pathways across the life course. We need to investigate whether childhood risk factors operate mainly through their effects on conventional adult risk factors, or whether they add independent risk or act interactively with later life factors to affect adult disease. Identification of pathways across the life course may have important policy implications, by highlighting the type and timing of interventions for maximum impact on health.

The following two sections introduce some of the childhood risk and protective factors that have been the subject of investigation in life course epidemiology and briefly outline some of the biological and social pathways that link childhood and adult health and disease.

1.2.1 Childhood risk and protective factors

The idea that childhood is important for adult health is not new in epidemiology or public health but was the prevailing model of health in the first half of the twentieth century. It was the rationale behind many of the maternal and child state welfare reforms that were instigated in the emerging industrial economies.[15,16] From the 1930s, as attention turned to the causes of adult chronic disease which lay behind the lack of improvement in middle-age mortality, an initial interest in the possible childhood origins of some of these chronic diseases gave way to an emphasis on adult risk factors.[17] In cardiovascular epidemiology, the adult lifestyle model dominated the post war era, with some notable exceptions.[18,19] In other research areas, such as adult respiratory disease,[20] and mental function,[21] early life sources of risk continued to be given attention.[5] A revival of interest in the role of early life factors in cardiovascular disease from the late 1970s stemmed first from the need to understand the natural history of adult risk factors (such as hypertension, smoking, fatty diets, and obesity). Secondly, and more importantly, it stemmed from ecological studies and imaginative historical cohort studies that linked poor childhood living conditions and impaired early growth to adult cardiovascular disease.

The research undertaken by David Barker and his research team at the MRC Environmental Epidemiology Unit in Southampton, England was particularly influential in raising the profile of early life factors during the 1980s and 1990s. They traced the whereabouts of hundreds of middle-aged and elderly British men and women for whom birth records had been kept by certain health visitors and hospitals between 1911 and 1944.[2,22] Various markers of poor fetal or infant body size (such as low weight at birth or at one year, or thinness or shortness at birth) were found to be associated with an increased risk of ischaemic heart disease, stroke, diabetes, respiratory disease and their associated adult risk factors such as high blood pressure and insulin resistance. According to Barker's fetal origins hypothesis,[2,23] environmental insults such as undernutrition during critical periods of growth and development have long-term effects on adult disease risk by 'programming' the structure or function of organs, tissues, or body systems.[24] A question of central importance for life course epidemiology and for public health is the extent to which the effects of programming are reversible or can be modified by later experience. In other words, how critical are critical periods?[5]

A life course approach incorporates, but is broader than, Barker's concept of 'biological programming'. It also examines whether different patterns of growth during childhood and adolescence are associated with later differential health risks. Distinguishing the effects of prenatal and postnatal growth on adult disease and assessing whether height or weight gain at particular stages of life modify the effect of impaired early growth are topics of current investigation. This was prompted by studies showing that the relationships between low birthweight (or ponderal index at birth) and increased risk of coronary heart disease, high blood pressure, and insulin resistance were particularly strong for overweight adults.[25–27] Although poor early growth has generally been identified as a health risk to date, the possible health risks associated with rapid growth, either *in utero* or in childhood, also need to be studied. Given the current epidemic of child and adult obesity in the developed and the developing world such research could have important public health implications for younger cohorts. The separate and joint effects of early growth and later body size are considered in relation to reproductive health (menarche and pregnancy in Chapter 2 and menopause in Chapter 4) breast cancer (Chapter 3), cardiovascular disease (Chapter 5), diabetes (Chapter 6), and musculoskeletal disorders (Chapter 7). Contributors discuss the possible underlying processes involved, for example maternal nutrition and genetic susceptibility.

There is also growing evidence, discussed in many of the chapters, that childhood social and economic factors have long-term effects on adult health independent of the later socioeconomic environment.[28–34] How do these factors leave enduring biological imprints and shape subsequent behaviour?[35–37] While some mechanisms operate through their effects on physical growth and maturation, others operate through effects on psychological and intellectual development. Childhood and adolescence are times of rapid accumulation of social and cognitive skills, habits, coping strategies, attitudes, and values. There is evidence of sensitive developmental stages in childhood when these skills and abilities are most easily acquired, although they may still be developed later with greater difficulty.[34,38] These abilities and skills strongly influence life course social and behavioural trajectories with implications for health in later life (see Chapters 8, 9, 11, 12, and 13).

1.2.2 Life course pathways to adult health and disease

The proponents of biological programming suggest that an adverse environment during rapid physical growth or development may lead to irreparable damage to some underlying structure and possibly its later function. Their focus is generally on risks during gestation or in the first few years of life. Those interested in psychosocial and behavioural development describe how childhood adversity may set into motion a 'chain of risk' where one bad experience tends to lead to another that leads to another in a cumulative way continuing into adulthood.[39] Protective chains may also occur where one advantage leads to another advantage and so on with long-term beneficial outcomes. These models promote adolescence and young adulthood as key life stages because many life transitions are negotiated during this time (decisions about education, further training, or personal relationships for example) which may act as key links in the lifetime chains of advantage and adversity. More general models of risk accumulation describe the long-term gradual damage to health from various environmental or behavioural insults individuals are exposed to over the life course.[40] Different types of life course models are discussed more fully elsewhere.[5,41]

Reproductive events, from puberty to pregnancy and menopause are markers of chronic disease risk and may form part of a chain of risk between early and adult life. In Chapter 2, Rich-Edwards examines earlier life influences on reproductive health such as pregnancy outcome, menstrual function, infertility, and polycystic ovary syndrome. She argues that the impact of early life factors may already be manifest in the health of young adults, although the effects may not come to clinical attention until middle-age. Pregnancy, due to its physiological stress, offers an interesting window into this process in young women. All the chapters on health outcomes review the role of reproductive events and try to distinguish between underlying biological and social processes.[42] Social determinants of sexual activity and reproduction are strong; childbearing and child rearing may impact on health by changing life trajectories and exposure to socioeconomic circumstances, stress and social support, as well as by altering physiological or psychological characteristics.[43] Timing of childbirth can also have an intergenerational effect on the adult health of offspring.[44]

We need to look to the endocrine system to understand the biological processes that underlie the links between indicators of childhood growth, reproductive events and later adult disease discussed in various chapters. Worthman argues that hormones play 'central roles in the physiological architecture of the human life course' mediating for example, the relationships between environmental, behavioural, and developmental factors and risks to adult health.[9] In Chapter 10 she outlines the life course trajectories of endocrine activity for women in western populations, with respect to a set of key endocrine axes, namely hypothalamo–pituitary–gonadal (HPG), hypothalamo–pituitary–adrenal (HPA), hypothal-amo–pituitary–thyroid (HPT), and weight regulation (lipostatic). Some hormones, such as the ovarian steroids, adrenal androgens, insulin-like growth factors and leptin, show consid-erable age related change. Although endocrine factors and the main functional pathways are nearly universal, the degree of individual variation may be very large. Worthman discusses the environmental, developmental, and behavioural factors that influence this variation and some of the consequences for women's health.

A life course perspective helps us understand better the ways in which conventional risk factors such as adult health behaviours and social class affect adult disease and how they may form part of lifetime chains of risk. First, it highlights the growing evidence that shows the effects of these risk factors vary by the timing[45] or duration[46–48] of exposure. Contributors address these questions when they investigate the relationships of exercise, diet, weight, and social position to adult health outcomes. Second, it draws attention to the lifelong processes that shape women's adult lives. Social, psychosocial, and biological chains of risk that link environment and behaviour in childhood, adolescence, and early adult life to adult social position, health damaging behaviours, or overweight and obesity are considered in Chapters 11, 13, and 14. In Chapter 12 what is known about life course influences on women's social relationships in the middle years is reviewed, including those that provide social support and those that involve care-giving, and are thus likely to impact on health. Sensitivity to the temporal as well as the current social context of women's lives (Sections 1.3.3 and 1.4.2) should guide policy on these conventional risk factors.

Early research into the childhood origins of disease probably underplayed the role of genetic factors in the development of disease risk. The growing genetic knowledge, specific-ally the development of the field of genetic epidemiology and of cheap and reliable methods to analyse DNA on large population samples, has opened up possibilities for studying the joint and interactive effects of genetic and environmental factors in studies of the life course. The role of genetic factors in the development of disease risk and possible genetic-environment interactions are discussed in several of the chapters.

1.3 Explaining patterns of disease using a life course perspective

The research findings on lifetime risk factors for chronic diseases reviewed in this book come mainly from individual-level population studies of women born in the first half of the twentieth century in what are now the established market economies. This raises a number of important questions. First, will the factors at each life stage that explain the development of disease risk in these cohorts also explain temporal trends? Second, what relevance do these findings have for women in less developed countries? Third, what relevance do they have for cohorts of women born in the second half of the twentieth century given the dramatic social changes that have affected women's lives?

1.3.1 Disease trends over time

Life expectancy has improved dramatically for the populations of the established market economies since the middle of the nineteenth century. There has also been a convergence in

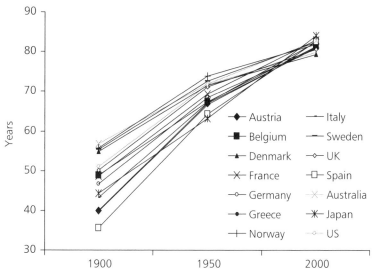

Fig. 1.2 Life expectancy in various industrial countries.[49]

life expectancy across these populations (Fig. 1.2).[49] In 1900 women in Australia and Scandanavia had the longest life expectancy at birth (55–56 years) and women in Austria, Greece, Spain, and Japan had the worst (44 years or less). In 2000 life expectancy had increased by about 30 years, the range was much narrower (79.3–84.1 years) and Japanese women had the best and Danish women the worst life expectancy at birth. The improvement in life expectancy has been due mainly to the decline of mortality from childhood infectious disease since the nineteenth century as health conditions, such as sanitation and nutritional standards, improved. There has been a time lag between the decline in child mortality and the decline in adult mortality. This raises a question about the extent to which improvements in childhood health (for example, in terms of fewer infections or better growth and development) that accompanied the decline in child mortality may have contributed to lower morbidity and mortality in adult life. Alternatively, better environmental conditions and changes in health care practices in adult life may have been responsible for the decline. This question is addressed further in Chapter 16 which discusses the decline of adult mortality in established market economies. Trends in various growth indicators (birthweight, height, and age at menarche) over the last 150 years are compared with long-term trends in breast cancer and cardiovascular diseases. We chose to examine patterns of growth because they are an important focus of current life course models and because 'the health implications of reaching reproductive and physical maturity at earlier ages, and achieving larger adult sizes, remain poorly understood.'[50]

1.3.2 Women in less developed countries

Many of the diseases that contribute most to death and disability among middle-aged women (45–59 years) in less developed countries are the same as those affecting women of this age in the established market economies, including cardiovascular disease, osteoarthritis, breast cancer, and depression.[1,51] Prevalence estimates are more uncertain because data are less available and often of poorer quality than in more developed countries. We do not yet know whether the factors at each life stage that explain the development of risk for these diseases in women living in established market economies can be generalized to women living in less developed countries, who may have very different life experiences. Davey Smith and Egger[52] argue that 'for different causes of death (or disease), and in different temporal and geographical situations, the determinants of mortality patterns (disease and health) will be distinct' (p. 1585). Tuberculosis, cervical cancer, and liver cirrhosis also contribute to the high disease burden among middle-aged women in less developed countries.[1] They provide other examples of 'life course' diseases, where infectious diseases acquired at younger ages are linked to adult chronic disease[53,54] (see Chapter 15). In addition, recent data are revealing the truly horrifying epidemic of human immunodeficiency virus (HIV) infection and acquired immunodeficiency syndrome (AIDS) on women in regions such as sub-Saharan Africa[55] which lies behind the rising mortality in young adult women in the 1990s from that region (see Chapter 17).

1.3.3 The impact of social change

The social, economic, and political status of women changed during the twentieth century although the pace of change varied widely across countries. Many of the changes will have affected particularly the life trajectories of women who were young in the post war period. These are the cohorts who are now beginning to reach middle-age. How will their life experiences, so different from the lives of their mothers and grandmothers (on whom the evidence for a life course model of health has so far been mainly based) change the prevailing patterns of health and disease in later life? For example, in established market economies women now have more opportunities in their working and personal lives, although the benefits have not been distributed equally across socioeconomic or ethnic groups. They are better educated and trained than previous cohorts and, partly because of this improvement in human capital, wage differentials between men and women, although still substantial, have declined.[56] There has been a striking increase in labour force participation, particularly in part-time work by married women.[57,58] Women are less likely to be married and more likely to be single or cohabiting.[59,60] Childbearing is becoming increasingly delayed, more women are remaining childless or having fewer children and the proportion of women's lives spent rearing their children has been reduced.[57,61,62] The increasing rates of divorce[60] and births outside marriage[63] have resulted in more single-mother households and these households have a high rate of poverty compared with two-parent households.[64] Higher divorce rates, changing patterns of family care, and the increase in life expectancy means that many older women live on their own, often in relative poverty.[65,66] Medical intervention is becoming increasingly sophisticated in postponing death, and possibly disability,[67,68] at least for those with access to high standards of health care. The benefits and costs of the mass 'natural experiments' of oral contraceptive use and hormone replacement therapy are still being assessed.[69–71] Trends in adult health behaviours and obesity (discussed in Chapters 13 and 14) are strongly related to lifetime socioeconomic circumstances and are affected by changing cultural norms and suggest a mixed impact on trends in women's health.

The long-term impact on health of perhaps less obvious changes that have occurred in the lives of women during childhood and adolescence is even harder to assess. The changing expectations of society towards women may bring extra pressures as well as extra opportunities, particularly in adolescence, perhaps leading to a greater uptake of risky health behaviours. There may be long-term effects on women's disease patterns of the recent trends in growth and age at menarche (discussed in Chapter 16) or in parental divorce. As yet, little is known about trends in other important risk factors, such as violence against girls and women. We do know from piecing together the evidence that intimate partner abuse, rape, and sexual assault of women is common.[72,73] The more limited evidence for physical, sexual, and emotional abuse and neglect of children suggests this is also widespread.[72] Prospective[74] as well as retrospective studies[75] demonstrate numerous long-term health consequences.

Short-term disruptions caused by wars, famine, and economic downturns can have long-term influences on social and health trajectories that vary according to age and thus play out in a cohort fashion.[21,76,77] Similarly, the cohort effects of a rapidly changing disease environment (as brought about, for example, by the epidemic of HIV infection) can be relatively easily observed with appropriate data (see Chapter 17). However, most of the social changes described above reflect long-term trends in market economies. Where strong and known relationships exist between risk factors and disease, for example between smoking and lung cancer, it may be possible to predict the future pattern of disease with some certainty. However the multifactorial causes of most chronic diseases, the distal nature of most social factors in relation to disease, and the possible interactions between risk factors complicate most predictions. We are only just beginning to learn about the changing psychosocial environment and how this may affect the secular trends in psychological distress[78] or health behaviours. How rapid or extensive social and political change in the context of continuing deprivation impacts differentially on the psychological and biological attributes of successive cohorts is still a challenge to be faced. In Chapter 17, Stein and her colleagues respond to this challenge by considering the effects of political liberation in South Africa on the life course of two different cohorts of women.

Thus a life course approach, with a focus on lifetime social as well as biological risk, encourages us to study social change and how it might affect the generalizability of epidemiological findings. At the simplest level it may mean that the relative importance of certain diseases, or certain causes of disease, will increase or diminish. Generalizability is also limited because risk factors are usually only markers of underlying disease processes and the meaning of these markers may change over time. For example the stress of being an immigrant may be different in areas where they represent a significant sized group in the population compared with areas where few immigrants live.[79] The impact of divorce for parents and for their children may vary according to whether divorce is a common event in a society. Even markers of biological risk like birthweight may change their meaning over time with the changing prevalence of different risk factors that cause low birthweight. Thus 'extrapolating from the past to the present and from one place to another can only be the start of the more difficult empirical task of understanding the particular factors which act together to produce the patterns seen in any one specific instance' (p. 1585).[52]

1.4 The study of women's lives and health experiences: challenges and opportunities

1.4.1 The availability of life course data on women

Life course epidemiology has studied women less than men. This partly reflects its original focus on cardiovascular disease. Epidemiological research into the aetiology of cardiovascular disease, although important to the health of both sexes, has paid little attention to women until recently. The early post war cohorts that were set up to investigate the role of proximal risk factors (such as hypertension or diabetes) and aspects of adult lifestyle on cardiovascular disease were generally limited to White middle-aged men.[17] Many were occupational cohorts so that, in an era when women were less likely to work than they are today, even when women were included their numbers were often small and they were unrepresentative of the general population. Many of these cohorts were also used for research on social variations in disease risk,[80] particularly in relation to the effects of social mobility, and later in relation to social inequalities in health as this became topical again in the 1980s.[81–84] Recently they have been used to study the childhood origins of adult chronic disease.[31,32,85,86] Historical cohorts used to investigate the fetal origins of adult chronic diseases (Section 1.2.1) also have fewer women than men and sometimes none at all,[6] partly because it is more time consuming to trace women who change their names on marriage.

Studies that have included women as well as men tend to analyse them separately and seldom formally test if risk factors have differential gender effects. True gender differences could provide clues to aetiology but interpretation of apparent differences from separate analyses can be misleading. The studies rarely have data on biological risk factors that are unique to women (such as age at menarche, menopause, and fertility history) and they seldom have good social data, especially of the kind that relates more to women's health (such as childhood sexual abuse or domestic violence). The historical cohorts usually have limited data on the intermediate period between infancy and middle-age. The cohort studies that began in adult life have to rely on retrospective recall of factors in childhood or young adult life, unless records can be linked to other sources of data. Thus, for certain stages of life, namely late childhood, adolescence, and early adult life, information is sparse, and yet these are times when women may be exposed to quite different biological risks and social environments than men with implications for later health.

Having recognized the need to study birth cohorts until death, the challenge is to develop the existing longitudinal data sets or set up new ones that can provide us with a life course perspective. The maturing of cohorts in continuing longitudinal studies originally investigating child health and development has already helped to foster a research focus on links between childhood experience and adult outcomes, including the long-term effects of physical growth, psychosocial development, and the childhood social environment. These include the US child development studies begun in the 1920s and 1930s,[87–89] the British birth cohort studies started in 1946,[90] 1958,[91] and 1970,[92] and the Dunedin birth cohort study begun in 1972–3.[93] There are also historical cohorts that are now being followed up with large numbers of women who are more representative of the general population than earlier historical cohorts.[94–96] It is essential that biological and social information on the adult lives of women in these cohorts, including their health and disease experiences and risk factors unique to women, is collected in sufficient depth to allow us to test life course (and not just early life) theories. Other sources of information are ongoing and newly set up longitudinal studies of adults where extra data might be extracted from past records or asked retrospectively[97] to enhance their potential to address life course theories.[98,99] The US Nurses' Health Study is an example of where this has been done sucessfully.[100] We also need to consider whether it is possible to enhance the longitudinal studies of women in midlife which were set up to study the menopause transition. Reviewing the research published to date will help to highlight the gaps in research and the most promising life course hypotheses that these new data could test.

1.4.2 Conceptual frameworks for the study of women's health: the need for a temporal perspective

In the second half of the nineteenth century scientists catalogued the biological differences between men and women, creating sharp boundaries between male and female.[101,102] Before that time, doctors were less likely to differentiate between the male and female ageing process. For example, 'climacteric' was commonly used to refer to the transition from one epoch of human life to another[103] rather than restricted to the female menopausal transition. Reproduction became the defining quality of femininity and the study of women's health focused on female reproductive processes, and the impact these processes were assumed to have on a woman's wider physical and mental health. The discovery of the sex hormones in the 1920s further contributed to the emphasis on biological differences, and increased the medicalization of women's health.

The women's health movement that was part of the second wave of feminism in the 1960s challenged this medicalization of women's health. Attention first focused on problems faced by women as consumers of medical care, particularly in regard to the control of women's fertility and the dissemination of health information.[104-106] Subsequently a social model of women's health began to compete with the medical or biological model as it was increasingly recognized that sources of risk for women's health were to be found in the nature of women's lives and their social and economic environment. In the social and psychological literature some researchers studying women's lives acknowledged the importance of a life course perspective,[107,108] described as the 'interweaving of many different dimensions of development and experience over the entire life-span of the individual' (p. 3).[107] However, the growing interest in gender inequalities in health, which usually meant the study of women's health in comparison to men's health, and in the health impact of women's social roles usually lacked a temporal perspective, certainly one that reached back into childhood.[109-114] These studies paralleled the revival of interest from the 1970s of the impact of socioeconomic conditions on health and disease, which also lacked a life course perspective.[117-122] In women's health research, there was little integration of social roles (the emphasis of North American research) and socioeconomic position (the emphasis of European research) until recently.[123-126]

One of the limitations of the social model of women's health has been the reliance on evidence from studies using aggregate measures of physical and mental health (such as self reported health or limiting longstanding illness) and all-cause mortality. Gradually studies with specific disease outcomes or using more finely graded markers of health and wellbeing have become more common. This partly reflects the successful efforts of feminist and professional advocates in putting women's health firmly on the political agenda, particularly in the US,[127,128] so that more research into women's health has been funded (for example the Women's Health Initiative).[129] Women are now more likely to be included in clinical trials and other research studies. Authors of recent textbooks on women's health reviewing the findings of these studies argue for the study of biological and social risk factors in integrated rather than competing models.[130,131] These textbooks and others[132,133] make reference to a life span perspective. However, this generally refers to the study of health and health problems at each life stage, rather than the study of how risks to later health may originate in early life and accumulate across the whole life course.

Our interdisciplinary life course approach thus complements and extends recent research on women's health. Contributors to this book focus on specific diseases and disorders and mediating mechanisms and actively investigate the interactive nature of social and biological risk processes that affect women's health and disease risk, rather than drawing false dichotomies between them. The role that reproductive factors play in women's health is rehabilitated and revised. By investigating how far women's health in middle and later life may be shaped by earlier social and biological experiences, a much-needed temporal perspective is added to current aetiological models of women's health.

In turn, the study of women's health will help to develop life course epidemiology. At the simplest level it tests the relevance of a life course approach to health outcomes that are unique to or more common in women. The investigation of gender and sex-specific developmental pathways to disease may provide clues to aetiology for both men and women. Biological transitions (such as puberty and menopause) are more distinct for women than for men or are unique to women (such as pregnancy) and social transitions to do with changes in social roles are, arguably, also more distinct. Thus, it may be easier to examine and model the intermediate links in the biological and social chains of risk that connect childhood to women's rather than men's health in adult life. Less is known about these intermediate links in life course epidemiology. Understanding pregnancy and continuity in pregnancy outcomes across generations also has a bearing on the health of the next generation, regardless of the sex of the offspring.

1.5 **Conclusions**

Life course epidemiology is the study of the contribution of biological and social factors acting independently, interactively, and cumulatively during gestation, childhood, adolescence, and adult life on health outcomes in later life. The purpose is to identify long-term risk and protective processes that explain variation in individual disease risk and changing patterns of disease over time or across populations. Contributors to this book apply a life course approach to the study of women's health. This complements and extends recent research models of women's health that also emphasize the interactive nature of biological and social risk processes on disease risk but pay less attention to a temporal perspective. By bringing together these two strands of research this book makes a unique contribution to interdisciplinary research, offers important new insights into the causes of women's health and provides challenges for future life course research.

References

1 **Murray CJL, Lopez AD**. *The global burden of disease: a comprehensive assessment of mortality and disability from diseases, injuries and risk factors in 1990 and projected to 2020*. WHO & World Bank. Cambridge, Mass.: Harvard University Press, 1996.

2 **Barker DJP**. *Mothers, babies and health in later life*. Edinburgh: Churchill Livingstone, 1998.

3 **Barker DJP**. *Fetal Origins of Cardiovascular and Lung Disease*. New York: Marcel Dekker, Inc., 2001.

4 **Kuh DL, Ben-Shlomo Y.** *A life course approach to chronic disease epidemiology: tracing the origins of ill-health from early to adult life*. Oxford: Oxford University Press, 1997.

5 **Ben-Shlomo Y, Kuh D.** A life course approach to chronic disease epidemiology: conceptual models, empirical challenges, and interdisciplinary perspectives. *Int J Epidemiol* 2002;**31**:285–93.

6 Leon D, Ben-Shlomo Y. Preadult influences on cardiovascular disease and cancer. In Kuh D, Ben-Shlomo Y, eds. *A life course approach to chronic disease epidemiology: tracing the origins of ill-health from early to adult life.* Oxford: Oxford University Press, 1997:45–77.

7 Cairns RB, Elder GH, Costello EJ. *Developmental Science.* Cambridge: Cambridge University Press, 1996.

8 Magnusson D. *The lifespan development of individuals: behavioral, neurobiological and psychosocial perspectives.* Cambridge: Cambridge University Press, 1996.

9 Panter-Brick C, Worthman CM. *Hormones, health and behavior.* Cambridge: Cambridge University Press, 1999.

10 Henry CJK, Ulijaszek. *Long-term consequences of early environment: growth, development and the lifespan perspective.* Oxford: Oxford University Press, 1996.

11 MacMichael AJ. Prisoners of the Proximate: loosening the constraints on epidemiology in an age of change. *Am J Epidemiol* 1999;**149**:887–97.

12 Elder GH, Jr. The life course and human development. In Damon W, Lerner RM, eds. *Handbook of Child Psychology Volume 1: Theoretical models of Human Development,* pp 939–91. New York: 1998, 1998.

13 Baltes PB, Lindenberger U, Staudinger UM. Life-span theory in developmental psychology. In Damon W, Lerner RM, eds. *Handbook of Child Psychology Volume 1: Theoretical models of Human Development,* pp 1029–143. New York: John Wiley & Sons, Inc., 1998.

14 Giele JZ, Elder GH, Jr. Life Course Research: Development of a Field. In Giele JZ, Elder GH, Jr., eds. *Methods of life course research: Qualitiative and quantitivae approaches.* Thousand Oaks, CA: Sage Publications, Inc., 1998:5–27.

15 Kuh D, Davey Smith G. When is mortality risk determined? Historical insights into a current debate. *Soc Hist Med* 1993;**6**:101–23.

16 Davey Smith G, Kuh D. William Ogilvy Kermack and the childhood origins of adult health and disease. *Int J Epidemiol* 2001;**30**:696–703.

17 Kuh D, Davey Smith G. The life course and adult chronic disease: an historical perspective with particular reference to coronary heart disease. In Kuh D, Ben-Shlomo Y, eds. *A life course approach to chronic disease epidemiology: tracing the origins of ill-health from early to adult life.* Oxford: Oxford University Press, 1997:15–44.

18 Abraham S, Collins G, Nordsieck M. Relationship of childhood weight status to morbidity in adults. *HSMHA Health Reports* 1971;**86**:273–84.

19 Osborn GR. Stages in development of coronary disease observed from 1,500 young subjects. Relationship of hypotension and infant feeding to aetiology. *Colloques Internationaux du Centre National de la Recherche Scientifique* 1967;**169**:93–139.

20 Reid DD. The beginnings of bronchitis. *Proc R Soc Med* 1969;**62**:311–6.

21 Stein Z, Susser M, Saenger G, Marolla F. *Famine and human development.* The Dutch Hunger Winter of 1944–45. New York: Oxford University Press, 1975.

22 Barker DJP. *Fetal and Infant Origins of Adult Disease.* London: British Medical Journal, 1992.

23 Barker DJP. Fetal origins of coronary heart disease. *Br Med J* 1995;**311**:171–4.

24 Lucas A. Programming by early nutrition in man. In Bock GR, Whelan J, eds. *The Childhood Environment and Adult Disease.* Chichester: John Wiley and Sons, 38–55.

25 Frankel S, Elwood P, Sweetnam P, Yarnell J, Davey Smith G. Birthweight, body mass index in middle age and incident coronary heart disease. *Lancet* 1996;**248**:1478–80.

26 Lithell HO, McKeigue PM, Berglund L, Mohsen R, Lithell U, Leon DA. Relationship of size at birth to non-insulin-dependent diabetes and insulin levels in men aged 50–60 years. *Br Med J* 1996;**312**:406–10.

27 Leon DA, Koupilova I, Lithell HO, Berglund L, Mohsen R, Vagero D, *et al.* Failure to realise growth potential in utero and adult obesity in relation to blood pressure in 50 year old Swedish men. *Br Med J* 1996;**312**:401–6.

28 Power C, Matthews S, Manor O. Inequalities in self rated health in the 1958 birth cohort: lifetime social circumstances or social mobility? *Br Med J* 1996;**313**:449–53.

29 Power C, Manor O, Fox AJ. *Health and Class: the Early Years.* London: Chapman Hall, 1991.

30 Kuh DJL,Wadsworth MEJ. Physical health status at 36 years in a British national birth cohort. *Soc Sci Med* 1993;**37**:905–16.

31 Blane D, Hart CL, Davey Smith G, Gillis CR, Hole DJ, Hawthorne WM. The association of cardiovascular risk factors with socioeconomic position during childhood and during adulthood. *Br Med J* 1996;**313**:1434–8.

32 Heslop P, Davey Smith G, Macleod J, Hart C. The socioeconomic position of employed women, risk factors and mortality. *Soc Sci Med* 2001;**53**:477–85.

33 Kreiger N, Chen JT, Selby JV. Class inequalities in women's health: combined impact of childhood and adult social class—a study of 630 US women. *Public Health* 2001;**115**:175–85.

34 Kuh D, Power C, Blane D, Bartley M. Social pathways between childhood and adult health. In Kuh D, Ben-Shlomo Y, eds. *A life course approach to chronic disease epidemiology: tracing the origins of ill-health from early to adult life.* Oxford: Oxford University Press, 1997:169–200.

35 Najman JM, Davey Smith G. The embodiment of class-related and health inequalities: Australian policies. *Aust J NZ Public Health* 2000;**24**:3.

36 Krieger N. A glossary for social epidemiology. *J Epidemiol Community Health* 2001;**55**: 693–700.

37 Seeman T. Developmental influences across the life span. *Ann NY Acad Sci* 1999;**896**:64–5.

38 Hertzman C, Wiens M. Child development and long-term outcomes: a population health perspective and summary of successful interventions. *Soc Sci Med* 1996;**43**:1083–95.

39 Rutter M. Pathways from childhood to adult life. *J Child Psychol Psychiatry* 1989;**30**:25–51.

40 Riley JC. *Sickness, recovery and death: a history and forecast of ill-health.* Basingstoke: Macmillan, 1989.

41 World Health Organization and the International Longevity Centre, UK. *The implications for training of embracing a life course approach to health.* Geneva: World Health Organization 2000.

42 Krieger N. Themes for social epidemiology in the 21st century: an ecosocial perspective. *Int J Epidemiol* 2001;**30**:668–77.

43 Olausson PO, Haglund B, Weitoft GR, Cnattingius S. Teenage childbearing and long-term socioeconomic consequences: a case study in Sweden. *Fam Plann Perspect* 2001;**33**:70–4.

44 Hardy JB, Shapiro S, Astone NM, Miller TL, Brooks-Gunn JHSC. Adolescent childbearing revisited: the age of inner-city mothers at delivery is a determinant of their children's self-sufficiency at age 27 to 33. *Pediatr* 1997;**100**:802–9.

45 Vanhala M, Vanhala P, Kumpusalo E, Halonen P, Takala J. Relation between obesity from childhood to adulthood and the metabolic syndrome: population based study. *Br Med J* 1998;**317**:319.

46 Power C, Manor O, Matthews S. The duration and timing of exposure: effects of socioeconomic environment on adult health. *Am J Public Health* 1999;**89**:1059–65.

47 Wamala SP, Lynch J, Kaplan GA. Women's exposure to early and later life socioeconomic disadvantage and coronary heart disease risk: the Stockholm Female Coronary Risk Study. *Int J Epidemiol* 2001;**30**:275–84.

48 Davey Smith G, Hart C, Blane D, Gillis C, Hawthorne V. Lifetime socioeconomic position and mortality: prospective observational study. *Br Med J* 1997;**314**:547–52.

49 National Research Council. *Preparing for an aging world: the case for cross-national research.* Washington, D.C.: National Academy Press, 2001.

50 **Worthman CM.** Epidemiology of human development. In Panter-Brick C, Worthman CM, eds. *Hormones, Health and Behavior.* Cambridge: Cambridge University Press, 1999:47–104.

51 **Alberti G.** Noncommunicable diseases: tomorrow's pandemics. *Bull World Health Organ* 2001;**79**:907.

52 **Davey Smith G, Egger M.** Commentary: Understanding it all—health, meta-theories, and mortality trends. *Br Med J* 1996;**313**:1584–5.

53 **Elo IT, Preston SH.** Effects of early-life conditions on adult mortality: a review. *Popul Index* 1992;**58**:186–212.

54 **Mosley WH, Gray R.** Childhood precursors of adult morbidity and mortality in developing countries: implications for health programs. In Gribble JN, Preston SH, eds. *The epidemiological transition*, National Academy Press, 1993.

55 **Salomon JA, Murray CJ.** Modelling HIV/AIDS epidemics in sub-Saharan Africa using seroprevalence data from antenatal clinics. *Bull World Health Organ* 2001;**79**:596–607.

56 **Joshi H, Paci P.** *Unequal Pay for Women and Men.* Massachusetts: Massachusetts Institute of Technology, 1998.

57 **Brewster KL, Rindfuss RR.** Fertility and women's employment in industrialized nations. *Annu Rev Sociol* 2000;**26**:271–96.

58 **Halsey HH, Webb J.** *Twentieth Century British Social Trends.* London: Macmillan, 2000.

59 **Coleman D, Salt J.** *The British population: patterns, trends and processes.* Oxford: Oxford University Press, 1992.

60 **Pearce D, Griffin T, Kelly J, Mikkelse L.** An overview of the population in Europe and North America. *Popul Trends* 1997;**89**:24–35.

61 **Coleman D.** Britain in Europe: international and regional comparisons of fertility levels and trends. In: Bhrolchain M, ed. *New perspectives on fertility in Britain.* Studies on medical and population subjects. No. 55. London, HMSO, 1993:67–93.

62 **Pearce D, Cantisani G, Laihonen A.** Changes in fertility and family sizes in Europe. *Popul Trends* 1999;**95**:33–40.

63 **Armitage B, Babb P.** Population Review: (4) Trends in fertility. *Popul Trends* 1996;**100**:7–13.

64 **Smith DJ.** Living conditions in the twentieth century. *Psychosocial Disorders in Young People: Time Trends and Their Causes*, Chichester: John Wiley & Sons Ltd, 1995.

65 **Evandrou M, Falkingham J.** Social security and the life course: developing sensitive policy alternative. In Arber S, Evandrou M, eds. *Ageing, Independence and the Life Course.* London: Jessica Kingsley Publishers, 1993:201–23.

66 **Parsons DO.** Poverty dynamics among mature women: evidence from the National Longitudinal Surveys 1967–1989. *National Longitudinal Surveys (NLS) Discussion Paper Series* 1995;25: http://stats.bls.gov/ore/pdf/nl950010.pdf.

67 **Robine J-M, Mormiche P, Sermet C.** Examination of the causes and mechanisms of the increase in disability-free life expectancy. *J Aging Health* 1998;**10**:171–91.

68 **Freedman VA, Martin LG.** Contribution of chronic conditions to aggregate changes in old-age functioning. *Am J Public Health* 2000;**90**:1759–60.

69 **Thorogood M, Villard-Mackintosh L.** Combined oral contraceptives: risks and benefits. *Br Med Bull* 1993;**49**:124–39.

70 WHO Scientific Group on Cardiovascular Disease and Steroid Hormone Contraception. *Cardiovascular disease and steroid hormone contraception: report of a WHO scientific group.* Geneva: WHO, 1998.

71 **Barrett-Connor E.** Hormone replacement therapy (HRT) risks and benefits. *Int J Epidemiol* 2001;**30**:423–6.

72 **Heise L, Pitanguy J, Germain A.** *Violence against women: the hidden health burden.* Washington, DC: World Bank, 1994.

73 **Alpert EJ.** Violence against women. In Ness R, Kuller L, eds. *Women in health and disease.* Oxford: Oxford University Press, 1998:112–29.

74 **Widom CS.** Childhood Victimization: Early Adversity and Subsequent Psychopathology. In Dohrenwend BP, ed. *Adversity, stress and psychopathology.* New York: Oxford University Press, 1998:81–95.

75 **Felitti VJ, Anda RF, Nordenberg D, Williamson DF, Spitz AM, Edwards V, *et al*.** Relationship of childhood abuse and household dysfunction to many of the leading causes of death in adults. *Am J Prev Med* 1998;**14**:245–58.

76 **Elder GHJ, Caspi A.** Economic stress in lives: developmental perspectives. *J Soc Issues* 1988;**44**:25–45.

77 **Mayer KA, Huinink J.** Age, period and cohort in the study of the life course: a comparison of classical A-P-C analysis with event history analysis or farewell to Lexis? In Magnusson D, Bergman LK, eds. *Data quality in longitudinal research.* Cambridge, MA: Cambridge University Press, 1990:211–32.

78 **Rutter M, Smith DJ.** *Psychosocial disorders in young people: time trends and their causes.* Chichester: John Wiley & Sons Ltd, 1995.

79 **Diez-Roux AV.** Bringing context back into epidemiology: variables and fallacies in multilevel analysis. *Am J Public Health* 1998;**88**:216–22.

80 **Davey Smith G.** Socioeconomic differentials. In Kuh D, Ben-Shlomo Y, eds. *A life course approach to chronic disease epidemiology: tracing the origins of ill-health from early to adult life.* Oxford: Oxford University Press, 1997:242–73.

81 **Rose G, Marmot MG.** Social class and coronary disease. *Br Heart J* 1981;**45**:13–9.

82 **Marmot MG, Shipley MJ, Rose G.** Inequalities in death—specific explanations of a general pattern? *Lancet* 1984;May 5:1003–6.

83 **Baker IA, Sweetnam PM, Yarnell JW, Bainton D, Elwood PC.** Haemostatic and other risk factors for ischaemic heart disease and social class: evidence from the Caerphilly and Speedwell studies. *Int J Epidemiol* 1988;**17**:759–65.

84 **Davey Smith G, Shipley MJ, Rose G.** The magnitude and causes of socioeconomic differentials in mortality: further evidence from the Whitehall Study. *J Epidemiol Community Health* 1990;**44**:265–70.

85 **Kaplan GA, Salonen JT.** Socioeconomic conditions in childhood and ischaemic heart disease during middle age. *Br Med J* 1990;**301**:1121–3.

86 **Lynch JW, Kaplan GA, Cohen RD, Kauhanen J, Wilson TW, Smith NL, *et al*.** Childhood and adult socioeconomic status a predictors of mortality in Finland. *Lancet* 1994;**343**:524–7.

87 **Eichorn DH, Haan N, Honzik MP, Mussen PH.** *Present and past in middle life.* London: Academic Press, 1981.

88 **Must A, Jacques PF, Dallal GE, Bajema CJ, Dietz WH.** Long-term morbidity and mortality of overweight adolescents. A follow-up of the Harvard Growth Study of 1922 to 1935. *N Engl J Med* 1992;**327**:1350–5.

89 **Schwartz JE, Friedman HS, Tucker JS, Tomlinson-Keasey C, Wingard DL, Criqui MH.** Sociodemographic and psychosocial factors in childhood as predictors of adult mortality. *Am J Public Health* 1995;**85**:1237–45.

90 **Wadsworth MEJ, Kuh DJL.** Childhood influences on adult health: a review of recent work in the British 1946 national birth cohort study, the MRC National Survey of Health and Development. *Paediat Perinat Epidemiol* 1997;**11**:2–20.

91 **Power C.** A review of child health in the 1958 cohort: National Child Development Study. *Paediat Perinat Epidemiol* 1992;**6**:91–110.

92 **Butler NR, Golding J, Howlett, BC,** eds. *From birth to five: a study of the health and behaviour of a national birth cohort*. Oxford: Pergamon, 1985.

93 **Silva PA, Stanton WR.** From child to adult. *The Dunedin Multidisciplinary Health and Development Study*. Auckland: Oxford University Press, 1996.

94 **Birch HG, Richardson SA, Baird D, Horobin G, Ilsley R.** *Mental subnormality in the community: a clinical and epidemiologic study*. Baltimore: Williams and Wilkins Co., 1970.

95 **Leon DA, Lithell HO, Vagero D, Koupilova I, Mohsen R, Berglund, L** *et al.* Reduced fetal growth rate and increased risk of ischaemic heart disease mortality in 15 thousand Swedish men and women born 1915–29. *Br Med J* 1998;**317**:241–5.

96 **Susser E, Terry MB, Matte T.** The birth cohorts grow up: new opportunities for epidemiology. *Paediat Perinat Epidemiol* 2000;**14**:98–100

97 **Berney LR, Blane DB.** Collecting retrospective data: accuracy of recall after 50 years judged against historical records. *Soc Sci Med* 1997;**45**:1519–25.

98 The Million Women Study Collaborative Group. The Million Women Study: design and characteristics of the study population. *Breast Cancer Res* 1999;**1**:73–80.

99 **Lawlor DA, Bedford C, Taylor M, Ebrahim S.** Geographic variation in cardiovascular risk factors and their control in older women: British Women's Heart and Health Study. *J Epid Community Health*, in press.

100 **Colditz GA, Manson JE, Hankinson SE.** The Nurses' Health Study: 20-year contribution to the understanding of health among women. *J Womens Health* 1997;**6**:49–62.

101 **Krieger N, Fee E.** Man-made Medicine and Women's Health: The biopolitics of sex/gender and race/ethnicity. *Int J of Health Serv* 1994;**24**:265–83.

102 **Moscucci O.** *The science of woman: gynaecology and gender in England 1800–1929*. Cambridge History of Medicine. Cambridge: Cambridge University Press,1990.

103 **Copland J.** *A Dictionary of Practical Medicine. Vol I*. London: Longman, Brown, Green, Longmans, & Roberts, 1858.

104 **Norsigian J.** The Women's Health Movement in the United States. In Moss KL, ed. *Man-made Medicine: Women's Health, Public Policy and Reform*. Durham and London: Duke University Press, 1996:79–98.

105 **Doyal L.** Women, health, and the sexual division of labor: a case study of the Women's Health Movement in Britain. *Int J Health Serv* 1983;**13**:373–87.

106 **Broom DH.** *Damned if we do: contradictions in women's health care*. Sydney: Allen & Unwin, 1991.

107 **Giele JZ.** *Women in the middle years*. New York: John Wiley & Sons, 1982.

108 **Rossi A.** Life-span theories and women's lives. *Signs: J Women Culture Soc* 1980;**6**:4–32.

109 **Nathanson CA.** Illness and the feminine role, a theoretical review. *Soc Sci Med* 1975;**9**: 57–62.

110 **Gove WR, Geerkin MR.** The effect of children and employment on the mental health of married men and women. *Soc Forces* 1977;**56**:66–76.

111 **Gove WR.** Gender differences in mental and physical illness among men and women. *Soc Sci Med* 1984;**19**:77–91.

112 **Verbrugge L.** The social roles of the sexes and their relative health and mortality. In Lopez A, Ruzicka L, eds. *Sex differentials in mortality trends, determinants and consequences*. Canberra: Australian National University Press, 1983:221–45.

113 **Verbrugge LM.** Role responsibilities, role burdens and physical health. In Crosby FJ, ed. *Spouse, Parent, Worker*. London: Yale University Press, 1987:154–166.

114 **Nathanson C.** Social roles and health status among women: the significance of employment. *Soc Sci Med* 1980;**14A**:463–71.

115 **Martikainen P.** Women's employment, marriage, motherhood and mortality: a test of the multiple role and role accumulation hypotheses. *Soc Sci Med* 1995;**40**:199–212.

116 **Weatherall R, Joshi H, Macran S.** Double burden or double blessing? Employment, motherhood and mortality in the Longitudinal Study of England and Wales. *Soc Sci Med* 1994;**38**:285–97.

117 **Black D, Morris JN, Smith C, Townsend P.** *Inequalities in Health: Report of a Research Working Group.* London: Department of Health and Social Security, 1980.

118 **Macran S, Clarke L, Sloggett A, Bethune A.** Women's socioeconomic status and self-assessed health: identifying some disadvantaged groups. *Sociol Health Illness* 1994;**16**:182–208.

119 **Kitagawa EM, Hauser PM.** *Differential mortality in the United States: a study in socioeconomic epidemiology.* Cambridge, MA.: Harvard University Press, 1973.

120 **Feinstein JS.** The relationship between socioeconomic status and health: a review of the literature. *Milbank Q* 1993;**71**:279–322.

121 **Kreiger N, Fee E.** Measuring social inequalities in health in the United States: a historical review, 1900–1950. *Int J Health Serv* 1996;**26**:391–418.

122 **Adler NE, Ostrove JM.** Socioeconomic status and health: what we know and what we don't. *Ann NY Acad Sci* 1999;**896**:3–15.

123 **Arber S.** Class, paid employment and family roles: making sense of structural disadvantage, gender and health status. *Soc Sci Med* 1991;**32**:425–36.

124 **Arber S.** Comparing inequalities in women's and men's health: Britain in the 1990s. *Soc Sci Med* 1997;**44**:773–87.

125 **Bartley M, Sacker A, Firth D, Pitzpatrick R.** Social position, social roles and women's health in England: changing relationships 1984 to 1993. *Soc Sci Med* 1999:**48**:99–115.

126 **Annandale E, Hunt K.** *Gender inequalities in health.* Buckingham: Open University Press, 2000.

127 **Seaman B, Wood SF.** Role of advocacy groups in research on women's health. In Goldman MB, Hatch MC. *Women and health.* New York: Academic Press, 2000:27–36.

128 **Goldman MB, Hatch MC.** State-of-the-art methods for women's health research. In Goldman MB, Hatch MC. *Women and health.* New York: Academic Press, 2000:37–49.

129 The Women's Health Initiative Study Group. Design of the Women's Health Initiative clinical trial and observational study. *Control Clin Trials* 1998;**19**:61–109.

130 **Ness R, Kuller L.** *Women in health and disease.* Oxford: Oxford University Press, 1998.

131 **Goldman MB, Hatch MC.** *Women and health.* New York: Academic Press, 2000.

132 **Allen KM.** *Women's health across the lifespan: a comprehensive perspective.* Janice Mitchell Phillips, 1997.

133 **Blechman EA, Brownell KD.** *Behavioural medicine and women: a comprehensive handbook.* New York: The Guilford Press, 1998.

Part II

Health, ageing, and disease

Chapter 2

A life course approach to women's reproductive health

Janet Rich-Edwards

Among the first indicators of vitality and health in a woman's life are patterns of menstruation, fertility, and pregnancy. This chapter explores the emerging evidence that adult reproductive function is shaped by intergenerational, *in utero*, and childhood factors, as well as adult environment. Social environment shapes women's reproductive health. For example, poor pregnancy outcomes, including low birthweight and preterm delivery, are more frequent among women at socioeconomic disadvantage. This birthweight gap between advantaged and disadvantaged women appears to be amplified with maternal age, suggesting a cumulative, weathering effect of hardship on women's health.

As a reflection of early life exposures, endocrine patterns, and health status in young adulthood, reproductive events offer insights into the risk of future chronic disease. Menstrual patterns and ovulatory disorders, including age at menarche, menstrual irregularity, polycystic ovarian syndrome and infertility, have been associated with subsequent risk of breast cancer, cardiovascular disease, and diabetes. The physiological stress of pregnancy may unmask latent risks of hypertension, diabetes, and heart disease. Both pregnancy complications and pregnancy outcomes (gestational duration and birthweight) may predict a mother's later morbidity and mortality. Further work is needed to quantify the value of reproductive factors for predicting chronic disease. A deeper understanding of the implications of reproductive health for overall health may offer new opportunities to change life course trajectories before they progress to chronic disease.

2.1 Introduction

'With the exception of the stomach, there is no organ that holds such numerous ramifications of sympathy with other organs as the womb.'

J. M. Good, *The Study of Medicine*, 1826, page 203[1]

For all their preoccupation with naming and cataloguing separate organ systems, physicians of the nineteenth century appreciated the integral association of women's reproductive function with overall health and disease processes. However, the twentieth century focus on detecting adult risk factors for chronic disease virtually blinded us to factors operating in the first half of life. In this search, menopause served as a retrospective horizon beyond which few investigators ventured. Now, through the broader lens of a life course approach, we are led back to examine the intimate associations of women's reproductive health with overall physical and mental health. The vitality and performance of the reproductive axis in early adulthood acts as a wayside marker: reproductive success or failure reflects childhood exposures; reproductive events among young women may also serve as sentinels of chronic disease in maturity. This chapter opens with a discussion of early life factors that shape women's reproductive health, with a focus on determinants of pregnancy outcome. The second half of the chapter presents evidence that the gynaecological and obstetric health status of young women reveals latent chronic disease processes.

2.2 Determinants of female reproductive health

Not all investigators overlooked the implications of early life exposures on women's reproductive health. In the 1940s, Baird and colleagues in Scotland observed that a woman's pregnancy outcomes were more closely related to the social class of her father than to that of her own husband. They and their colleagues in Aberdeen also noted that women born during the Great Depression were more likely to bear low birthweight infants than women born in more prosperous times.[2] In the 1980s, Emanuel and Valanis furthered this approach, arguing that pregnancy outcome is not merely an acute condition lasting ten lunar months, but depends upon the preconceptional vitality of the mother and possibly her forebears.[3,4]

The female reproductive axis is highly sensitive to the physical and social environment throughout life. In fact, there is a premium on reproductive responsiveness: menstruation, pregnancy, and lactation are valuable, but physiologically expensive functions that are not critical to survival. The optimal system is one that can respond with agility to shifts in environmental resources and stressors.[5] However, a completely plastic system, requiring rapid remodelling of the reproductive axis, is inefficient. Thus, the growing girl must commit to a physiological fulcrum from which to respond; the optimal 'set point' is probably customized during development by incorporating information from the early environment. Variation in adult reproductive function around such a set point reflects influence of current environment. Evidence of environmental impact on the reproductive axis can be drawn from patterns of menarche, menstruation, and menopause across geography and time.

2.2.1 Place and time

In the 1980s, the 'typical' woman began to menstruate at age 14, bore her first live child at age 22, and underwent natural menopause at age 50, according to an international WHO collaborative study of 19 000 women in 13 study sites in the developed and developing world.[6] Behind this composite profile lies considerable geographic variation in the reproductive lives of women: for example the reproductive career of a typical woman in Chang Mai, Thailand is six years shorter than that of a typical Australian woman. Across the study sites, the median age at menarche ranged from 13 to 16 years, while the median age at menopause ranged from 49 to 52 years. Although menarche came later to girls in Asia and Africa than to girls in industrialized nations, no such geographic pattern was apparent for age at menopause. Ethnographic studies of 'natural fertility' populations also provide some perspective on the range of female reproductive careers. Among the Dogon of Mali, a non-contracepting, breastfeeding population, visits to the menstrual hut indicate that menstruation is a rare event for women during the peak childbearing years of age 20 to 34.[7] The typical Dogon woman menstruates only 100 times during her life, compared with approximately 300 cycles for a typical mother of three in the West.

Geographic variation in age at menarche and menopause could reflect both genetic and environmental influences on reproduction. However, time trends within populations reveal potent environmental influences on reproductive development. Although there is only slight evidence of a small increase in age at menopause (Chapter 4),[8,9] there has been a strong and well-documented fall in the mean age at menarche in developed countries in the last century, at a rate of 3 to 4 months per decade, which may now be levelling off.[10] Frisch and colleagues have argued that increasing adiposity among girls triggers earlier menarche.[11] However, rising energy intake may not be responsible for the entire trend. Observing that the dropping age at menarche in the modern era has paralleled falling rates of morbidity and mortality, Ellison proposed that the menarcheal trends may be attributed to improved hygiene, medical care and workload as well as to enhanced nutrition. Thus the demographic transition, by reducing the energy costs of survival, may have contributed to a positive energy balance and accelerated growth. Figure 2.1 demonstrates the striking correlation ($r=0.95$) between mean menarcheal age and infant mortality rates in Scandinavia from 1800 to 1950.[12]

The pattern evident in Fig. 2.1 is reminiscent of Anders Forsdahl's observations that adult mortality is better correlated with infant mortality rates at the time of one's birth than at the time of one's death.[13] Patterns such as these imply that conditions during early development may leave an enduring imprint on the body, whether or not that childhood

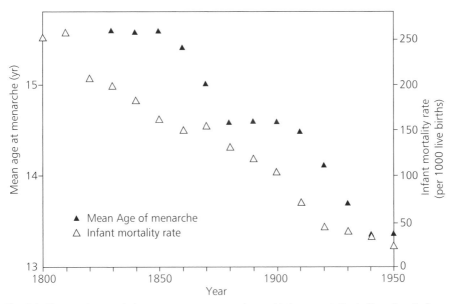

Fig. 2.1 The secular trends in mean age at menarche and infant mortality in Scandinavia from 1800 to 1950.[12]

environment persists into adulthood. Although the fall in menarcheal age lags 30 years behind the fall in infant mortality, too long a gap to suggest that infant conditions affected age at menarche, the pattern prompts speculation that perinatal conditions may affect the next generation of daughters. Thus, a girl born in an era of improved nutrition and hygiene may bear daughters whose sexual maturation is accelerated. In this light, it is interesting to examine evidence that *in utero* factors may determine the reproductive health of daughters and perhaps granddaughters.

2.2.2 Of grandmothers, mothers, and daughters: intergenerational and intrauterine influences on female reproductive function

In pregnancy outcomes, as in other family traits, the apple falls close by the roots. Across generations of a family, there is a tendency to repeat pregnancy outcomes, especially birthweight.[14–16] It has been estimated that 12% of fetal growth restriction in the developed world is attributable to the 'effect' of the mother's own birthweight on that of her offspring (only 3% of preterm births were attributed to preterm in the previous generation).[17] Although by 18 months of age, a child's height is equally determined by the heights of its mother and father,[10] the infant's size at birth is better predicted by the mother's birthweight than by the father's birthweight. This phenomenon of 'catch-up' or 'catch-down' growth in infancy indicates that maternal factors constrain or promote fetal growth, as demonstrated by classic cross-breeding experiments in animals.[18] The determinants of fetal growth, including growth factors, placental function, gestational diabetes, maternal diet, and maternal pelvic size, reflect both genetic and environmental influences acting throughout the mother's life. The strong tendency for women to repeat pregnancy outcomes (such as birthweight and gestational duration) even in the face of changing adult social circumstances and state-of-the-art prenatal care, suggests that a woman carries an intrinsic or stable trait that was set long before sperm meets egg.[19]

Such 'set points' may be determined in the womb. A mother's own *in utero* experience might programme her future reproductive performance by determining the quality of the ova she carries into adulthood, the vascularization of her uterus, or the setting of the intricate hormonal mechanisms necessary for successful conception and pregnancy.[20] In other words, the growth restricted female fetus may make physiological sacrifices during development that compromise her own ability as an adult to bear a normal birthweight child. Although attractive, this hypothesis of *in utero* 'programming' of pregnancy outcome is largely untested. To date, the only information relating human pregnancy outcome to mother's intrauterine environment is derived from the 'natural' experiments of diethylstilboestrol administration and wartime famine, reviewed below. First we review the evidence of genetic and *in utero* determinants of age at menarche and menstrual function.

Age at menarche is a good example of the joint genetic and environmental control of female reproduction. Consistent correlations in menarcheal age of approximately 0.30 have been reported between mothers and daughters as well as between sisters.[21] Monozygotic twins have higher correlations in menarcheal age than do dizygotic twins; the higher correlation could reflect shared genes or a shared placenta. In their study of over 600 twins, Sneider and colleagues estimated the genetic contribution to age at menarche at 45%; this still leaves over half of the variance to environment, which is consistent with the secular trend.[21,22]

Birthweight appears to be correlated with menarcheal age, although in a surprising direction: menarche comes later to girls of higher birthweight.[23] An explanation of this paradox may be that adrenarche is exaggerated among children who were small for gestational age, perhaps indicating earlier or more sensitive activation of the hypothalamic–pituitary–adrenal (HPA) axis.[24,25] Given this profile, we might expect polycystic ovary syndrome (PCOS),[26] an endocrine disorder characterized by androgen excess and oligomenorrhoea, to be more prevalent among women born of low birthweight. However, the only study to investigate perinatal risk factors for PCOS reported more PCOS among those born of high birthweight or after a prolonged gestation.[26] Several factors may explain these associations: higher risk of obesity among large infants, fetal exposure to high levels of testosterone in late pregnancy, or a common genetic determinant of both PCOS and fetal growth.[27,28] PCOS is a highly heterogeneous condition: its subtypes may be differently related to fetal exposures. These studies, which require replication, contribute indirect evidence of fetal programming of sexual maturation and function in adulthood.

More direct evidence that the *in utero* environment shapes the adult reproductive axis comes from animal experiments demonstrating that the cyclic gonadotropin release essential to female fertility is programmed by fetal exposure to steroid hormones.[29] Women exposed *in utero* to diethylstilboestrol (DES), a potent oestrogen previously used to avert miscarriage, are themselves at increased risk of poor pregnancy outcomes, including miscarriage, ectopic pregnancy, stillbirth, and preterm birth.[30,31] However, *in utero* DES exposure does not affect age at menarche, and there is conflicting evidence regarding its effect, if any, on fertility and menstrual patterns.[30,31]

It has been claimed that maternal diet during pregnancy may also programme adult health outcomes of offspring.[32] However, there are as yet few human data to support the hypothesis that variations in maternal diet affect maturation rates, menstrual patterns, or pregnancy outcomes of daughters. Among the horrors of World War II were the acute famines endured by civilians in Europe. During the winter of 1945, food rations in the western Netherlands fell below 1000 calories per day for four months; average birthweight plummeted, and infant mortality soared.[33] Seven hundred girls born in Amsterdam during the Dutch Hunger Winter have been traced to examine the long-term effects of *in utero* exposure to famine. Although daughters born to women exposed to the famine while pregnant had normal age at menarche and no apparent menstrual perturbations in adulthood, their offspring (the grandchildren) did experience higher perinatal mortality.[20] Mothers whose own birthweights were depressed by *in utero* famine exposure also tended to bear offspring of reduced birthweight. In other words, nutrition of the first generation affected the birthweight of the third generation by determining the birthweight of the second generation, a demonstration of intergenerational phenotypic transmission.[34] In Guatamala, daughters of women fed a high energy, high protein supplement during pregnancy underwent menarche at the same age as daughters of women who were fed a low energy, no-protein supplement.[35] While the results of such natural and intentional experiments do not preclude an effect of maternal prenatal diet (especially micronutrients) on daughter's menstrual cycling and fertility, they yield no support for that idea.

Although animal experiments demonstrate that hormonal manipulation *in utero* can 'programme' the female reproductive axis, there are to date only a handful of reports that hint at fetal determinants of age at menarche, PCOS, and pregnancy outcomes in humans. More work needs to be done to replicate early findings, as well as to identify direct physiological mechanisms through which the female reproductive axis may be programmed *in utero*.

2.2.3 **Growth and body habitus**

2.2.3.1 Menarche and menstruation

Although height, weight, and adiposity are all strongly associated with the onset of menarche, vigorous debate persists as to whether menarche is synchronized with skeletal maturation or the attainment of critical weight.[36] Furthermore, it is unknown which determinants of prepubertal growth—genes, diet, activity, hormones, or infections—affect the timing of menarche. For example, data are inconsistent regarding the contribution, if any, of calorie intake and diet composition on the timing of menarche among adequately nourished girls.[37] Nor is there agreement regarding the relevant 'critical period' for determining menarche: diet and body size recorded before age six years may predict menarcheal age as well as those factors recorded much closer to puberty.[37]

Among mature women, extremes of adiposity are related to irregular menstrual cycling and risk of ovulatory disorder infertility.[38] However, several studies have shown that adult weight gain or loss, where appropriate, can improve fertility outcomes.[39–41] Although intensive physical training of athletes may temporarily disrupt menstrual cycling, lower levels of vigorous activity may promote regular reproductive functioning and fertility, particularly if they help maintain optimal weight.[42]

2.2.3.2 Pregnancy

Pregnancy outcomes are also related to maternal body habitus. A mother's height and prepregnant weight are positively associated with the fetal growth rate of her offspring, although the association of birthweight with maternal weight is strongest among lean mothers. Low prepregnant weight is also a predictor of increased risk of preterm delivery.[17] Certainly, weight gain during the third trimester of pregnancy is positively associated with fetal growth, especially where women are chronically undernourished.[17]

2.2.3.3 Menopause

As reviewed in Chapter 4, associations of age at menopause with such factors as birthweight,[26,43,44] height,[45] and menarcheal age,[45–47] are generally weak or non-existent among well-nourished women. However, some studies suggest that slower growth in early childhood and chronic malnourishment may be related to earlier age at menopause. In adulthood, very lean women or those who are dieting may have earlier menopause.[9,48]

Height, and to some extent adiposity, are determined in childhood (see Chapter 14). Thus the associations of these factors with menstrual cycling, fertility, and pregnancy outcome are further evidence of the importance of childhood environment on reproductive health. Nevertheless, changes in physical activity and energy intake in adulthood clearly affect fertility and pregnancy outcome. Thus, the female reproductive axis is highly sensitive to alterations in energy balance in childhood and thoughout the reproductive years.

2.2.4 **Stress, socioeconomic status, and weathering**

Good, in 1826, remarked upon the 'close chain of sympathy that prevails between the brain and the sexual organs, from the time of the development of the latter to their becoming torpid and superannuated on the cessation of the catemenia'(p. 161).[1] More recent observations and experiments demonstrate the integration of the female reproductive system with the HPA axis.[49] At each level of the reproductive system, products of the HPA stress response determine the frequency and amplitude of the hormones that govern menstrual cycling and pregnancy. Hypothalamic corticotropin-releasing hormone (CRH), the first hormone in the fight-or-flight response, regulates secretion of gonadotropin-releasing hormone. Cortisol inhibits ovulation. Extrahypothalamic CRH (produced by the ovaries, endometrium, and placenta) may regulate ovulation, menstruation, ovum implantation, and trigger labour and delivery. Of current research interest is the association of placental CRH levels with the risk of preterm delivery, suggesting that physiological and psychological stressors may set the 'placental clock' towards early delivery.[50–52] Thus, there is ample physiological basis for the observation that stress, by activating the HPA system, affects menstruation, fertility, and pregnancy outcome (Fig. 2.2).

2.2.4.1 Menarche, menstruation, and menopause

There is surprisingly little data on stress and age at menarche, perhaps due to the difficulty of measuring stressors in childhood. However, it is clear that war delays menarche. During World War II, girls in the Netherlands, Finland, Germany, Belgium, and Japan (but apparently not in Norway) showed delays of several months in mean menarcheal age (see citations in Van Noord[53]). In more recent history, girls deported from Srebrenica underwent menarche 16 months later than girls from peaceful areas of unoccupied Bosnia and Herzegovina.[54] There is some evidence from World War II that the delays in menarche are not exclusively due to nutritional deprivation accompanying war. The eight-month delay in the mean age of menarche in the Netherlands from 1940 to 1945 was similar before, during, and after the time-limited famine of the Dutch Hunger Winter of 1944–1945.[53] Thus, it is certainly plausible that psychological stress of war affects the onset of reproductive life.

Once established, menstrual cycles and fertility are sensitive to psychological state. Current depression is associated with reduced chances of conceiving with *in vitro* fertilization.[55,56] Two recent trials of group therapy showed dramatic improvements in conception rates for women having difficulty becoming pregnant.[57,58] Finally, a few studies have indicated that psychosocial stress and lower socioeconomic status may be associated with

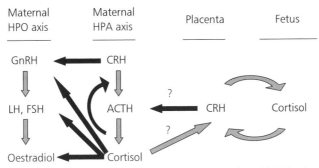

Fig. 2.2 Interactions of the maternal hypothalamic–pituitary–adrenal (HPA) axis with maternal hypothalamic–pituitary–ovarian (HPO) axis, placenta, and fetus. Adapted from Chrousos et al., 1998[49] and Majzoub JA, Karalis KP 1999.[50]

earlier age at menopause, suggesting that stress may shorten a reproductive career at its beginning or its end.[9,48]

2.2.4.2 Stress and pregnancy outcome

As methods for measuring psychosocial stress improve, the evidence grows that stress and distress hinder fetal growth and shorten pregnancy, while social support and fulfilling intimate relationships buffer the impact of stress on pregnancy outcome.[59,60] Perceived stress, anxiety, and depression during pregnancy appear to reduce birthweight and/or increase the risk of preterm delivery.[61,62] Although checklists of negative life events have been associated with spontaneous abortion of chromosomally normal fetuses,[63–65] they do not appear to predict the outcome of established pregnancies (perhaps because event inventories fail to measure women's emotional responses).[61] Poor family functioning,[66,67] household role stress[68] and, less consistently, work-related stress,[61] have been related to pregnancy outcomes. Evidence is also mounting that exposure to interpersonal and community violence and the threat of such violence may affect pregnancy outcome.[52,69] As studies improve their identification and measurement of stressors and stress responses most salient to women of childbearing age, estimates of the effect of psychosocial stress on reproductive outcomes are likely to rise.

Low socioeconomic status may be construed as an 'upstream' stressor that induces psychological and physiological stress responses.[70] Indeed, socioeconomic status is among the strongest and most consistent predictors of both fetal growth restriction and preterm delivery. As Kramer and colleagues have documented, the 'poor fare poorly' in highly stratified societies, such as the US, but also in more equitable societies with universal health care, as in Europe and Canada.[70] Cigarette smoking, low gestational weight gain, short stature, bacterial vaginosis, and psychosocial stress are implicated as the mediators between poverty and pregnancy outcome.[70] Although this list may completely enumerate the inner workings of the 'black box' between socioeconomic status and pregnancy outcome, far more work is needed to confirm, detail, and quantify these associations in a variety of populations. To date, no study has measured enough of these presumed mediators of poverty to 'explain away' the powerful predictor of socioeconomic status.

In the US, a stark racial/ethnic gap in risk of prematurity, low birthweight, and neonatal mortality has persisted for generations: African American women bear more than twice the risk of these outcomes compared with White women.[71,72] Although largely unexamined in other countries with sizeable ethnic minorities, this phenomenon is not unique to the US.[70] For example, in the economically depressed East London, women of African and West Indian descent are more likely to bear low birthweight infants than European White mothers.[73] Although genetic differences might underlie disparate birthweight distributions, especially where adult body size distributions differ, the very high mortality among infants of any race/ethnicity born in the 'tail' of extreme preterm (less than 28 weeks) and low birthweight (below 1500 g) belies their characterization as normal, healthy variants. Furthermore, migrant studies consistently show that foreign-born Africans living in the US have a lower risk of low birthweight than US-born African Americans.[4,74–77] Similarly, there exists a 'Latina paradox', that, despite their lower socioeconomic standing, Mexican immigrants to the US have better birth outcomes than do Mexican American women.[78,79] Such studies are not immune to the 'healthy immigrant' bias, but some have shown that the risk of low birthweight rises with duration or residence in the US and markers of acculturation.[80–82]

Many attempts to understand ethnic disparities in terms of maternal education, income, and health habits have failed to explain more than a third of the gap in low birthweight and preterm birth. This may be due partially to inadequate measurement of current socioeconomic position: even the most deluxe studies rarely include measures more sensitive than maternal education, household income, and dependence on public assistance. Newer studies should take into account financial security (wealth), economic obligations to family and friends, housing stability, and local living costs, among others. The persistent racial/ethnic gap also suggests unmeasured stressors that are unique to minority status: one study has shown associations between African American mothers' self-reported exposure to racism and risk of very low birthweight, and other tests of this hypothesis are imminent.[52,83] Also, in our failure to measure poverty and other stressors in childhood, we may be missing a critical window for the development of stress responses and future reproductive health.[84] A cumulative effect of stress across the life course is suggested by data showing that the racial/ethnic gap in risk of poor pregnancy outcome increases with maternal age.

2.2.4.3 Cumulative stress and 'weathering'

Geronimus coined the 'weathering hypothesis' to explain the observation that prevalence of many diseases increases faster with age for African Americans compared to White Americans.[85] Using birth certificates from the state of Michigan, Geronimus demonstrated that the risk of delivering a low birthweight infant increases rapidly with maternal age for Black, but not White, mothers.[86] Figure 2.3 shows risk of low birthweight by maternal

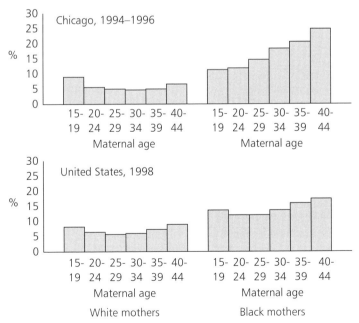

Fig. 2.3 Percent of low birthweight (<2500 gm) births by maternal age, singleton births to Black and White mothers in Chicago (1994–1996) and the US (1998). All data are derived from birth certificates in Chicago[88] and the US.[87]

ethnicity and age in the US. The risk of delivering a low birthweight infant begins to rise at age 30 for White women and age 20 for Black women.[87] Data from Chicago indicate that this divergence may be particularly pronounced in urban areas.[88] However, in this analysis, adjustment for the interactions of age with other risk factors eliminated most of the ethnic divergence in age slopes. In other words, the risk of delivering a low birthweight infant rose more quickly with maternal age for women at social and economic disadvantage, regardless of ethnicity.

These age trajectories suggest that hardships may act cumulatively to age women prematurely, jeopardizing their reproductive health. However, these observations are all founded on cross-sectional data; longitudinal studies linking sequential births to the same mother are needed to definitively demonstrate 'weathering'. Eventually, studies may reveal intergenerational transmission of 'weathering' such that the embodied stresses of poverty and discrimination in one generation are passed on as somatic legacy to the next generation. This may seem a grim prospect, but it also implies that improving the health of today's girls and young women may yield benefits in future decades.

2.3 Reproductive health as a sentinel of chronic disease

New evidence indicates that reproductive health in early adulthood is a marker for underlying propensities and ongoing chronic disease processes.[45,89,90] Furthermore, some reproductive choices, such as the decision to defer childbearing, may alter the course of chronic disease. In this section, I only mention the implications of menstrual characteristics and reproductive choices for breast cancer and cardiovascular disease (more fully reviewed in Chapters 3 and 5), and focus more on associations of pregnancy complications and pregnancy outcomes as predictors of chronic disease and mortality.

2.3.1 Menstrual function and fertility as predictors of chronic disease

As markers of the cumulative exposure to cyclic reproductive steroids, age at menarche and menopause, as well as menstrual patterns and fertility, may have multiple—and sometimes competing—implications for later health and disease. Early menarche[91] and late menopause confer higher risk of breast cancer.[92] In contrast, age at menarche has little bearing on cardiovascular risk, and only premature age at menopause is associated with significantly higher risk of heart disease.[92] Some, but not all, studies indicate that rapid establishment of regular cycles after menarche[93–95] and regular cycles throughout reproductive life[96–98] predict higher breast cancer risk. On the other hand, data from the US Nurses' Health Study indicate that women with regular cycles have lower risks of hypertension, diabetes, coronary heart disease and possibly ischaemic stroke.[99–101] Women with PCOS bear a 40–50% elevated risk of cardiovascular disease, primarily through the higher risks of obesity, glucose intolerance, hyperlipidaemia, and hypertension that may accompany PCOS.[102,103] Both a twofold increase and twofold decrease in risk of breast cancer have been reported among women with PCOS.[104,105]

Although these studies generally support the hypothesis that increased exposure to ovulatory cycles promotes breast cancer and protects against cardiovascular disease, their findings are not unanimous, and most reported associations are modest. The confusion may stem from the difficulty of accurately measuring lifetime menstrual characteristics by questionnaire, a necessity in studies large enough to detect associations with chronic disease events.

2.3.2 Age at first pregnancy and parity as predictors of chronic disease

As discussed in Chapter 3, nulliparity and late age at first pregnancy are established predictors of increased risk of breast cancer, although it is uncertain whether subsequent births affect breast cancer risk.[96] Teenage motherhood or bearing more than four or five children in one's life have been associated with a modestly increased risk of coronary heart disease; however, these associations seem likely to be confounded by socioeconomic status.[106] Nevertheless, parity's association with weight gain and central fat deposition, both potent risk factors for cardiovascular disease that are difficult to reverse, highlights the critical importance of the reproductive years for laying the foundation for health after menopause.

2.3.3 Complications of pregnancy as predictors of chronic disease

Pregnancy puts a physiological stress on the body that can unmask underlying propensity for chronic disease. Pregnancy complications such as gestational diabetes mellitus, gestational hypertension, and preeclampsia portend later type 2 diabetes, chronic hypertension, and endothelial dysfunction. Some characteristics of pregnancy may predict breast cancer risk.

Worldwide, hypertensive disorders of pregnancy, comprised of preeclampsia/eclampsia and gestational hypertension, affect 5–10% of pregnancies.[107] Preeclampsia is accompanied by low levels of maternal oestrogens and growth factors and high levels of CRH, alpha-fetoprotein (AFP), and testosterone during pregnancy.[108] Several retrospective studies indicate that women whose pregnancies were complicated by preclampsia/eclampsia or gestational hypertension bear higher risk of coronary heart disease incidence and mortality long after they have stopped childbearing.[107,109] Similarly, women with a history of gestational diabetes mellitus are at increased risk of future type 2 diabetes mellitus.[110,111] Most women who develop hypertensive disorders of pregnancy or gestational diabetes have no apparent risk factors for coronary heart disease before their pregnancies. Most of these complications of pregnancy remit at delivery. Thus, when such complications arise in pregnancy, they may be the first warning that a woman is at increased risk for future cardiovascular disease. A postpartum oral glucose tolerance test for gestational diabetics and blood pressure monitoring among those with hypertension in pregnancy will help identify the women at highest risk of future diabetes and hypertension.[111–113]

Investigations are just beginning into whether pregnancy complications predict future breast cancer risk. Two reports of increased breast cancer risk among women who bore preterm infants need to be replicated.[114,115] However, several conditions of pregnancy associated with preterm delivery have been inversely associated with breast cancer risk, including raised AFP levels,[116,117] preeclampsia, and placental anomalies.[118] These conditions are marked by high levels of CRH and testosterone. Thus, further work is needed to reconcile studies showing positive associations of breast cancer with preterm delivery, but inverse associations with the risk factors for preterm delivery.

The work investigating pregnancy complications as predictors of remote maternal outcomes has just begun. Future studies should quantify the long-term implications for maternal health of carrying pregnancies characterized by neural tube defects (associated with folic acid deficiency), elevations in AFP, placental compromise, or aberrant levels of biomarkers for fetal maturation, gestational length, and birthweight, including CRH, insulin-like growth factors, and oestriol.

2.3.4 Pregnancy outcomes: intimations of mortality?

A series of studies in Scotland, England, and Finland by Davey Smith and colleagues has documented consistent associations between the birthweight and gestational age of a woman's offspring and the length of her own lifespan.[119–121] Overall, mothers of large infants tend to live longer lives. This is especially true of cardiovascular mortality: these studies estimate that every kilogram decrease in offspring birthweight is associated with a twofold higher risk of cardiovascular mortality in the mother. Conversely, the data from Finland suggest that delivery of larger infants may be associated with an increased risk of breast cancer mortality.[120] Interestingly, these studies indicate that the associations between offspring size and later mortality exist even after adjustment for known pregnancy complications.

What do these data tell us? Certainly, factors in the parents' adult lives, such as smoking, could influence both the birthweight of their children and their own future risk of disease. However, adjustment for adult social class and lifestyle risk factors (such as smoking) appears to do little to dampen the associations of offspring birthweight with maternal longevity. Alternatively, the correlation between a woman's pregnancy outcomes and her mortality is plausible evidence that early life exposures of girls and young women set the course for lifelong health, determining both pregnancy outcomes and risk of disease in maturity. Thus, pregnancy outcome acts as a wayside marker, revealing the accumulated influence of genes and early environment. This explanation would account for the stronger associations of offspring birthweight with maternal mortality than with paternal mortality. In truth, these explanations are not mutually exclusive: the correlations between offspring birthweight and mortality of the mothers probably reflect accumulating and correlated exposures before, during, and after the pregnancy.

In summary, many lines of evidence suggest that the reproductive lives of women provide glimpses into future health. A smoothly functioning reproductive axis, marked by regular menstruation and uncomplicated pregnancy, portends lower risk of cardiovascular disease. On the other hand, many reproductive features associated with inefficient reproduction and lower lifelong oestrogen levels—later age at menarche, irregular cycles, ovulatory infertility, and preeclampsia—are associated with lower breast cancer risk. Further work to quantify the degree of absolute risk associated with different reproductive patterns would indicate whether women's reproductive characteristics can be used to identify women at high risk of certain chronic diseases. This information might be used to tailor health advice to women, from early in their lives, rather than waiting for the first signs of chronic disease to emerge at menopause.

2.4 Conclusions and policy implications

Age at menarche, menstrual function, fertility, pregnancy outcome, and age at menopause are known to be sensitive to a woman's *immediate* environment. Evidence is now growing that reproductive health also reflects cumulative environmental exposures across the life course, some of which date back to childhood, fetal life, and perhaps even the lives of her mother and grandmother. Furthermore, the correlations between menstrual patterns and pregnancy outcomes with later cardiovascular disease, cancer, and mortality may reveal early life antecedents of chronic disease. In particular, pregnancy complications and birth outcomes may unmask previously unsuspected chronic disease processes in their early stages, possibly offering opportunities for earlier and more effective intervention.

Much of the work presented in this chapter is new, and derived from studies that need to be replicated in different populations. It is critical to determine whether reproductive characteristics are risk factors for chronic disease in their own right, or whether they merely reflect earlier exposures in childhood and adolescence that are direct determinants of chronic disease. For example, if irregular cycles predict cardiovascular disease, is that because irregular cycles represent cumulative hormone exposures, or because they reveal fetal or childhood factors that determine both reproductive function and cardiovascular disease? The answers to such questions imply different points of intervention. It is also incumbent upon researchers to identify mediators and interventions to counteract deleterious exposures incurred *in utero* or in childhood. For example, would women whose HPA axes were shaped by childhood trauma benefit from stress management programmes during pregnancy, or is the die already cast?

Although many questions remain, the twentieth century evidence has borne out Good's nineteenth century observation of the 'extensive sympathy which the sexual organs maintain with every other part of the system'.[1] Vitality in the reproductive axis reflects harmony in the psyche and body. A society which determines and invests in the optimal nutrition, health, and well-being of its girls reaps the rewards in the vitality of its future grandmothers, mothers, daughters, and sons.

Acknowledgements

The work on this chapter was supported by the March of Dimes Birth Defects Foundation.

Commentary on 'A life course approach to women's reproductive health'

Susan Morton

It is fitting that one of the first chapters in this book should examine a life course approach to women's reproductive health as this raises the underlying and critically important question of when does the life course of a woman begin? This chapter elegantly details how a woman's reproductive life from menarche to menopause is both shaped by her early life experiences and offers an insight into her likely future health status. Pregnancy outcomes in particular reflect a woman's physical and social development from early life to adulthood and unmask latent risk factors for the development of later chronic diseases, especially cardiovascular disease[107,109] and diabetes mellitus.[110,111] Further the timing of a woman's first pregnancy and number of subsequent pregnancies may modify her risk of breast cancer,[93] and the fetal growth of her offspring may predict her own mortality.[118-120] Additionally her own intrauterine development may influence her adult reproductive capacity and outcomes.[14-16] These complex and intergenerational relationships suggest that a life course approach to a woman's reproductive health should probably begin before she was conceived.

The strength of evidence linking temporally distant early events with later reproductive function remains variable with many of the underlying biological mechanisms still to be elucidated or validated. In particular much of the evidence in support of intrauterine programming of reproductive function is derived from unfortunate natural experiments involving drug-use in pregnancy, war, or famine, which are not generalizable to the conditions under which most pregnancies currently occur. Further, evidence that has been accredited as direct may in fact not be so. For example the increased risk of poor reproductive outcomes in the daughters of mothers who took diethylstilboestrol (DES) for threatened abortion might represent evidence of an intergenerational continuity in maternal risk of poor pregnancy outcomes, either genetically or environmentally mediated, rather than a direct programming effect by the artificial hormone in pregnancy. Similarly whilst acute, severe famine, as experienced in the Dutch Hunger Winter, caused a small reduction in average offspring birthweight, a recent meta-analysis of randomized controlled trials of maternal dietary supplementation in pregnancy, under more normal nutritional conditions, has shown disappointingly small increases in average birthweight of less than 50 g, even in previously undernourished women.[122] Animal experiments may suggest that alteration of maternal diet in pregnancy has direct effects on offspring size but this is not yet conclusive for humans. In human pregnancy maternal nutrition is not equivalent to fetal nutrition because of the complex interactions that exist between mother and infant largely mediated by the functionally complex human placenta.[123] Even when biological pathways are well understood they may not fully explain the relationships that we see between size at birth and later reproductive function, as in the example of polycystic ovarian syndrome (PCOS) outlined in this chapter. However as the author points out the life course approach to reproductive health allows for the modification of intrauterine programming by early life and adult life environmental influences.

The impact of stress in early and adult life, both physiological and psychological, has recently emerged as such a potential modifier of adult reproductive health. Whilst plausible biological mechanisms do exist which link stimulation of the hypothalamic–pituitary–adrenal (HPA) axis with the hormonal control of fertility and reproduction (hypothalamic–pituitary–ovarian axis), the measurement of stress itself is complex and is especially so in childhood. Much of the supposition to date is therefore based on stress measurement gathered through retrospective personal report, which is subject to recall bias in particular. Other factors known to be strongly associated with reproductive outcomes are also extremely difficult to measure accurately. Social class categorization for women is particularly problematic. Aside from lack of agreement over appropriate occupational codes for women is the determination of the time point in her life at which the socioeconomic environment has the greatest impact. It may well be a woman's very early life socioeconomic environment that is most influential in setting her trajectory of reproductive health throughout middle and later life, as postulated almost half a century ago by Baird and colleagues.[2] In addition to understanding individual determinants of reproductive health further work is required to understand the ethnic differences seen in population health, as clearly demonstrated for American women in this chapter. No study to date has been able to offer an adequate explanation for these differences in pregnancy outcomes using known individual risk factors.

Elucidating the underlying biological mechanisms responsible for accumulation of risk has important implications for possible interventions. Establishing when a critical or sensitive period occurs currently depends more on when data have been collected than time points that are necessarily biologically or socially appropriate for intervention. The temptation to intervene in pregnancy to improve maternal and infant health is strong but it should be tempered by the growing knowledge that the full benefit, or indeed harm, of such short-term measures may not be evident for several generations.

The emerging evidence that the physiological stress of pregnancy may unmask the potential for later adult chronic disease also offers a potential opportunity for intervention to delay or ameliorate these problems. Rich-Edwards summarizes the current research in this interesting area and rightly suggests that more work is needed to decide whether pregnancy is an appropriate place to intervene or indeed begin monitoring women at risk, or whether the intervention needs to occur earlier in her life course. Further it may be difficult to intervene in pregnancy when the conditions being unmasked, especially preeclampsia, are themselves complex and their natural progression poorly predictable.

Rich-Edwards has presented a compelling and well-documented collection of research in support a life course approach to women's reproductive health. There is growing evidence that reproduction function is indeed both determined by early life experiences and capable of adaptation to current environmental influences. Further reproductive patterns may offer an early glimpse into risks for future health and therefore offer new opportunities to intervene to prevent or lessen chronic disease morbidity. However caution is required until a causative link is established rather than an association which unmasks intergenerational continuities in reproductive trajectories. For in the gender adapted words of William Wordsworth it does seem ever more apparent that 'The child is the *mother* of the *woman*.' (Wordsworth 1770–1850)

References

1 **Good JM**. *The Study of Medicine*. 1826.

2 **Baird D**. The epidemiology of low birth weight: changes in incidence in Aberdeen. *J Biosoc Sci* 1974;**6**:323–41.

3 **Emanuel I**. Maternal health during childhood and later reproductive performance. *Ann NY Acad Sci* 1986;**477**:27–39.

4 **Valanis BM, Rush D**. A partial explanation of superior birth weights among foreign-born women. *Soc Biol* 1979;**26**:198–210.

5 **Ellison PT, Panter-Brick C, Lipson SF, O'Rourke MT**. The ecological context of human ovarian function. *Hum Reprod* 1993;**8**:2248–58.

6 **Morabia A, Costanza MC**. World Health Organization Collaborative Study of Neoplasia and Steroid Contraceptives. International variability in ages at menarche, first livebirth, and menopause. *Am J Epidemiol* 1998;**148**:1195–1205.

7 **Strassman BI**. New paradigms for the female reproductive system. Menstrual cycling and breast cancer: an evolutionary perspective. *J Women's Health* 2001;**8**:193–202.

8 Flint M. Is there a secular trend in age of menopause? *Maturitas* 1978;**1**:133–9.

9 Khaw KT. Epidemiology of the menopause. *Br Med Bull* 1992;**48**:249–61.

10 Tanner JM. *Fetus into Man. Physical growth from conception to maturity*. Cambridge, MA. Harvard University Press, 1990.

11 Frisch RE. Body fat, menarche, fitness and fertility. *Prog Reprod Biol Med* 1990;**14**:1–26.

12 Ellison PT. Morbidity, mortality, and menarche. *Hum Biol* 1981;**53**:635–43.

13 Forsdahl A. Are poor living conditions in childhood and adolescence an important risk factor for arteriosclerotic heart disease? *Br J Prev Soc Med* 1977;**31**:91–5.

14 Klebanoff MA, Graubard BI, Kessel SS, Berendes HW. Low birthweight across generations. *J Am Med Assoc* 1984;**252**:2423–7.

15 Wang X, Zuckerman B, Coffman GA, Corwin MJ. Familial aggregation of low birthweight among whites and blacks in the United States. *N Engl J Med* 1995;**333**:1744–9.

16 Emanuel I, Filakti H, Alberman E, Evans SWJ. Intergenerational studies of human birthweight from the 1958 birth cohort. Evidence for a multigenerational effect. *Br J Obstet Gynaecol* 1992;**99**:67–74.

17 Kramer MS. Determinants of low birth weight: methodological assessment and meta-analysis. *Bull World Health Organ* 1987;**65**:663–737.

18 Walton A, Hammond J. The maternal effects on growth and conformation in Shire horse-Shetland pony crosses. *Proc R Soc Lond [Biol]* 1938;**125**:311–34.

19 Bakketieg LS, Hoffman HJ, Harley EE. The tendency to repeat gestational age and birth weight in successive births. *Am J Obstet Gynecol* 1979;**135**:1086–103.

20 Lumey LH, Stein AD. *In utero* exposure to famine and subsequent fertility: the Dutch Famine Birth Cohort Study. *Am J Public Health* 1997;**87**:1962–6.

21 Treloar SA, Martin NG. Age at menarche as a fitness trait: nonadditive genetic variance detected in a large twin sample. *Am J Hum Genet* 1990;**47**:137–48.

22 Snieder H, MacGregor AJ, Spector TD. Genes control the cessation of a woman reproductive life: a twin study of hysterectomy and age at menopause. *J Clin Endocrinol Metab* 1998;**83**:1875–80.

23 Cooper C, Kuh D, Egger P, Wadsworth M, Barker D. Childhood growth and age at menarche. *Br J Obstet Gynaecol* 1996;**103**:814–7.

24 Ibanez L, Potau N, Marcos MV, deZegher F. Exaggerated adrenarche and hyperinsulinism in adolescent girls born small for gestational age. *J Clin Endocrinol Metab* 1999;**84**:4739–41.

25 Clark P, Hindmarsh PC, Shiell AW, Law CM, Honan JW, Barker DJP. Size at birth and adreno-corticol function in childhood. *Clin Epidemiol* 1996;**45**:721–6.

26 Cresswell JL, Egger P, Fall CH. Is the age of menopause determined *in utero*? *Early Hum Dev* 1997;**49**:143–8.

27 Waterworth DM, Bennett ST, Gharani N, McCarthy MI, Hague S, Batty S, Conway GS, White D, Todd JA, Franks S, Williamson R. Linkage and association of insulin gene VNTR regulatory polymorphism with polycystic ovary syndrome. *Lancet* 1997;**349**:986–90.

28 Edozien L. Length of gestation and polycystic ovaries in adulthood. *Lancet* 1998;**351**:295–6.

29 Barraclough CA, Gorski RA. Evidence that the hypothalamus is responsible for androgen-induced sterility in the female rat. *Endocrinol* 1961;**68**:68–79.

30 Golden RJ, Noller KL, Titus-Ernstoff L, Kaufman RH, Mittendorf R, Stillman R, Reese EA. Environmental endocrine modulators and human health: an assessment of the biological evidence. *Crit Rev Toxicol* 1998;**28**:109–227.

31 Goldberg JM, Tommaso F. Effect of diethylstilbestrol on reproductive function. *Fertil Steril* 1999;**72**:1–7.

32 Barker DJP. *Mothers, babies, and disease in later life*. London: BMJ Publishing Group, 1994.

33 Stein AD, Ravelli ACJ, Lumey LH. Famine, third-trimester pregnancy weight gain, and intrauterine growth: the Dutch Famine Birth Cohort Study. *Hum Biol* 1995;**67**:135–50.

34 Stein AD, Lumey LH. The relationship between maternal and offspring birthweights after maternal prenatal famine exposure: the Dutch Famine Birth Cohort Study. *Hum Biol* 2000;**72**:641–54.

35 Ramakrishnan U, Barnhart H, Schroeder DG, Stein AD, Martorell R. Early childhood nutrition, education and fertility milestones in Guatemala. *J Nutr* 1999;**129**:2196–202.

36 Ellison PT. Skeletal growth, fatness, and menarcheal age: a comparison of two hypotheses. *Hum Biol* 1982;**54**:269–81.

37 Berkey CS, Gardner JD, Frazier AL, Colditz GA. Relation of childhood diet and body size to menarche and adolescent growth in girls. *Am J Epidemiol* 2000;**152**:446–52.

38 Kato I, Toniolo P, Koenig KL, Shore RE, Zeleniuch-Jacquotte A, Akhmedkhanov A, Riboli E. Epidemiologic correlates with menstrual cycle length in middle aged women. *Eur J Epidemiol* 1999;**15**:809–14.

39 Bates GW, Whitworth NS. Effect of body weight reduction on plasma androgens in obese, infertile women. *Fertil Steril* 1982;**4**:406–9.

40 Harlass FE, Plymate SR, Fariss BL, Belts RP. Weight loss is associated with correction of gonadotropin and sex steroid abnormalities in the obese anovulatory female. *Fertil Steril* 1984;**42**:649–52.

41 Kiddy DS, Hamilton-Fairley D, Bush A, Short F, Anyaoku V, Reed MJ, Franks S. Improvement in endocrine and ovarian function during dietary treatment of obese women with polycystic ovary syndrome. *Clin Endocrinol* 1992;**36**:105–11.

42 Rich-Edwards JW, Spiegelman D, Garland M, Hertzmark E, Hunter DJ, Colditz GA, Willett WC, Wand H, Manson JE. Physical activity, body mass index, and ovulatory disorder infertility. *Epidemiol* 2002;**13**:184–90.

43 Hardy R, Kuh D. Reproductive characteristic risk factors and the age at inception of the perimenopause in a British National Cohort. *Am J Epidemiol* 1999;**149**:612–20.

44 Treloar SA, Sadrazden S, Do KA, Martin NG, Lambalk CB. Birthweight and age at menopause in Australian female twin pairs: exploration of the fetal origin hypothesis. *Hum Reprod* 2000;**15**:55–9.

45 Van Noord P, Dubas J, Corland M, Boersma H, te Velde E. Age at natural menopause in a population-based screening cohort: the role of menarche, fecundity, and lifestyle factors. *Fertil Steril* 1997;**68**:95–102.

46 Parazzini F, Negri E, La Vecchia C. Reproductive and general lifestyle determinants of age at menopause. *Maturitas* 1992;**15**:141–9.

47 Parazzini F, Tavani A, Ricci E, La Vecchia C. Menstrual and reproductive factors and hip fractures in post menopausal women. *Maturitas* 1996;**24**:191–6.

48 Bromberger JT, Matthews KA, Kuller LH, Wing RR, Meilahn EN, Plantinga P. Prospective study of the determinants of age at menopause. *Am J Epidemiol* 1997;**145**:124–33.

49 Chrousos GP, Torpy DJ, Gold PW. Interactions between the hypothalamic-pituitary-adrenal axis and the female reproductive system: clinical implications. *Ann Intern Med* 1998;**129**:229–40.

50 Majzoub JA, Karalis KP. Placental corticotropin-releasing hormone: Function and regulation. *Am J Obstet Gynecol* 1999;**180**:S242–6.

51 McLean M, Bisits A, Davies J, Woods R, Lowry P, Smith R. A placental clock controlling the length of human pregnancy. *Nat Med* 1995;**1**:460–3.

52 Rich-Edwards JW, Krieger N, Majzoub J, Zierler S, Lieberman E, Gillman MW. Maternal experiences of racism and violence as predictors of preterm birth: rationale and study design. *Pediatr Perinat Epidemiol* 2001;**15**:124–35.

53 Van Noord P, Kaaks R. The effect of wartime conditions and the 1944–45 Dutch Famine on recalled menarcheal age in participants of the DOM breast cancer screening project. *Ann Human Biol* 1991;**18**:57–70.

54 Tahirovic HF. Menarcheal age and the stress of war: an example from Bosnia. *Eur J Pediatr* 1998;**157**:978–80.

55 Demyttenaere K, Bonte L, Gheldorf M, Vervaeke M, Meuleman C, Vanderschuerem D, D'Hooghe T. Coping style and depression level influence outcome in in vitro fertilization. *Fertil Steril* 1998;**69**:1026–33.

56 Thiering P, Beaurepaire J, Jone M, Saunders D, Tennant C. Mood state as predictor of treatment outcome after in vitro fertilization/embryo transfer technology. *J Psychosom Res* 1993;**37**:481–91.

57 Domar A, Auttermeister P, Friedman R. The relationship between distress and conception in infertile women. *J Am Med Wom Assoc* 1999;**54**:196–8.

58 Domar AD, Clapp D, Slawsby E, Dusek J, Kessel B, Freizinger M. The impact of group psychological interventions on pregnancy rates in infertile women. *Fertil Steril* 2000;**73**:805–11.

59 Lobel M. Conceptualizations, measurements, and effects of prenatal maternal stress on birth outcomes. *J Behav Med* 1994;**17**:225–72.

60 McLean DE, Hatfield-Timajchy K, Wingo PA, Floyd RL. Psychosocial measurement: implications for the study of preterm delivery in black women. *Am J Prev Med* 1993;**9** (6 suppl):39–67.

61 Hoffman S, James SA, Siegel E. Stress, social support and pregnancy outcome: a reassessment based on recent research. *Paediatr Perinat Epidemiol* 1996;**10**:380–405.

62 Hoffman S, Hatch MC. Depressive symptomatology during pregnancy: evidence for an association with decreased fetal growth in pregnancies for lower social class women. *Health Psychol* 2000;**19**:535–43.

63 Boyles SH, Ness RB, Grisso JA, Markovic N, Bromberger J, CiFelli D. Life event stress and the association with spontaneous abortion in gravid women at an urban emergency department. *Health Psychol* 2000;**19**:510–14.

64 Heugebauer R, Kline J, Stein Z, Shrout P, Warburton D, Susser M. Association of stressful life events with chromosomally normal spontaneous abortion. *Am J Epidemiol* 1996;**143**:588–96.

65 O'Hare T, Creed F. Life events and miscarriage. *Br J Psych* 1995;**167**:799–805.

66 Ramsey CN, Abell TD, Baker LC. The relationship between family functioning, life events, family structure, and the outcome of pregnancy. *J Fam Pract* 1985;**22**:521–7.

67 Reeb KA, Graham AV, Zyzanski SJ, Kitson GC. Predicting low birthweight and complicated labor in urban black women: a biopsychosocial perspective. *Soc Sci Med* 1987;**25**:1321–7.

68 Pritchard DW, Teo Mfphm PYK. Preterm birth, low birthweight and the stressfullness of the household role for pregnant women. *Soc Sci Med* 1994;**38**:89–96.

69 Collins JW, David RJ, Symons R, Handler A, Wall S, Andes S. African-American mothers' perception of their residential environment, stressful life events, and very low birthweight. *Epidemiol* 1998;**9**:286–9.

70 Kramer MS, Seguin L, Lydon J, Goulet L. Socioeconomic disparities in pregnancy outcome: why do the poor fare so poorly? *Pediatr Perinat Epidemiol* 2000;**14**:194–210.

71 Guyer B, Martin JA, MacDorman MF, Anderson RN, Strobino DM. Annual summary of vital statistics-1996. *Pediatrics* 1997;**100**:905–18.

72 Kleinman JC, Kessel SS. Racial differences in low birth weight. Trends and risks factors. *N Engl J Med* 1987;**317**:749–53.

73 Collins JW, Derrick M, Hilder L, Kempley S. Relation of maternal ethnicity to infant birthweight in East London, England. *Ethn Dis* 1997;**7**:1–4.

74 National Center for Health Statistics. *Factors associated with low birth weight*. United States, 1976. Vital Health Stat [21] No. 37, Hyattsville, MD, 1980.

75 Friedman DJ, Cohen BB, Mahan CM, Lederman RI, Vezina RJ, Dunn VH. Maternal ethnicity and birthweight among Blacks. *Ethn Dis* 1993;**3**:255–69.

76 Pallotto EK, Collins JW, David RJ. Enigma of maternal race and infant birth weight: a population-based study of US-born Black and Caribbean-born Black women. *Epidemiol* 2000;**151**:1080–5.

77 David RJ, Collins JW, Jr. Differing birth weight among infants of U.S.-born blacks, African-born blacks, and U.S.-born whites. *N Engl J Med* 1997;**337**:1209–14.

78 Fuentes-Afflick E, Hessol NA, Perez-Stable EJ. Testing the epidemiologic paradox of low birth weight in Latinos. *Arch Pediatr Adolesc Med* 1999;**153**:147–53.

79 Singh G, Yu S. Adverse pregnancy outcomes: differences between US- and foreign-born women in major US racial and ethnic groups. *Am J Public Health* 1996;**86**:837–43.

80 Guendelman S, English PB. Effect of United States residence on birth outcomes among Mexican immigrants: an exploratory study. *Am J Epidemiol* 1995;**142**:S30–8.

81 Cobas JA, Balcazr H, Benen MB, Keith VM, Chong Y. Acculturation and low-birthweight infants among Latino women: a reanalysis of HANES data with structural equation models. *Am J Public Health* 1996;**86**:394–6.

82 Scribner R, Dwyer JL. Acculturation and low birthweight among Latinos in the Hispanic HANES. *Am J Public Health* 1989;**79**:1263–7.

83 Collins JW, David RJ, Symons R, Handler A, Wall SN, Dwyer L. Low-income African-American mothers' perceptions of exposure to racial discrimination and infant birth weight. *Epidemiol* 2000;**11**:337–9.

84 Horan DL, Hill LD, Schulkin J. Childhood sexual abuse and preterm labor in adulthood: an endocrinological hypothesis. *Women's Health Issues* 2000;**10**:27–33.

85 Geronimus AT. The weathering hypothesis and the health of African-American women and infants: evidence and speculation. *Ethn Dis* 1992;**2**:207–21.

86 Geronimus AT. Black/white differences in the relationship of maternal age to birthweight: a population-based test of the weathering hypothesis. *Soc Sci Med* 1996;**42**:589–97.

87 Ventura SJ, Martin JA, Curtin SC, Mathews TJ, Park MM. *Births: Final data for 1998*. National Vital Statistics Reports 2000;**48**:1–100.

88 Rich-Edwards JW, Buka SL, Kindlon DJ, Earls JE. *Novel uses of birth certificate data to monitor inequalities in maternal and child health*. Presented at the American Public Health Association annual meeting, 1999, Washington, DC.

89 Sowers MFR, LaPietra MT. Menopause: its epidemiology and potential association with chronic diseases. *Epidemiol Rev* 1996;**17**:287–301.

90 Windham GC, Elkin EP, Swan SH, Waller KO, Fenster L. Cigarette smoking and effects on menstrual function. *Obstet Gynecol* 1999;**93**:59–65.

91 Ursin G, Bernstein L, Pike MC. Cancer Surveys: Advances and Prospects in Clinical, Epidemiological and Laboratory Oncology. In: Doll R, Fraumeni JF, Jr., Muir CS, eds. *Trends in Cancer Incidence and Mortality*. Cold Spring Harbor: Cold Spring Harbor Laboratory Press, 1994:241–64.

92 Hsieh C, Trichopoulos D, Katsouyanni K, Yuasa S. Age at menarche, age at menopause, height and obesity as risk factor for breast cancer: associations and interactions in an international case-control study. *Int J Cancer* 1990;**46**:796–800.

93 Butler LM, Potischman NA, Newman B, Millikan RC, Brogan D, Gammon MD, Swanson CA, Brinton LA. Menstrual risk factors and early-onset breast cancer. *Cancer Causes Control* 2000;**11**:451–8.

94 Titus-Ernstoff L, Longnecker MP, Newcomb PA, Dain B, Greenberg ER, Mittendorf R, Stampfer M, Willett W. Menstrual factors in relation to breast cancer risk. *Cancer Epidemiol Biomarkers Prev* 1998;**7**:783–9.

95 Rockhill B, Moorman PG, Newman B. Age at menarche, time to regular cycling, and breast cancer. *Cancer Causes Control* 1998;**9**:447–53.

96 Kelsey JL, Gammon MD, John EM. Reproductive factors and breast cancer. *Epidemiol Rev* 1993;**15**:36–47.

97 Klip H, Burger CW, Kenemans P, van Leeuwen FE. Cancer risk associated with subfertility and ovulation induction: a review. *Cancer Causes Control* 2000;**11**:319–44.

98 Garland M, Hunter DJ, Manson JE, Stampfer MJ, Spiegelman D, Speizer F, Willett WC. Menstrual cycle characteristics and history of ovulatory infertility in relation to breast cancer risk in a large cohort of US women. *Am J Epidemiol* 1998;**147**:636–43.

99 Solomon CG, Hu FB, Dunaif A, Rich-Edwards JW, Willet WC, Hunter DJ, Colditz GA, Speizer FE, Manson JE. Long or highly irregular menstrual cycles as a marker of risk of type 2 diabetes mellitus: a prospective study. *J Am Med Assoc* 2001;**285**:2421–6.

100 Rich-Edwards JW, Solomon CG, Dunaif A, Colditz GA, Hunter DJ, Stampfer MJ, Spiegelman D, Willett WC, Manson JE. *Associations of menstrual cycle characteristics with risk of hypertension in adult women.* Presented at the Sixth Annual Congress on Women's Health, Washington DC, 1998.

101 Solomon CG, Hu F, Willet W, Dunaif A, Rich-Edwards J, Stampfer MJ. Menstrual cycle irregularity and risk for future cardiovascular disease. *J Clin Endocrinol Metab*, in press.

102 Pierpont T, McKeigue PM, Issacs AJ, Wild SH, Jacobs HS. Mortality of women with polycystic ovary syndrome at long-term follow-up. *J Clin Epidemiol* 1998;**51**:581–6.

103 Wild S, Pierpont T, McKeigue P, Jacobs H. Cardiovascular disease in women with PCOS at long-term follow-up: a retrospective cohort study. *Clin Endocrinol* 2000;**52**:595–600.

104 Coulam CB, Annegers JF, Kranz JS. Chronic anovulation syndrome and associated neoplasia. *Obstet Gynecol* 1983;**61**:403–7.

105 Gammon MD, Thompson WD. Polycystic ovaries and the risk of breast cancer. *Am J Epidemiol* 1989;**129**:865–73.

106 Ness RB, Harris T, Cobb J, Flegal KM, Kelsey JL, Balanger A, Stunkard AJ, D'Agostino RB. Number of pregnancies and the subsequent risk of cardiovascular disease. *N Engl J Med* 1993;**328**:1528–33.

107 Zhang J, Zeisler J, Hatch MC, Berkowitz G. Epidemiology of pregnancy-induced hypertension. *Epidemiol Rev* 1997;**19**:218–32.

108 Innes KE, Byers TE. Preeclampsia and breast cancer risk. *Epidemiol* 1999;**10**:722–32.

109 Jonsdottir LS, Arngrimsson R, Geirsson RT, Sigvaldason H, Sigfusson N. Death rates from ischemic heart disease in women with a history of hypertension in pregnancy. *Acta Obstet Gynecol Scand* 1995;**74**:772–6.

110 Mestman JH, Anderson GV, Guadalupe V. Follow-up study of 360 subjects with abnormal carbohydrate metabolism during pregnancy. *Obstet Gynecol* 1972;**39**:421–5.

111 Dornhorst A, Rossi M. Risk and prevention of type 2 diabetes in women with gestational diabetes. *Diabetes Care* 1998;**21** Suppl 2:B43–9.

112 Kjos SL, Peters RK, Xiang A, Henry OA, Montoro M, Buchanan TA. Predicting future diabetes in Latino women with gestational diabetes. Utility of early postpartum glucose tolerance testing. *Diabetes* 1995;**44**:586–91.

113 Chelsey LC, Annitto JE, Cosgrove RA. The remote prognosis of eclamptic women. Sixth periodic report. *Am J Obstet Gynecol* 1975;**124**:446–59.

114 Ekbom A, Hsieh C, Lipworth L, Adami HQ, Trichopoulos D. Intrauterine environment and breast cancer risk in women: a population-based study. *J Natl Cancer Inst* 1997;**89**:71–6.

115 Hsieh C, Lambe M, Trichopoulos D, Adami HO, Ekbom A. Delivery of premature newborns and maternal breast-cancer risk. *Lancet* 1999;**353**:1239.

116 Richardson BE, Hulka BS, Peck JL, Hughes CL, van de Berg BJ, Christianson RE, Calvin JA. Levels of maternal serum alpha-fetoprotein (AFP) in pregnant women and subsequent breast cancer risk. *Am J Epidemiol* 1998;**148**:719–27.

117 Melbye M, Wohlfahrt J, Lei U, Norgaard-Pedersen B, Mouridsen HT, Lambe M, Michels KB. Alpha-fetoprotein levels in maternal serum during pregnancy and maternal breast cancer incidence. *J Natl Cancer Inst* 2000;**92**:1001–5.

118 Cohn BA, Cirillo PM, Christianson RE, van de Berg BJ, Siiteri PK. Placental characteristics and reduced risk of maternal breast cancer. *J Natl Cancer Inst* 2001;**93**:1133–40.

119 Davey-Smith G, Hart C, Ferrell C, Upton M, Hole D, Hawthorne V, Watt G. Birth weight of offspring and mortality in the Renfrew and Paisley study: prospective observational study. *Br Med J* 1997;**315**:1189–93.

120 Davey-Smith G, Whitley E, Gissler M, Hemminki E. Birth dimensions of offspring, premature birth, and the mortality of mothers. *Lancet* 2000;**356**:2066–7.

121 Davey-Smith G, Harding S, Rosato M. Relation between infants' birth weight and mothers' mortality: prospective observational study. *Br Med J* 2000;**320**:839–40.

122 Kramer MS. *Balanced Protein/Energy Supplementation in Pregnancy (Cochrane Review)*. The Cochrane Library. Issue 4. Oxford: Update Software, 1999.

123 Harding JE. The nutritional basis of the fetal origins of adult disease. *Int J Epidemiol* 2001;**30**:15–23.

Chapter 3

Breast cancer aetiology: where do we go from here?

Isabel dos Santos Silva and Bianca L. De Stavola

Evidence has been growing in the last few years in support of the hypothesis that early life exposures may be as important in the aetiology of breast cancer as those acting in adult life. Associations have been reported, although not always consistently across all studies, between breast cancer risk and various *in utero* exposures. In particular, the evidence points to a positive association between birthweight and breast cancer risk at premenopausal, but not postmenopausal, ages. Rapid childhood growth as indicated by leg length, adult height, and the timing of menarche has also been associated with an increase in the risk of breast cancer. Support for the role of prenatal and postnatal growth rates is also provided by evidence of a positive association between adult serum levels of insulin-like growth factors and subsequent risk of breast cancer. Though there are still many unanswered questions regarding the role of early life exposures on breast cancer risk, and how they may interact with the established adult risk factors, these findings imply the need for research and preventative efforts to shift from adult to early life.

3.1 Introduction

More than three decades of epidemiological studies have identified various adult risk factors for breast cancer. In recent years, however, epidemiological research has raised the possibility that factors operating *in utero* and in early life may be as important in the aetiology of this tumour as those acting in adult life. In this chapter, we begin by reviewing briefly the established adult risk factors for breast cancer. We will then assess the evidence linking breast cancer with childhood and prenatal exposures. Finally, we will consider the aetiology of breast cancer in a life course framework in which risk factors occurring at each life stage are linked to investigate possible pathways from early life events to adulthood and subsequent occurrence of breast cancer.

3.2 Adult risk factors

The overwhelming evidence for a strong association between reproductive and menstrual factors and breast cancer risk provides indirect evidence for the involvement of female sex hormones in the aetiology of the disease. Breast cancer risk appears to be determined in large part by the cumulative exposure of breast epithelium to oestrogens and, possibly, progesterone. Most of this exposure is accumulated during the years of active ovarian function. For example, the fact that the rate of increase in breast cancer incidence dramatically slows down around the age of 50 years, the average age of menopause, suggests that cyclic production of relatively large amounts of sex hormones by the ovaries is implicated in the aetiology of breast cancer. This is supported by the fact that women who experience natural menopause before age 45 have only half the risk of those whose menopause occurs after age 55.[1] More direct evidence comes from prospective studies showing that high levels of serum oestrogens, particularly at postmenopausal ages, are associated with increased risks of subsequent breast cancer.[2–5]

Age at birth of first child has also been considered as an important risk factor for breast cancer since the large international study by MacMahon et al.[6] The risk in women first bearing a child before age 20 was estimated to be one-third of that of women first bearing after age 34; in contrast, the risk associated with a first birth after age 34 exceeded that associated with nulliparity. Subsequent studies have also shown a protective effect of high parity that is independent of the effect of age at first birth.[7,8] Moreover, women within three years of their last childbirth were found to have a significantly increased risk of breast cancer relative to women whose last birth was ten or more years earlier; this effect persisted after adjusting for parity and age at first birth.[8] Thus, it appears from these findings that pregnancy has a dual effect on breast cancer—a short-term increase in risk followed by a long-term protective effect. Pregnancy is associated with very high levels of oestrogens, progesterone, and prolactin. These high hormone levels induce cell differentiation as well as cell proliferation and this could explain the biphasic effect of pregnancy on breast cancer. Within the two-stage model proposed by Moolgavkar et al.,[9] pregnancy may act as an anti-initiator by reducing the pool of susceptible stem cells through differentiation, and as a promoter by inducing proliferation of cells which have already suffered malignant transformation. There is also some evidence that the decreased risk of breast cancer associated with early first full-term pregnancy is mediated, at least in part, by long-term alterations in levels of sex-hormone binding globulin (SHBG): SHBG levels are permanently raised after a first full-term pregnancy,[10] with a consequent reduction in the amount of circulating free oestrogens readily available to receptors in the breast tissue.

Prolonged breastfeeding delays the re-establishment of ovulation following a complete pregnancy and could therefore protect against breast cancer. The evidence in support of this hypothesis has been largely inconsistent partly because most studies have been conducted in populations where the lifetime duration of breastfeeding of most women is rather short. In contrast, a strong protective effect of breastfeeding was reported by a population-based case-control study conducted in China,[11] where breastfeeding is usually carried out for much longer. In this study,[11] women who breastfed for a total of more than nine years had only 37% (95% confidence interval (CI): 14% to 98%) of the breast cancer risk of those who breastfed for a total of less than three years, after adjusting for parity and age at first birth. This association was independent of age or menopausal status.

The role of sex hormones in the aetiology of breast cancer is also supported by recent pooled reanalyses of individual data from more than 50 epidemiological studies on the use of exogenous sex hormones.[12,13] Postmenopausal hormone replacement therapy (HRT) seems to be associated with an excess of breast cancer risk in current and recent users.[12]

Oral contraceptive use has only a small effect on breast cancer risk, which is to increase the risk in current and recent users.[13]

The effect of adiposity can also be seen within the context of the female sex hormones hypothesis. Most studies showed a positive association between body mass index (BMI) and postmenopausal breast cancer risk, although the relative risks found in cohort studies[14] are much closer to the null value than those found in case-control studies.[15,16] In post-menopausal women, the extraglandular conversion of androstenedione to oestrone and then oestradiol in adipose tissue accounts for 90% of circulating oestradiol.[17] Moreover, increased weight is not only associated with higher postmenopausal oestrogen levels but also with reduced levels of SHBG and, therefore, with greater tissue availability of oestrogens.[18] For premenopausal breast cancer, however, the relationship of obesity with breast cancer is inverted. A recent meta-analysis[19] concluded that there was an inverse association of BMI with premenopausal breast cancer, which was stronger in cohort than case-control studies. This protective effect of obesity in younger women could not be adequately explained by difficulties in detection of tumours in heavy women. It could, however, be due to the association of premenopausal obesity with anovulation and progesterone deficiency.[20] Most of the studies that have examined the relationship between weight and breast cancer risk relied on anthropometric measurements taken at a particular time (generally, early or mid-adulthood). In case-control studies, data on anthropometric variables are usually collected some time after the cases have been diagnosed (and are, therefore, potentially susceptible to have been affected by the disease itself). In cohort studies, anthropometric measurements are usually taken at an adult baseline, with no account of changes through life. This approach is clearly inappropriate because most women experience marked body size fluctuations throughout life.[21] This limitation has been highlighted by recent research (based on recall data) suggesting that weight gain may be an important risk factor for post-menopausal breast cancer,[22–26] and in some studies this effect was shown to be independent of BMI.[23,26]

Breast density, as ascertained from mammograms, is also a well-established risk factor for breast cancer, which is being increasingly used as an intermediate marker for this tumour in many epidemiological studies.[27,28] Several studies have reported the magnitude of the breast cancer risk associated with increasing breast density, after adjusting for reproductive and anthropometric factors, to be about a fourfold to sixfold rise when density is measured on a continuous scale as percentage of breast density.[27] It is a twofold to fourfold increase when density is measured using the qualitative classification proposed by Wolfe.[29] Little is known about the relationship between levels of endogenous oestrogens and mammographic features. Preliminary results from the US Nurses' Health Study showed a positive correlation between free percentage oestradiol and percentage of breast density.[30] Indirect support for a role of endogenous oestrogens in determining high-density patterns is also provided by studies showing that breast density increases with the use of oestrogen replacement therapy [31,32] and decreases with the administration of tamoxifen[33] or hormonal contraceptive regimens designed to suppress ovarian function.[34]

3.3 Early life risk factors

One of the most striking features in breast cancer epidemiology is the marked international variability of the disease. The incidence of this cancer varies more than fivefold around the world,[35] with highest rates in western countries. This variability cannot be explained by genetic factors, since the risk of breast cancer in migrants from low- to high-incidence areas shifts to that of the adopted country suggesting that its aetiology is determined largely by environmental or behavioural factors.[36] Further support comes from studies showing gradients in risk with socioeconomic status within ethnically homogeneous populations, with risk rising from lower to higher social groups in most populations.[37]

Hoel et al.[38] showed that the much higher rates of breast cancer in the US than in Japan could not be explained by differences in age at first birth, nulliparity, or age at menopause, but were correlated with differences in age at menarche and postmenopausal weight. Both age at menarche and postmenopausal weight are thought to be influenced by nutritional factors. Thus, diet has been regarded as a primary suspect for the marked international variability in breast cancer incidence.

Findings from animal[39] and ecological studies[40] support positive associations between dietary factors, particularly high fat intake, and breast cancer risk but individual-based epidemiological studies have produced rather inconsistent results, except for a positive association with alcohol intake.[41] But most of these studies focused on diet in adult life. The critical vulnerability period may occur early in life[42] since both adult height and age at menarche, which are associated with breast cancer risk and are established by the end of childhood, seem to be influenced by nutritional status early in life. Migrant studies also indicate that factors in early life make a more substantial contribution to breast cancer development than those in later life.[36]

Only four studies have so far examined the relationship between recalled adolescent diet and breast cancer risk. The first[43] reported an inverse association, although not statistically significant, between dietary fat intake during adolescence and breast cancer risk; in this study, increasing total fibre intake was also associated with a statistically significant increased risk of breast cancer but only in postmenopausal women. The second study[44] found a statistically significant positive association between childhood consumption of visible fat on meat and risk of premenopausal breast cancer; in contrast, childhood consumption of whole milk or vegetable oils were inversely related to the risk of postmenopausal and premenopausal breast cancer, respectively. The third study asked premenopausal women about their diet at ages 12–13 years.[45] High intake of fruit and vegetables appeared protective whereas high intake of chicken or high-fat meat were associated with slight increases in risk, though these findings were of borderline statistical significance. The fourth study was conducted within the US Nurses' Health Study and was based on recalled diet during high school.[46] High intakes of fibre, methionine, monounsaturated fat or eggs had a protective effect amongst postmenopausal women. In the only study to have so far assessed prospectively the role of diet in early life there was no relationship between energy intake and breast cancer mortality, but the number of breast cancer deaths was too small (only 26) for any conclusion to be drawn.[47] A few studies, based on self or maternal reports, have shown a protective effect of having been breastfed, particularly for premenopausal breast cancer, but these findings have not been confirmed by others.[48]

Hypotheses relating to childhood and adolescence diet are difficult to test directly in humans because recorded measures of dietary intake at young ages are scarce and reports by adults of their dietary intake in the distant past are unlikely to be sufficiently valid. As an alternative approach to assess the role of early diet on breast cancer risks, many studies have used anthropometric indicators as markers of early nutrition. In particular, adult height has been used as a rough proxy measure for childhood energy intake. Adult height is correlated positively with international breast cancer rates,[49] thus suggesting that childhood and adolescent energy intake may influence breast cancer risk decades later. In Japan, for instance, a substantial increase in average height occurred during the twentieth century,[50] presumably due to improved nutrition, which preceded the secular increase in breast cancer incidence.[51] A strong positive association between height and breast cancer risks was found among Norwegian women who reached puberty during World War II, a period when there was a large inter-individual variability in energy intake as some geographic areas were more affected by food shortages than others.[52,53] These findings would be consistent with the hypothesis that caloric restriction during adolescence may have favourable long-term consequences on breast cancer risk. A recent study,[54] however, found no evidence that breast cancer risk was associated with caloric restriction, as measured by proxy markers such as father's job and area of residence, among Dutch women who experienced puberty during World War II.

Individual-based studies have also confirmed the association between adult height and risk of breast cancer. In most of these studies, adult height was positively associated with breast cancer risk,[16] and this association persisted even after adjusting for age at menarche and reproductive history.[55,56] A recent review[57] concluded that the few studies that did not show an association between height and breast cancer tended to rely on self reported height, and hence, it is possible that non-differential exposure misclassification might have accounted for their negative findings. Similarly, a pooled analysis of seven cohort studies[14] found a positive relationship between height and both premenopausal and postmenopausal breast cancer, but the test for linear trend across the height categories was significant for postmenopausal women only.

It is unclear by what mechanism height is a predictor of breast cancer risk. Adult height is probably not a risk factor in itself, but it may be a marker of exposure to nutritional factors and growth early in life. As mentioned in Chapter 2, the relationship between childhood growth and age at menarche is well-documented, with peak-height velocity preceding menarche by about 1.2 years[58] and a critical body mass being thought to be required for onset of menarche.[59] Age at menarche appears to be inversely related to high energy intake[60] and body size.[61,62] A younger age at menarche is associated with an increased risk of breast cancer independently of other established risk factors.[63,64] An approximate 20% decrease in breast cancer risk results from each year that menarche is delayed.[65] Women with early menarche will be exposed to a larger cumulative number of monthly cycles of oestrogens, which might directly increase the risk of malignancy. Early menarche may also lead to higher levels of oestrogens throughout the reproductive life.[66] Teenage girls from populations with low breast cancer rates have both later menarche and a lower cumulative total number of ovulatory cycles for a fixed number of years since menarche, than do girls from high risk populations.[67] However, there is no relationship between age at peak height velocity, or its magnitude, and final adult height.[58] Moreover, the effect of adult height on breast cancer risk seems to be, at least in part, independent of that of age at menarche.[55,56] As a possible explanation for the influence of adult height on breast cancer risk, height may be just an indirect marker for mammary gland size and, by inference, a rough indicator of the number of ductal stem cells at risk of malignant transformation.[68]

Few investigations have attempted to examine changes in height during puberty and breast cancer risk later in life.[22,69,70] In one of these studies,[69] age when a woman reached her final adult height was found to be an important predictor of breast cancer at young ages, independent of age at menarche. In the US Nurses' Health Study,[70] early menarche, extremely lean body mass at age 10 years, and taller adult height were predictive of higher peak-height growth velocities during adolescence and of elevated breast cancer risk later in life. These studies, though, were forced to rely on the women's ability to recall their size in the distant past. Some investigators have tried to overcome this limitation by using adult anthropometric indicators supposed to reflect more closely preadolescent growth. Leg length, often estimated as sitting height-to-standing height ratio, is one such indicator as most of the pre-pubertal increases in height are due to increases in leg length,[71] but few studies have so far examined its relationship with breast cancer risk. In a large population-based case-control study in the US there was no relationship between adult sitting-to-standing height ratio and breast cancer risk in women aged under 45 years.[56] In another small case-control study,[72] there was no association between adult height and breast cancer risk but the cases had statistically significant longer legs than controls. In the Boyd Orr prospective study there was a positive association between leg length measured in childhood and mortality from breast cancer, but the association was statistically significant only for those women whose leg length was measured in the pre-pubertal period, that is, before age 8 years.[71] The importance of childhood growth on the aetiology of breast cancer has been corroborated by more recent findings based on a British cohort of about 2000 girls born immediately after World War II and for whom height and weight were measured throughout childhood. The magnitude of their growth rates early in childhood, between ages two and seven years, appeared to be strongly associated with premenopausal breast cancer, even after the effect of other early life factors and adulthood reproductive factors were accounted for.[73]

Support for the role of early nutrition and growth on breast cancer aetiology also comes from an endocrinological perspective. Better nutrition accelerates growth hormone release which, in turn, increases levels of insulin-like growth factors (IGFs). IGFs are important in determining the rate of growth throughout fetal and childhood development. The adolescent growth spurt involves stimulation by growth hormone, insulin, IGFs, and sex steroid hormones, and it has been suggested that the combination of IGFs and sex steroids result in mitogenic effects on developing mammary tissue in adolescence and a concomitant increased risk of epithelial atypia and carcinogenesis.[74] Four case-control studies[75–78] have so far examined the relationship between serum levels of IGF-1, and one of its binding proteins (IGFBP-3) and breast cancer risk. With one exception,[78] all have found adult serum levels of IGF-1 and/or IGF-1:IGFBP-3 ratios to be associated with an increased risk. In addition, two prospective studies[79,80] investigated pre-diagnostic serum IGF-1 concentrations in relation to subsequent breast cancer risk. The first, a case-control study nested within the US Nurses' Health Study cohort,[79] found a higher risk among premenopausal women who were in the top third of serum IGF-1 concentration than among those in the lowest third (odds ratio (OR)=2.33; 95% CI: 1.06–5.16). This association became stronger when adjustment was made for levels of the carrier protein IGFBP-3 (OR=2.88; 95% CI: 1.21–6.85). No association between levels of IGF-1 and breast cancer incidence was observed among postmenopausal women. The second prospective study was a nested case-control study conducted within the New York University Women's Health Study.[80] Similarly to the US Nurses' Health Study, the risk of breast cancer increased with increasing serum levels of IGF-1 in premenopausal women, particularly in those aged under 50 years, but not in postmenopausal women. In contrast to the US Nurses' Health Study, however, the association of risk with IGF-1 became weaker after adjusting for IGFBP-3. In the US Nurses' Health Study there was also an association between IGF-1 and breast density, which was confined to premenopausal women.[81]

IGFs are involved in the control of mitogenesis, cell-cycle regulation, cell survival, and cell transformation. IGF-1 not only stimulates cell proliferation but also inhibits apoptosis in many tissue types. Hence, it is not surprising that the epidemiological data, although limited, support the hypothesis that higher plasma IGF-1 levels would affect breast density and, possibly via this pathway, higher rates of breast cancer. However, it is not clear whether adult serum levels of IGF-1 and IGFBP-3 are associated with an increased breast cancer risk in their own right, or only indirectly through their potential correlation with levels during the periods of fetal and childhood growth. In cross-sectional population measurements, mean IGF-1 and IGFBP-3 concentrations in the blood rise with age from birth to puberty and then decline,[82] but there are no longitudinal data to determine whether girls with high levels in childhood go on to have high levels in adulthood.

3.4 Prenatal origins of breast cancer

In recent years it has been suggested that breast cancer may originate *in utero*.[83] Trichopoulos suggested that *in utero* exposure to high levels of oestrogens might increase the risk of breast cancer later in life on the basis of four assumptions: (1) endogenous oestrogens are important breast cancer risk factors; (2) exposures that act postnatally can also act prenatally; (3) levels of endogenous oestrogens are at least ten times higher during pregnancy than during other periods of adult life; and (4) there is wide inter-individual variation in the levels of pregnancy oestrogens and this variability is probably related to exogenous factors.

This hypothesis was a useful starting point which has sparked a considerable amount of work into the prenatal and perinatal origins of breast cancer. As it is not possible currently to test this hypothesis using biological data on oestrogen levels experienced by women while *in utero* many decades ago, epidemiological research has so far relied on indirect markers of exposure to high or low levels of pregnancy oestrogens. Birthweight is one such marker. Eight studies[84–91] have so far examined the relationship between birthweight and breast cancer (Table 3.1). These studies differed in terms of their design, source of birthweight data (birth records, self-report, or maternal report) and ability to control for other perinatal factors, maternal characteristics, and adult life risk factors. Findings from four of these studies[86,87,90,91] support the hypothesis that high birthweight is associated with an increased risk of breast cancer, particularly at premenopausal ages. The first one,[86] a pooled analysis of data from two population-based case-control studies, revealed a J-shaped association at premenopausal ages (Table 3.1), with small (<2500 g) and heavy babies (>4000 g) being at an increased risk of developing breast cancer later in life relative to babies who were average (2500–2999 g). At postmenopausal ages, however, breast cancer risk decreased with increasing birthweight although the test for trend was only borderline significant. A J-shaped association between birthweight and breast cancer risk in very young women (aged 14 to 37 years) was also reported by Innes *et al.*[91] The third study,[87] a case-control study nested within the US Nurses' Health Study, showed a strong relationship between birthweight (as reported by the nurses themselves or by their mothers) and risk of breast cancer later in life. Women who weighed less than 2500 g at birth had about half the risk of women who weighed 4000 g or more, after adjusting for age at diagnosis, parity, age at first birth, age at menarche, adult BMI and family history of breast cancer (Table 3.1). This association was particularly strong at premenopausal ages. The fourth study,[90] conducted within a nationally representative cohort of British women born immediately after World War II who have been followed up since then, confirmed the positive association between birthweight and breast cancer risk, which was again particularly strong at premenopausal ages (Table 3.1; Fig. 3.1). This association was not affected by other perinatal and later life factors, but was strengthened by tallness in childhood.[90] The other four studies in Table 3.1 did not show any association between birthweight and breast cancer.

A causal association between birthweight and breast cancer later in life has some biological plausibility. There is a direct correlation between birthweight, birth length, and mammary gland development. Low birthweight babies and short babies have a rudimentary breast morphology whereas heavy and long babies have well-developed breasts.[92] Chinese and Japanese American newborns on average weigh about 150 g less than White American newborns.[93] Thus, this difference could accommodate some of the contrast in breast cancer rates between western countries and Japan and China. It is not clear, however, whether birthweight is a risk factor for breast cancer because it is a measure of the rate of fetal growth or because it captures other aspects of the *in utero* environment. This issue was recently examined in a Swedish cohort of about 6000 women born in the Uppsala Academic Hospital between 1915–29.[94] Detailed and complete data were available on a large number of perinatal characteristics that were routinely recorded at the time of birth including various measures of birth size and gestational age. This allowed investigation on whether size at birth may influence breast cancer risk later in life and, if so, whether this effect may be explained by variations in the rate of fetal growth. There were positive and strong associations for birthweight, birth length and head circumference and premenopausal (Table 3.2), but not postmenopausal, breast cancer risk, which became stronger after adjusting for gestational

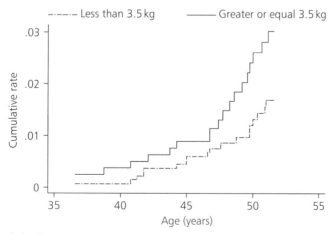

Fig. 3.1 Cumulative breast cancer incidence rates by birthweight in the Medical Research Council National Survey of Health and Development (cohort size = 2221, 37 breast cancer cases).[90]

Table 3.1 Birthweight and breast cancer risk

Author, year	Study design	No. breast cancer cases/controls	Birthweight (g)	RR*	Comments
Le Marchand et al., 1988 (84)	Population-based case-control study	153 cases 461 controls	*All ages* 1162–2948 2949–3340 3341–4451 P=0.41‡	1.00† 0.65 0.76	Birthweight data obtained from birth records. No adjustment was made for maternal factors, other birth characteristics or adult risk factors.
Ekbom et al., 1992 (85)	Population-based case-control study	458 cases 1197 controls	*All ages* <2500 2500–2999 3000–3499 3500–3999 ≥4000 P=0.25‡	1.18 1.00† 1.29 1.47 1.23	Birthweight data obtained from birth records. Relative risks adjusted for maternal characteristics but not for gestational age or adult risk factors.
Sanderson et al., 1996 (86)	2 population-based case-control studies	746 cases 960 controls	*Ages 21–45 yrs* <2500 2500–2999 3000–3499 3500–3999 ≥4000 P=0.06‡	1.3 1.0† 1.3 1.2 1.7	Self reported birthweight. Relative risks adjusted for subject's age, menopausal status and maternal smoking.
		401 cases 439 controls	*Ages 50–64 yrs* <2500 2500–2999 3000–3499 3500–3999 ≥4000 P=0.06‡	0.9 1.0† 1.1 0.8 0.6	Self reported birthweight. Relative risks adjusted for subject's age, menopausal status and maternal smoking.

Michels et al., 1996 (87)	Case-control study nested within the US Nurses' Health Study	582 cases 1569 controls	All ages		Birthweight reported by mothers.
			<2500	0.55	Relative risks not adjusted for maternal factors or other perinatal characteristics but adjusted for adult risk factors.
			2500–2999	0.66	
			3000–3499	0.68	
			3500–3999	0.86	The relation between breast cancer and birthweight was more marked at ages under 45 (P for trend=0.05) and 45–50 years (P=0.03) than at older ages (P=0.18).
			≥ 4000	1.00†	
				P=0.008‡	
			Ages <45 yrs.		
			<2500	0.51	
			2500–2999	0.62	
			3000–3499	0.61	
			3500–3999	0.89	
			≥4000	1.00†	
				P=0.05‡	
Ekbom et al., 1997 (88)	Enlargement of the initial study by Ekbom et al., 1992	1068 cases 2727 controls	All ages		Birthweight data obtained from birth records.
			<2500	0.80	Relative risks adjusted for maternal factors and for some perinatal characteristics but not for gestational age. No adjustment for adult risk factors.
			2500–2999	1.00†	
			3000–3499	1.00	
			3500–3999	0.99	
			≥4000	1.04	No evidence of interaction with age at diagnosis.
				P=0.56‡	
Sanderson et al., 1998 (89)	Two population-base case-control studies among women under the age of 45 years	510 case mothers 436 control mothers	Age under 45 yrs.		Birthweight data reported by mothers.
			<2500	1.2	Further adjustment for maternal factors, other perinatal characteristics and adult risk factors did not affect the results.
			2500–2999	1.0†	
			3000–3499	1.0	
			3500–3999	1.0	
			≥4000	1.3	
				P=n/a‡	

Table 3.1 (*Cont.*)

Author, year	Study design	No. breast cancer cases/controls	Birthweight (g)	RR*	Comments
De Stavola et al., 2000 (90)	Representative cohort of British women born in 1946	37 cases 2221 women in the cohort	*All ages* <3000 3000–3499 3500–3999 ≥4000 P=0.09‡	1.00† 1.05 1.76 2.02	Birthweight data obtained from birth records. Relative risk adjusted for age only but further adjustment for birth characteristics, and childhood and adulthood risk factors did not affect the results. Data on gestational age not available in this study.
			Premenopausal <3000 3000–3499 3500–3999 ≥4000 P=0.03‡	1.00† 1.99 3.26 5.65	Women were still too young to allow separate examination of the association at postmenopausal ages.
Innes et al., 2000 (91)	Population-based case-control study	484 cases 2870 controls	*Ages 14–37 years* <1500 1500–2499 2500–3499 3500–4499 ≥4500 P=n/a‡	3.00 1.54 1.00† 1.08 3.10	Birthweight data obtained from birth records. Relative risks adjusted for gestational age, maternal and paternal age, preeclampsia, abruptio placentae, multifetal gestation, birth order, race/ethnicity.

*Relative risks (RR) as estimated by odds ratios in case-control studies and rate ratios in cohort studies.

†Taken as the baseline category.

‡P-value for linear trend across the various birthweight categories.

n/a not given in the paper.

age. Further simultaneous adjustments showed that for the same ponderal index and gestational age, a 2 cm increase (equal to one standard deviation (SD)) in birth length was associated with a 31% (95% CI: 2% to 67%) increase in breast cancer risk at premenopausal ages. Similarly, for the same ponderal index and gestational age, an increase in head circumference of 1.4 cm (equal to 1 SD) was associated with a 33% (11% to 61%) increase in risk. In contrast, after adjusting for birth length or head circumference ponderal index had no effect on breast cancer risk at premenopausal ages. For a similar birth length (or head circumference), an increase in 1 week of gestational age was associated with a 12% (-24% to 0%) decrease in risk. These results were not affected by further adjustment for maternal characteristics and adult breast cancer risk factors. These findings point towards the rate of fetal growth, as measured by birth length and head circumference adjusted for gestational age, rather than achieved birth size, being the critical factor in determining breast cancer risk perhaps as a result of *in utero* exposure to high levels of oestrogens, IGFs,

Table 3.2 Birth characteristics and premenopausal breast cancer risk in a Swedish cohort of women born in the Uppsala Academic Hospital between 1915–29 and followed up until the end of 1998 (cohort size = 5420, 67 premenopausal breast cancer cases)

Birth characteristic	Category	N*	No. breast cancers	HR† (95% CI)	P-value for trend
Birthweight (g)	<3000	999	9	1	
	3000–3499	2134	21	1.34 (0.60, 2.96)	
	3500–3999	1691	26	2.21 (0.97, 5.05)	
	≥4000	583	11	2.90 (1.16, 7.27)	0.007
Birth length (cm)	<49.5	1508	11	1	
	49.5–50.9	1296	18	2.16 (1.01, 4.64)	
	51.0–51.9	1030	14	2.30 (1.04, 5.07)	
	52.0–53.4	1147	18	2.93 (1.39, 6.19)	
	≥53.5	432	6	2.89 (1.07, 7.80)	0.005
Ponderal index (kg/m³)	<24.7	1313	16	1	
	24.7–26.2	1379	15	0.84 (0.41, 1.72)	
	26.3–27.9	1292	14	0.83 (0.39, 1.74)	
	≥28.0	1429	22	1.18 (0.59, 2.35)	0.61
Placental weight (g)	<570	1418	14	1	
	570–649	1244	11	0.91 (0.41, 2.00)	
	650–749	1382	21	1.61 (0.82, 3.17)	
	≥750	1369	21	1.63 (0.82, 3.24)	0.07
Head circumference (cm)‡	<34.0	1396	8	1	
	34.0–34.9	1564	19	2.49 (1.10, 5.61)	
	35.0–35.4	1017	16	3.41 (1.43, 8.13)	
	≥35.5	1278	22	4.17 (1.79, 9.69)	0.001

*Total numbers do not always add up to 5420 due to missing data.

†Hazard ratios (HR) and 95% confidence intervals (95% CI) estimated using a stratified Cox regression survival model with gestational age treated as a continuous variable and strata defined by period of birth (1915–19, 1920–24, 1925–29). Robust standard errors were used to take into account correlations among siblings.

‡Occipito-frontal circumference.

and other growth factors. Alternatively, or additionally, fetal growth could be associated with breast cancer through its association with postnatal growth rates, but this could not be assessed in this study.

More generally, the role of other *in utero* exposures in determining breast cancer risk has been the subject of a recent review.[48] The authors concluded that overall the data were consistent with maternal preeclampsia or eclampsia being associated with a reduced risk of breast cancer while having been born a twin was associated with an increased risk and interpreted these factors as possible markers of exposure to, respectively, low and high pregnancy oestrogen levels.[48] The relationships with gestational age, maternal age, and birth order were regarded as inconsistent.

3.5 Life course perspective

The preceding sections strongly suggest that the aetiology of breast cancer is complex with aetiological factors acting at (and accumulating through) different stages of life, extending from the prenatal period to late adulthood. The recent shift of focus from adult to early life risk factors, however, has been mainly achieved using traditional analytical methods, that is by estimating the effect of early life factors while adjusting, when possible, for well-known adult risk factors. This approach does not account for the time ordering in which these exposures occur and does not examine the likely causal relationships and interactions between them. For a full understanding of the aetiology of this cancer, a life course perspective—and not just the collection of life course data—is required. Studies should be focused on identifying 'pathways of disease' and on establishing how prenatal and early life risk factors interact with those operating in adulthood. For instance, is fetal growth a risk factor for premenopausal breast cancer in its own right, or merely a marker of postnatal growth? Is an early age at menarche causally related to breast cancer because it increases exposure of the breast to endogenous oestrogens, or is it only indirectly associated with it through its own association with pre-pubertal growth rates? To what extent can the effects of rapid prenatal and postnatal growth be counterbalanced by changes in body size in adult life? If a life course perspective of the aetiology of breast cancer is sought, these and other related questions need to be addressed. How best to do that is the subject of current methodological research[95] as early life and adult risk factors, as well as breast cancer incidence, need to be modelled jointly to determine how they relate to each other. Once these issues are resolved, the insights given by a life course approach would—hopefully—allow identification of appropriate points for intervention. The challenge is open for both epidemiologists and statisticians alike, as complex relationships need to be disentangled.

3.6 Conclusions

The evidence reviewed in this chapter is in favour of the hypothesis that prenatal and early life exposures may be as important in the aetiology of breast cancer, particularly at premenopausal ages, as those occurring in adult life. Strong associations have been reported, although not always consistently across studies, for birthweight and other proxy measures of *in utero* exposures. There is also evidence that early nutrition and rapid prenatal and postnatal growth may affect breast cancer development. These findings would argue for the need to shift the focus of breast cancer research and prevention to early life. Further prospective studies with measurements taken throughout the prenatal period and childhood should thus be conducted to identify the mechanisms that link early nutrition and growth to hormonal profiles and development of breast cancer later in life. Population-based preventive strategies focused on early life are likely to follow as known genetic factors account for only about 10% of all breast cancer cases[51] and most established adult life risk factors are not amenable to change.

Commentary on 'Breast cancer aetiology: where do we go from here?'

Nancy Potischman

Many years of epidemiological research have identified a consistent set of breast cancer risk factors. The list of established risk factors varies slightly across investigators but generally includes those mentioned in the chapter for adult and adolescent time periods. Additional established risk factors, which may or may not be related to an oestrogenic mechanism, include family history of breast cancer, alcohol consumption, socioeconomic status, body fat distribution, and smoking. Estimates of the attributable risk related to established factors indicate that they account for only approximately 50% of the disease.[96–98] *In utero* and early life factors have recently emerged as potential risk factors but have not been included in this estimate of attributable risk.

With a large proportion of breast cancer risk yet to be identified, authors[96–98] have called for new research strategies to breast cancer research. Thus, the introduction of the life course approach is timely and potentially useful in refining our understanding of risk factors. These relationships can be considered as independently causal, cumulatively causal, a clustering of correlated risk factors, or related to each other through effect modification. The authors of this chapter have contributed an excellent first review of the life course approach and demonstrated its necessity and relevance to breast cancer research. Several issues would benefit from further elaboration.

For example the established risk factors tend to be independent of one another in standard statistical analyses. Yet, an important question regarding confounding of prenatal and postnatal risk factors by risk factors later in life remains unanswered. Studies that have evaluated this issue have found little or no confounding by established risk factors.[87,90,94] Such findings are important for record linkage studies that rely on birth registries and cancer registries for their data. In these studies, maternal pregnancy characteristics and the child's birth characteristics can be obtained but adult risk factor data are lacking. There is a need to use methods that take time ordering into account to explore the relationships among all risk factors further.

Additionally, few investigators have examined effect modification of the early life factors by later risk factors. A recent paper[90] is an excellent example of how effect modification can elucidate and refine our hypotheses about the associations among risk factors. The authors demonstrated that the risk associated with birthweight is modified by height attained at age seven but not at age two or fifteen. In addition, the attained height at age seven was negatively correlated with age at menarche, indicating a possible biological link between risk and birthweight, rate of early growth, and age at menarche. Similar types of analyses evaluating effect modification of the birthweight association with risk factors from later in life would be useful. Such analyses may aid in the interpreting the meaning of the birthweight effect, and would be amenable to new statistical approaches.[95]

Given the new focus on establishing prenatal and postnatal risk factors, high birthweight has not been shown definitively to be associated with a high oestrogen environment. A recent review of the fetal origins hypothesis noted that maternal and child research has identified a variety of determinants of birthweight and recommends evaluating rate of intrauterine growth and other factors instead of birthweight.[99] In addition, an ecological study showed higher pregnancy oestrogens and lower birthweights for Chinese compared with American women,[100] clearly contradicting the oestrogen-birthweight hypothesis. Further, although the original *in utero* hypothesis[83] was focused on oestrogens, new data suggest that androgens may be important risk factors to consider.[3,101,102] Evaluating breast cancer risk factors for early time periods is an evolving field, whose results will take us further into complex biological explanations of risk factors and may cause us to modify our hypotheses.

The casual reader may not appreciate the difficulty in using the life course approach to study relatively rare diseases, such as breast cancer, compared with more common diseases, such as cardiovascular disease. Cohort studies including a lifetime of risk factors are not large enough to generate reasonable numbers of cases, as evidenced by the 37 cases in the only cohort study published to date.[90] Case-control studies are limited in the amount of early information available from adult subjects, and data from mothers are problematic because many mothers are missing from the sample obtained. Record linkage studies are the most productive sources of new results, but have been limited to data from one time period, usually birth information. Thus, data sources with large numbers of subjects and information across the life cycle are needed. Only with this type of data can the life course approach be attempted with confidence in the observed risk factor associations.

References

1 Trichopoulos D, MacMahon B. Menopause and breast cancer risk. *J Natl Cancer Inst* 1972;**48**:605–13.

2 Toniolo PG, Levitz M, Zeleniuch-Jacquotte A, Banerjee S, Koening KL, Shore RE, *et al*. A prospective study of endogenous estrogens and breast cancer in postmenopausal women. *J Natl Cancer Inst* 1995;**87**:190–7.

3 Berrino F, Muti P, Micheli A, Bolelli G, Krogh V, Sciajno R, *et al*. Serum sex hormones levels after menopause and subsequent breast cancer. *J Natl Cancer Inst* 1996;**88**:291–6.

4 Thomas HV, Key TJ, Allen DS, Moore JW, Dowsett M, Fentiman IS, *et al*. A prospective study of endogenous hormone concentrations and breast cancer risk in premenopausal women. *Br J Cancer* 1997;**75**:1075–9.

5 Thomas HV, Key TJ, Allen DS, Moore JW, Dowsett M, Fentiman IS, *et al*. A prospective study of endogenous hormone concentrations and breast cancer risk in postmenopausal women. *Br J Cancer* 1997;**76**:401–5.

6 MacMahon B, Cole P, Lin TM, Lowe CR, Mirra AP, Ravnihar B, *et al*. Age at first birth and breast cancer risk. A summary of an international study. *Bull World Health Organ* 1970;**43**:209–21.

7 Albrektsen G, Heuch I, Tretli S, Kvale G. Breast cancer incidence before age 55 in relation to parity and age at first and last births: a prospective study of one million Norwegian women. *Epidemiology* 1994;**5**:604–11.

8 Leon DA, Carpenter LM, Broeders MJ, Gunnarskog J, Murphy MF. Breast cancer in Swedish women before age 50: evidence of a dual effect of completed pregnancy. *Cancer Causes Control* 1995;**6**:283–91.

9 Moolgavkar SH, Day NE, Stevens RG. Two-stage model for carcinogenesis: epidemiology of breast cancer in females. *J Natl Cancer Inst* 1980;**65**:559–69.

10 Bernstein L, Pike MC, Ross RK, Judd HL, Brown JB, Henderson BE. Estrogen and sex-hormone binding globulin levels in nulliparous and parous women. *J Natl Cancer Inst* 1985;**74**:741–5.

11 Yuan J-M, Yu MC, Ross RK, Gao Y-T, Henderson BE. Risk factors for breast cancer in Chinese women in Shangai. *Cancer Res* 1988;**48**:1949–53.

12 Collaborative Group on Hormonal Factors in Breast Cancer (CGHFBC). Breast cancer and hormonal replacement therapy: collaborative reanalysis of data from 51 epidemiological studies of 52 705 women with breast cancer and 108 411 women without breast cancer. *Lancet* 1997;**350**:1047–59.

13 Collaborative Group on Hormonal Factors in Breast Cancer (CGHFBC). Breast cancer and hormonal contraceptives: collaborative reanalysis of individual data on 53 297 women with breast cancer and 100 239 women without breast cancer from 54 epidemiological studies. *Lancet* 1996;**347**:1713–27.

14 van den Brandt PA, Spiegelman D, Yaun S-S, Adami H-O, Beeson L, Folsom AR, *et al*. Pooled analysis of prospective cohort studies on height, weight, and breast cancer risk. *Am J Epidemiol* 2000;**152**:514–27.

15 Hunter DJ, Willett WC. Diet, body size, and breast cancer. *Epidemiol Rev* 1993;**15**:110–32.

16 Hunter DJ, Willett WC. Nutrition and breast cancer. *Cancer Causes Control* 1996;**7**:56–68.

17 Grodin JM, Siiteri PK, MacDonald PC. Source of estrogen production in postmenopausal women. *J Clin Endocrinol Metab* 1973;**36**:207–14.

18 Siiteri PK, Hanmmond GL, Nisker JA. Increased availability of serum estrogens in breast cancer: a new hypothesis. In: Pike MC, Siiteri PK, Welsch CW, eds. *Hormones and Breast Cancer*, Banbury Report 8. Cold Spring Harbor, New York: Cold Spring Harbor Laboratory, 1981:87.

19 Ursin G, Longnecker MP, Haile RW, Greenland S. A meta-analysis of body mass index and risk of premenopausal breast cancer. *Epidemiology* 1995;**6**:137–41.

20 Pike MC, Spicer DV, Dahmoush L, Press MF. Estrogens, progestogens, normal breast cell proliferation, and breast cancer risk. *Epidemiol Rev* 1993;**15**:17–35.

21 Ballard-Barbash R. Anthropometry and breast cancer. Body size—a moving target. *Cancer* 1994;**74**:1090–100.

22 Brinton LA, Swanson CA. Height and weight at various ages and risk of breast cancer. *Ann Epidemiol* 1992;**2**:597–609.

23 Ballard-Barbash R, Schatzkin A, Taylor PR, Kahle LL. Association of change in body mass with breast cancer. *Cancer Res* 1990;**50**:2152–5.

24 Folsom AR, Kaye SA, Prineas RJ, Potter JD, Gapstur SM, Wallace RB. Increased carcinoma of the breast associated with abdominal adiposity in postmenopausal women. *Am J Epidemiol* 1990;**131**:794–803.

25 Le Marchand L, Kolonel LN, Earle ME, Mi M-P. Body size at different periods of life and breast cancer risk. *Am J Epidemiol* 1988;**128**:137–52.

26 Trentham-Dietz A, Newcomb PA, Storer BE, Longnecker MP, Baron J, Greenberg ER, *et al*. Body size and risk of breast cancer. *Am J Epidemiol* 1997;**145**:1011–19.

27 Byrne C, Schairer C, Wolfe J, Parekh N, Salane M, Brinton LA, *et al*. Mammographic features and breast cancer risk: effects with time, age, and menopause status. *J Natl Cancer Inst* 1995;**87**:1622–9.

28 Byrne C. Studying mammographic density: implications for understanding breast cancer. *J Natl Cancer Inst* 1997;**89**:531–3.

29 Whitehead J, Carlile T, Kopecky KJ, Thompson DJ, Gilbert FI, Present AJ, *et al*. The relationship between Wolfe's classification of mammograms, accepted breast cancer risk factors, and the incidence of breast cancer. *Am J Epidemiol* 1985;**122**:994–1006.

30 Byrne C, Hankinson S, Colditz G, Pollack M, Speizer F. A cross-sectional study of mammographic density and plasma hormones. *Am J Epidemiol* 1999;**149(Suppl)**:S48 (abstract).

31 Kaufman Z, Garstin WI, Hayes R, Michell MJ, Baum M. The mammographic parenchymal patterns of women on hormonal replacement therapy. *Clin Radiol* 1991;**43**:389–92.

32 Berkowitz JE, Gatewood OM, Goldblum LE, Gayler BW. Hormonal replacement therapy: mammographic manifestations. *Radiology* 1990;**174**:199–201.

33 Ursin G, Pike MC, Spicer DV. Can mammographic densities predict effects of tamoxifen on the breast? *J Natl Cancer Inst* 1996;**88**:128–9.

34 Spicer DV, Ursin G, Parisky YR, Pearce JG, Shoupe D, Pike A, *et al*. Changes in mammographic densities by a hormonal contraceptive designed to reduce breast cancer risk. *J Natl Cancer Inst* 1994;**86**:431–6.

35 Whelan SL, Parkin DM, Masuyer E (eds). *Patterns of Cancer in Five Continents*. IARC Scientific Publication No. 102. Lyon: International Agency for Research on Cancer, 1990.

36 Shimizu H, Ross RK, Bernstein L, Yatani R, Henderson BE, Mack TM. Cancer of the prostate and breast among Japanese and white immigrants in Los Angeles. *Br J Cancer* 1991;**63**:963–6.

37 Kogevinas M, Pearce N, Susser M, Boffetta P (eds). *Social Inequalities and Cancer*. IARC Scientific Publications, 138. Lyon: International Agency for Research on Cancer, 1997.

38 Hoel DG, Wakabayashi T, Pike MC. Secular trends in the distribution of the breast cancer risk factors—menarche, first birth, menopause, and weight—in Hiroshima and Nagasaki, Japan. *Am J Epidemiol* 1983;**118**:78–89.

39 Tannenbaum A, Silverstone H. Nutrition in relation to cancer. *Adv Cancer Res* 1953;**1**:4517.

40 Armstrong BK, Doll R. Environmental factors and cancer incidence and mortality in different countries with special reference to dietary practices. *Int J Cancer* 1975;**15**:617–31.

41 World Cancer Research Fund (WCRF). *Food, Nutrition and the Prevention of Breast Cancer: A Global Perspective*. Washington: American Institute for Cancer Research, 1997: 252–87.

42 de Waard F, Trichopoulos D. A unifying concept of the aetiology of breast cancer. *Int J Cancer* 1988;**41**:666–9.

43 Pryor M, Slattery M, Robison L, Egger M. Adolescent diet and breast cancer in Utah. *Cancer Res* 1989;**49**:2161–7.

44 Hislop T, Coldman A, Elwood J, Brauer G, Kan L. Childhood and recent eating patterns and risk of breast cancer. *Cancer Det Prev* 1986;**9**:47–58.

45 Potischman N, Weiss HA, Swanson CA, Coates RJ, Gammon MD, Malone KE, *et al*. Diet during adolescence and risk of breast cancer among young women. *J Natl Cancer Inst* 1998;**90**:226–33.

46 Frazier L, Angell J, Willett W, Speizer F, Colditz G. Adolescent diet and risk of breast cancer. *Am J Epidemiol* 1997;**145(Suppl)**:S46 (abstract).

47 Frankel S, Gunnell D, Peters T, Maynard M, Davey Smith G. Childhood energy intake and adult mortality from cancer: the Boyd Orr Cohort Study. *Br Med J* 1998;**316**:499–504.

48 Potischman N, Troisi R. *In-utero* and early life exposures in relation to risk of breast cancer. *Cancer Causes Control* 1999;**10**:561–73.

49 Gray GE, Pike MC, Henderson BE. Breast cancer incidence and mortality rates in different countries in relation to known risk factors and dietary practices. *Br J Cancer* 1979;**39**:1–7.

50 Matsumoto K, Kudo Y, Takeuchi H, Takeda S. Secular trend in age of maximum increment in mean height of Japanese children born from 1887–1965. *Wakayama Medical Reports* 1980;**23**:99–106.

51 Ursin G, Bernstein L, Pike MC. Breast cancer. In: Doll R, Fraumeni JF Jr, Muir CS, eds. *Trends in Cancer Incidence and Mortality. Cancer Surveys.* Volume 19/20. New York: Cold Spring Harbor Laboratory Press, 1994:241–64.

52 Vatten LJ, Kvinnsland S. Body height and risk of breast cancer. A prospective study of 23,831 Norwegian women. *Br J Cancer* 1990;**61**:881–5.

53 Tretli S, Gaard M. Lifestyle changes during adolescence and risk of breast cancer: an ecologic study of the effect of World War II in Norway. *Cancer Causes Control* 1996;**7**:507–12.

54 Dirx MJM, van den Brandt PA, Goldbohm A, Lumey LH. Diet in adolescence and the risk of breast cancer: results of the Netherlands Cohort Study. *Cancer Causes Control* 1999;**10**:189–99.

55 De Stavola BL, Wang DY, Allen DS, Giaconi J, Fentiman IS, Reed MJ, *et al.* The association of height, weight, menstrual and reproductive events with breast cancer: results from two prospective studies on the island of Guernsey (United Kingdom). *Cancer Causes Control* 1993;**4**:331–40.

56 Swanson CA, Coates RJ, Schoenberg JB, Malone KE, Gammon MD, Stanford JL, *et al.* Body size and breast cancer risk among women under age 45 years. *Am J Epidemiol* 1996;**143**:698–706.

57 Wang DY, De Stavola BL, Allen DS, Fentiman IS, Bulbrook RD, Hayward JL, *et al.* Breast cancer is positively associated with height. *Breast Cancer Res Treatment* 1997;**43**:123–8.

58 Tanner JM. *Foetus into Man. Physical Growth from Conception to Maturity.* Second edition. Ware, England: Castlemead Publications, 1989.

59 Frisch RE. Body fat, menarche, fitness and fertility. *Hum Reprod* 1987;**2**:521–33.

60 Petridou E, Syrigou E, Toupadaki N, Zavitsanos X, Willet W. Determinants of age at menarche as early life predictors of breast cancer risk. *Int J Cancer* 1996;**68**:193–8.

61 Moisan J, Meyer F, Gingras S. A nested case-control study of the correlates of early menarche. *Am J Epidemiol* 1990;**132**:953–61.

62 Frisch RE, Gotz-Welbergen AV, McArthur JW, Albright T, Witschi J, Bullen B, *et al.* Delayed menarche and amenorrhea of college athletes in relation to age of onset of training. *J Am Med Assoc* 1981;**246**:1559–63.

63 Hsieh CC, Trichopoulos D, Katsouyanni K, Yuasa S. Age at menarche, age at menopause, height and obesity as risk factors for breast cancer: associations and interactions in an international case-control study. *Int J Cancer* 1990;**46**:796–800.

64 Kelsey JL, Gammon MD, John EM. Reproductive factors and breast cancer. *Epidemiol Rev* 1993;**15**:36–47.

65 Henderson BE, Pike MC, Bernstein L, Ross RK. Breast cancer. In: Schottenfeld D, Fraumeni Jr JF, eds. *Cancer Epidemiology and Prevention.* Second Edition. Oxford: Oxford University Press, 1996:1022–39.

66 Bernstein L, Pike MC, Ross RK, Henderson BE. Age at menarche and oestrogen concentrations of adult women. *Cancer Causes Control* 1991;**2**:221–5.

67 MacMahon B, Trichopoulos D, Brown J, Andersen AP, Aoki K, Cole P, *et al.* Age at menarche, probability of ovulation and breast cancer risk. *Int J Cancer* 1982;**29**:13–6.

68 Trichopoulos D, Lipman RD. Mammary gland mass and breast cancer risk. *Epidemiology* 1992;**3**:523–6.

69 Li CI, Malone KE, White E, Daling JR. Age when maximum height is reached as a risk factor for breast cancer among young US women. *Epidemiology* 1997;**8**:559–65.

70 Berkey CS, Frazier AL, Gardner JD, Colditz GA. Adolescence of breast carcinoma risk. *Cancer* 1999;**85**:2400–9.

71 Gunnell D, Davey Smith G, Frankel S, Nanchahal K, Braddon FE, Pemberton J, *et al*. Childhood leg length and adult mortality: follow up of the Carnegie (Boyd Orr) survey of diet and health in pre-war Britain. *J Epidemiol Community Health* 1998;**52**:142–52.

72 Modina R, Borsellino G, Poma S, Baroni M, Di Nubila B, Sacchi P. Breast carcinoma and skeletal formation. *Eur J Cancer* 1992;**28A**:1068 (abstract).

73 dos Santos Silva I, De Stavola B, McCormack V, Kuh D, Hardy R, Wardsworth MEJ. Childhood growth, adult size and risk of breast cancer, in preparation.

74 Stoll BA, Vatten LJ, Kvinnsland S. Does physical maturity influence breast cancer risk? *Acta Oncol* 1994;**33**:171–6.

75 Peyrat JP, Bonneterre J, Hecquet B, Vennin P, Louchez MM, Fournier C, *et al*. Plasma insulin-like growth factor-I (IGF-I) concentrations in human breast cancer. *Eur J Cancer* 1993;**29A**:492–7.

76 Bruning PF, van Doorn J, Bonfrer JM, Van Noord PA, Korse CM, Linders TC, *et al*. Insulin-like growth factor-binding protein 3 is decreased in early-stage operable premenopausal breast cancer. *Int J Cancer* 1995;**62**:266–70.

77 Bohlke K, Cramer DW, Trichopoulos D, Mantzoros CS. Insulin-like growth factor-I in relation to premenopausal ductal carcinoma in situ of the breast. *Epidemiology* 1998;**9**:570–3.

78 Petridou E, Papadiamantis Y, Markopoulos C, Spanos E, Dessypris N, Trichopoulos D. Leptin and insulin growth factor I in relation to breast cancer (Greece). *Cancer Causes Control* 2000;**11**:383–8.

79 Hankinson SE, Willett WC, Colditz GA, Hunter DJ, Michaud DS, Deroo B, *et al*. Circulating concentrations of insulin-like growth factor-I and risk of breast cancer. *Lancet* 1998;**351**:1393–6.

80 Toniolo P, Brunning PF, Akhmedkhanov A, Bonfrer JM, Koening KL, Lukanova A, *et al*. Serum insulin-like growth factor-I and breast cancer. *Int J Cancer* 2000;**88**:828–32.

81 Byrne C, Colditz GA, Willett WC, Speizer FE, Pollak M, Hankinson SE. Plasma insulin-like growth factor I, IGF-binding protein 3, and mammographic density. *Cancer Res* 2000;**60**:3744–8.

82 Juul A, Bang P, Hertel NT, Main K, Dalgaard P, Jorgensen K, *et al*. Serum insulin-like growth factor-I in 1030 healthy children, adolescents, and adults: relation to age, sex, stage of puberty, testicular size, and body mass index. *J Clin Endocrinol Metab* 1994;**78**:744–52.

83 Trichopoulos D. Hypothesis: does breast cancer originate in utero? *Lancet* 1990;**335**:939–40.

84 Le Marchand L, Kolonel LN, Myers BC, Mi M-P. Birth characteristics of premenopausal women with breast cancer. *Br J Cancer* 1988;**57**:437–9.

85 Ekbom A, Trichopoulos D, Adami H-O, Hsieh C-C, Lan S-J. Evidence of prenatal influences on breast cancer risk. *Lancet* 1992;**340**:1015–18.

86 Sanderson M, Williams MA, Malone KE, Stanford JL, Emanuel I, White E, *et al*. Perinatal factors and the risk of breast cancer. *Epidemiology* 1996;**7**:34–7.

87 Michels KB, Trichopoulos D, Robins JM, Rosner BA, Manson JE, Hunter DJ, *et al*. Birthweight as a risk factor for breast cancer. *Lancet* 1996;**348**:1542–6.

88 Ekbom A, Hsieh C-C, Lipworth L, Adami H-O, Trichopoulos D. Intrauterine environment and breast cancer risk in women: a population-based study. *J Natl Cancer Inst* 1997;**88**:71–6.

89 Sanderson M, Williams MA, Daling JR, Holt VL, Malone KE, Self SG, *et al*. Maternal factors and breast cancer risk among young women. *Pediatr Perinat Epidemiol* 1998;**12**:397–407.

90 De Stavola BL, Hardy R, Kuh D, dos Santos Silva I, Wadsworth M, Swerdlow AJ. Birthweight, childhood growth and risk of breast cancer in a British birth cohort. *Br J Cancer* 2000;**83**:964–8.

91 Innes K, Byers T, Schymura M. Birth characteristics and subsequent risk for breast cancer in very young women. *Am J Epidemiol* 2000;**152**:1121–8.

92 Anbazhagan R, Nathan B, Gusterson BA. Perinatal influences and breast cancer. *Lancet* 1992;**340**:1477–8.

93 Wang X, Guyer B, Paige DM. Differences in gestational age-specific birthweight among Chinese, Japanese and White Americans. *Int J Epidemiol* 1994;**23**:119–128.

94 McCormack VA, dos Santos Silva I, De Stavola BL, Leon D, Mohsen R, Lithell HO. Foetal growth and subsequent risk of breast cancer: results from a long-term follow-up of a Swedish cohort of over 5000 women, submitted.

95 De Stavola BL, Mann V, Hardy R, McCormack V, dos Santos Silva I, Kuh D, *et al*. Life course modelling of birthweight, childhood growth and breast cancer risk. The International Society for Clinical Biostatistics, ISCB. 22nd Annual Conference, Abstract O:65, p. 104. August 19–23, 2001, Stockholm, Sweden.

96 Madigan MP, Ziegler RG, Benichou J, Byrne C, Hoover RN. Proportion of breast cancer cases in the United States explained by well-established risk factors. *J Natl Cancer Inst* 1995;**87**:1681–5.

97 Tavani A, Braga C, La Vecchia C, Negri E, Russo A, Francheschi S. Attributable risks for breast cancer in Italy: Education, family history and reproductive and hormonal factors. *Int J Cancer* 1997;**70**:159–63.

98 Brinton LA, Benichou J, Gammon MD, Brogan DR, Coates R, Schoenberg JB. Ethnicity and variation in breast cancer incidence. *Int J Cancer* 1997;**73**:349–55.

99 Rasmussen KM. The 'fetal origins' hypothesis: Challenges and opportunities for maternal and child nutrition. *Annu Rev Nutr* 2001;**21**:73–95.

100 Lipworth L, Hsieh C-C, Wide L, Ekbom A, Yu SZ, Yu GP, *et al*. Maternal pregnancy hormone levels in an area with a high incidence (Boston, USA) and in an area with a low incidence (Shanghai, China) of breast cancer. *Br J Cancer* 1999;**79**:7–12.

101 Hankinson SE, Willett WC, Manson JE, Colditz GA, Hunter DJ, Spiegelman D, *et al*. Plasma sex steroid hormone levels and risk of breast cancer in postmenopausal women. *J Natl Cancer Inst* 1998;**90**:1292–9.

102 Dorgan JF, Longcope C, Stanczyk FZ, Stephenson HE Jr, Hoover RN. Plasma sex steroid hormone levels and risk of breast cancer in postmenopausal women. *J Natl Cancer Inst* 1999;**91**:380–1.

Chapter 4

Menopause and gynaecological disorders: a life course perspective

Rebecca Hardy and Diana Kuh

A developmental life course perspective has been largely absent from studies of reproductive ageing and of women's health experiences and treatment choices during the menopause transition. The purpose of this chapter is to show the relevance of such an approach. Age at menopause has a genetic component, and the main adult risk factors are cigarette smoking and nulliparity. Little is known about the factors that affect the initial follicle reserve and atresia before menarche. New research that examines the relationship between early growth and development and age at menopause suggests there may be common hormonal or nutritional pathways.

The decision to undergo hysterectomy for benign conditions is part of a social process related to education, childbearing status, and attitude to health care, all of which may be shaped by earlier experiences. Uterine fibroids and endometriosis are two of the most common indications for hysterectomy; both have been linked to markers of oestrogen exposure and endometriosis is also related to exposure to menstrual flow. It remains unclear whether cumulative exposure to oestrogen or exposure during a susceptible period is most important.

Although vasomotor symptoms are largely driven by hormonal changes occurring during menopause, psychological symptoms at this time are affected by earlier adversity and individual characteristics, operating independently or interactively with current life stress. There may be a group of women who are more psychologically vulnerable to changes, hormonal or social, during the menopause transition. Hormone replacement therapy use is becoming more tailored to individual preferences and risk profiles for chronic diseases, and both are shaped by earlier experiences.

4.1 Introduction

The final cessation of menstruation, menopause, is the most prominent marker of reproductive ageing and has biological and social implications for women's health in midlife and beyond. Earlier menopause is associated with an increased risk of osteoporosis (Chapter 7) and a later menopause with an increased risk of breast cancer (Chapter 3). Cardiovascular risk is raised in women who have undergone bilateral oophorectomy and may also be raised by hysterectomy or early natural menopause (Chapter 5). Societal and individual attitudes to loss of fertility and ageing may also affect health and well-being of women during and after the menopause transition.

Unlike most systems that age slowly and continue to function until death, the loss of reproductive function occurs in middle life. The most reliable estimates indicate that the median age at menopause in the western industrialized countries has been approximately 50–52 years from the 1960s through to the more current studies,[1–4] but there is wide variation among women (Fig. 4.1). In developing countries, the median age has been found to be 48 years or younger,[5–9] although methodological problems could account for at least some of this apparent earlier transition. Although the final menstrual period is a precisely defined marker of cessation of reproductive life, the biological and endocrinological changes take place gradually in the preceding years with associated decline in fertility. The phase directly prior to the last menstrual period, known as the perimenopause, is often characterized by irregular menstrual cycles and occurrence of hot flushes and cold sweating. The inception of the perimenopause is poorly defined,[10] although serial measurements of hormonal concentrations in a large US longitudinal study should help to refine the definition of the stages of the menopause transition.[11]

Some women do not experience a natural menopause, but instead undergo a hysterectomy or bilateral oophorectomy. Hysterectomy rates vary by geographical location, even across regions within a country, and time.[12–16] Rates have been highest in the US where more than one in three women have been found to undergo a hysterectomy before the age of 60 years.[17,18] The figure is approximately one in five in the UK.[15] Hysterectomy is rare before the age of 25 years and rates steadily increase up to the age of 40–50 years and decline in the postmenopausal years (Fig. 4.1).

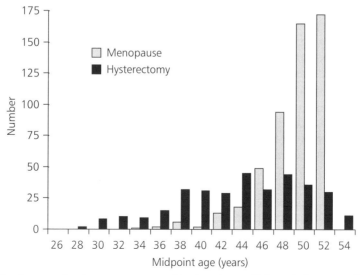

Fig. 4.1 Number experiencing menopause and hysterectomy within each 2-year age band in a birth cohort of 1572 British women followed until age 54.

The menopause has long been seen as a time of worsening health by women[19,20] and as a medical condition by physicians.[21,22] With the isolation of the sex hormones in the mid 1920s and the subsequent development of techniques for measuring blood levels of oestrogen,[23] menopause became viewed as an oestrogen deficiency state which could be 'treated' by hormone replacement, retaining the woman's 'femininity' and preventing distressing menopausal symptoms.[24] This medicalization of the menopause has been criticized[25,26] and an alternative sociocultural perspective focuses on women's accounts of the menopausal transition and places them in relation to their changing social situation in midlife. Evidence of differing experiences of symptoms at the menopause in different cultures,[27,28] has helped inform the view that the 'disease' is a socially constructed concept. Both medical and social models focus on tackling the immediate consequences, whether physical, psychological, or social, of the menopause and the negotiation of the change, rather than taking a long-term life course perspective.

This chapter reviews the factors at each stage of life that affect timing of the menopause, common urogenital disorders and the decision to have a hysterectomy, and the level of symptomatology experienced during the menopause transition and the decision to take hormone replacement therapy (HRT). In particular, we consider whether developmental processes or early life experiences influence these outcomes in addition to genetic and adult social and biological factors. Studying factors associated with natural menopause particularly in populations where hysterectomy and HRT use are common poses methodological challenges. These have been discussed elsewhere[29,30] and will not be considered in this chapter.

4.2 Timing of the menopause

4.2.1 Cause of menopause

A woman is born with an exhaustible and non-renewable supply of ovarian follicles. In the early stages of embryo development primordial germ cells migrate to the site of the future ovary where they multiply until around five months gestation, after which the number of ovarian follicles decreases both *in utero* and during early postnatal life. Follicles (each of which surrounds an oocyte) are then lost throughout a woman's reproductive life through ovulation. A study of the ovaries of women undergoing hysterectomy showed that those with regular menstrual cycles had a 10-fold greater supply of follicles compared with women of the same age experiencing irregularity.[31] A comparison of these data with those obtained from younger women suggests a dramatic acceleration in follicular depletion in the decade before menopause, while in postmenopausal women the ovary is largely devoid of follicles.[31] The prevailing view holds that the exhaustion of the pool of growing ovarian follicles triggers the menopause and that any hypothalamic–pituitary changes are a consequence of reduced ovarian function. A more recent alternative view proposes that age related changes to the central nervous system are the trigger and that the exhaustion of the ovarian follicles is a consequence of the alteration of the neural signal.[32]

According to estimates from the US between 0.3% and 0.9% of women undergo a premature menopause,[33,34] generally regarded as occurring before the age of 40 years, a disorder which appears heterogeneous and aetiologically distinct from menopause occuring at more typical ages. Genetic factors, such as the carrying of one X chromosome with a fragile X permutation, exposure to ionizing radiation, chemotherapy, certain viral agents, enzymatic defects, and immune disturbances have all been implicated.[35]

4.2.2 **Risk factors for age at menopause**

4.2.2.1 Genetic

Associations between mothers' and daughters' age at menopause have been observed[36,37] and twin studies provide estimates of heritability ranging from 31–63%.[38–40] Although the genetic effect may be considerable, there remains scope for the influence of environmental factors.

4.2.2.2 Fetal development and childhood

The peak number of follicles attained as well as the number retained at birth could be the most important determinant of age at menopause,[41,42] but little is known about the factors that influence either, or the rate of follicular atresia in postnatal life prior to ovulation.[42] A number of pathways have been suggested through which prenatal factors could influence fertility including interference with normal germ cell formation and migration or acceleration of prenatal follicular attrition.[43] It is biologically plausible that the apparently large individual variation in follicles at birth could be a result of intrauterine growth, as well as chance processes[42] and genetic factors. Direct evidence of variations in follicles at birth are limited, with two studies by the same team[44,45] comparing the volume percentages of primordial follicles in the ovaries of severely growth retarded fetuses with normal size fetuses producing conflicting findings. The first study showed much lower percentages in the four growth retarded fetuses compared with their matched controls, but the other slightly larger study showed no difference between the two groups. Epidemiological studies have also been few. A twin study from Australia[46] found no evidence that the heavier twin had a later menopause. In a cohort of British women aged 40–42 years for whom detailed birth measurements were available, the 12 who had undergone an early menopause were significantly shorter at birth and had a significantly greater ponderal index than the other women.[47] Two British cohort studies observed no association between birthweight and age at menopause, but did find that heavier weight at one year[47] and at two years[48] was associated with a later menopause. Whether these findings represent a prenatal or early postnatal effect of growth on reproductive ageing remains to be elucidated.

In a study based in New Guinea[6] women with severe and prolonged malnourishment (and small height and weight) had a median age at menopause of 43.6 years compared with a group in the same region with better nourishment who had a median age of 47.3 years. This, together with the fact that women from developing countries may have an earlier menopause than those from developed countries (Section 4.1), suggests a role for chronic malnourishment, possibly acting prenatally through maternal undernutrition or postnatally through poor childhood growth.

Hormonal influences may underlie the association between poorer cognitive function in childhood[49] and early adolescence[50] and an earlier age at menopause. Findings from the 1946 British birth cohort show that 61% of women who had been in the lowest third of the cognitive score distribution during childhood had reached menopause by the age of 53 years compared with only 48% who had been in the top third (Fig. 4.2). The possibility of this association being explained by social factors was unlikely as both studies carried out adequate adjustment. Brain development and reproductive ageing may both be influenced by ovarian steroids operating from early life onwards, perhaps through a similar effect on neuron and oocyte loss.[42]

A few other studies have tested hypotheses relating to intrauterine programming of reproductive ageing. Handedness, a characteristic thought to be influenced by the intrauterine endocrine environment, was investigated but not found to be related to age at menopause.[51]

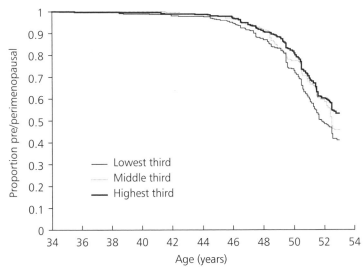

Fig. 4.2 Survivor functions for age at menopause (up to 53 years) by thirds of cognition score distribution at age 8 years. MRC National Survey of Health and Development.

It has also been proposed that when the maternal menstrual cycle is irregular at conception, meaning that the maturational state of the oocyte at ovulation may not be optimal, there is a higher risk of ovarian maldevelopment in the daughter[43] which could lead to subfecundity and also influence menopausal age. Risk factors for this 'oocyte over-ripeness' therefore include particularly young or old maternal age, short birth interval and month of birth (since there is a suggestion that menstrual function varies seasonally), but findings have been inconsistent.

4.2.2.3 Age at menarche and reproductive factors

One hypothesis which has received attention is that the age of menopause will depend on the rate of depletion of oocytes during a woman's reproductive life[52–54] where fewer ovulatory cycles result in a later menopause.[53] Late menarche indicates delayed onset of ovulatory cycles[55] and pregnancy and oral contraceptive (OC) use contribute to periods of anovulation and would all thus be expected to delay the onset of the menopause. Most studies have shown no association between menarcheal age and menopausal age,[52,56–60] and those studies indicating an effect have not been consistent in direction.[4,53,54] Parity, on the other hand, has shown a consistent association with age at menopause. Nulliparous women have an earlier menopause than parous women[52,53,56,58,60–62] and an increasing age at menopause with increasing number of pregnancies[52–54,56] is also likely. Sensitivity analyses, with restriction to children born to women under the age of 35 years, suggest the findings are unlikely to be a result of a greater number of fertile years among women with more children. There has been little consistency in findings relating to OC use,[53,54,56,61,63] although some do provide support for the oocyte depletion hypothesis.[56,61] Women with a history of irregular and long menstrual cycles will have, on average, fewer ovulatory cycles in a given time and would thus be expected to have a later menopause and this has been supported.[52–54,56]

Since relatively small numbers of oocytes are preserved during the short periods of anovulation due to the factors considered, the hypothesis is too simplistic. Only in the case of unilateral oophorectomy, the removal of one ovary and therefore half of the oocytes, would the loss be large enough to influence age at menopause and this has been borne out.[53,54] There is evidence that follicle-stimulating hormone influences the rate of follicular depletion, and therefore the longer the follicle-stimulating hormone is suppressed, during pregnancy for example, the greater the likelihood that menopause will be delayed. That the size of the initial follicle reserve may influence a women's whole reproductive life, determining menstrual characteristics and fertility as well as age at menopause is also a possibility. Both menstrual cycle length and the rate of follicular atresia may be influenced by the pituitary gland,[52] thus short menstrual cycles may be a manifestation of pre-existing oocyte depletion.[53]

4.2.2.4 Adult social and behavioural factors

Of all lifestyle factors investigated, only cigarette smoking has consistently been observed to be related to an earlier menopause[1,3,4,30,50,57,60,62,64,65] (by approximately 2 years[65]), probably due to the toxic effect of smoking on the follicles leading to faster rates of atresia.[66]

Although widely investigated, findings relating to socioeconomic status have been inconsistent,[1,3,4,30,50,56,62,65,67] perhaps due to the different levels of adjustment for confounding variables as well as the different measures of socioeconomic status used. The idea that cumulative stress, perhaps related to lower socioeconomic status or other lifestyle factors, influences menopause remains a possibility. Bromberger *et al.*[1] hypothesized that dysfunction of the hypothalmus may play a role in the cessation of menses and observed, in a US study, that psychosocial stress, in terms of life events, was associated with early menopause in African-American women. This would be consistent with suggestions that there is a relationship between the hypothalamic–pituitary–adrenal (HPA) axis and reproduction throughout life (Chapter 2). An association between early menopause and medically treated depression was observed in a case-control study, although the direction of any mechanism remained unclear.[68] Most studies have observed no association between BMI or weight and age at menopause in the developed countries.[1,4,30,56,57,62,64,67,69] It may be that it is only extreme underweight or extreme restriction of calorie intake which is a risk for early menopause. Women who reported being on a weight reduction diet, for example, were found to have an earlier menopause than others.[1]

4.2.3 Secular variation

Data appear to suggest a secular increase in the age at menopause in developed countries between the mid-nineteenth and mid-twentieth centuries, with trends varying by country.[70] Methodological problems in determining a summary measure for age at menopause, with early estimates tending to be means, rather than the more appropriate median, and being from recalled menopausal ages have however prompted others to argue that there is a lack of clear evidence for any trend.[67] It is unclear how both the increased use of HRT and the number of hysterectomy operations have influenced more recent estimates. This lack of a clear secular trend contrasts with the striking secular decline in the average age at menarche (Chapter 16). The absence of an association between menarcheal and menopausal age at the individual level makes it unclear whether any secular trend in menopause would be expected and in which direction any such trend should be. The rates of the important environmental risk factors for early menopause, cigarette smoking and nulliparity, increased during the twentieth century (see Chapters 13 and 16) and may have masked any secular increase in age at menopause, due for example, to improved childhood growth and nutrition.

4.3 Hysterectomy and gynaecological disorders

4.3.1 Pathways to hysterectomy

There are two categories of risk factor at the individual level for hysterectomy; the gynaecological diseases and clinical symptoms for which hysterectomy is a possible treatment and the woman's characteristics which may influence preference for a type of treatment (Fig. 4.3). Additionally, there are factors relating to the health care providers' practice and policy, but these will not be considered here. Uterine leiomyomas (or 'fibroids') and endometriosis are two of the most common disorders treated by hysterectomy. Their incidence and prevalence are not easy to determine because definitive diagnosis is through surgical examination and so many cases remain undetected. Epidemiological studies of the risk factors for both diseases are therefore also prone to bias due to problems with selection of the control group as well as case ascertainment.

Fibroids are benign neoplasms of uterine smooth muscle and frequently cause symptoms such as excessive menstrual bleeding and pelvic pain. Rates increase with age through the reproductive years[71-74] and decline in the postmenopausal years.[71,73] Rates appear to be

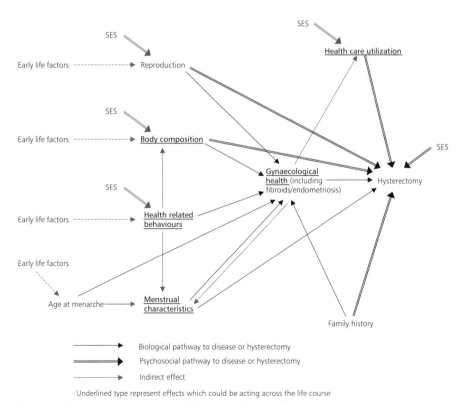

Fig. 4.3 Pathways to hysterectomy: a life course framework.

higher among Black than White women across all ages[72–74] and have been shown to peak at an earlier age (35–39 years) in Blacks compared with Whites (40–44 years).[72]

Endometriosis is the presence of functioning endometrial glands and stroma outside of the uterus, probably the result of transportation of menstrual blood containing endometrial tissue back from the uterus into the peritoneal cavity. Once endometrium is located outside the uterus growth must be stimulated, possibly by oestrogens or growth factors. Symptoms include premenstrual spotting, heavy menstrual bleeding, and menstrual cramps. Endometriosis is only found after menarche, appears to increase during the menstrual years with studies showing a peak around 35–45 years of age,[74–76] and the risk decreases considerably after menopause.[77] White women have been shown to have higher rates than Black women in some studies,[74,78] and Asian women had the highest prevalence of all in one study.[79]

4.3.2 Risk factors for fibroids, endometriosis, and hysterectomy

4.3.2.1 Genetic

Twin studies suggest a genetic component of risk for both fibroids[38,39,80] and endometriosis.[80–82] This genetic component of risk for gynaecological disease, together with evidence of heritability for menorrhagia, explains much of the high degree of heritability in hysterectomy where heritability estimates range between 56% and 59%.[38,83] The familial clustering of hysterectomy may also include a social component since preference for treatment may be influenced by the prior experiences of relations.

4.3.2.2 Age at menarche and menstrual characteristics across the life course

Menstrual characteristics that increase oestrogen levels may promote the growth of fibroids and development of endometriosis. A protective effect of late menarche on the development of fibroids has been indicated by a number of epidemiological studies.[84–86] This may be because women with an early menarche have higher levels of oestradiol[87,88] and, on average, a greater lifetime exposure to ovulatory cycles and thus to oestrogen. There is only weak evidence for such an effect on endometriosis.[89–91] Short cycle length (usually under 28 days) or frequent menstrual cycles[79,91–95] and long duration of flow[91,93] have been shown to be associated with an increased risk of endometriosis. As well as indicators of increased exposure to oestrogen, such characteristics may be indicative of retrograde menstruation. A study carried out in Japan suggested that women who developed fibroids were more likely than controls to report regular menstrual cycle patterns during their teenage years.[96]

There is some evidence of continuity in gynaecological health across the life course.[97] Associations of endometriosis with heavy menstrual flow, dysmenorrhoea[91,93,98] and other gynaecological problems[90] as well as with medical procedures,[90] must be interpreted with caution as although these characteristics are potential precursors of endometriosis they may also indicate pre-existing disease. A prospective study in the UK did, however, observe that pelvic inflammatory disease sufferers had a much higher subsequent diagnosis of endometriosis than non-sufferers.[99] Women who have hysterectomies are also more likely to have reported a history of troublesome premenstrual complaints and more dilatation and curettage procedures.[100] A long history of gynaecological complaints may lead to hysterectomy and those having a hysterectomy for relief of menstrual complaints may have been at higher risk of subsequent fibroid or endometriosis development.

4.3.2.3 Socioeconomic status across the life course

With few exceptions,[101] women with less education and lower socioeconomic status have been found to have a higher prevalence of hysterectomy than other women.[18,100,102–107] In a British birth cohort, women from a manual social class of origin, defined by father's occupation, were at greater risk of hysterectomy at all ages up to 50 years than those from a non manual class of origin.[108] The same study observed that the inverse adult social class gradient was particularly strong at younger ages (below 40 years).[107] This study suggests that the factors associated with the early environment may influence the risk of gynaecological problems and the age at which they first occur. Consistent with these findings, hysterectomy for menstrual bleeding is more common in women of lower socioeconomic status.[15,101,109] Paradoxically, studies have tended to show an increased risk of fibroids[101,110,111] and possibly endometriosis[90,112] in women of higher socioeconomic status. Although this may be due to detection bias, given the evidence for continuity in gynaecological symptoms (see Section 4.3.2.2.), women of lower socioeconomic status may undergo hysterectomy at an earlier stage of disease development than other women.

Patient treatment preference and participation in the treatment decision making process is also implicated. Women of a higher socioeconomic status may be more respected by health professionals and therefore be given more choice and information regarding treatment. More highly educated women and those in professional social classes were found to be more likely than other women to express their preference for treatment of menstrual disorder, and to prefer drug treatment as opposed to surgery.[113]

4.3.2.4 Body composition

Heavy women appear to have lower levels of progestin than lighter women[114] suggesting that they have excess oestrogen unopposed by progesterone,[115] whereas a tendency to store body fat peripherally may be related to a higher ratio of oestrogens to androgens.[116,117] Increasing BMI has generally been associated with increasing risk of fibroid development[71,118] and an Italian study observed a low risk among underweight women ($<20 \text{ kg/m}^2$) compared with others.[119] Weight gain during adulthood (since age 18 years) was identified as the important aspect in relation to fibroid development in one US study.[118] Results of studies for endometriosis have been inconclusive.[91,98,117] However, tall women have been found to have an increased risk of endometriosis[91,98] which may be a result of tall women having higher follicular-phase plasma-oestradiol levels than shorter women.[120]

The increased risk of hysterectomy among women of high BMI[103,104,121] may be determined by the influence of body composition on fibroids and other gynaecological symptoms. Overweight is more common in those of lower socioeconomic status, both in terms of current and childhood status (Chapter 14), and hence there may also be some confounding with treatment decision making (see Section 4.3.2.3.).

4.3.2.5 Reproductive factors

Generally, parous women have a lower risk of fibroids than nulliparous women[71,85,86,96,111,119] with risk decreasing with increasing numbers of children.[71,85,86,96,111,119] Nulliparous women have higher oestradiol levels than parous women,[122] whereas among pregnant women levels of free oestradiol and total oestradiol are lower in women in a second pregnancy than a first.[123] Increasing parity would also be expected to reduce the risk of endometriosis as it decreases the number of menstrual cycles as well as influencing hormones and this is supported by most[79,90,94,124] but not all[76] studies. Separating out the potential effects of childbearing from those of fertility is an important but difficult task. In a US cohort where the effects of infertility were controlled for, parity and history of infertility were found to exert independent effects on fibroid risk.[86] The association of induced and spontaneous abortions with both fibroids[85,119] and endometriosis[124,125] remains unclear.

Use of OCs would be expected to decrease the risk of both fibroids and endometriosis by reducing oestrogen levels and menstrual flow. The lack of a consistent effect for both fibroids[71,84,85,110,126] and endometriosis[76,79,95,124,127] may be, at least in part, due to methodological issues. For example, OC use may mask or be related to the symptoms of disease such as dysmenorrhoea and infertility. One study suggested that there was an increased risk of fibroids only among women who had first used OCs at ages 13–16 years.[86] This was interpreted as evidence that early first sexual intercourse, and therefore early exposure to sexually transmitted diseases, may play a role in disease development. Other studies suggest that various gynaecological disorders are more common in women with a history of sexual abuse.[128,129]

Women who have consciously decided that they have completed their family may be less likely to resist hysterectomy as a treatment option. In one study, those who had their first child before the age of 21 years had a higher risk of surgery than women who had their first child at older ages[103] and women who have previously been sterilized appear more likely than others to have a hysterectomy.[130–132] Corroborative evidence comes from a study of a sample of women referred for menstrual disorders which found nulliparous women and non-sterilized parous women saw the reproductive consequences of hysterectomy as less acceptable than others.[133] However, an increased hysterectomy rate among sterilized women compared with non-sterilized women who had also completed their families (women whose husbands had undergone vasectomy),[132] suggests that other pathways are also operating, such as a differential preference for surgical intervention. The fact that women of higher socioeconomic status are more likely than other women to delay having children, may explain some of the socioeconomic gradient in hysterectomy. The biological and social effects of nulliparity on hysterectomy risk could therefore be acting in opposing directions.

4.3.2.6 Health related behaviour across the life course

Strenuous exercise[134] and cigarette smoking[135] have been shown to decrease endogenous oestrogen levels. On balance, however, the evidence for cigarette smoking is not convincing for premenopausal women and hence more indirect mechanisms are likely. Former college athletes were less likely to report benign uterine tumours (most of which would have been fibroids) than non-athletes[136] and women who take part in strenuous regular exercise appear to have a lower risk of endometriosis than other women.[90,91,98] Cigarette smoking has generally been associated with decreased risk of fibroids,[71,84,85,119] whereas for endometriosis the estimated effects suggest a decreased risk although findings have tended not to be statistically significant.[90–92,98] In two studies, a decreased risk of endometriosis was observed only among those who began smoking as teenagers[91,93] suggesting a possible critical period for exposure. In addition, a high intake of red meat and low intake of green vegetables, fruit and fish have been associated with increased fibroid risk,[137] consistent with the finding that vegetarians have decreased plasma concentrations of oestrogen in comparison with women who eat meat.[138] It is not yet clear whether these health behaviours affect gynaecological disease directly or through their relationships with age at menarche, menstrual characteristics and body composition (Fig. 4.3) or both. The pathways to hysterectomy are likely to be even more complex because of the social patterning of behaviours with, for example, higher social class women being less likely to smoke, thus conferring greater risk of disease, but also being more likely to resist hysterectomy.

4.3.2.7 Health care use

As well as women undergoing hysterectomy operations having had an excess of prior gynaecological problems and treatment, they may also have experienced more prior non-gynaecological treatment and surgery and use of prescription medications.[100] This raises the possibility that there is a group of women more prone to surgery and medical intervention than others. Greater contact with a health professional may mean that the possibility of a hysterectomy is more likely to be discussed, and perhaps encouraged.

4.4 A life course perspective on symptomatology during the menopausal transition and HRT use

4.4.1 Continuity or change in symptom reporting?

A focus of the first longitudinal studies to follow general population samples of middle-aged women through the menopausal transition was to clarify which symptoms were directly due to biological changes associated with the menopause.[139–143] Vasomotor symptoms are strongly related to the stage of menopause[67,140,141,143,144] but there is far less consensus for psychological symptoms.[139,140,142–144] Symptoms attributed to the menopause may be a result of concurrent life events,[145–148] since the age at which women reach the menopause is also a life stage when they are more likely to suffer the illness or death of a spouse, become a carer for elderly parents, and experience children leaving home. Irrespective of whether symptoms are directly related to the menopause, the level of symptom reporting in midlife has been high.

Psychological symptoms provide a good example of how there may be continuity across the life course as well as an accumulation of risk from earlier life leading to symptoms around the time of the menopause (Chapter 8).[149] Urinary incontinence is a further example of a common midlife problem that is associated with social and biological factors at various stages of the life course.[150] Findings from a British birth cohort study showed that women who reported symptoms of urge incontinence were more likely to have suffered from childhood enuresis. Shared common origins could be bladder instability or a failure to learn to achieve normal bladder control at the time of 'potty training' or psychological distress.[150]

Women experiencing poor health around the time of the menopause have often experienced poorer health in earlier life.[148,149,151] A possible subgroup of women who are susceptible to poor psychological health at the menopause has been observed;[143,144] premenstrual tension and experience of hot flushes when menstruating regularly have been associated with occurrence of vasomotor symptoms at menopause.[152] The possibility of interactions between the menopausal transition and earlier life factors as well as concurrent social stressors has been considered in only a few studies.[144,153] Results from a study of Australian women suggest that the menopausal transition acted as a vulnerability factor, amplifying the negative effects of job loss, poor perception of own health, and number of daily hassles.[153]

4.4.2 Life course aspects of hormone replacement therapy use

Women started taking HRT in the 1930s and by the 1960s it was fashionable in the US and UK. In the US the prescription rate gradually increased throughout the late 1960s and early 1970s with a peak around 1975 followed by a rapid decline and low levels of usage throughout the 1980s.[154,155] The drop corresponds to the reporting of studies showing a raised risk of endometrial cancer in women using solely oestrogen preparations.[156] In the UK there was a similar pattern over this period, although with lower rates.[157] The 1980s saw the publication of findings indicating that HRT users had a lower risk of coronary heart disease than non-users,[158] triggering new interest in HRT as a preventive medication. HRT has gained in popularity since the 1980s and, as yet, its use does not seem to have been affected by the less favourable results for cardiovascular disease outcomes in the clinical trials compared with the observational studies (Chapter 5). A recent study found that 45% of a cohort of British women had tried HRT before the age of 50 years.[159] Its popularity may in part be due to the ageing of the baby boom cohort who, as the first generation to have access throughout their reproductive lives to the contraceptive pill, may see the use of hormonal preparations in midlife as a natural extension of earlier pill use and reflect a willingness to use medication as a preventive measure.[159] Certainly a relationship between prior use of OCs and HRT use has generally been observed.[159–162]

All studies show greater use of HRT among women who have had a hysterectomy[159,163–167] for whom there are clear treatment benefits. Many earlier studies of the characteristics of HRT users who had not had hysterectomies, indicated that women who took HRT were healthier than other women.[161,163,164,166] There is evidence that the characteristics of women who are more likely to use HRT are changing and that the characteristics may be different in Europe compared with the US. More recent and British based studies[159,162] have suggested that a 'healthy user' effect is no longer apparent, at least in younger cohorts. Further follow-up of these cohorts is required to determine characteristics of long-term users.

The accumulating evidence relating to the long-term benefits and costs of HRT on health and disease and the reluctance of substantial numbers of women to commit themselves to its long-term use suggests a new approach is needed. In what has been described, perhaps rather optimistically, as a 'paradigm shift',[168] medical practitioners are being encouraged to tailor HRT prescribing to an individual woman's risk and hormonal profile rather than suggest HRT is a panacea for all middle-aged and older women.[168,169] Given that risk factors at various life stages have already been identified for breast cancer, cardiovascular disease, and osteoporosis (Chapters 3, 5, and 7), this approach should, by implication, have a life course perspective. Understanding the potential interactions between these risk factors and HRT use on later health is also of importance.

4.5 Conclusions

Currently there is intriguing, but sparse and indirect, evidence of early life influences on age at menopause. Given the lack of understanding regarding the influence on initial ovarian follicle reserve and initial atresia this research is worth pursuing further. The impact of adult life factors (such as cigarette smoking) on age at menopause may be greater in women with a small initial oocyte reserve. With delayed childbearing becoming more common in western countries, and assuming that the distribution in age at menopause mirrors the distribution in fertility decline, understanding the factors relating to timing of the menopause will help to identify those women at risk of fertility problems at an early age.[170]

Research suggests that oestrogen plays an important role in the development of fibroids and, to a lesser extent, endometriosis. The similarity between the risk factors for fibroids and those for breast cancer (see Chapter 3) also provides support for this hypothesis. It is unclear whether it is cumulative exposure to oestrogen or exposure at a vulnerable stage of life (for example around the age at menarche) that is most important. The evidence relating to individual markers of hormonal status is not entirely consistent possibly due to the methodological problems of defining cases and controls for these diseases. For endometriosis, exposure to menstrual flow may be a more important risk factor than exposure to oestrogen, but again it is uncertain whether it is long duration of exposure or exposure at particular time points which is critical. More research is warranted on the relationship between early sexual experience or abuse and gynaecological disorders. Both the biological indications and the social preference for hysterectomy may have their origins earlier in life, and be reflected in a woman's gynaecological history and previous use of health care.

Longitudinal studies should investigate whether there may be subgroups of women whose characteristics make them particularly susceptible to hormonal changes or psychosocial stress during the menopausal transition. A life course perspective would encourage attention to such possible interactions between earlier and later life, whereas investigating the life course characteristics of women who experience an easy transition could highlight successful strategies. The strategies a woman chooses to negotiate the menopause, including the decision to use HRT, need to be highly informed and tailored to her disease risk profile and her individual preferences; both are likely to have been shaped by earlier experiences.

Commentary on 'Menopause and gynaecological disorders: a life course perspective'

Sybil Crawford and Catherine Johannes

Hardy and Kuh present an excellent case for the relevance of a developmental life course approach in examining the menopause, its accompanying symptoms and treatment, and factors leading to hysterectomy for benign conditions. Whereas most literature focuses on midlife events related to menopause, the authors aptly point out that early life events, even prenatal ones may affect the age of menopause and gynaecological health in general.

Timing of the menopause has been linked to a number of health conditions, including cancer, heart disease, bone loss, and depression. Age at menopause affects cumulative exposure to endogenous oestrogen, and thus risk for hormonally-mediated diseases or conditions. A life course approach is appropriate because age at menopause is determined by the number of follicles attained prenatally and by the subsequent rate of follicular depletion, well before the final menstrual period.

Hardy and Kuh summarize premenopausal factors affecting the follicle pool. Studies of prenatal factors are sparse, although maternal and childhood nutrition may influence follicular reserve. Reproductive factors affecting depletion of oocytes through ovulation include parity and cycle length/number of ovulatory cycles. Other factors are unilateral oophorectomy and suppression of follicle-stimulating hormone, for example during pregnancy. Important behavioural influences include smoking, stress and depression, and extreme underweight or restriction of calorie intake.

Future research might focus on a life course approach regarding these behavioural influences. For example, studies consistently have found that smokers reach menopause 1–2 years earlier than non-smokers, but results vary regarding current versus past smoking or a dose–response relationship. Conceptual models to be explored include critical exposure periods, whether later influences interact with exposure during a critical period, whether risk accumulates with exposure over time, or whether early exposure sets off a chain of later risk.

The authors present a complex array of interrelated factors that may lead to hysterectomy, both from a biological and social perspective (Fig. 4.3). Hysterectomy for benign conditions is a condition well-suited for a life course approach because of the many variables that enter into the decision to undergo surgery. If medical indications alone determined the risk of hysterectomy, then the wide variation in rates between countries, within regions of a country, or among levels of social strata would be unlikely. Risk factors for the two leading medical indications for hysterectomy, uterine leiomyomas and endometriosis, are reviewed as well as health-related behaviours, social and economic status, and health care use. The factors that have a direct impact on the risk of leiomyomas and endometriosis are almost all affected by socioeconomic status, and all could be determined by early life factors. These conditions themselves also lead to increased health care usage, a direct risk factor for hysterectomy. A full understanding would require a life course approach to determine true temporal sequence of events and the impact of social factors.

Hardy and Kuh note that vasomotor symptoms have been linked consistently to the menopause transition, but attribution of other symptoms is less clear. One role of menopause may be to magnify the effect of other factors, including concurrent stressors. The utility of a life course approach is suggested by evidence that premenopausal factors, such as premenstrual syndrome, are associated with menopausal symptoms. Avis and colleagues, for example, found negative attitudes toward menopause while still premenopausal predicted greater frequency of vasomotor symptoms during the menopause transition.[171]

Secular trends in HRT use during the past five decades have resulted in quite different patterns of use by birth cohort. Women entering the menopause now may be more likely to use HRT because of their past experience with oral contraceptives. Recent availability of effective medications other than HRT for the prevention of osteoporosis and cardiovascular disease, changes in HRT preparations, and impending results from clinical trials about the effectiveness of HRT will continue to modify usage patterns. Regional and ethnic variation in HRT use and the well-described 'healthy-user effect' also suggest the utility of a life course approach to hormone therapy.

In addition to the outcomes examined by Hardy and Kuh, a similar life course approach could be applied to diseases or conditions affected by menopause, such as low bone density, treating the transition to menopause as an influence rather than an outcome (Chapter 7). A life course approach could examine whether the menopause-associated acceleration in bone loss is related to peak bone mass from an earlier critical period.

Current literature leaves many gaps in knowledge regarding the impact of early life events on menopause, hysterectomy, and other gynaecological conditions. In particular, research is needed on determinants of the initial follicle reserve and the rate of loss over time, and factors that influence hormone levels. Factors not discussed in detail in this chapter that may be relevant to a life course approach are chronic diseases, environmental exposures, and dietary factors other than malnutrition. A recent report links type I diabetes with earlier age of menopause independent of other known factors.[172] Exposures to chemicals in the environment or ingested in the diet at critical periods in life could also affect hormone levels and subsequent disease risk.

References

1 Bromberger JT, Matthews KA, Kuller LH, Wing RR, Meilahn EN, Planting P. Prospective study of the determinants of age at menopause. *Am J Epidemiol* 1997;**145**:124–33.

2 McKinlay SM. The normal menopause transition: an overview. *Maturitas* 1996;**23**:137–45.

3 Luoto R, Kaprio J, Uutela A. Age at menopause and sociodemographic status in Finland. *Am J Epidemiol* 1994;**139**:64–76.

4 Do K-A, Treloar SA, Pandeya N, Purdie D, Green AC, Heath AC, *et al*. Predictive factors of age at menopause in a large Australian twin study. *Hum Biol* 1998;**70**:1073–91.

5 Rizk DEE, Bener A, Ezimokhai M, Hassan M, Micallef R. The age and symptomatology of natural menopause among United Arab Emirates women. *Maturitas* 1998;**29**:197–202.

6 Scragg RFR. Menopause and reproductive span in rural Niugini. *Proceedings of the annual symposium of the Papua New Guinea Medical Society, Port Moresby, Papua New Guinea*, pp 126–44. Port Moresby: Papua New Guinea Medical Society, 1973.

7 Kwawukume EY, Ghost TS, Wilson JB. Menopausal age of Ghanaian women. *Int J Gynecol Obstet* 1993;**40**:151–5.

8 Garrido-Latorre F, Lazcano-Ponce EC, Lopez-Carillo L, Hernandez-Avila M. Age of natural menopause among women in Mexico City. *Int J Gynecol Obstet* 1996;**53**:159–66.

9 Gonzales GF, Villena A, De La Cruz D. Age of natural menopause among women in Lima City, Peru. *Int J Gynecol Obstet* 1997;**57**:69–72.

10 Brambilla D, McKinlay SM, Johannes CB. Defining the perimenopause for application in epidemiologic investigations. *Am J Epidemiol* 1994;**140**:1091–5.

11 Sowers M, Crawford SL, Sternfeld B, Morganstein D, Gold EB, Greendale A, *et al*. SWAN: A multicenter, multiethnic, community-based cohort study of women and the menopausal transition. In Lobo RA, Kelsey J, Marcus R, eds. *Menopause: Biology and Pathobiology*, pp 175–88. San Diego: Academic Press, 2000.

12 Vuorma S, Teperi J, Hurskainen R, Keskimaki I, Kujansuu E. Hysterectomy trends in Finland in 1987–1995: a register based analysis. *Acta Obstet Gynecol Scand* 1998;**77**:770–6.

13 Coulter A, McPherson K, Vessey M. Do British women undergo too many or too few hysterectomies? *Soc Sci Med* 1988;**27**:987–94.

14 McPherson K, Wennberg JE, Hovind OB, Clifford P. Small area variations in the use of common surgical procedures; within and between England and Wales, Canada and the United States of America. *Soc Sci Med* 1982;**15A**:273–88.

15 Vessey MP, Villard-Mackintosh L, McPherson K, Coulter A, Yeates D. The epidemiology of hysterectomy: findings in a large cohort study. *Br J Obstet Gynaecol* 1992;**99**:402–7.

16 Lepine LA, Hillis SD, Marchbanks PA, Koonin LM, Morrow B, Kieke BA, *et al.* Hysterectomy Surveillance—United States, 1980–1993. *CDC Surveillance Summaries, August 8, 1997. MMWR* 1997;46 (No.SS-4):1–15, Atlanta: CDC, 1997.

17 Pokras R, Hufnagel VG. Hysterectomies in the United States, 1965–1984. *Vital and Health Statistics, Vol 13(92)*, Washington, DC. DHHS publication PHS 88–1753: National Center for Health Statistics, 1987.

18 Marks NF, Shinberg DS. Socioeconomic differences in hysterectomy: the Wisconsin longitudinal study. *Am J Public Health* 1997;**87**:1507–14.

19 Avis NE, McKinlay SM. A longitudinal analysis of women's attitudes toward the menopause: results from the Massachusetts Women's Health Study. *Maturitas* 1991;**13**:65–79.

20 Avis NE. Women's perception of the menopause. *Eur Menopause J* 1996;**3**:80–4.

21 Ballard KD, Kuh D, Wadsworth MEJ. The role of the menopause in women's experiences of the 'change of life'. *Sociol Health Illness* 2001;**23**:397–424.

22 Cowan G, Warren LG, Young JL. Medical perceptions of menopausal symptoms. *Psychol Women Q* 1985;**9**:3–14.

23 Moscucci O. Medicine, age and gender: the menopause in history. *J Br Menopause Soc* 1999;**5**:149–53.

24 Wilson RA. *Feminine Forever*. New York: Mayflower-Dell, 1966.

25 Greer G. *The Change: women, ageing and the menopause*. London: Penguin Books, 1991.

26 Komesaroff P, Rothfield P, Daly J. *Reinterpreting menopause: cultural and philosophical issues*. London: Routledge, 2001.

27 Lock M. Contested meanings of the menopause. *Lancet* 1991;**337**:1270–2.

28 Martin MC, Block JE, Sanchez SD, Arnaud CD, Beyene Y. Menopause without symptoms: the endocrinology of menopause among rural Mayan Indians. *Am J Obstet Gynecol* 1993;**168**:1839–43.

29 Crawford SL. Epidemiology: methodologic challenges in the study of the menopause. In Lobo RA, Kelsey J, Marcus R, eds. *Menopause: Biology and Pathobiology*, pp 159–74. San Diego: Academic Press, 2000.

30 Hardy R, Kuh D, Wadsworth M. Smoking, body mass index, socioeconomic status and the age at menopause transition in a British national cohort. *Int J Epidemiol* 2000;**29**:845–51.

31 Richardson SJ, Senika V, Nelson JF. Follicular depletion during the menopause transition: evidence for accelerated loss and ultimate exhaustion. *J Clin Endocrinol Metab* 1987;**65**:1231–7.

32 Wise PM, Krajnak KM, Kashon ML. Menopause: the aging of multiple pacemakers. *Science* 1996;**273**:67–70.

33 Aimen J, Smentek C. Premature ovarian failure. *Obstet Gynecol* 1986;**67**:604–6.

34 Coulam CB, Adamson SC, Annegers JF. Incidence of premature ovarian failure. *Obstet Gynecol* 1986;**67**:604–6.

35 Rebar RW. Premature ovarian failure. In Lobo RA, Kelsey J, Marcus R, eds. *Menopause: Biology and Pathobiology*, pp 135–46. San Diego: Academic Press, 2000.

36 Torgerson DJ, Thomas RE, Reid DM. Mothers' and daughters' menopausal ages: is there a link? *Eur J Obstet Gynecol* 1997;**74**:63–6.

37 Cramer DW, Xu H, Harlow BL. Family history as a predictor of early menopause. *Fertil Steril* 1995;**64**:740–5.

38 Sneider A, MacGregor AJ, Spector TD. Genes control the cessation of a woman's reproductive life: a twin study of hysterectomy and age at menopause. *J Clin Endocrinol Metab* 1998;**83**:1875–80.

39 Treloar SA, Do K-A, Martin NG. Genetic influences on the age at menopause. *Lancet* 1998;**352**:1084–5.

40 Do K-A, Broom BM, Kuhnert P, Duffy DL, Todorov AA, Treloar SA, *et al*. Genetic analysis of the age at menopause by using estimating equations and Bayesian random effects models. *Stat Med* 2000;**19**:1217–35.

41 Ginsberg J. What determines the age at menopause? The number of ovarian follicles seems the most important factor. *Br Med J* 1991;**302**:1288–9.

42 Finch CE, Kirkwood TBL. *Chance, Development and Aging*. Oxford: Oxford University Press, 2000.

43 Smits L, Zeilhuis G, Jongbloet P, Bouchard G. The association of birth interval, maternal age and season of birth with the fertility of daughters: a retrospective, cohort study based on family reconstitutions from nineteenth and early twentieth century Quebec. *Paediat Perinat Epidemiol* 1999;**13**:408–20.

44 De Bruin JP, Dorland M, Bruinse HW, Spliet W, Nikkels PGJ, te Velde ER. Fetal growth retardation as a cause of impaired ovarian development. *Early Hum Dev* 1998;**51**:39–46.

45 De Bruin JP, Nikkels PGJ, Bruinse HW, van Haaften M, Looman CWN, te Velde ER. Morphometry of human ovaries in normal and growth-restricted fetuses. *Early Hum Dev* 2001;**60**:179–92.

46 Treloar SA, Sadrzadeh S, Do K-A, Martin NG, Lambalk CB. Birth weight and age at menopause in Australian female twin pairs: exploration of the fetal origin hypothesis. *Hum Reprod* 2000;**15**:55–9.

47 Cresswell JL, Egger P, Fall CHD, Osmond C, Fraser RB, Barker DJP. Is the age of menopause determined in-utero? *Early Hum Dev* 1997;**49**:143–8.

48 Hardy R, Kuh D. Does early growth influence timing of menopause? Evidence from a British cohort study. *Hum Reprod*, in press.

49 Richards M, Kuh DL, Hardy R, Wadsworth MEJ. Lifetime cognitive function and timing of natural menopause. *Neurology* 1999;**53**:308–14.

50 Shinberg DS. An event history analysis of age at last menstrual period: correlates of natural and surgical menopause among midlife Wisconsin women. *Soc Sci Med* 1998;**46**:1381–96.

51 Pavia M, Hsieh CC, Ekbom A, Adami HO, Trichopoulos D. Handedness, age at menarche, and age at menopause. *Obstet Gynecol* 1994;**83**:579–582.

52 Whelan EA, Sandler DP, McConnaughey DR, Weinberg CR. Menstrual and reproductive characteristics and age at natural menopause. *Am J Epidemiol* 1990;**131**:625–32.

53 Cramer DW, Xu H, Harlow BL. Does 'incessant' ovulation increase risk for early menopause? *Am J Obstet Gynecol* 1995;**172**:568–73.

54 Hardy R, Kuh D. Reproductive characteristics and the age at inception of perimenopause in a British national cohort. *Am J Epidemiol* 1999;**149**:612–20.

55 Apter D, Vihko R. Early menarche, a risk factor for breast cancer, indicates early onset of ovulatory cycles. *J Clin Endocrinol Metab* 1983;**57**:82–6.

56 Stanford JL, Hartge P, Brinton LA, Hoover RN, Brookmeyer R. Factors influencing the age at natural menopause. *J Chron Dis* 1987;**11**:995–1002.

57 Willett W, Stampfer MJ, Bain C, Lipnick R, Speizer F, Rosner B, *et al*. Cigarette smoking, relative weight, and menopause. *Am J Epidemiol* 1983;**117**:651–8.

58 Benjamin F. The age of menarche and of the menopause in white South African women and certain factors influencing these times. *S Afr Med J* 1960;**34**:316–20.

59 McKinlay S, Jefferys M, Thompson B. An investigation of the age at menopause. *J Biosoc Sci* 1972;**4**:161–73.

60 van Noord PA, Dubas JS, Dorland M, Boersma H, te Velde E. Age at natural menopause in a population-based screening cohort: the role of menarche, fecundity, and lifestyle factors. *Fertil Steril* 1997;**68**:95–102.

61 van Keep PA, Brand PC, Kegert PH. Factors affecting the age at menopause. *J Biosoc Sci* 1979;(Suppl.)**6**:37–55.

62 Torgerson DJ, Avenell A, Russell IT, Reid DM. Factors associated with onset of menopause in women aged 45–49. *Maturitas* 1994;**19**:83–92.

63 Brambilla DJ, McKinlay SM. A prospective study of factors affecting age at menopause. *J Clin Epidemiol* 1989;**42**:1031–9.

64 Cramer DW, Harlow BL, Xu C, Barbieri R. Cross-sectional and case-controlled analyses of the association between smoking and early menopause. *Maturitas* 1995;**22**:79–87.

65 McKinlay S, Bifano N, McKinlay J. Smoking and age at menopause in women. *Ann Intern Med* 1985;**103**:350–6.

66 Westhoff C, Murphy P, Heller D. Predictors of ovarian follicle number. *Fertil Steril* 2000;**74**:624–8.

67 McKinlay S, Brambilla D, Posner J. The normal menopause transition. *Am J Hum Biol* 1992;**4**:37–46.

68 Harlow BL, Cramer DW, Annis KM. Association of medically treated depression and age at natural menopause. *Am J Epidemiol* 1995;**141**:1170–6.

69 Sherman B, Wallace R, Bean J, Schlabaugh L. Relationship of body weight to menarcheal and menopausal age: implications for breast cancer risk. *J Clin Endocrinol Metab* 1981;**52**:488–93.

70 Flint M. Is there a secular trend in age at menopause? *Maturitas* 1978;**1**:133–9.

71 Ross RK, Pike MC, Vessey MP, Bull D, Yeates D, Casagrande JT. Risk factors for uterine fibroids: reduced risk associated with oral contraceptives. *Br Med J* 1986;**293**:359–62.

72 Marshall LM, Spiegelman D, Barbieri RL, Goldman MB, Manson JE, Colditz GA *et al.* Variation in the incidence of uterine leiomyoma among premenopausal women by age and race. *Obstet Gynecol* 1997;**90**:967–73.

73 Wilcox LS, Koomin LM, Pokras R, Strauss LT, Xia Z, Peterson HB. Hysterectomy in the United States 1988–1990. *Obstet Gynecol* 1994;**83**:549–55.

74 Velebil P, Wingo PA, Xia Z, Wilcox LA, Peterson HB. Rates of hospitalization for gynecologic disorders among reproductive-age women in the United States. *Obstet Gynecol* 1995;**86**:764–9.

75 Housten DE, Noller KL, Melton LJ, Selwyn BJ, Hardy RJ. Incidence of pelvic endometriosis in Rochester, Minnesota. *Am J Epidemiol* 1987;**125**:959–69.

76 Vessey MP, Villard-Mackintosh L, Painter R. Epidemiology of endometriosis in women attending family planning clinics. *Br Med J* 1993;**306**:182–4.

77 Holt VL, Jenkins J. Endometriosis. In Goldman MB, Hatch MC, eds. *Women and Health*, pp 226–39. New York: Academic Press, 2000.

78 Kirshon B, Poindexter AN, Fast J. Endometriosis in multiparous women. *J Reprod Med* 1989;**34**:215–7.

79 Sangi-Haghpeykar H, Poindexter AN. Epidemiology of endometriosis among parous women. *Obstet Gynecol* 1995;**85**:983–92.

80 Hadfield RM, Mardon HJ, Barlow DH, Kennedy SH. Endometriosis in monozygotic twins. *Fertil Steril* 1997;**68**:941–2.

81 Treloar SA, O'Connor DT, O'Connor VM, Martin NG. Genetic influences on endometriosis in an Australian twin sample. *Fertil Steril* 1999;**71**:701–10.

82 Moen MH. Endometriosis in monozygotic twins. *Acta Obstet Gynecol Scand* 1994;**73**:59–62.

83 Treloar SA, Martin NG, Dennerstein L, Raphael B, Heath AC. Pathways to hysterectomy: insights from longitudinal twin research. *Am J Obstet Gynecol* 1992;**167**:82–8.

84 Romieu I, Walker AM, Jicks S. Determinants of uterine fibroids. *Post Market Surveill* 1991;**5**:119–33.

85 Lumbiganon P, Rugpao S, Phandhu-fung S, Luopaiboon M, Vudhikamraksa N, Werawatakul Y. Protective effect of depot-medroxyprogesterone acetate on surgically treated uterine leionmyomas: a multicentre case-control study. *Br J Obstet Gynaecol* 1996;**103**:909–14.

86 Marshall LM, Spiegelman D, Goldman MB, Manson JE, Colditz GA, Barbieri RL, *et al*. A prospective study of reproductive factors and oral contraceptive use in relation to the risk of terine leiomyomata. *Fertil Steril* 1998;**70**:432–9.

87 MacMahon B, Trichopoulos D, Brown J, Andersen AP, Cole P, DeWaard F, *et al*. Age at menarche, urine estrogens and breast cancer risk. *Int J Cancer* 1982;**30**:427–31.

88 Apter D, Reinila M, Vihko R. Some endocrine characteristics of early menarche, a risk factor for breast cancer, are preserved into adulthood. *Int J Cancer* 1989;**44**:783–7.

89 Parazzini F, LaVecchia C, Franceschi S, Negri E, Cecchetti G. Risk factors for endometrioid, mucinous and serous benign ovarian cysts. *Int J Epidemiol* 1989;**18**:108–12.

90 Moen MH, Schei B. Epidemiology of endometriosis in a Norwegian county. *Acta Obstet Gynecol Scand* 1997;**76**:559–62.

91 Cramer DW, Wilson E, Stillman RJ, Berger MJ, Belisle S, Schiff I, *et al*. The relation of endometriosis to menstrual characteristics, smoking and exercise. *J Am Med Assoc* 1986;**255**:1904–8.

92 Matorras R, Rodiquez F, Piuoan JI, Ramon O, Gutierrez de Teran G, Rodrigues-Escudero F. Epidemiology of endometriosis in infertile women. *Fertil Steril* 1995;**63**:34–8.

93 Darrow SL, Vena JE, Batt RE, Zielezny MA, Michalek AM, Selman S. Menstrual cycle characteristics and the risk of endometriosis. *Epidemiology* 1993;**4**:135–42.

94 Gruppo Italiano per lo Studio dell' endometriosi. Risk factors for pelvic endometriosis in women with pelvic pain or infertility. *Eur J Obstet Gynecol Reprod Biol* 1999;**83**:195–9.

95 Italian Endometriosis Study Group. Oral contraceptive use and risk of endometriosis. *Br J Obstet Gynaecol* 1999;**106**:695–9.

96 Sato F, Miyake H, Nishi M, Mori M, Kudo R. Early normal menstrual cycle pattern and the development of uterine leiomyomas. *J Wom Health Gend Based Med* 2000;**9**:299–302.

97 Gardner J. Adolescent menstrual characteristics as predictors of gynaecological health. *Ann Hum Biol* 1983;**10**:31–40.

98 Signorello LB, Harlow BL, Cramer DW, Spiegelman D, Hill JA. Epidemiologic determinants of endometriosis: a hospital-based case-control study. *Ann Epidemiol* 1997;**7**:267–74.

99 Buchan H, Vessey M, Goldacre M, Fairweather J. Morbidity following pelvic inflammatory disease. *Br J Obstet Gynaecol* 1993;**100**:558–62.

100 Dennerstein L, Shelley J, Smith AMA, Ryan M. Hysterectomy experience among mid-aged Australian women. *Med J Aust* 1994;**161**:311–3.

101 Luoto R, Keskimaki I, Reunanen A. Socioeconomic variations in hysterectomy: evidence from a linkage study of the Finnish hospital discharge register and population census. *J Epidemiol Community Health* 1997;**51**:67–73.

102 Kjerulff K, Langenberg P, Guzinski G. The socioeconomic correlates of hysterectomies in the United States. *Am J Public Health* 1993;**83**:106–8.

103 Meilahn EN, Matthews KA, Egeland G, Kelsey SF. Characteristics of women with hysterectomy. *Maturitas* 1989;**11**:319–29.

104 Progetto Menopausa Italia Study Group. Determinants of hysterectomy and oophorectomy in women attending menopause clinics in Italy. *Maturitas* 2000;**36**:19–25.

105 Kuh D, Stirling S. Socioeconomic variation in admission for diseases of female genital system and breast in a national cohort aged 15–43. *Br Med J* 1995;**311**:840–3.

106 Treloar SA, Do K-A, O'Connor VM, O'Connor DT, Yeo MA, Martin NG. Predictors of hysterectomy: an Australian study. *Am J Obstet Gynecol* 1999;**180**:945–54.

107 Marshall SF, Hardy RJ, Kuh D. Socioeconomic variations in hysterectomy up to age 52: national population based prospective cohort study. *Br Med J* 2000;**320**:1579.

108 Marshall S, Hardy R, Kuh D. Changes with age in the socioeconomic gradient in hysterectomy: findings from a national cohort. *J Epidemiol Community Health* 2000;**54**:782.

109 Brett KM, Marsh JV, Madans JH. Epidemiology of hysterectomy in the United States: Demographic and reproductive factors in a nationally representative sample. *J Wom Health* 1997;**6**:309–16.

110 Chiaffarino F, Parazzini F, La Vecchia C, Marsico S, Surace M, Ricci E. Use of oral contraceptives and uterine fibroids: results from a case-control study. *Br J Obstet Gynaecol* 1999;**106**:857–60.

111 Parazzini F, LaVecchia C, Negri E, Cecchetti G, Fedele L. Epidemiologic characteristics of women with uterine fibroids: a case-control study. *Obstet Gynecol* 1988;**72**:853–7.

112 Beral V, Rolfs R, Joesoef MR, Aral S, Cramer DW. Primary infertility: characteristics of women in North America according to pathological findings. *J Epidemiol Community Health* 1994;**48**:576–9.

113 Coulter A, Peto V, Doll H. Patients' preferences and general practitioners' decisions in the treatment of menstrual disorders. *Fam Pract* 1994;**11**:67–74.

114 Westhoff C, Gentile G, Lee J, Zacur H, Heilbig D. Predictors of ovarian steriod secretion in reproductive-age women. *Am J Epidemiol* 1996;**144**:381–8.

115 Schwartz SM, Marshall LM. Uterine Leiomyomata. In Goldman M, Hatch M, eds. *Women and Health*, pp 240–52. New York: Academic Press, 2000.

116 Rebuffe-Scrive M. Steroid hormones and distribution of adipose tissue. *Acta Med Scand Suppl* 1988;**723**:143–6.

117 McCann SE, Freudenheim JL, Darrow SL, Batt RE, Zielezny MA. Endometriosis and body fat distribution. *Obstet Gynecol* 1993;**82**:545–9.

118 Marshall LM, Spiegelman D, Manson JE, Goldman MB, Barbieri RL, Stampfer MJ, *et al.* Risk of uterine leiomyomata among premenopausal women in relation to body size and cigarette smoking. *Epidemiology* 1998;**9**:511–7.

119 Parazzini F, Negri E, La Vecchia C, Chatenond L, Ricci E, Guarnerio P. Reproductive factors and risk of uterine fibroids. *Epidemiology* 1996;**7**:440–2.

120 Dorgan JF, Reichman ME, Judd JT, Brown C. The relation of body size to plasma levels of estrogens and androgens in premenopausal women. *Cancer Causes Control* 1995;**6**:3–8.

121 Settnes A, Jorgensen T. Hysterectomy in a Danish cohort. Prevalence, incidence and socio-demographic characteristics. *Acta Obstet Gynecol Scand* 1996;**75**:274–80.

122 Bernstein L, Pike MC, Ross RK, Judd HL, Brown JB, Henderson BE. Estrogen and sex hormone-binding globulin levels in nulliparous and parous women. *J Natl Cancer Inst* 1985;**74**:741–5.

123 Panagiotopoulou K, Katsouyanni K, Petridou E, Garas Y, Tzonou A, Trichopoulos D. Maternal age, parity and pregnancy estrogens. *Cancer Causes Control* 1990;**1**:119–24.

124 Parazzini F, Ferraroni M, Fedele L, Bocciolone L, Rubessa S, Riccardi A. Pelvic endometriosis: reproductive and menstrual risk factors at different stages in Lombardy, northern Italy. *J Epidemiol Community Health* 1995;**49**:61–4.

125 Darrow SL, Selman S, Batt RE, Zielezny MA, Vena JE. Sexual activity, contraception, and reproductive factors in predicting endometriosis. *Am J Epidemiol* 1994;**140**:500–9.

126 Parazzini F, Negri E, La Vecchia C, Fedele L, Rabaiotti M, Luchini L. Oral contraceptive use and risk of uterine fibroids. *Obstet Gynecol* 1992;**79**:430–3.

127 Kirshon B, Poindexter III AN, Fast J. Endometriosis in multiparous women. *J Reprod Med* 1989;**34**:215–7.

128 Lampe A, Solder E, Ennemoser A, Schubert C, Rumpold G, Sollner W. Chronic pelvic pain and previous sexual abuse. *Obstet Gynecol* 2000;**96**:929–33.

129 Golding JM, Wilsnack SC, Learman LA. Prevalence of sexual assault history among women with common gynecologic symptoms. *Am J Obstet Gynecol* 1998;**179**:1013–9.

130 **Goldhaber MK, Armstrong MA, Golditch IM, Sheehe PR, Petitti DB, Friedman GD**. Long-term risk of hysterectomy among 80,007 sterilized and comparison women at Kaiser Permanente, 1971–1987. *Am J Epidemiol* 1993;**138**:508–21.

131 **Templeton AA, Cole S**. Hysterectomy following sterilization. *Br J Obstet Gynaecol* 1982;**89**:845–8.

132 **Hillis SD, Marchbanks A, Ratliff Tylor L, Peterson HB**, for the US Collaborative Review of Sterilization Working Group. Higher hysterectomy risk for sterilized than nonsterilized women: findings from the US Collaborative Review of Sterilization. *Obstet Gynecol* 1998;**91**:241–6.

133 **Warner P**. Preferences regarding treatments for period problems: relationship to menstrual and demographic factors. *J Psychosom Obstet Gynecol* 1994;**15**:93–110.

134 **Boyden BR, Pamenter RW, Stanforth PR, Rotkis TC, Wilmore JH**. Sex steroids and endurance running in women. *Fertil Steril* 1983;**39**:629–32.

135 **MacMahon B, Trichopoulos D, Cole P, Brown J**. Cigarette smoking and urinary estrogens. *N Engl J Med* 1982;**307**:1062–5.

136 **Wyshak G, Frisch RE, Albright NL, Albright TE, Schiff I**. Lower prevalence of benign diseases of the breast and benign tumours of the reproductive system in former college athletes compared to non-athletes. *Br J Cancer* 1986;**54**:841–5.

137 **Chiaffarino F, Parazzini F, La Vecchia C, Chatenoud L, Di Cintio E, Marisico S**. Diet and uterine myomas. *Obstet Gynecol* 1999;**94**:395–8.

138 **Goldin BR, Adlercreutz H, Gorbach SL, Warram JH, Dwyer JT, Swenson L, *et al***. Estrogen excretion patterns and plasma levels in vegetarian and omnivorous women. *N Engl J Med* 1982;**307**:1542–7.

139 **Avis NE, Brambilla D, McKinlay SM, Vass K**. A Longitudinal Analysis of the Association between Menopause and Depression Results from the Massachusetts Women's Health Study. *Ann Epidemiol* 1994;**4**:214–20.

140 **Holte A**. Influences of natural menopause on health complaints: A prospective study of healthy Norwegian women. *Maturitas* 1992;**14**:127–41.

141 **Hunter MS**. Somatic Experience of the Menopause: A Prospective Study. *Psychosom Med* 1990;**52**:357–67.

142 **Kaufert PA, Gilbert P, Tate R**. The Manitoba Project: a re-examination of the link between menopause and depression. *Maturitas* 1992;**14**:143–55.

143 **Matthews KA, Wing RR, Kuller LH, Meilahn EN, Kelsey SF, Costello EJ *et al***. Influences of natural menopause on psychological characteristics and symptoms of middle-aged healthy women. *J Consult Clin Psychol* 1990;**58**:345–51.

144 **Hardy R, Kuh D**. Change in psychological and vasomotor symptom reporting during the menopause. *Soc Sci Med*, in press.

145 **Winokur G**. Depression in the menopause. *Am Journal Psychiatry* 1973;**130**:92–3.

146 **Greene JG, Cooke DJ**. Life stress and symptoms at the climacterium. *Br J Psychiatry* 1980;**136**:486–91.

147 **Holte A, Mikkelsen A**. Psychosocial determinants of climacteric complaints. *Maturitas* 1991;**13**:205–15.

148 **Dennerstein L, Smith AMA, Morse C, Burger H, Green A, Hopper J, *et al***. Menopausal symptoms in Australian women. *Med J Aust* 1993;**159**:232–6.

149 **Kuh D, Hardy R, Rodgers B, Wadsworth MEJ**. Early life factors in relation to psychological distress in midlife. *Soc Sci Med*, in press.

150 **Kuh D, Cardozo L, Hardy R**. The pattern and predictors of incontinence in women during middle life. *J Epidemiol Community Health* 1999;**53**:453–8.

151 **Kuh DL, Wadsworth M, Hardy R**. Women's health in midlife: the influence of the menopause, social factors and health in earlier life. *Br J Obstet Gynaecol* 1997;**104**:923–33.

152 **Hunter M.** The South-East England longitudinal study of the climacteric and postmenopause. *Maturitas* 1992;**14**:117–26.

153 **Dennerstein L, Lehert P, Burger H, Dudley E.** Mood and menopausal transition. *J Nerv Ment Dis* 1999;**187**:685–91.

154 **Kennedy Dl, Baum C, Forbes MB.** Noncontraceptive estrogens and progestins: use patterns over time. *Obstet Gynecol* 1985;**65**:441–6.

155 **Wysowski DK, Golden L, Burke L.** Use of menopausal estrogens and medroxyprogesterone in the United States, 1982–1992. *Obstet Gynecol* 1995;**85**:6–10.

156 **Ziel HK, Finkle WD.** Increased risk of endometrial carcinoma among users of conjugated oestrogens. *N Engl J Med* 1975;**293**:1167–70.

157 **Hunt K, Vessey M.** Long-term effects of postmenopausal hormone therapy. *Br J Hospital Med* 1987;**38**:450–60.

158 **Bush TL, Barrett-Connor E.** Non-contraceptive estrogen use and cardiovascular disease. *Epidemiol Rev* 1985;**7**:80–104.

159 **Kuh D, Hardy R, Wadsworth M.** Social and behavioural influences on the uptake of hormone replacement therapy among younger women. *Br J Obstet Gynaecol* 2000;**107**:731–9.

160 **Moorhead T, Hannaford P, Warskyj M.** Prevalence and characteristics associated with use of hormone replacement therapy in Britain. *Br J Obstet Gynaecol* 1997;**104**:290–7.

161 **Hemminki E, Malin M, Topo P.** Selection to postmenopausal therapy by women's characteristics. *J Clin Epidemiol* 1993;**46**:211–9.

162 **Lancaster T, Surman G, Lawrence M, Mant D, Vessey M, Thorogood M, *et al*.** Hormone replacement therapy: characteristics of users and non-users in a British general practice cohort identified through computerised prescribing records. *J Epidemiol Community Health* 1995;**49**:389–94.

163 **Johannes CB, Crawford SL, Posner JG, McKinlay SM.** Longitudinal patterns and correlates of hormone replacement therapy use in middle-aged women. *Am J Epidemiol* 1994;**140**:439–51.

164 **Derby CA, Hume AL, McFarland Barbour M, McPhillips JB, Lasater TM, Carleton RA.** Correlates of postmenopausal estrogen use and trends through the 1980s in two Southeastern New England communities. *Am J Epidemiol* 1993;**137**:1125–35.

165 **Grodstein F, Stampfer MJ, Manson JE, Colditz GA, Willett WC, Rosner B, *et al*.** Postmenopausal estrogen and progestin use and the risk of cardiovascular disease. *N Engl J Med* 1996;**335**:453–61.

166 **Marks NF, Shinberg DS.** Socioeconomic status differences in hormone therapy. *Am J Epidemiol* 1998;**148**:1–13.

167 **Cauley JA, Cummings SR, Black DM, Mascioli SR, Seeley DG.** Prevalence and determinants of estrogen use in a population study. *AmJ Obstet Gynecol* 1990;**163**:1438–44.

168 **Santoro NF, Col NF, Eckman MH, Wong JB, Pauker SG, Cauley JA, *et al*.** Hormone replacement therapy—where are we going? *J Clin Endocrinol Metab* 1999;**84**:1798–812.

169 National Heart, Lung and Blood Institute, NIH Office of Research on Women's Health, Giovanni Lorenzini Medical Science Foundation. Best Clinical Practices. Chapter 13 from the International Position Paper on *Women's health and menopause: a comprehensive approach*. March 2002 [online] Available at http://www.nhlbi.nih.gov/health/prof/heart/other/wm-menop.htm

170 **te Velde ER, Scheffer GJ, Dorland M, Broekmans FJ, Fauser BCJM.** Developmental and endocrine aspects of normal ovarian aging. *Mol Cell Endocrinol* 1998;**145**:67–73.

171 **Avis NE, Crawford SL, McKinlay SM.** Psychosocial, behavioral, and health factors related to menopause symptomatology. *Women's Health: Res Gender Behav Pol* 1997;**3**:103–20.

172 **Dorman JS, Steenkiste AR, Strotmeyer ES, Burke JP, Kuller LH, Swoh CK.** Menopause in type 1 diabetic women: Is it premature? *Diabetes* 2001;**50**:1857–62.

Chapter 5

A life course approach to coronary heart disease and stroke

Debbie A. Lawlor, Shah Ebrahim, and
George Davey Smith

Classical adult risk factors have similar relative risks for coronary heart disease and stroke in women and men, though absolute coronary risk is lower for women. Diabetes, glucose intolerance, and the insulin resistance syndrome appear to be stronger risk factors for coronary disease in women than men. As in men, there is an inverse association between birthweight and risk of coronary heart disease, stroke, and hypertension in women. Poor infant nutrition and accelerated growth in later life are also associated with coronary heart disease and stroke risk in women. The underlying mechanisms for these associations are unclear but plausibly include genetic, environmental, and socioeconomic factors acting across the life course.

Hormone replacement therapy may not reduce coronary heart disease risk, although endogenous oestrogen may play a role in the aetiology of heart disease in women. Proxy measures of oestrogen exposure, such as age at menarche, menstrual pattern, parity, and age at menopause show inconsistent associations with cardiovascular disease. However, no assessment of the effects of lifetime exposure to endogenous oestrogen has been made.

There is insufficient knowledge about the earlier life course determinants of cardiovascular disease in women to merit changes to current preventive health policies.

5.1 Introduction

Coronary heart disease (CHD) is the main cause of death in women in most industrialized countries.[1–3] Due to women's longer life expectancy the absolute number of women dying of CHD is similar to that of men. Worldwide in 1996 there were 16.7 million deaths from CHD, 8.7 million of which were in women.[3] Stroke is also an important cause of death, accounting for over 12 million deaths worldwide per year, more than half of which are in women.[2,3] In industrialized countries between 15–30% of women over the age of 60 have symptomatic CHD and a further 4–10% have suffered a stroke.[1,2,4,5] More than 50% of women with CHD or stroke are severely disabled by their symptoms and globally these conditions are a substantial contributor to disabled life expectancy, second only to mental health.[6] Women are the main providers of care to disabled heart disease or stroke patients, either as family or professional carers.[7]

5.1.1 Sex differences in CHD and stroke occurrence

The ratio of male to female CHD mortality varies temporally, geographically, and with age.[8–11] The twentieth century CHD 'epidemic' only affected men in most industrialized countries,[9] as illustrated in data from England and Wales (Fig. 5.1). The post World War II increase in the sex ratio of CHD mortality was experienced by all age groups at the same time, indicating an environmental insult, affecting predominantly men, and occurring some time prior to the late 1940s.[9] Sex differences in smoking, hypertension, or alcohol consumption are unlikely explanations, since mortality from stroke, which shares these risk factors, does not show the same pattern (Fig. 5.2).[9] Diagnostic bias or use of non-specific or other circulatory diagnostic categories in women do not appear to explain these trends either.[9]

The sex difference in CHD mortality and incidence varies between countries from little or no difference in China and Cuba to much larger differences in Western Europe.[8,9] Women's CHD mortality rates correlate more strongly with men from the same country than with women from different countries.

The decrease in the sex difference in CHD mortality with increasing age is due to a slowing of the male rate rather than a postmenopausal increase in female rates.[10,11] For breast

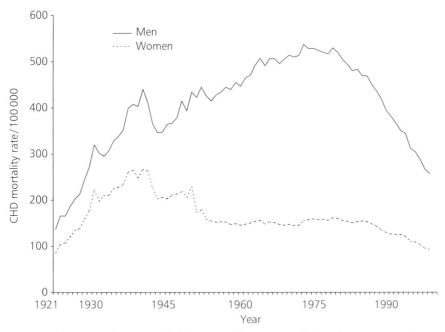

Fig. 5.1 Secular trends in age standardized mortality rates per 100 000 from coronary heart disease for men and women, 1921–1998, England and Wales.[9]

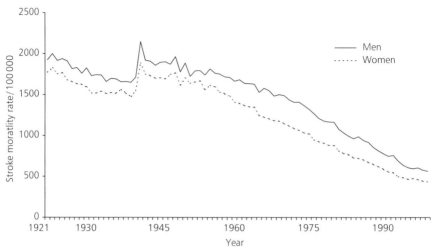

Fig. 5.2 Secular trends in age standardized mortality rates per 100 000 from stroke for men and women 1921–1998, England and Wales.[9]

cancer, there is an obvious postmenopausal slowing of the rate of increase which is not seen in CHD. These secular, geographical and age related trends, which cannot be explained solely by a cardioprotective effect of oestrogen in women, highlight the importance of environmental factors in determining sex differences in CHD occurrence.[9] The decline, in both sexes, in stroke mortality over the last century (Fig. 5.2) cannot be fully explained by treatment of hypertension, lifestyle changes, or competing risk from CHD.[12]

5.2 Sex differences in effects and distributions of adult risk factors

5.2.1 Assessing sex differences

The exclusion of women from earlier aetiological studies on the assumption that findings would equally apply to women[13] limits causal understanding and assessment of the reasons for sex differences in the occurrence of CHD. Although recent studies have included women and men, sex differences have often been poorly analysed. Valid conclusions about sex differences in risk factor effects depend upon identical measurements, outcomes and analyses being used in both sexes; adequate numbers of women and men being included in the study and formal tests of statistical interaction being performed.[14,15] Post-hoc subgroup analyses of sex are common but 'interesting' sex differences in findings are more likely to be presented than concordant results.[15]

5.2.2 Classical adult risk factors

Most prospective studies have found that the classical adult risk factors—smoking,[4,16–19] hypertension,[4,16–18] cholesterol,[4,16–18,20] obesity,[21–23] and physical inactivity[24,25]—have similar relative risks for CHD and stroke in women and men. Since the age specific absolute risk of CHD is lower in women compared with men, the extra cases (absolute risk) associated with each of these risk factors is lower in women than in men. In women, as with men, the risk associated with smoking returns to levels similar to those found in non-smokers within five years of smoking cessation.[26,27] In clinical trials of treatment for hypertension,[28] isolated systolic hypertension,[29] secondary prevention of CHD with statins[30] and aspirin[31] the relative effect in women is similar to that in men. There is a similar J-shaped curve for the relationship between alcohol consumption and CHD risk in women and men.[32] Moderate alcohol consumption in both sexes may also protect against ischaemic stroke.[33] Binge drinking is associated with increased risk of both stroke and CHD, though fewer studies have looked specifically at the effect of binge drinking in women.[34] Levels of these classical risk factors vary between the sexes and with age but these differences do not appear to explain the sex difference in CHD occurrence.[18]

5.2.3 Diabetes and the insulin resistance syndrome

Inconsistent sex differences in the association between diabetes and CHD have been reported,[16,35–38] but a meta-analysis of all prospective cohort studies found that diabetes had a greater impact in women than men (relative risk 2.54 (95% confidence interval (CI) 2.08, 3.09) in women and 1.76 (1.51, 2.05) in men, $p=0.004$ comparison between men and women).[39] Other components of the insulin resistance syndrome—a clustering of CHD risk factors in individuals including, glucose intolerance, obesity, insulin resistance, high blood pressure, and dyslipidaemia[40]—show sex differences in their effect on cardiovascular disease. Low levels of high-density lipoprotein cholesterol (HDLc) and an excess of very low-density lipoprotein cholesterol (LDLc) particles appear to be more detrimental to women than men.[41] Insulin resistance has been found to be a stronger predictor of large vessel arterial stiffness, a possible precursor of CHD and stroke, in women compared with men.[42]

5.2.4 Abdominal obesity

Abdominal obesity may lead to the insulin resistance syndrome, and is a stronger predictor of CHD risk than general obesity.[43] In most Caucasian populations not only is the mean waist–hip ratio (a proxy indicator of abdominal obesity) for men greater than that for women, the distributions of waist–hip ratio in women and men do not overlap.[44] In one large prospective study it was concluded that the sex difference in CHD risk could be largely explained by the sex difference in body fat distribution because the sex difference in CHD incidence disappeared after adjustment for waist–hip ratio.[45] As the distributions of waist–hip ratio do not overlap, waist–hip ratio acts as a proxy for any other sex-varying factor, making these results difficult to interpret. If waist–hip ratio showed a continuous linear relationship with CHD risk, independently of sex, then a marked difference in the distribution of central obesity could explain sex differences in CHD occurrence (Fig. 5.3).

5.2.5 Dietary fat

Animal studies[46] and a trial in humans[47] have found that women increase levels of the cardio-protective high-density lipoprotein cholesterol (HDLc) in response to a diet high in saturated fat to a much greater extent than men. In trials of low fat diets that have reported sex-specific responses some,[48–51] but not all,[52–54] show a more detrimental effect on HDLc levels in women compared with men. Most of these trials are small and did not have an *a priori* hypothesis regarding a sex difference, and so further studies are required to clarify this issue. If women do respond differently to dietary fat this may have important implications for the provision of dietary public health messages. It would also contribute to sex differences, and trends in sex differences in CHD.[9]

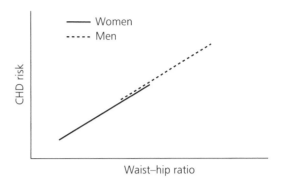

Fig. 5.3 Hypothetical situation in which relationship between waist hip ratio and CHD is continuous across both sexes.

5.3 Early life influences

5.3.1 Tracking of risk factors through the life course

High blood pressure, adverse lipid profiles and obesity have been shown to persist (track) from childhood to adulthood in women and men (see Chapter 14).[55–58] Behavioural risk factors such as smoking, diet, and inactivity are also established fairly early on in life and 'track' throughout the life course (see Chapter 13).[59,60]

5.3.2 Birth size and coronary heart disease and stroke risk

Birth size is inversely associated with both CHD and stroke risk.[61] Table 5.1 shows a summary of the studies that have reported sex-specific associations between birth size and CHD and stroke events and in women only, although most studies do not report sex specific findings (often stating that no sex differences have been found). The inverse association between birthweight and both CHD and stroke risk is found in women and men. Among these studies, losses to follow-up in the Hertfordshire cohort[62,63] may have led to selection bias,[64] and use of self report in the US Nurses Health Study[65] may have diluted effects due to misclassification bias.[66,67] However, a consistent direction of effect is seen in all, and is confirmed in one of the methodologically strongest studies from Uppsala.[68] In the Helsinki cohorts, shortness at birth in women, and thinness at birth in men, respectively are associated with greatest CHD risk.[69,70] Different patterns of growth may be associated with programming (Section 5.3.4) of different metabolic risk factors. Investigators of the Helsinki studies suggested that shortness (female pattern) is associated with persistent liver changes resulting in increased cholesterol and fibrinogen levels and thinness (male pattern) with increased insulin resistance. However, the same investigators, using a UK cohort, have also concluded that low birthweight in women is more strongly associated with insulin resistance than in men.[71]

5.3.3 Birth size and hypertension risk

Low birthweight is associated with increased blood pressure in later life.[72] Table 5.2 shows a summary of the studies that have reported sex-specific associations. Some studies suggest that the association between birthweight and blood pressure in childhood is stronger for women than for men.[76] However, a meta-analysis of mixed sex studies found no differences in the systolic blood pressure and birthweight relationship between men and women, neither in childhood/adolescence nor in adulthood.[91]

5.3.4 Mechanisms underlying the association between birth size and later CHD, stroke, and hypertension risk

Three theories may explain the underlying mechanisms of the associations between early life growth patterns and later life CHD and stroke. They are not mutually exclusive and a number of different pathways may act in the association. In one, poor intrauterine nutrition leads not only to small birth size but also, depending upon the timing (or critical period), it 'programmes' selective changes in body composition, cell size and number, hormonal axes and metabolism leading to increased adult disease risk.[61] A second theory suggests that specific genetic factors influence both birth size and later adult disease risk.[92] Finally, socioeconomic factors acting across the life course may be the explanation, as birthweight may be a marker of family socioeconomic circumstances during gestation, with cumulative socioeconomic conditions throughout the life course influencing heart disease and stroke risk.[93] It is difficult to disentangle the role of socioeconomic factors. Simple adjustments for social class or educational level may be too crude, since socioeconomic factors at any stage in the life course are strongly associated with behavioural risk factors such as smoking, diet, and physical activity.

Programming theory suggests that the primary prevention of heart disease and stroke may depend upon changing the body composition and diets of young women.[94] The effects on offspring cardiovascular disease risk and risk factors of maternal weight and diet before and during pregnancy are contradictory. Those born during the Dutch famine of 1944, and whose mothers were under-nourished during pregnancy, have increased glucose intolerance, an atherogenic lipid profile but normal blood pressure when compared with those born immediately before or after the famine.[95–97] People born during the 1941 siege of Leningrad do not have increased CHD risk[98] and cohorts born in the 1860s Finnish famine had similar adult survival rates to those born immediately before and after the famine.[99] Prospective studies assessing the association between maternal nutritional intake during pregnancy and heart disease, stroke, or risk factors in offspring have also found inconsistent results.[100,101] Higher intakes of carbohydrates, fats and protein during pregnancy were associated with higher adult blood pressure and glucose intolerance in the offspring of a cohort from Aberdeen,[102,103] but weight gain during pregnancy was not associated with systolic blood pressure at age 17 in an Israeli cohort.[81]

Genetic and non-genetic influences may be distinguished in twin studies in which differences in outcomes between dizygotic (non-identical) twins may be due to genetic and/or non-genetic factors, whereas differences between monozygotic (identical) twins, who share the same genetic background, must be the result of non-genetic factors.[104] In four studies of dizygotic twin pairs blood pressure in adolescence and early adult life was on average higher in the lower birthweight twin.[105–107] Since maternal nutrition both during and before pregnancy is the same for both twins these findings suggest that maternal nutrition is not the key influence in the birthweight blood pressure association. Some support for programming is provided by two of these studies as both the lower birthweight dizygotic and monozygotic twin[105,106] tended to have the highest systolic blood pressure. In the larger of these studies, the method of analysis may have influenced the findings, as a reanalysis showed that the relationship only held up for dizygotic twins,[107] and was consistent with two further twin studies using medical record or maternal (rather than self-reported) assessment of birthweight.[107,108] The lack of association in monozygotic twins and association in dizygotic twins suggests that genetic influences may be involved in the birthweight

Table 5.1 Cohort studies of association between birth size and coronary heart disease & stroke with sex specific results

Study	Number included in final analysis (% eligible)	Period of birth	Exposure (source)	Outcome	Number of cases	Age at death or follow-up	Results	Adjustment for:
Hertfordshire, UK[62][63]	♀ 5585 (60) ♂ 10141 (79)	♀ 1923–30 ♂ 1911–30	Birthweight (medical records)	CHD mortality	♀ 88 ♂ 853	♀ 20–69 ♂ 20–81	♀ Inverse p_{trend} not significant at 5% level ♂ Inverse $p_{trend} < 0.05$	Crude
Uppsala, Sweden[68]	♀ 6351 ♂ 7012 2.7% not traced (sex specific loss not provided)	♀ 1915–29 ♂ 1915–29	Birthweight (medical records)	CHD mortality	♀ 187 ♂ 679	♀ 29–80 ♂ 29–80	♀ 0.83 (0.62–1.10) ♂ 0.77 (0.67–0.90) Rate ratio associated with 1000 g increase in birthweight	Childhood and adulthood socio-economic circumstances
Nurses Health Study, US[65]	♀ 79297 (61)	1921–46	Birthweight (self report by adults)	Non-fatal CHD events	889	30–71	5% (0%–9%) Regression coefficient – % decrease in risk for every 454 g increase in weight (95% confidence interval)	Numerous potential confounders[a]
Helsinki, Finland [69,70]	♀ 3447 (93) ♂ 3641 (92)	1924–33	Birthweight (medical records)	♀ CHD event (fatal or non fatal) ♂ CHD mortality	279 310	62–71	♀ Inverse $p_{trend} = 0.08$ ♂ Inverse $p_{trend} = 0.05$	Gestational age

Study	Cohort N (%)	Birth years	Exposure	Outcome	N	Age	Association	Confounders
Helsinki, Finland [69,70]	♀ 3447 (93) ♂ 3641 (92)	1924–33	Birth length (medical records)	♀ CHD event (fatal or non fatal) ♂ CHD mortality	279 310	62–71	♀ Inverse $p_{trend} = 0.001$ ♂ No association	Gestational age
Helsinki, Finland [69,70]	♀ 3447 (93) ♂ 3641 (92)	1924–33	Ponderal index (medical records)	♀ CHD event (fatal or non fatal) ♂ CHD mortality	279 310	62–71	♀ No association ♂ Inverse $p_{trend} < 0.0001$	Gestational age
Uppsala, Sweden [68]	♀ 6351 ♂ 7012 2.7% not traced (sex specific loss not provided)	♀ 1915–29 ♂ 1915–29	Birthweight (medical records)	Stroke mortality	♀ 105 ♂ 113	♀ 29–80 ♂ 29–80	♀ 0.84 (0.57–1.24) ♂ 0.71 (0.49–1.03) Rate ratio associated with 1000 g increase in birthweight	Childhood and adulthood socio-economic circumstances
Nurses Health Study, US [65]	♀ 79297 (61)	1921–46	Birthweight (self report by adults)	Non-fatal stroke	364	30–71	11% (5%–18%) Regression coefficient – % decrease in risk for every 454 g increase in weight (95% confidence Interval)	Numerous potential confounders[a]

♀ Female; ♂ Male; CHD Coronary Heart Disease.

[a] *maternal* – smoking, diabetes and weight; *childhood* – social class; *adult* – social class, hypertension, diabetes, body mass index, waist hip ratio, smoking, alcohol, physical activity, saturated fat consumption, aspirin use, ethnic group.

p_{trend} p-value for test for trend across groups of exposure.

Table 5.2 Cohort studies of association between birth size and systolic blood pressure with sex specific or female only results

Study	N	Period of birth	Source of birth weight	Age at follow-up (years)	Regression of SBP on birth weight (95% confidence interval) or direction of association if regression not presented	Adjusted for:
Law et al, 1993 UK [73]*	♀ 646 ♂ 698	1975–1977	Medical records	1	♀ 1.30 (−0.80, 3.40) ♂ −0.60 (−2.60, 1.40)	Current ponderal index
Law et al, 1993 UK [73]*	♀ 584 ♂ 631	1975–1977	Medical records	3	♀ −1.60 (−3.40, −0.30) ♂ −1.50 (−3.30, 0.20)	Current BMI
Law et al, 1993 UK [73]*	♀ 506 ♂ 560	1975–1977	Medical records	7	♀ −2.10 (−4.00, −0.30) ♂ −1.50 (−3.20, 0.20)	Current BMI
Law et al, 1993 UK [73]*	♀ 218 ♂ 227	1975–1977	Medical records	10	♀ −2.30 (−4.80, 0.20) ♂ −0.80 (−3.10, 1.50)	Current BMI
Whincup et al, 1999 UK [74]	♀ 889 ♂ 971	1991–1992	Medical records	3	♀ −1.98 (−2.98, −0.98) ♂ −1.86 (−2.74, −0.98)	Age, current height and BMI
Whincup et al, 1989 UK [75]	♀ 1802 ♂ 1789	1980–1983	Medical records	5–7	♀ −2.00 (−2.80, −1.30) ♂ −1.60 (−2.30, −0.80)	Current BMI
Taylor et al, 1997 UK [76]	♀ 1442 ♂ 1568	1973–1976	Parental report + medical records for 52%	8–11	♀ −2.54 (−3.60, −1.48) ♂ −0.64 (−1.58, 0.30)	Current ponderal index, town, person who measured blood pressure, age

Study	Sample size	Birth year	Data source	Age	Association	Adjustments
Donker et al, 1997 [77]	♀ 701 ♂ 745	2 groups born: 1973–1974 1976–1980	Medical records or birth certificates	7–11	♀ No association ♂ No association (Inverse association with diastolic BP in black boys only)	Age, current weight and height
Barker et al, 1989 UK [78]	♀ 4834 ♂ 5087	1970	Medical records	10	♀ inverse ♂ inverse	Current weight and height
Taittonen et al, 1996 Finland [79]*	♀ 259 ♂ 246	Not given	Medical records	6	♀ −0.94 (−1.91, 0.04) ♂ −1.84 (−2.82, −0.86)	Current BMI
Taittonen et al, 1996 Finland [79]*	♀ 287 ♂ 250	Not given	Medical records	12	♀ −0.58 (−1.58, 0.41) ♂ −1.92 (−2.85, −0.98)	Current BMI
Taittonen et al, 1996 Finland [79]*	♀ 181 ♂ 148	Not given	Medical records	18	♀ −2.50 (−3.50, −1.50) ♂ −2.05 (−3.14, −0.96)	Current BMI
Rabbia et al, 1999 Italy [80]	♀ 650 ♂ 660	1977–1978	Medical records	12–14	♀ −0.27 (−1.9, 1.33) ♂ −0.07 (−1.6, 1.53)	Current weight, height, heart rate, age, sport, TV, stage of sexual development, familial risk of hypertension, parental cultural level, maternal risk of fetal distress
Laor et al, 1997 Jerusalem [81]	♀ 4149 ♂ 6684	1974–1976	Medical records	17	♀ −0.73 (−1.51, 0.05) ♂ −0.94 (−1.54, −0.33)	Gestational age, current BMI, height, birth order, ethnic origin, social status, mother's educational attainment and weight gain and body mass index during pregnancy

Table 5.2 (*Cont.*)

Study	N	Period of birth	Source of birth weight	Age at follow-up (years)	Regression of SBP on birth weight (95% confidence interval) or direction of association if regression not presented	Adjusted for:
Seidman et al, 1991 Jerusalem [82]	♀ 12846	1964–1971	Medical records	17	♀ weak inverse	Current BMI
	♂ 19734				♂ weak inverse	
Stocks et al, 1999 UK [83]	♀ 783	1971–79	Parental report	18–25	♀ −1.97 (−3.75, −0.18)	Current BMI, height and age
	♂ 572				♂ −0.70 (−2.70, 1.31)	
Macintyre et al, 1991 UK [84]	♀ 425	1971–1972	Parental report	15	♀ 0.63 (−1.23, 2.50)	Current BMI, weight, height, room temperature, season, social class, housing, smoking, drinking, exercise, heart rate, mother's height
	♂ 413				♂ −0.45 (−2.12, 1.22)	
Kolacek et al, 1993 Croatia [85]	♀ 251	1968–1969	Parental report	18–23	♀ −0.52 (−1.0, −0.1)	Current BMI
	♂ 214				♂ −0.34 (−0.69, 0.0)	
Moore et al, 1999 Australia [86]	♀ 287	1975–1976	Medical records	20	♀ −4.6 (−6.4, −2.9)	Current BMI
	♂ 297				♂ −2.6 (−4.4, −0.7)	
Wadsworth et al, 1985 UK [87]	♀ 1553	1946	Medical records	36	♀ −2.0 (−3.5, −0.4)	Current BMI, parental history of hypertension, childhood and current socio-economic class
	♂ 1396				♂ −2.3 (−3.8, −0.8)	

Study	n	Year of birth	Blood pressure method	Age	Effect estimate	Adjustment
Law et al, 1993 UK [73]	♀ 116 ♂ 123	1939–1943	Medical records	46–50	♀ −2.7 (−10.5, 5.1) ♂ −2.8 (−9.3, 3.7)	Current BMI
Law et al, 1993 UK [73]	♀ 103 ♂ 117	1935–1938	Medical records	59–63	♀ −3.4 (−13.6, 6.8) ♂ −3.4 (−9.1, 2.3)	Current BMI
Law et al, 1993 UK [73]	♀ 203 ♂ 426	♀ 1923–1930 ♂ 1920–1930	Medical records	59–63	♀ −2.7 (−8.8, 3.4) ♂ −3.0 (−6.9, 0.9)	Current BMI
Law et al, 1993 UK [73]	♀ 116 ♂ 123	♀ 1923–1930 ♂ 1920–1930	Medical records	64–71	♀ −5.5 (−12.2, 1.2) ♂ −4.9 (−8.8, −1.0)	Current BMI
Hennessy et al, 1997 UK [88]	♀ 3172	1958	Medical records	33	No association with self reported hypertension	
Curhan et al, 1996 US [89]	♀ 92940	1947–1964	Self report in categories	27–44	−0.35 (−0.41, −0.29)	Current BMI, age and parental history of hypertension
Curhan et al, 1996 US [89]	♀ 71100	1921–1946	Self report in categories	46–71	−1.39 (−1.49, −1.26)	Current BMI, age and parental history of hypertension
Yarbrough et al, 1998 US [90]	♀ 303	Not given	Self report	50–84	1.41 (p > 0.10)	Current BMI and age

♀ Female; ♂ Male; BMI Body Mass Index; * repeated measures in the same cohort.

and systolic blood pressure relationship, since removal of genetic variation removes the association. One twin study has looked at the association with CHD risk.[109] In this study, within both monozygotic and same sex dizygotic twin pairs birthweight, birth length, ponderal index and head circumference were not associated with acute myocardial infarction, suggesting that genetic factors or early childhood environmental factors are involved in the birthweight CHD association. In this study hospital records of birth details were used and checked to ensure that measurements were attributed to the correct twin. However, only 40 monozygotic and 72 dizygotic twin pairs were included and this study has been criticized for being under powered.[110]

The influence of genetic factors are also suggested by the finding of an inverse association between a child's birthweight and the mother's risk of CHD.[111–113] Since the child's birthweight cannot influence its mother's CHD risk through intrauterine nutrition, an intergenerational factor must be involved—genetic factors are one plausible explanation. This intergenerational effect may also be explained by generally healthier mothers giving birth to larger babies and being at lower risk of heart disease themselves. The general health of the mother and offspring birthweight may both be determined by a number of factors including socioeconomic position and nutrition across her own life course. However, the relationship was not removed by controlling for mother's size and other CHD risk factors, including socioeconomic circumstances. Age at menarche and menstrual pattern, which may be related both to CHD risk[114] and offspring's birthweight,[115] were not controlled for and remain possible explanatory factors. Furthermore, the child's birthweight also predicts, but not as strongly, the father's cardiovascular disease risk.[113,116] As father's risk cannot be explained by confounding due to maternal health behaviour or menstrual pattern, this provides further support for the genetic theory, but the stronger association for mothers suggests other factors are involved. Taken together, the findings suggest that both genetic factors and life course factors determining the general health of the mother explain these intergenerational effects.

5.3.5 Growth and nutrition in infancy and childhood

5.3.5.1 Infant feeding

An association between breastfeeding in infancy and heart disease or stroke risk was first proposed in the 1960s following post-mortem evidence of atherosclerosis in children who had been wholly artificially fed.[117] This observation was not confirmed in subsequent studies.[118,119] Investigators of the Hertfordshire historical cohort have reported that standardized mortality ratios for cardiovascular disease before the age of 65 were greater among those who were exclusively bottle-fed than those who were breastfed during the first year of life in both women and men.[62,63] However, these findings were not confirmed in a Californian cohort of children followed up for 65 years from 1922.[120] The relevance of these findings to contemporary cohorts is limited given the significant changes in modern formula milks and feeding practices.

In both historical and contemporary cohorts, breastfeeding in infancy has been shown to be associated with favourable lipid profiles, lower levels of glucose, and lower blood pressure in later childhood or adulthood.[121] A recent study of blood pressure in 13–16 year-olds who had been born prematurely and were involved in a randomized controlled trial of different feeding interventions at birth found that the 66 children who had been assigned banked breast milk had a mean arterial blood pressure that was 4 mmHg less than the

64 who were assigned preterm formula milk.[122] The size of this effect was similar in girls and boys. Since the preterm formula milk used in this study was similar in nutritional content to breast milk the investigators suggested that non-nutrient factors found in breast milk, such as hormones, may be responsible for the effect on blood pressure.

Prolonged breastfeeding beyond four months has been reported to be associated with brachial arterial stiffness in both sexes.[123] However, of 1526 individuals invited to participate in this study, only 28% agreed to do so and participant report of maternal recall of type and duration of infant feeding was used to determine the exposure; these factors may have lead to bias. There is no *a priori* reason for the hypothesis, which further weakens its credibility.

5.3.5.2 Height and leg length

Short stature in adulthood is associated with both CHD and stroke risk in women and men[124–127] and a recent study of skeletal remains from the ninth century suggests that tall stature has been associated with greater chances of survival for many centuries.[128] The underlying pathway for this association is unclear but controlling for adult risk factors, such as smoking, body mass index, cholesterol, blood pressure levels, and adult socioeconomic position attenuates, but does not remove, the association.[124,127] Further, the association is not a reflection of the birthweight and adult cardiovascular disease relationship.[127]

Leg length appears to be the component of height most strongly associated with increased cardiovascular risk.[129] Leg length reflects nutrition, socioeconomic position and possibly infection in childhood; thus these factors may explain the association.[129,130] Interruption of growth at any stage in the life course leads to relatively short legs and long torso.[131,132] This is particularly so in the prepubertal period when the main growth period of limbs occurs.[133] Preliminary analysis of the British Women's Heart and Health Study has found leg length to be inversely associated with prevalent CHD and stroke.[134] The inverse association between height, and in particular leg length, and CHD and stroke risk suggest that environmental factors acting during childhood are associated with CHD and stroke risk.

5.3.5.3 Accelerated postnatal growth

The relationship between small birth size and increased CHD risk may be stronger or only present among individuals who are above average size in later life. These results suggest that the effect of small birth size on CHD and stroke risk is increased by relatively accelerated postnatal growth (centile crossing). It is not clear whether accelerated growth at a particular time in the life course or at any stage is detrimental to those born small at birth. Among women in the Hertfordshire cohort the highest cardiovascular disease death rates occurred in those with below average birthweight but above average weight at one year.[62] In men there was no increased risk associated with centile crossing in the first year of life. Indeed the highest rates of cardiovascular disease deaths were among those with below average birthweight and below average weight at one year. In the Helsinki cohort the effects of small birth size on risk were increased by accelerated growth, occurring some time in the first seven years of life, in both women and men.[69] A recent analysis of the men only in this cohort suggests that low weight gain in infancy (up to one year of age) is associated with increased CHD risk, irrespective of birthweight. This indicates the possible importance of postnatal nutrition on coronary risk. After the age of one, rapid weight gain (centile crossing) was associated with increased CHD risk but only in those who were thin at birth.[135] In a systematic review 13 out of 16 studies found that the effect of small birth size on systolic blood pressure in later life was greatest in those who were relatively larger in later life in both women and men.[72] Programming may lead to permanently reduced cell numbers in specific tissues. Accelerated postnatal growth then increases risk either because overgrowth of the limited number of cells affects their function or because large body size exerts an excessive metabolic demand on the limited number of cells.[135] However, the apparent effects of postnatal growth could reflect the fact that at a given birthweight an individual who is taller or heavier in later life is more likely to have been growth retarded as a fetus than someone who is shorter in later life.

5.4 Factors unique to women

The associations between a number of factors that are unique to women reflecting female sex hormone exposure or other biological or social factors, and CHD or stroke risk have rarely been assessed using a life course approach. Attempts to combine age at menarche, menstrual history, parity and age at menopause to give an indication of lifetime exposure to endogenous oestrogens have not been made. Further, although the decreased occurrence of CHD in women compared with men during the reproductive years has been widely assumed to be due to a cardioprotective effect of oestrogen, the association between indicators of oestrogen exposure and CHD have rarely been assessed. For example, a Medline search from 1966 to the present combining the exploded terms 'breast neoplasm' and 'menarche' produces 327 hits whereas combining the exploded term 'cardiovascular disease' with 'menarche' produces only 35 hits. Few studies have examined the interaction between measures of oestrogen exposure and other CHD or stroke risk factors, particularly early life risk factors.

5.4.1 Endogenous oestrogen

In postmenopausal women with angina, serum oestrone levels are not associated with angiographic evidence of coronary artery disease or lipid profiles.[136,137] Nor do baseline levels of oestrone or oestradiol predict either CHD or total cardiovascular disease mortality over 20 years of follow-up.[138] Although these studies used a single measure of post-menopausal oestrogen, this is justified since there is minimal individual variation in oestrogen levels in postmenopausal women. No difference in premenopausal endogenous oestrogen (as measured by a single baseline 24-hour urinary excretion) was found in women with CHD and age matched controls.[139] A true protective effect of lifetime exposure to endogenous oestrogen cannot be ruled out from the negative findings of these single measure studies.

5.4.2 Age at menarche

Earlier age at menarche may reflect a greater lifetime exposure to oestrogen and is associated with increased breast cancer risk, a known oestrogen dependent condition (see Chapter 3). If oestrogen is cardioprotective then a late menarche may be associated with increased CHD risk. However, two studies that have assessed this association found that late age at menarche, assessed retrospectively in adulthood was weakly associated with a decreased CHD risk. In a small hospital case-control study menarcheal age over 15 compared with under 12 had an age adjusted relative risk of 0.61 (95% CI 0.33, 1.12).[140] In the US Nurses'

Health Study, with over 700 000 women-years of follow-up, menarcheal age at 16 was weakly associated with decreased CHD risk, compared with menarcheal age at 13, after controlling for socioeconomic and other known risk factors, including weight (relative risk (95% CI) 0.8 (0.4, 1.6)).[141] In the US Nurses' Health Study, self report was found to be accurate when compared with medical records of age at menarche in a subgroup, and late menarcheal age has been shown to be associated with decreased breast cancer risk, as expected, in this group suggesting that misclassification bias is unlikely to explain the results. The authors of the US Nurses' Health Study conclude that their results indicate that current oestrogen exposure (e.g. postmenopausal hormone replacement) is more important in determining CHD risk than past (or premenopausal) exposure. However, the results from both these studies are imprecise, no further studies of the association have been conducted, and results in the US Nurses' Health Study may be biased by the use of self report of likely confounding factors such as weight.

5.4.3 Polycystic ovary syndrome

Polycystic ovary syndrome (PCOS) is a heterogenous group of disorders involving altered ovarian function and characterized by chronic anovulation, hirsutism, obesity, and high circulating levels of androgens.[142] PCOS is associated with insulin resistance, dyslipidaemia, abdominal obesity, hypertension, and an increased risk of diabetes.[143] It has been predicted that women with PCOS should be at a seven fold increased risk of CHD due to these adverse risk factors.[143] Direct assessment of the risk of cardiovascular disease found no increase in CHD but an increased risk of stroke.[144] Two possible explanations for this unexpected finding were proposed. First, the risk factors associated with PCOS may not predict heart disease in women to the same extent as in men, which is implausible as CHD risk factors operated similarly in women and men. Alternatively, women with PCOS may be protected from the detrimental effects of the risk factors by some other factor, possibly unopposed oestrogen. Although progestogen levels are low in women with PCOS, so too are oestrogen levels and a protective effect of unopposed oestrogen in women with PCOS seems unlikely. Thus the PCOS findings remain an enigma.

5.4.4 Parity

A number of case-control and cross-sectional studies have found parity to be associated with increased risk of cardiovascular disease and several theories have been suggested to explain this association.[145–150] Pregnancy may 'reset' ovarian function leading to permanently lower premenopausal oestrogen levels and therefore lifetime exposure.[151] Parity is also associated with general obesity, upper abdominal obesity, glucose intolerance, dyslipidaemia, and hypertension. High progestogen and cortisol levels during pregnancy may result in permanent changes in these metabolic risk factors and hence increased cardiovascular disease risk.[145] How much of these associations are due to residual confounding, particularly due to socioeconomic factors, the hormonal effects of pregnancy or the effects of lifestyle changes (for example in diet or physical activity) related to child rearing is unclear. Six prospective studies have looked at the association between parity and CHD, stroke or all-cause mortality risk (Table 5.3). Only the Cancer Prevention Study did not show a relationship of increasing CHD or stroke risk with number of pregnancies and/or live births which was attributed to residual socioeconomic confounding explaining the positive findings of other studies.[153] Perhaps a more plausible explanation is that the effect is

Table 5.3 Cohort studies of the association between parity and CHD or stroke risk

Study	Number	Outcome	Number of events	Results	Adjusted for:
Framingham US [152]	2375	Total cardiovascular disease events (fatal and non-fatal)	527	relative risk (95% CI) 6 or more pregnancies compared with none total CVD 1.5 (1.1, 2.0) CHD 1.7 (1.2, 2.4)	Age, education, BMI, systolic blood pressure, cholesterol, smoking, glucose intolerance, left ventricular hypertrophy
NHANES 1 US [152]	2533	Total CHD events (fatal and non-fatal)	604	relative risk (95% CI) 6 or more pregnancies compared with none 1.3 (1.0, 1.8)	Age, education, BMI, systolic blood pressure, cholesterol, smoking, glucose intolerance, left ventricular hypertrophy
CPS II	585445	CHD mortality	4787	relative risk (95% CI) 6 or more live births compared with none 0.94 (0.83, 1.08)	Age, hypertension, smoking, lung disease, diabetes, employment status, education, exercise, body mass index, hormone replacement use, index of vegetable consumption
ONS longitudinal study UK [154]	108352	All cause and cause specific mortality	567 CHD deaths 276 stroke deaths	Linear trend towards increasing CHD and stroke mortality with increasing parity from 0 to 5 or more e.g. for women in manual social classes standardised mortality rates for CHD increased from 113 for women with no children to 149 for those with 5 or more	Age, social class
Dutch Civil Servants [155]	1200 women	CHD mortality	Not provided	*Women:* relative risk (95% CI) 4 or more children compared with none 2.5 (1.0, 5.8) 4 or more pregnancies compared with none 1.4 (0.6, 3.3)	Age, systolic blood pressure, cholesterol, BMI, income, smoking

	1048 husbands		*Husbands:* 4 or more children compared with none 1.6 (0.9, 2.6)	
Nurse's Health Study US [140]	119963 women	CHD events (fatal or non-fatal)	308	relative risk (95% confidence interval) 1 or more pregnancies (lasting at least 6 months) compared with none 1.2 (0.8, 1.8) No significant trend among parous women only with number of pregnancies	Age and 'multiple cardiovascular risk factors' not detailed

CI confidence interval; CHD coronary heart disease; BMI body mass index.

real but the Cancer Prevention Study did not detect any effect because of misclassification bias associated with the higher socioeconomic position and younger age at recruitment of women, many of whom may not have completed their families. Among Dutch civil servants, a stronger effect with number of children rather than number of pregnancies was found which would be consistent with social, behavioural, or emotional factors associated with raising children.[155] This view is supported by the moderate increase in CHD mortality in fathers associated with greater number of children in this study.[155]

5.4.5 Use of hormonal contraception

Oral contraceptives cause a small increase in the risk of CHD but this is confined to women with known risk factors, in particular those who smoke.[156,157] The oral contraceptive pill is also associated with increased risk of stroke and this risk is further increased in smokers, women with high blood pressure, and with higher doses of oestrogen or progestogen.[12] Low dose pills are associated with only slightly increased risk in non-smoking, normotensive women.

5.4.6 Age at menopause

A number of observational studies have assessed the association between early age at menopause and increased CHD or stroke risk and produced conflicting results.[112] Many did not control for important confounding factors, in particular smoking and socioeconomic position. In the US Nurses' Health Study[158] there was no association between age at menopause and CHD risk, for a naturally occurring menopause, after controlling for adult risk factors, including smoking and socioeconomic position. However, women who had had a bilateral oophorectomy and who were not taking oestrogen replacement had twice the risk of CHD compared with premenopausal women, but those taking oestrogen replacement had a similar risk to premenopausal women.[158]

Several studies have reported adverse effects of the menopause on lipid profiles, blood pressure, and obesity.[159] Since these factors all vary with age it is difficult to distinguish a discrete effect of the menopause from age-related effects. Patterns of change in lipids, blood pressure, body mass index, smoking, alcohol consumption, and exercise have been monitored in an ongoing longitudinal study of 150 women as they passed through the menopause.[160] Changes over a six-year period were modelled with reference to the final menstrual period. Although all risk factor levels changed over the six-year span only HDLc was dependent on the final menstrual period. There was a significant decrease in HDLc levels following the menopause, which was counterbalanced by an equal increase in the year before the menopause.[160]

5.4.7 Hormone replacement therapy

Trials in the 1960s and 1970s to prevent CHD in men by giving them high doses of oestrogen had to be stopped early because of increased mortality amongst those taking oestrogen.[161] In studies of male to female transsexuals long-term oestrogen treatment in biological men appears to have favourable effects on lipid profiles and endothelial dependent vasodilation but has no effect on systemic arterial compliance or blood pressure.[162,163]

Numerous observational studies have investigated the effect of hormone replacement therapy (HRT) on both CHD and stroke risk in postmenopausal women. These have been summarized in several meta-analyses that have reported a risk reduction in the range of

20–50%.[114,164] Observational studies tend to exaggerate the true effect of HRT because women who take HRT are likely to be thinner, non-smokers, more physically active, free from diabetes or hypertension, and from higher socioeconomic groups.[164]

A meta-analysis of HRT trials found an increased risk of total cardiovascular disease events (including peripheral vascular disease) associated with HRT use—pooled odds ratio 1.34 (95% CI 0.55, 3.30).[165] Although the investigators concluded that their findings were not consistent with an effect of HRT seen in observational studies, the confidence intervals are consistent with an effect of this size. The Postmenopausal Estrogen/ Progestin Interventions Trial (PEPI), a randomized controlled trial of the effect of hormone replacement on cardiovascular disease risk factors, found favourable improvements in the lipid profiles and post-load glucose levels of women who were assigned to hormone use.[166] In the Heart and Estrogen/progestin Replacement Study (HERS), a randomized controlled trial of the effect of hormone replacement in secondary prevention, there was no overall effect of HRT at four years follow-up for CHD, stroke or peripheral vascular disease.[167] However, during the first year of follow-up there was a 50% increase in total CHD and stroke events among the hormone treated group compared with the placebo group, counter-balanced by a slightly decreased risk in the final study year. These changes in risk may represent a chance finding and were not defined as an *a priori* hypothesis. HRT may cause an early increase as a result of 'harvesting' of the most vulnerable cases. Alternatively real and opposing effects of HRT may occur in different subgroups at different times.[168] A more recent secondary prevention trial found no effect of either oestrogen alone or oestrogen plus progestogen when compared with placebo on the progression of coronary atheroma.[169]

Randomized controlled trials to assess the effect of HRT in healthy women have begun.[170,171] In the Women's Health Initiative trial 27 348 women, aged between 50 and 79 and with no history of any form of cardiovascular disease, have been randomized to receive either hormone replacement or placebo. The trial is intended to run for 11 years with final results being available in 2005. Early safety monitoring in this trial found a slight increase in risk associated with hormone use in the first two years but conclusions regarding the effectiveness of hormone replacement in primary prevention of CHD and stroke must await the final results of these trials.

5.5 Social factors across the life course

5.5.1 Socioeconomic position across the life course

CHD and stroke mortality and morbidity vary both between and within countries by geographic region and socioeconomic position. In England and Wales the socioeconomic gap in CHD and stroke risk has increased since the 1930s among women and is wider for women than men. In addition, there has been a consistent relationship over time between low socioeconomic position and increased cardiovascular disease risk in women, whereas in men risk appeared to be greatest in those from the higher socioeconomic classes in the earlier half of the century (Table 5.4). Adult area-based and individually assigned socioeconomic indicators make independent contributions to cardiovascular disease mortality in both women and men.[172] In a prospective study of men a trend of increasing cardiovascular disease risk was found with increases in a cumulative score of poor socioeconomic position across the life course.[93] Recent studies have shown the same to be true in women.[173,174] Swedish women who experienced poor socioeconomic circumstances in both childhood

Table 5.4 Cardiovascular disease by social class among women and men 1931–1991 for England and Wales: Standardized Mortality Ratios

	Women						Men					
	I	II	IIIn	IIIm	IV	V	I	II	IIIn	IIIm	IV	V
All Cardiovascular Disease												
1931	67	84	99		110	117	102	102	96		100	106
1951	87	80	101		108	110	123	102	102		86	102
1961	65	77	103		109	145	92	92	104		98	121
1971	62	77	86	121	125	147	86	89	110	106	110	118
1981	54	63	84	119	140	191	69	80	102	108	113	151
1991							65	72	106	123	121	186
CHD												
1931	157	126	93		85	88	237	147	96		67	67
1951	102	86	101		104	105	147	110	105		79	89
1961	69	81	103		107	143	98	95	106		96	112
1971	58	77	81	125	123	146	88	91	114	107	108	111
1981	46	63	80	122	144	192	71	82	105	109	112	144
1991							63	73	107	125	121	182
Stroke												
1931	75	90	101		107	109	112	106	96		100	106
1951	101	96	101		102	101	124	104	102		86	102
1961	68	80	104		108	140	86	89	104		98	121
1971	76	84	93	116	124	139	80	86	110	106	110	118
1981	62	62	87	116	135	179	62	72	102	108	113	151
1991							70	67	106	123	121	186

Sources for calculating SMRs: The Registrar-General's Decennial Supplement England & Wales Occupational Mortality – 1931; 1951; 1961; 1970–1972; 1979–80, 1982–83 & Drever F & Whitehead M (eds) Health Inequalities Series Decennial Supplement No 15, 1997. All available from the Office of National Statistics, London.

For women social class is for Married Women and based on Husband's Occupation. 1931 data for ages 20–65; 1951, 1981, 1991 data for ages 20–64; 1961, 1971 data for ages 15–64. IIIn – Social class III non-manual; IIIm – Social class III manual; prior to 1971 social class III was not split into these sub-categories. Comparable data for women for 1991 not available.

and adulthood had four times the risk of developing premature CHD than those who did not suffer disadvantage at either time.[174]

The mechanisms underlying the association between poor socioeconomic position and increased disease risk are the subject of much debate.[175,176] Behavioural risk factors such as smoking, poor diet and physical inactivity are more common in the most disadvantaged groups. Adjustment for these risk factors reduces the association between socioeconomic position and CHD and stroke risk but does not completely remove it. There is agreement that the direct effects of poverty at an individual level (e.g. inability to buy good food), and at a societal level, (e.g. living in an area with little investment in housing, transport infrastructure, and community facilities) are important pathways in the association.[175,176] Poverty, and its associated factors, will tend to operate in different ways in childhood, adolescence, and adulthood, but will combine to increase CHD and stroke risk.

There is disagreement over the role of relative poverty in the association. In addition to the direct effects of poverty, relative poverty has adverse health consequences because of the emotional stress of recognition of a relatively inferior position.[176] The resulting emotional stress is believed to affect physiological processes, in particular neuroendocrine pathways, which are postulated to cause increased cardiovascular disease. The importance of this debate lies in its implications. If relative poverty plays a substantial role in the association between poverty and disease outcomes, then providing the poorest members of society with adequate incomes and material structures to afford a 'healthy' life would be insufficient to reduce their risk to that of more affluent members of society, if relative differences remained. Unpicking the direct effects of poverty from associated behavioural risk factors and subtle psychological effects of absolute and relative material disadvantage is difficult in epidemiological studies. A further challenge is to examine the health effects of such experiences as they accumulate over the life course.

5.5.2 Work outside the home

Work outside the home, in general, does not appear to be detrimental to women's cardiovascular health.[177] However, as with men, women in lower social grades of work are at increased disease risk.[178–180] Low socioeconomic position is associated with low levels of job control and work variety, which in turn are linked with CHD risk. This is interpreted as indicating a clear psychosocial pathway.[176] However, the association between job control and CHD risk may be explained by residual confounding, reverse causality or reporting bias, and the pathway linking these may still be the direct effects of poverty which lead to both low job status and increased CHD risk.

5.5.3 Social networks

In men social ties (or networks) appear beneficial to cardiovascular health but in women the results appear less consistent.[181] In both the North Karelia and Evans County prospective studies no association was observed between number of social ties and CHD or stroke risk in women, whereas strong associations were observed among men.[182,183] Gender differences in reporting of social ties could explain these results. A large Swedish study found a U-shaped relationship between number of social ties and CHD risk in both women and men.[184] The increased risk with number of social ties was particularly strong among elderly people. Social ties may increase or decrease in response to declines in health prior to a clinical event, and although social ties data were collected prospectively, their apparent strong detrimental effect among elderly people suggests that reverse causality may explain the association. It is also possible that quality rather than quantity of social ties is important. For women, more so than men, increased numbers of social ties, including marriage, family, religious and other community ties may reflect increased roles, in particular caring roles, that increase stress and CHD risk.[185]

5.6 Conclusions and policy implications

The main classical cardiovascular risk factors have the same effects in women as they do in men and preventive treatments that lower risk factors—antihypertensive drugs, aspirin, and cholesterol lowering drugs—work equally well in both sexes. Diabetes and the insulin resistance syndrome may confer greater risk to women than men. Women may be protected from coronary heart disease by a number of interacting factors including a more favourable fat distribution, a less adverse response to dietary saturated fats, and endogenous oestrogens. Research examining the cumulative lifetime exposure to endogenous oestrogens and CHD and stroke risk would be particularly valuable. Low birthweight, poor infant nutrition and accelerated postnatal growth are all associated with CHD and stroke risk in both women and men. It would be simplistic to consider that solely promoting good maternal and child health would be an adequate health policy for the control of CHD and stroke. The effect of manipulation of early life development on cardiovascular disease is not known. As knowledge accumulates our understanding of the complex pattern of causation operating from early to late life will deepen. Policy makers should not interpret this evidence as indicating that women are responsible—at an individual level—for the cardiovascular health of the entire population and promote 'victim-blaming'[186] of all fertile women and mothers.

Commentary on 'A life course approach to coronary heart disease and stroke.'

Catherine Law

The authors highlight the massive burden of disease that coronary heart disease and stroke represent for women worldwide. In contrast, knowledge of the causes and prevention of these diseases is incomplete, particularly for women, and even more so for women living in developing countries. Much research on women has concentrated on describing the differences from the epidemiology of disease in men, rather than describing, *a priori*, what affects women's chances of getting disease. As the authors discuss, even this limited literature may be hard to interpret, as it is prone to publication bias, making 'interesting' differences more likely to be reported than similarities. Furthermore, the differences may be interpreted in contexts that are more applicable to one gender. For example, the association of work related stress to coronary heart disease (CHD) in women is documented only for work outside the home in developed countries (Section 5.5.2). But the hypothesis that psychosocial stress relating to job control and satisfaction leads to CHD might be equally applicable to work inside the home, or to work in developing countries.

Despite the emphasis in the published literature on differences, it is the similarities that I find striking. For women, as for men, reduced growth in fetal life and infancy, accelerated growth in later childhood, and adult lifestyle factors such as smoking, obesity, and physical inactivity are all associated with cardiovascular disease (CVD). Biological risk factors such as hypertension predict CVD in women and their reduction lowers that risk. Exceptions are insulin resistance and lipid levels, where adverse profiles may have disproportionately high impact on CVD in women compared with men (Sections 5.2 and 5.3).

A life course perspective seems especially relevant to the study of CVD in women, because women influence the health of their children through intergenerational, environmental, and genetic factors. Women's health, itself a legacy of the past, casts shadow or light forward into the next generation and beyond. Perhaps more than for other 'adult' diseases, there is evidence which links CVD with different parts of the life course from fetal life to old age. The biggest gaps occur when joining the different parts up. This may be far more complex than simple summation across the years. Biological risk factors are most likely to be programmed at a critical period early in life, perhaps before birth or in very early childhood. The effect of later exposures may depend on the nature and magnitude of early experience, not simply on adding later exposure to it.[187] Critical periods may also occur in relation to psychological and social development, for example, in critical periods for learning.[188]

The authors' full description of the associations of CVD with life course variables also exposes glaring gaps in our understanding of the mechanisms which underlie these associations. We lack evidence on factors acting in fetal life other than maternal nutrition, and even for this information is limited. The role of lifetime exposure to endogenous oestrogen has not been explored, despite its potential importance to clinical practice in fertility control and postmenopausal hormone replacement therapy. Cardiovascular disease is an important determinant of socioeconomic inequalities in health, but the roles of absolute and relative poverty, and the effects of disadvantage at societal and individual level remain matters of debate and conflicting evidence.[189]

Arguably, the only importance in understanding the causes of CVD and the similarities and differences between men and women is in using that knowledge for prevention. Here lies the biggest gap in the evidence, for interventions to prevent cardiovascular disease have tended to take wholly adult approaches, often from a medical intervention model such as screening or pharmaceutical approaches. But the evidence from a life course approach suggests interventions which address factors in pregnancy, childhood, adolescence, and young adult life should also be evaluated.

The authors conclude that fertile women and mothers should not be the subject of 'victim-blaming' for the cardiovascular health of the population. Instead, I suggest the evidence be used to positively promote the health of women and children, which is justified for its short-term as well as for any long-term benefits.[190] I agree with the authors that 'it would be simplistic to consider that solely promoting good maternal and child health would be an adequate health policy for control of CHD and stroke'. But it might be a good place to start.

References

1 **Petersen S, Mockford C, Rayner M**. *Coronary heart disease statistics*. British Heart Foundation statistics database 1999. London: British Heart Foundation, 1999.

2 **Rayner M, Petersen S**. *European cardiovascular disease statistics*. London: British Heart Foundation, 2000.

3 **World Health Organisation** *World Health Statistics Annuals 1996*. Geneva: World Health Organisation, 1996.

4 **Hart CL, Hole DJ, Davey Smith G**. Risk factors and 20-year stroke mortality in men and women in the Renfrew/Paisley study in Scotland. *Stroke* 1999;**30**:1999–2007.

5 **Bonita R, Beaglehole R, Asplund K**. The worldwide problem of stroke. *Curr Opin Neurol* 1994;**7**:5–10.

6 **Lopez AD, Murray CC**. The global burden of disease, 1990–2020. *Nat Med* 1998;**4**:1241–3.

7 **Ebrahim S, Nouri F**. Caring for stroke patients at home. *Int Rehabil Med* 1987;**8**:171–3.

8 **Zhang XH, Sasaki S, Kesteloot H**. The sex ratio of mortality and its secular trends. *Int J Epidemiol* 1995;**24**:720–729.

9 **Lawlor DA, Ebrahim S, Davey Smith G**. Sex matters: secular and geographical trends in sex differences in ischaemic heart disease mortality. *Br Med J* 2001;**323**:541–5.

10 **Tunstall-Pedoe H**. Myth and paradox of coronary risk and the menopause. *Lancet* 1998;**351**:1425–7.

11 **Tracy RE**. Sex difference in coronary disease: two opposing views. *J Chron Dis* 1966;**19**:1245–51.

12 **Ebrahim S, Harwood R**. *Stroke. Epidemiology, evidence and clinical practice*. Oxford: Oxford University Press, 2000.

13 **Khaw KT**. Where are the women in studies of coronary heart disease? *Br Med J* 1993;**306**:1145–6.

14 **Sterne JAC, Davey Smith G**. Shifting the evidence—what's wrong with significance tests? *Br Med J* 2001;**322**:226–31.

15 **Brookes ST, Whitley E, Peters TJ, Mulheren PA, Egger M, Davey Smith G**. Subgroup analysis in randomised controlled trials: quantifying the risks of false-positives and false-negatives. *Health Technol Assess* **2001**;5:1–56.

16 **Kannel WB, Wilson PW**. Risk factors that attenuate the female coronary disease advantage. *Arch Intern Med* 1995;**155**:57–61.

17 **Hart CL, Hole DJ, Davey Smith G**. Comparison of risk factors for stroke incidence and stroke mortality in 20 years of follow-up in men and women in the Renfrew/Paisley Study in Scotland. *Stroke* 2000;**31**:1893–6.

18 **Isles CG, Hole DJ, Hawthorne VM, Lever AF**. Relation between coronary risk and coronary mortality in women of the Renfrew and Paisley survey: comparison with men. *Lancet* 1992;**339**:702–6.

19 **Prescott E, Hippe M, Schnohr P, Hein HO, Vestbo J**. Smoking and risk of myocardial infarction in women and men: longitudinal population study. *Br Med J* 1998;**316**:1043–7.

20 **Castelli WP, Garrison RJ, Wilson PW, Abbott RD, Kalousdian S, Kannel WB**. Incidence of coronary heart disease and lipoprotein cholesterol levels. The Framingham Study. *J Am Med Assoc* 1986;**256**:2835–8.

21 Dorn JM, Schisterman EF, Winkelstein W, Jr., Trevisan M. Body mass index and mortality in a general population sample of men and women. The Buffalo Health Study. *Am J Epidemiol* 1997;**146**:919–31.

22 Hubert HB, Feinleib M, McNamara PM, Castelli WP. Obesity as an independent risk factor for cardiovascular disease: a 26-year follow-up of participants in the Framingham Heart Study. *Circulation* 1983;**67**:968–77.

23 Manson JE, Colditz GA, Stampfer MJ, Willett WC, Rosner B, Manson RR, Speizer FE, Hennekens CH. A prospective study of obesity and risk of coronary heart disease in women. *N Engl J Med* 1990;**322**:882–9.

24 Berlin JA, Colditz GA. A meta-analysis of physical activity in the prevention of coronary heart disease. *Am J Epidemiol* 1990;**132**:612–28.

25 Andersen LB, Schnohr P, Schroll M, Hein HO. All-cause mortality associated with physical activity during leisure time, work, sports, and cycling to work. *Arch Intern Med* 2000;**160**:1621–8.

26 Kawachi I, Colditz GA, Stampfer MJ, Willett WC, Manson JE, Rosner B, Speizer FE, Hennekens CH. Smoking cessation and decreased risk of stroke in women. *J Am Med Assoc* 1993;**269**:232–6.

27 Kawachi I, Colditz GA, Stampfer MJ, Willett WC, Manson JE, Rosner B, Speizer FE, Hennekens CH. Smoking cessation and time course of decreased risks of coronary heart disease in middle-aged women. *Arch Intern Med* 1994;**154**:169–75.

28 Kjeldsen SE, Kolloch RE, Leonetti G, Mallion JM, Zanchetti A, Elmfeldt D, Warnold I, Hansson L. Influence of gender and age on preventing cardiovascular disease by antihypertensive treatment and acetylsalicylic acid. The HOT study. Hypertension Optimal Treatment. *J Hypertens* 2000;**18**:629–42.

29 SHEP Cooperative Research Group. Prevention of stroke by antihypertensive drug treatment in older persons with isolated systolic hypertension. Final results of the Systolic Hypertension in the Elderly Program (SHEP). *J Am Med Assoc* 1991;**265**:3255–64.

30 Ebrahim S, Davey Smith G, McCabe C, Payne N, Pickin M, Sheldon TA, Lampe F, Sampson F, Ward S, Wannamethee G. What role for statins? A review and economic model. *Health Technol Assess* 1999;**3**:1–96.

31 Antiplatelet Trialists' Collaboration. Collaborative overview of randomised trials of antiplatelet therapy–I: Prevention of death, myocardial infarction, and stroke by prolonged antiplatelet therapy in various categories of patients. *Br Med J* 1994;**308**:81–106.

32 Corrao G, Rubbiati L, Bagnardi V, Zambon A, Poikolainen K. Alcohol and coronary heart disease: a meta-analysis. *Addiction* 2000;**95**:1505–23.

33 Sacco RL, Elkind M, Boden-Albala B, Lin IF, Kargman DE, Hauser WA, Shea S, Paik MC. The protective effect of moderate alcohol consumption on ischemic stroke. *J Am Med Assoc* 1999;**281**:53–60.

34 Britton A, McKee M. The relation between alcohol and cardiovascular disease in Eastern Europe: explaining the paradox. *J Epidemiol Community Health* 2000;**54**:328–32.

35 Barrett-Connor EL, Cohn BA, Wingard DL, Edelstein SL. Why is diabetes mellitus a stronger risk factor for fatal ischemic heart disease in women than in men? The Rancho Bernardo Study. *J Am Med Assoc* 1991;**265**:627–31.

36 Heyden S, Heiss G, Bartel AG, Hames CG. Sex differences in coronary mortality among diabetics in Evans County, Georgia. *J Chron Dis* 1980;**33**:265–73.

37 Kleinman JC, Donahue RP, Harris MI, Finucane FF, Madans JH, Brock DB. Mortality among diabetics in a national sample. *Am J Epidemiol* 1988;**128**:389–401.

38 Folsom AR, Szklo M, Stevens J, Liao F, Smith R, Eckfeldt JH. A prospective study of coronary heart disease in relation to fasting insulin, glucose, and diabetes. The Atherosclerosis Risk in Communities (ARIC) Study. *Diabetes Care* 1997;**20**:935–42.

39 Lee WL, Cheung AM, Cape D, Zinman B. Impact of diabetes on coronary artery disease in women and men: a meta-analysis of prospective studies. *Diabetes Care* 2000;**23**:962–8.

40 Liese AD, Mayer-Davis EJ, Haffner SM. Development of the multiple metabolic syndrome: an epidemiologic perspective. *Epidemiol Rev* 1998;**20**:157–72.

41 Jacobs DR, Jr., Mebane IL, Bangdiwala SI, Criqui MH, Tyroler HA. High density lipoprotein cholesterol as a predictor of cardiovascular disease mortality in men and women: the follow-up study of the Lipid Research Clinics Prevalence Study. *Am J Epidemiol* 1990;**131**:32–47.

42 Giltay EJ, Lambert J, Elbers JM, Gooren LJ, Asscheman H, Stehouwer CD. Arterial compliance and distensibility are modulated by body composition in both men and women but by insulin sensitivity only in women. *Diabetologia* 1999;**42**:214–21.

43 Lapidus L, Bengtsson C. Regional obesity as a health hazard in women–a prospective study. *Acta Medica Scandinavica—Supplementum* 1988;**723**:53–9.

44 Barrett-Connor E. Sex differences in coronary heart disease. Why are women so superior? The 1995 Ancel Keys Lecture. *Circulation* 1997;**95**:252–64.

45 Larsson B, Bengtsson C, Bjorntop P, *et al*. Is abdominal body fat distribution a major explanation for the sex difference in the incidence of myocardial infarction? The study of men born in 1913 and the study of women, Goteborg, Sweden. *Am J Epidemiol* 1992 **135**:266–73.

46 Wilson TA, Nicolosi RJ, Lawton CW, Babiak J. Gender differences in response to a hypercholesterolemic diet in hamsters: effects on plasma lipoprotein cholesterol concentrations and early aortic atherosclerosis. *Atherosclerosis* 1999;**146**:83–91.

47 Clifton PM, Nestel PJ. Influence of gender, body mass index, and age on response of plasma lipids to dietary fat plus cholesterol. *Arterioscler Thromb* 1992;**12**:955–62.

48 Walden CE, Retzlaff BM, Buck BL, Wallick S, McCann BS, Knopp RH. Differential effect of National Cholesterol Education Program (NCEP) Step II diet on HDL cholesterol, its subfractions, and apoprotein A-I levels in hypercholesterolemic women and men after 1 year: the beFIT Study. *Arterioscler Thromb Vasc Biol* 2000;**20**:1580–7.

49 Walden CE, Retzlaff BM, Buck BL, McCann BS, Knopp RH. Lipoprotein lipid response to the National Cholesterol Education Program step II diet by hypercholesterolemic and combined hyperlipidemic women and men. *Arterioscler Thromb Vasc Biol* 1997;**17**:375–82.

50 Wood PD, Stefanick ML, Williams PT, Haskell WL. The effects on plasma lipoproteins of a prudent weight-reducing diet, with or without exercise, in overweight men and women. *N Engl J Med* 1991;**325**:461–6.

51 Cobb M, Greenspan J, Timmons M, Teitelbaum H. Gender differences in lipoprotein responses to diet. *Ann Nutr Metab* 1993;**37**:225–36.

52 Geil PB, Anderson JW, Gustafson NJ. Women and men with hypercholesterolemia respond similarly to an American Heart Association step 1 diet. *J Am Diet Assoc* 1995;**95**:436–41.

53 Ginsberg HN, Kris-Etherton P, Dennis B, Elmer PJ, Ershaw A, Lefevre M, Pearson T, Rohein P, Ramakrshnan R, Reed R, Steward K. Effects of reducing dietary saturated fatty acids on plasma

lipids and lipoproteins in healthy subjects: the DELTA Study, protocol 1. *Arterioscler Thromb Vas Biol* 1998;**18**:441–9.

54 Stefanick ML, Mackey S, Sheehan M, Ellsworth N, Haskell WL, Wood PD. Effects of diet and exercise in men and postmenopausal women with low levels of HDL cholesterol and high levels of LDL cholesterol. *N Engl J Med* 1998;**339**:12–20.

55 Lauer RM, Mahoney LT, Clarke WR. Tracking of blood pressure during childhood: the Muscatine Study. *Clin Exp Hypertens* 1986;**8**:515–37.

56 Clarke WR, Schrott HG, Leaverton PE, Connor WE, Lauer RM. Tracking of blood lipids and blood pressures in school age children: the Muscatine study. *Circulation* 1978;**58**:626–34.

57 Webber LS, Srinivasan SR, Wattigney WA, Berenson GS. Tracking of serum lipids and lipoproteins from childhood to adulthood. The Bogalusa Heart Study. *Am J Epidemiol* 1991;**133**:884–99.

58 Vanhala M, Vanhala P, Kumpusalo E, Halonen P, Takala J. Relation between obesity from childhood to adulthood and the metabolic syndrome: population based study. *B Med J* 1998; **317**:319

59 Kuh DJL, Cooper C. Physical activity at 36 years: patterns and childhood predictors in a longitudinal study. *J Epidemiol Community Health* 1992;**46**:114–9.

60 Health Education Authority. *Tomorrow's young adults.* London: Health Education Authority, 1992.

61 Godfrey KM, Barker DJ. Fetal nutrition and adult disease. *Am J Clin Nutr* 2000;**71**:1344S–1352S.

62 Osmond C, Barker DJ, Winter PD, Fall CH, Simmonds SJ. Early growth and death from cardiovascular disease in women. *Br Med J* 1993;**307**:1519–24.

63 Barker DJ, Winter PD, Osmond C, Margetts B, Simmonds SJ. Weight in infancy and death from ischaemic heart disease. *Lancet* 1989;**2**:577–80.

64 Joseph KS, Kramer MS. Review of the evidence on fetal and early childhood antecedents of adult chronic disease. *Epidemiol Rev* 1996;**18**:158–74.

65 Rich-Edwards JW, Stampfer MJ, Manson JE, *et al.* Birth weight and risk of cardiovascular disease in a cohort of women followed up since 1976. *Br Med J* 1997;**315**:396–400.

66 Kemp M, Gunnell D, Maynard M, Davey Smith G, Frankel S. How accurate is self reported birth weight among the elderly? *J Epidemiol Community Health* 2000;**54**:639–40.

67 Andersson SW, Niklasson A, Lapidus L, Hallberg L, Bengtsson C, Hulthen L. Poor agreement between self-reported birth weight and birth weight from original records in adult women. *Am J Epidemiol* 2000;**152**:609–16.

68 Leon DA, Lithell HO, Vagero D, Koupilova I, Mohsen R, Berglund L, Lithell UB, Mckeigue PM. Reduced fetal growth rate and increased risk of death from ischaemic heart disease: cohort study of 15 000 Swedish men and women born 1915–29. *Br Med J* 1998;**317**:241–5.

69 Forsen T, Eriksson JG, Tuomilehto J, Osmond C, Barker DJ. Growth in utero and during childhood among women who develop coronary heart disease: longitudinal study. *Br Med J* 1999;**319**:1403–7.

70 Forsen T, Eriksson JG, Tuomilehto J, Teramo K, Osmond C, Barker DJ. Mother's weight in pregnancy and coronary heart disease in a cohort of Finnish men: follow up study. *Br Med J* 1997;**315**:837–40.

71 Fall CH, Osmond C, Barker DJ, Clark PM, Hales CN, Stirling Y, Meade TM. Fetal and infant growth and cardiovascular risk factors in women. *Br Med J* 1995;**310**:428–32.

72 Huxley RR, Shiell AW, Law CM. The role of size at birth and postnatal catch-up growth in determining systolic blood pressure: a systematic review of the literature. *J Hypertens* 2000;**18**:815–31.

73 Law CM, de Swiet M, Osmond C, Fayers PM, Barker DJ, Cruddas AM, Fall CH. Initiation of hypertension in utero and its amplification throughout life. *Br Med J* 1993;**306**:24–7.

74 Whincup PH, Bredow M, Payne F, Sadler S, Golding J. Size at birth and blood pressure at 3 years of age. The Avon Longitudinal Study of Pregnancy and Childhood (ALSPAC). *Am J Epidemiol* 1999;**149**:730–9.

75 Whincup PH, Cook DG, Shaper AG. Early influences on blood pressure: a study of children aged 5–7 years. *Br Med J* 1989;**299**:587–91.

76 Taylor SJ, Whincup PH, Cook DG, Papacosta O, Walker M. Size at birth and blood pressure: cross sectional study in 8–11 year old children. *Br Med J* 1997;**314**:475–80.

77 Donker GA, Labarthe DR, Harrist RB, Selwyn BJ, Wattigney W, Berenson GS. Low birth weight and blood pressure at age 7–11 years in a biracial sample. *Am J Epidemiol* 1997;**145**:387–97.

78 Barker DJ, Osmond C, Golding J, Kuh D, Wadsworth ME. Growth in utero, blood pressure in childhood and adult life, and mortality from cardiovascular disease. *Br Med J* 1989;**298**: 564–7.

79 Taittonen L, Nuutinen M, Turtinen J, Uhari M. Prenatal and postnatal factors in predicting later blood pressure among children: cardiovascular risk in young Finns. *Pediatr Res* 1996;**40**:627–32.

80 Rabbia F, Veglio F, Grosso T, Nacca R, Martini G, Riva P, di Cella SM, Schiavane D, Chiandussi L. Relationship between birth weight and blood pressure in adolescence. *Prev Med* 1999;**29**:455–9.

81 Laor A, Stevenson DK, Shemer J, Gale R, Seidman DS. Size at birth, maternal nutritional status in pregnancy, and blood pressure at age 17: population based analysis. *Br Med J* 1997;**315**:449–53.

82 Seidman DS, Laor A, Gale R, Stevenson DK, Mashiach S, Danon YL. Birth weight, current body weight, and blood pressure in late adolescence. *Br Med J* 1991;**302**:1235–7.

83 Stocks NP, Davey Smith G. Blood pressure and birthweight in first year university students aged 18–25. *Public Health* 1999;**113**:273–7.

84 Macintyre S, Watt G, West P, Ecob R. Correlates of blood pressure in 15 year olds in the west of Scotland. *J Epidemiol Community Health* 1991;**45**:143–7.

85 Kolacek S, Kapetanovic T, Luzar V. Early determinants of cardiovascular risk factors in adults. B. Blood pressure. *Acta Paediatr* 1993;**82**:377–82.

86 Moore VM, Cockington RA, Ryan P, Robinson JS. The relationship between birth weight and blood pressure amplifies from childhood to adulthood. *J Hypertens* 1999;**17**:883–8.

87 Wadsworth ME, Cripps HA, Midwinter RE, Colley JR. Blood pressure in a national birth cohort at the age of 36 related to social and familial factors, smoking, and body mass. *BMJ (Clin Res Ed)* 1985;**291**:1534–38.

88 Hennessy E, Alberman E. The effects of own fetal growth on reported hypertension in parous women aged 33. *Int J Epidemiol*. 1997;**26**:562–70.

89 Curhan GC, Chertow GM, Willett WC, *et al*. Birth weight and adult hypertension and obesity in women. *Circulation* 1996;**94**:1310–5.

90 Yarbrough DE, Barrett-Connor E, Kritz-Silverstein D, Wingard DL. Birth weight, adult weight, and girth as predictors of the metabolic syndrome in postmenopausal women: the Rancho Bernardo Study. *Diabetes Care* 1998;**21**:1652–8.

91 Lawlor DA, Ebrahim S, Davey Smith G. Is there a sex difference in the association between birth weight and systolic blood pressure in later life. *Am J Epidemiol* 2002, in press.

92 Hattersley AT, Tooke JE. The fetal insulin hypothesis: an alternative explanation of the association of low birthweight with diabetes and vascular disease. *Lancet* 1999;**353**:1789–92.

93 Davey Smith G, Hart C, Blane D, Gillis C, Hawthorne V. Lifetime socioeconomic position and mortality: prospective observational study. *Br Med J* 1997;**314**:547–52.

94 Barker DJ. Early growth and cardiovascular disease. *Arch Dis Child* 1999;**80**:305–7.

95 Roseboom TJ, van der Meulen JH, Ravelli AC, van Montfrans GA, Osmond C, Barker DJ, Bleker OP. Blood pressure in adults after prenatal exposure to famine. *J Hypertens* 1999;**17**: 325–30.

96 Roseboom TJ, van der Meulen JHP, Osmond C, Barker DJP, Ravelli ACJ, Bleker OP. Plasma lipid profiles in adults after prenatal exposure to the Dutch famine. *Am J Clin Nutr* 2000;**72**:1101–6.

97 Ravelli AC, van der Meulen JH, Michels RP, Osmond C, Barker DJ, Hales CN, Bleker OP. Glucose tolerance in adults after prenatal exposure to famine. *Lancet* 1998;**351**:173–7.

98 Stanner SA, Bulmer K, Andres C, Lantseva OE, Borodina V, Poteen VV, Yudkin JS. Does malnutrition in utero determine diabetes and coronary heart disease in adulthood? Results from the Leningrad siege study, a cross sectional study. *Br Med J* 1997;**315**:1342–8.

99 Kannisto V, Christensen K, Vaupel JW. No increased mortality in later life for cohorts born during famine. *Am J Epidemiol* 1997;**145**:987–94.

100 Godfrey K, Robinson S, Barker DJ, Osmond C, Cox V. Maternal nutrition in early and late pregnancy in relation to placental and fetal growth. *Br Med J* 1996;**312**:410–4.

101 Mathews F, Yudkin P, Neil A. Influence of maternal nutrition on outcome of pregnancy: prospective cohort study. *Br Med J* 1999;**319**:339–43.

102 Shiell AW, Campbell DM, Hall MH, Barker DJ. Diet in late pregnancy and glucose-insulin metabolism of the offspring 40 years later. *Br J Obstet Gynaecol* 2000;**107**:890–5.

103 Campbell DM, Hall MH, Barker DJ, Cross J, Shiell AW, Godfrey KM. Diet in pregnancy and the offspring's blood pressure 40 years later. *Br J Obstet Gynaecol* 1996;**103**:273–80.

104 Phillips DI. Twin studies in medical research: can they tell us whether diseases are genetically determined? *Lancet* 1993;**341**:1008–9.

105 Dwyer T, Blizzard L, Morley R, Ponsonby AL. Within pair association between birth weight and blood pressure at age 8 in twins from a cohort study. *Br Med J* 1999;**319**:1325–9.

106 Poulter NR, Chang CL, MacGregor AJ, Snieder H, Spector TD. Association between birth weight and adult blood pressure in twins: historical cohort study. *Br Med J* 1999;**319**:1330–3.

107 IJzerman RG, Stehouwer CD, Boomsma DI. Evidence for genetic factors explaining the birth weight-blood pressure relation : analysis in twins. *Hypertension* 2000;**36**:1008–12.

108 Zhang J, Brenner RA, Klebanoff MA. Differences in birth weight and blood pressure at age 7 years among twins. *Am J Epidemiol* 2001;**153**:779–82.

109 Hubinette A, Cnattingius S, Ekbom A, de Faire U, Kramer M, Lichtenstein P. Birthweight, early environment, and genetics: a study of twins discordant for acute myocardial infarction. *Lancet* 2001;**357**:1997–2001.

110 **Poulter NR**. Commentary: Birthweights, maternal cardiovascular events, and Barker hypothesis. *Lancet* 2001;**357**:1990–1.

111 **Davey Smith G, Harding S, Rosato M**. Relation between infants' birth weight and mothers' mortality: prospective observational study. *Br Med J* 2000;**320**:839–40.

112 **Davey Smith G, Whitley E, Gissler M, Hemminki E**. Birth dimensions of offspring, premature birth, and the mortality of mothers. *Lancet* 2000;**356**:2066–7.

113 **Davey Smith G, Hart C, Ferrell C, Upton M, Hole D, Hawthorne V, Watt G**. Birth weight of offspring and mortality in the Renfrew and Paisley study: prospective observational study. *Br Med J* 1997;**315**:1189–93.

114 **Barrett-Connor E, Bush TL**. Estrogen and coronary heart disease in women. *J Am Med Assoc* 1991;**265**:1861–7.

115 **Petridou E, Trichopoulos D, Revinthi K, Tong D, Papathoma E**. Modulation of birthweight through gestational age and fetal growth. *Child Care Health Dev* 1996;**22**:37–53.

116 **Rasmussen F, Sterne JAC, Davey Smith G, Tynelius P, Leon DA**. Fetal growth is associated with parents' cardiovascular mortality. *Am J Epidemiol* 2001;**153(Suppl)**:S98. (Abstract)

117 **Osborn GR**. Stages in development of coronary disease observed from 1,500 young subjects. Relationship of hypotension and infant feeding to aetiology. *Colloques Internationaux du Centre National de la Recherche Scientifique* 1967;**169**:93–139.

118 **Burr ML, Beasley WH, Fisher CB**. Breast feeding, maternal smoking and early atheroma. *Eur Heart J* 1984;**5**:588–91.

119 **Cowen DD**. Myocardial infarction and infant feeding. *Practitioner* 1973;**210**:661–3.

120 **Wingard DL, Criqui MH, Edelstein SL, Tucker J, Tomlinson-Keasey C, Schwartz JE, Friedman HS**. Is breast-feeding in infancy associated with adult longevity? *Am J Public Health* 1994;**84**:1458–62.

121 **Ravelli AC, van der Meulen JH, Osmond C, Barker DJ, Bleker OP**. Infant feeding and adult glucose tolerance, lipid profile, blood pressure, and obesity. *Arch Dis Child* 2000;**82**: 248–52.

122 **Singhal A, Cole JT, Lucas A**. Early nutrition in preterm infants and later blood pressure: two cohorts after randomised trials. *Lancet* 2001;**357**:413–9.

123 **Leeson CP, Kattenhorn M, Deanfield JE, Lucas A**. Duration of breast feeding and arterial distensibility in early adult life: population based study. *Br Med J* 2001;**322**:643–7.

124 **McCarron P, Hart CL, Hole D, Davey Smith G**. The relation between adult height and haemorrhagic and ischaemic stroke in the Renfrew/Paisley study. *J Epidemiol Community Health* 2001;**55**:404–5.

125 **D'Avanzo B, La Vecchia C, Negri E**. Height and the risk of acute myocardial infarction in Italian women. *Soc Sci Med* 1994;**38**:193–6.

126 **Palmer JR, Rosenberg L, Shapiro S**. Stature and the risk of myocardial infarction in women. *Am J Epidemiol* 1990;**132**:27–32.

127 **Rich-Edwards JW, Manson JE, Stampfer MJ, Colditz GA, Willett WC, Rosner B, Speizer FE, Hennekens CH**. Height and the risk of cardiovascular disease in women. *Am J Epidemiol* 1995;**142**:909–17.

128 **Gunnell D, Rogers J, Dieppe P**. Height and health: predicting longevity from bone length in archaeological remains. *J Epidemiol Community Health* 2001;**55**:505–7.

129 Davey Smith G, Gunnell D, Sweetnam P, Yarnell J, Elwood P. Leg length, insulin resistance and coronary heart disease risk: the Caerphilly study. *J Epidemiol Community Health* 2001;**55**:867–872.

130 Gunnell D, Davey Smith G, Ness AR, Frankel S. The effects of dietary supplementation on growth and adult mortality: a re-analysis and follow-up of a pre-war study. *Public Health* 2000;**114**:109–16.

131 Leitch I. Growth and Health. *Br J Nutr* 1951;**5**:142–51.

132 Mitchell HS. Nutrition in relation to stature. *J Am Diet Assoc* 1962;**40**:521–4.

133 Gerver WJ, De Bruin R. Relationship between height, sitting height and subischial leg length in Dutch children: presentation of normal values. *Acta Paediatr* 1995;**84**:532–5.

134 Taylor M, Lawlor DA, Bedford C, Ebrahim S. Leg length and cardiovascular risk factors in British women: the British Women's Heart and Health Study. *Proceedings of the 5th International conference on preventive cardiology. Osaka, Japan, May 2001.* 2001; (Abstract)

135 Eriksson JG, Forsen T, Tuomilehto J, Osmond C, Barker DJP. Early growth and coronary heart disease in later life: longitudinal study. *Br Med J* 2001;**322**:949–53.

136 Cauley JA, Gutai JP, Glynn NW, Paternostro-Bayles M, Cottington E, Kuller LH. Serum estrone concentrations and coronary artery disease in postmenopausal women. *Arterioscler Thromb* 1994;**14**:14–8.

137 Cauley JA, Gutai JP, Kuller LH, Powell JG. The relation of endogenous sex steroid hormone concentrations to serum lipid and lipoprotein levels in postmenopausal women. *Am J Epidemiol* 1990;**132**:884–94.

138 Barrett-Connor E, Goodman-Gruen D. Prospective study of endogenous sex hormones and fatal cardiovascular disease in postmenopausal women . *Br Med J* 1995;**311**:1193–6.

139 Gorgels WJ, Graaf Y, Blankenstein MA, Collette HJ, Erkelens DW, Banga JD. Urinary sex hormone excretions in premenopausal women and coronary heart disease risk: a nested case-referent study in the DOM-cohort. *J Clin Epidemiol* 1997;**50**:275–81.

140 La Vecchia C, Decarli A, Franceschi S, Gentile A, Negri E, Parazzini F. Menstrual and reproductive factors and the risk of myocardial infarction in women under fifty-five years of age. *Am J Obstet Gynecol* 1987;**157**:1108–12.

141 Colditz GA, Willett WC, Stampfer MJ, Rosner B, Speizer FE, Hennekens CH. A prospective study of age at menarche, parity, age at first birth, and coronary heart disease in women. *Am J Epidemiol* 1987;**126**:861–70.

142 Franks S. Polycystic ovary syndrome. *N Engl J Med* 1995;**333**:853–61.

143 Dahlgren E, Janson PO, Johansson S, Lapidus L, Oden A. Polycystic ovary syndrome and risk for myocardial infarction. Evaluated from a risk factor model based on a prospective population study of women. *Acta Obstetricia et Gynecologica Scandinavica* 1992;**71**: 599–604.

144 Wild S, Pierpoint T, McKeigue P, Jacobs H. Cardiovascular disease in women with polycystic ovary syndrome at long term follow-up: a retrospective cohort study. *Clin Endocrinol* 2000;**52**:595–600.

145 Ness RB, Schotland HM, Flegel KM, Shofer FS. Reproductive history and coronary heart disease risk in women. *Epidemiol Rev* 1994;**16**:298–314.

146 Winkelstein W, Rekate A. Age trend of mortality from coronary artery disease in women and observations on the reproductive patterns of those affected. *Am Heart J* 1964;**67**:481–8.

147 **Bengtsson C, Rybo G, Westerberg H**. Number of pregnancies, use of oral contraceptives and menopausal age in women with ischaemic heart disease, compared to a population sample of women. *Acta Medica Scandinavica—Supplementum* 1973;**549 (suppl)**:75–81.

148 **Beard CM, Fuster V, Annegers JF**. Reproductive history in women with coronary heart disease. A case-control study. *Am J Epidemiol* 1984;**120**:108–14.

149 **Beard CM, Griffin MR, Offord KP, Edwards WD**. Risk factors for sudden unexpected cardiac death in young women in Rochester, Minnesota, 1960 through 1974. *Mayo Clin Proc* 1986;**61**:186–91.

150 **Beral V**. Long term effects of childbearing on health. *J Epidemiol Community Health* 1985;**39**:343–6.

151 **Bernstien L, Pike MC, Ross RK, Judd HL, Brown JB, Henderson BE**. Estrogen and sex hormone-binding globulin levels in nulliparous and parous women. *J Natl Cancer Inst* 1985;**74**:741–5.

152 **Ness RB, Harris T, Cobb J, Flegal KM, Kelsey JL, Balanger A, Stunkard AJ, D'Agostino RB**. Number of pregnancies and the subsequent risk of cardiovascular disease. *N Engl J Med* 1993;**328**:1528–33.

153 **Steenland K, Lally C, Thun M**. Parity and coronary heart disease among women in the American Cancer Society CPS II population. *Epidemiology* 1996;**7**:641–3.

154 **Green A, Beral V, Moser K**. Mortality in women in relation to their childbearing history. *Br Med J* 1988;**297**:391–5.

155 **Dekker JM, Schouten EG**. Number of pregnancies and risk of cardiovascular disease. *N Engl J Med* 1993;**329**:1893–4.

156 **WHO Collaborative Study of Cardiovascular Disease and Steroid Hormone Contraception**. Acute myocardial infarction and combined oral contraceptives: results of an international multicentre case-control study. *Lancet* 1997;**349**:1202–9.

157 **Dunn N, Thorogood M, Faragher B, de Caestecher L, MacDonald TM, McCallum C, Thomas S, Mann R**. Oral contraceptives and myocardial infarction: results of the MICA case- control study. *Br Med J* 1999;**318**:1579–83.

158 **Colditz GA, Willett WC, Stampfer MJ, Rosner B, Speizer FE, Hennekens CH**. Menopause and the risk of coronary heart disease in women. *N Engl J Med* 1987;**316**:1105–10.

159 **Kuller LH, Meilahn EN, Cauley JA, Gutai JP, Matthews KA**. Epidemiologic studies of menopause: changes in risk factors and disease. *Exp Gerontol* 1994;**29**:495–509.

160 **Do KA, Green A, Guthrie JR, Dudley EC, Burger HG, Dennerstein L**. Longitudinal study of risk factors for coronary heart disease across the menopausal transition. *Am J Epidemiol* 2000;**151**:584–93.

161 **The Coronary Drug Project Research Group**. The Coronary Drug Project. Findings leading to discontinuation of the 2.5-mg day estrogen group. *J Am Med Assoc* 1973;**226**:652–7.

162 **New G, Duffy SJ, Harper RW, Meredith IT**. Long-term oestrogen therapy is associated with improved endothelium- dependent vasodilation in the forearm resistance circulation of biological males. *Clin Exp Pharmacol Physiol* 2000;**27**:25–33.

163 **New G, Berry KL, Cameron JD, Harper RW, Meredith IT**. Long-term oestrogen treatment does not alter systemic arterial compliance and haemodynamics in biological males. *Coron Artery Dis* 2000;**11**:253–9.

164 Barrett-Connor E, Grady D. Hormone replacement therapy, heart disease, and other considerations. *Ann Rev Public Health* 1998;**19**:55–72.

165 Hemminki E, McPherson K. Value of drug-licensing documents in studying the effect of postmenopausal hormone therapy on cardiovascular disease. *Lancet* 2000;**355**:566–9.

166 Espeland MA, Marcovina SM, Miller V, Wood PD, Wasilayskas C, Sherwin R, Schrott H, Bush TL. Effect of postmenopausal hormone therapy on lipoprotein(a) concentration. PEPI Investigators. Postmenopausal Estrogen/Progestin Interventions. *Circulation* 1998;**97**:979–86.

167 Hulley S, Grady D, Bush T, Furberg C, Herrington D, Riggs B, Vittinghoff E. Randomized trial of estrogen plus progestin for secondary prevention of coronary heart disease in postmenopausal women. Heart and Estrogen/progestin Replacement Study (HERS) Research Group. *J Am Med Assoc* 1998;**280**:605–13.

168 Herrington DM. The HERS trial results: paradigms lost? Heart and Estrogen/progestin Replacement Study. *Ann Intern Med* 1999;**131**:463–6.

169 Herrington DM, Reboussin DM, Brosnihan KB, Sharp PC, Shumaker SA, Snyder TE, Furberg CD, Kowalchuk GJ, Strickey TD. Effects of estrogen replacement on the progression of coronary-artery atherosclerosis. *N Eng J Med* 2000;**343**:522–9.

170 The Women's Health Initiative Study Group. Design of the Women's Health Initiative clinical trial and observational study. The Women's Health Initiative Study Group. *Control Clin Trials* 1998;**19**:61–109.

171 Wren BG. Megatrials of hormonal replacement therapy. *Drugs Aging* 1998;**12**:343–8.

172 Davey Smith G, Hart C, Watt G, Hole D, Hawthorne V. Individual social class, area-based deprivation, cardiovascular disease risk factors, and mortality: the Renfrew and Paisley Study. *J Epidemiol Community Health* 1998;**52**:399–405.

173 Heslop P, Davey Smith G, Macleod J, Hart C. The socioeconomic position of women, risk factors and mortality. *Soc Sci Med* 2001;**53**:477–85.

174 Wamala SP, Lynch J, Kaplan GA. Women's exposure to early and later life socioeconomic disadvantage and coronary heart disease risk: the Stockholm Female Coronary Risk Study. *Int J Epidemiol* 2001;**30**:275–84.

175 Lynch JW, Davey Smith G, Kaplan GA, House JS. Income inequality and mortality: importance to health of individual income, psychosocial environment, or material conditions. *Br Med J* 2000;**320**:1200–4.

176 Marmot M, Wilkinson RG. Psychosocial and material pathways in the relation between income and health: a response to Lynch *et al. Br Med J* 2001;**322**:1233–6.

177 Haynes SG, Feinleib M. Women, work and coronary heart disease: prospective findings from the Framingham heart study. *Am J Public Health* 1980;**70**:133–41.

178 Marmot MG, Davey Smith G, Stansfeld S, Patel C, North F, Head J, White I, Brunner E, Feeney A. Health inequalities among British civil servants: the Whitehall II study. *Lancet* 1991;**337**:1387–93.

179 Bosma H, Peter R, Siegrist J, Marmot M. Two alternative job stress models and the risk of coronary heart disease. *Am J Public Health* 1998;**88**:68–74.

180 Marmot MG, Bosma H, Hemingway H, Brunner E, Stansfeld S. Contribution of job control and other risk factors to social variations in coronary heart disease incidence. *Lancet* 1997;**350**:235–9.

181 House JS, Landis KR, Umberson D. Social relationships and health. *Science* 1988;**241**:540–5.

182 **Kaplan GA, Salonen JT, Cohen RD, Brand RJ, Syme SL, Puska P.** Social connections and mortality from all causes and from cardiovascular disease: prospective evidence from eastern Finland. *Am J Epidemiol* 1988;**128**:370–80.

183 **Schoenbach VJ, Kaplan BH, Fredman L, Kleinbaum DG.** Social ties and mortality in Evans County, Georgia. *Am J Epidemiol* 1986;**123**:577–91.

184 **Orth-Gomer K, Johnsson JV.** Social network interaction and mortality. A six year follow-up study of a random sample of the Swedish population. *J Chron Dis* 1987;**40**:949–57.

185 **Orth-Gomer K, Chesney MA.** Social stress/strain and heart disease in women. In: Julian DG, Wenger NK, eds. *Women and Heart Disease*. London: Martin Dunitz, 1997:407–20.

186 **Ryan W.** *Blaming the Victim*. London: Orbach and Chambers, 1971.

187 **Barker DJP, Forsen T, Uutela A, Osmond C, Eriksson JG.** Size at birth and resilience to the effects of poor living conditions in adult life: longitudinal study. *Br Med J* 2001;**323**:1273–6.

188 **Sylva K.** The impact of early learning on children's later development. In: Ball C, ed. Start right: the importance of early learning. London: Royal Society of Arts, 1994:84–96.

189 **Whitehead M, Diderichsen F.** Social capital and health: tip-toeing through the minefield of evidence. *Lancet* 2001;**358**:165–6.

190 Independent Inquiry into Inequalities in Health. *Report of the Independent Inquiry into Inequalities in Health*. London: The Stationery Office, 1998.

Chapter 6

A life course approach to diabetes

Helen M. Colhoun and Nish Chaturvedi

The most important determinants of type 2 diabetes risk in women, as in men, are obesity and genetic factors. Although the sex ratio of diabetes varies across countries, women are not consistently at higher risk of diabetes than men except where their obesity levels are much greater. Studies in children and adults are consistent with the idea that impaired fetal growth is associated with an increased risk of diabetes in adulthood in women. Although this may be attributable at least in part to an intrauterine rather than genetic effect, it has not been demonstrated conclusively. However, the well-documented effect of maternal diabetes in pregnancy on future risk of diabetes in offspring is strong evidence that programming of metabolism occurs *in utero*. Through the life course, aspects of lifestyles that affect diabetes risk include physical activity and dietary patterns, and these in turn are subject to strong social determinants. Further risk factors specific to women include parity through its effects on body mass index, and, possibly, progestin exposure. Gestational diabetes and, possibly, longer menstrual cycle are risk markers of future development of diabetes. Mainly because of rising obesity, the risk of type 2 diabetes is set to rise exponentially over the next few decades in women and in men and is now an emerging problem in children. Exposure to diabetes *in utero* is an important factor in the emergence of type 2 diabetes in children. Reductions in body mass index in women of fertile age in countries where obesity is increasing are particularly important for preventing the rise of type 2 diabetes in adults and children.

6.1 Introduction

Diabetes is a metabolic disorder of multiple aetiology characterized by chronic hyperglycaemia (high blood glucose). Type 2 diabetes is the commonest form of diabetes and is generally characterized by an older age of onset, does not necessarily require insulin therapy, and has resistance to the effects of insulin as a major feature accompanied by beta cell (the insulin secreting cells of the pancreas) failure.[1] Diabetes can be diagnosed on the basis of a raised fasting blood glucose or raised glucose after ingestion of a standard glucose load (a glucose tolerance test).[1] When resistance to the effects of insulin is present, insulin secretion by the pancreas is initially increased, so that fasting plasma insulin levels and insulin levels after a test meal or glucose ingestion are elevated. Plasma glucose levels can remain normal during this compensated phase of disease development. Eventually the pancreatic beta cell fails or decompensates so that insulin levels fall or are inadequate and blood glucose rises. In some patients with type 2 diabetes, beta cell failure rather than insulin resistance may be the main defect. There are many different methods for assessing whether insulin resistance and beta cell failure exist and these have been reviewed elsewhere.[2] The incidence of type 2 diabetes increases with age. The prevalence has been increasing and is expected to double over the next 25 years.[3,4] The greatest increase is now being seen in the restructuring countries, particularly Asia and is driven by increasing obesity and a reduction in physical activity. There are striking ethnic differences in diabetes risk, with groups such as the Pima Indians, Nauruans, Mexican Americans, South Asians, and African Americans being of highest risk compared with populations of European descent. Rates of diabetes can thus vary from greater than 50% in the Pima Indians, to around 5% in European populations.[5] There is no consistent sex difference in diabetes prevalence worldwide.[5] In the US, the age standardized rate of diagnosed diabetes in women versus men is 0.87 among non-Hispanic Whites (p=non-significant), 1.25 for non-Hispanic Blacks (p=0.04) and 1.41 for Hispanic Whites (p=0.003).[6] In populations where there is an excess in women it is explained by higher levels of obesity amongst the women.[7,8] The relationship of socioeconomic status to diabetes incidence varies between different cultures and reflects prevailing socioeconomic patterns of obesity and physical activity. In the US and Western Europe diabetes prevalence is currently highest in those in less advantaged social strata.[9] The socioeconomic class gradients in diabetes in Western Europe and the US are greater for women than men consistent with the greater socioeconomic differences in obesity in women than men.[10] The gradients observed today in Western Europe have not always been present, arguing against a role for relative social position itself rather than the factors it correlates with at any time. In the early twentieth century diabetes was more common among men in the higher than lower social classes but there was little gradient in women.[10] In developing countries a reverse socioeconomic pattern is seen, with more affluent members of society having the highest rates of diabetes. In general, epidemiological data fit the hypothesis that, as developing countries become more affluent, diabetes emerges as a problem for the most affluent initially but later the socioeconomic trends are reversed.[9]

This chapter focuses specifically on determinants of type 2 diabetes in women and girls from conception through the life course. Although we consider each part of the life course in discrete sections, risks in one part of life can increase the probability of exposure to further risks or can create susceptibility to risks in later parts of life (amplification). For example being underweight at birth might increase the probability of overfeeding in infancy or increase the effects of obesity on diabetes risk in later life. Some of the risk factors considered are specific to women and some are not. Obesity, the main modifiable determinant of diabetes risk is considered separately in Chapter 14. There are important sex differences in the effect of diabetes on risk of complications, particularly cardiovascular disease and these are considered in Chapter 5.

6.2 Genetic determinants of diabetes risk

Type 2 diabetes clusters in families with first degree relatives of an affected person having a fourfold risk compared with the general population.[11] A genetic contribution is suggested by the excess concordance among monozygotic compared with dizygotic twins,[12,13] ethnic differences in risk that do not disappear with migration to low risk areas[14] and risk that is proportional to the degree of ethnic admixture (i.e. among mixed race individuals, the proportion of one's genes that are from one ethnic group or another) between high and low risk populations.[15] The genetic basis of a number of rarer forms of diabetes that often present clinically as type 2 diabetes has now been elucidated.[16] For type 2 diabetes studies have identified regions of the genome harbouring potential susceptibility loci.[16] In one region finer mapping has identified the calpain-10 gene as a susceptibility locus in Mexican Americans.[17] No sex specific effects have been reported for either linked regions or the calpain-10 gene. Associations have been reported between type 2 diabetes and having a particular variant (the class III allele at the variable number of tandem repeats (VNTR) locus) in the insulin gene.[18,19] However this variant (the Class III allele) has also been reported to be associated with larger head circumference, length, and weight (200 g higher) at birth whereas lower size at birth is associated with increased risk of diabetes in adulthood (Section 6.4.1). Thus the nature of any relationship between this variant and diabetes risk and the mechanism of action of this relationship is not clear. Further data are needed before a role for this genetic variant in type 2 diabetes risk can be confirmed.

6.3 Parent of origin effects on diabetes risk

6.3.1 Excess maternal transmission of diabetes

A number of epidemiological studies have reported an excess of maternal compared with paternal history of type 2 diabetes among diabetes patients, or a greater proportion of affected offspring in women than men with diabetes.[20–24] The most detailed analysis of parental transmission is from the Kaiser Permanente Diabetes Register.[23] Here siblings of a diabetic patient whose mother also had diabetes had an odds ratio of 2.9 of having diabetes themselves compared with siblings of diabetic patients with no parents affected. The odds ratio where the father had diabetes was 2.4 and was significantly lower than if the mother had diabetes. Women with diabetes were more likely to have diabetic offspring than men (3.4% versus 2.2%) with female and male offspring being equally affected.

6.3.2 Potential explanations of excess maternal transmission

6.3.2.1 Bias

It is important to consider potential explanations of excess maternal transmission here as it has sometimes been interpreted as strong evidence of the effect of the intrauterine environment on diabetes (Table 6.1). An obvious explanation is bias arising from differences in

Table 6.1 Potential explanations of apparent excess of maternal versus paternal history of diabetes in diabetic offspring

- non-response or ascertainment bias
- mistaken paternity
- sex-specific assortative mating (affected women more likely to have affected mates than affected men)
- mitochondrial inheritance
- genetic imprinting – e.g., a disease causing allele in an imprinted gene or loss of usual imprinting
- intrauterine environment
- greater sharing of postnatal environment between offspring and mothers than between offspring and fathers

parental lifespan, sex differences in detection of diabetes, sex-specific assortative mating or more missing paternal than maternal diabetes status data. In the Kaiser Permanente Study, a validation substudy suggested that these were not important sources of bias. Furthermore excess maternal transmission has been observed where parental information is almost complete, as in the Pima Indians.[25,26] Non-paternity bias might however make some contribution and has not been addressed.

6.3.2.2 Mitochondrial inheritance

Some potential genetic explanations of the excess maternal transmission should also be considered including mitochondrial inheritance. Most genetic material (DNA) is inherited from our parents through chomosomes but in addition we inherit some DNA from cellular bodies called mitochondria. All mitochondrial DNA is inherited from the mother rather than the father, and therefore any disease causing genes in mitochondria will be transmitted from mothers to offspring. Men who inherit these genes from their mothers cannot in turn transmit the disease gene to offspring because their mitochondrial DNA is not passed on. The plausibility of a partly mitochondrial basis for diabetes is suggested by the fact that the rare syndrome of Maternally Inherited Diabetes and Deafness (MIDD) results from mutations in the mitochondrial leucyl tRNA gene.[27] An association between a more common mitochondrial polymorphism (the 16189 variant T → C transition in the first hypervariable region of mitochondrial DNA) and insulin resistance has been reported in men[28] and in the Avon Longtitudinal Study of Pregnancy and Childhood was associated with birthweight.[29]

6.3.2.3 Genomic imprinting

Genomic imprinting might also explain a parent of origin effect. Humans inherit two complete sets of chromosomes, one from each parent, and usually both the maternal and paternal allele at any given genetic locus is expressed. However, some genes are imprinted, that is only one allele is expressed in a parent of origin specific manner (i.e. either the maternal allele is always expressed and the paternal silent or vice versa).[30] Thus a disease causing allele in an imprinted gene will cause a parent of origin pattern of disease transmission. Importantly, many of the genes that are known to be ordinarily imprinted are involved in fetal and placental growth and development[31,32] including insulin and insulin-like growth factor II.[33] There is increasing recognition of the importance of fetal growth to adult diabetes risk so that imprinting is a plausible explanation of excess maternal transmission.

6.3.2.4 Excess sharing of maternal versus paternal environment

A greater effect of maternal than paternal risk of diabetes on offspring might be because of the greater degree of shared intrauterine or postnatal environment. Theoretically the effect of excess sharing of maternal postnatal environment could be quantified by comparing rates of diabetes in offspring of diabetic mothers separated from their mothers at birth with rates of those not separated, matched for degree of shared paternal environment. However such studies are ethically and logistically problematic and have not been done. Regarding shared intrauterine environment, there is an increasing body of evidence that persisting abnormalities of metabolism may be set by influences early in life notably in the intrauterine period. The inverse association between birthweight and glucose intolerance or diabetes in middle-aged adults has been confirmed in several different study populations,[34,35] but until recently, women were under-represented in these cohorts. Some of the more recent studies have included women, but not reported their findings separately.[36] There are now several published studies which report the association between birthweight and adult (i.e. middle-aged) glucose intolerance in women and these are described below.

6.4 The effect of intrauterine environment on diabetes risk in women

6.4.1 Relationship between measures of size at birth and diabetes risk in studies in adults

6.4.1.1 Glucose intolerance

As in men, studies of women show an inverse association between birthweight and adult diabetes incidence and prevalence (Table 6.2).[37–39] The largest of these studies yielded only 185 cases, which may account for the lack of statistical significance compared with men. But maternal or gestational diabetes can often result in a large baby, which in turn is at greater risk of diabetes (Section 6.4.2). This accounts for the U-shaped association between birthweight and adult diabetes observed in some studies,[40] particularly when the risk of gestational diabetes is high.[36]

As in male cohorts, interactions with adult obesity were observed, so that small babies who grew into obese women were at greatest risk.[37,40] This catch-up growth (accelerated growth of low birthweight babies in childhood) appears to be greater for women than men. For example, in a Finnish cohort childhood body mass index (BMI) (between the ages of 7 and 15 years) was strongly related to adult diabetes only in women.[39] Unfortunately, adult BMI was not available in this study, so that the relative contributions of childhood and adult obesity, and catch-up growth in childhood on adult diabetes could not be assessed.

It is unclear whether the associations between measures of early life influences and adult glucose intolerance are stronger or weaker in women than in men, or dependent upon the early life measure in question. It appears unlikely that there are marked sex differences in the effect of birthweight and adult glucose intolerance, though many of these studies were probably too underpowered to demonstrate an interaction.

The existence of an inverse association with birthweight may be due to confounding by many factors, a key factor being social class at birth or in early childhood. This may not be well measured so that simple statistical adjustment may not adequately control for differences. Previous studies have all claimed little impact of social class in early life on the association between birthweight and adult diabetes.[38,39,41] Further, the Rancho Bernardo study, based in a socially homogenous geographical area of California, is largely restricted to an affluent population in late adulthood, therefore making confounding by social class a less likely explanation for such findings.[37]

The association between low birthweight and adult glucose intolerance was more marked for women with no parental history of diabetes, compared to those with at least one parent with diabetes.[40] This stronger association in women with no parental history of diabetes may be due to the elimination of genetic factors or a diabetic intrauterine environment in this subgroup, which may otherwise blur the association between early life influences and adult diabetes.

Whereas the study of Pima Indians reflected findings in European populations,[36] data from South India demonstrated no relationship between birthweight and adult diabetes,

Table 6.2 Studies reporting associations between size at birth and glucose homeostasis in middle age women

Study location	N of women	Age	Measure of size at birth	Measure of glucose intolerance	Relationship
Rancho Bernardo, USA[37]	303	50–84	Birthweight*	New and known DM	Inverse
Nurses Health, USA[40]	69526	46–71	Birthweight*	Known DM	U-shaped
Hertfordshire, UK[38]	297	60–71	Birthweight, weight at one year	New and known DM	Inverse
Preston, UK[41]	126	46–54	Birthweight, Placental weight, Head circumference, Birth length, Ponderal index	IGT and new DM	Inverse
Helsinki, Finland[39]	3447	64–73	Birthweight, birth length, ponderal index, placental weight	Treated DM	Inverse
Adelaide, Australia[44]	78	Mean 20 years	Birthweight, birth length	Glucose and insulin response to IVGTT	None
San Antonio, US[43]	228	25–64	Birthweight	Fasting and 2 hr glucose and insulin	Inverse
Pimas, Arizona, US[36]	1179 men and women	20–39	Birthweight	New and known diabetes	U-shaped
Mysore, India[42]	244	39–60	Birthweight, birth, length, ponderal index, head circumference	Known and new DM	None with birthweight, positive association with ponderal index, and inverse with birth length

* Self report.

even though numbers were relatively large.[42] Although the sexes were combined here, approximately 50% were women, and no indication is given that there is a gender difference in these relationships. One possible explanation is that 96% of birthweights in this cohort fell below the mean for a comparator UK population, and therefore may fall outside the range where an inverse association may be expected.

In summary, the inverse association between birthweight and adult glucose intolerance in men is also applicable to women, and is of approximately the same strength.

6.4.1.2 Associations between size at birth and glucose and insulin levels in studies of adults

There are also reports of associations between early life measures and glucose, insulin, and measures of insulin resistance. Low birthweight was associated with elevated fasting and post-challenge glucose, and with elevated insulin levels, the latter a surrogate for elevated insulin resistance in European,[37,38] and Mexican American women.[43] Interestingly, both in Hertfordshire and in Mexican Americans, no such association between fasting values and birthweight were observed for men.[38,43] The stronger associations described previously for women in the Preston study were also observed for other measures of early growth and markers of insulin resistance, including two-hour post-load glucose and insulin.[41]

A study of young Australian adults however showed that whilst men who were shorter or lighter at birth were insulin resistant at age 20 years they also had greater glucose effectiveness, indicating compensation for insulin resistance. This compensation may attenuate with age resulting in the emergence of glucose intolerance in the men. In contrast measures of birth size were unrelated to measures of insulin sensitivity (low levels of insulin sensitivity being related to a greater degree of glucose intolerance) in women in whom current BMI was the main determinant.[44]

However, in complete contrast to the above, the data from Mysore showed that fasting insulin and 32–33 split proinsulin were only inversely related to birthweight in men.[42] The insulin increment at 30 minutes (a measure of insulin sensitivity) was not related to birthweight or length, but was inversely related to ponderal index (birth length/birthweight[3], a measure of thinness at birth) in both men and women. In a multivariate model with both birthweight and length however, mean insulin increment fell with decreasing length and increasing weight.

Thus the mechanism of an association between early growth and diabetes remains unclear, and could be due either to insulin resistance, beta cell failure, or a combination of the two, and may vary by ethnicity. Clearly any such association is also modified by adult obesity.

6.4.1.3 Associations between size at birth and glucose and insulin in studies of children

Several studies have examined the relationship of size at birth to various indices of glucose homeostasis in childhood including fasting and post-load glucose and insulin (Table 6.3). The extent to which childhood measures of glucose and insulin track into adult life and predict adult diabetes needs to be evaluated. In adults, inappropriately raised fasting insulin levels are generally indicative of resistance to the effects of insulin with the pancreatic beta cell producing more insulin to compensate. However, in children fasting insulin is correlated with current height and may be more of a marker of maturation or growth rather than insulin resistance.[45] Fairly low tracking correlations have been reported for glucose ($r=0.30$) and insulin ($r=0.36$) across 3–5 years of follow-up in young subjects.[46–48] As frank diabetes is not common in children most of the studies of the role of size at birth have examined glucose and insulin levels fasting or after a glucose load, higher levels of which may indicate glucose intolerance and insulin resistance respectively. In some a measure of insulin resistance was formally estimated using a standard modelling equation (the HOMA model).

Table 6.3 Studies of size at birth and aspects of glucose homeostasis in children

Law CM (1995)[49]	Salisbury, UK	123 girls; 127 boys	7.7 years
Forrester TE (1996)[50]	Jamaica		
Whincup (1997)[45]	England & Wales	539 girls; 595 boys	11 years
Crowther NJ (1998)[53]	South Africa	73 girls; 79 boys	7 years
Bavdekar (1999)[52]	Pune, India	221 girls; 256 boys	8.5 years
Dabelea (1999)[54]	Arizona Pimas	3061 girls & boys	5–29 years

The main findings from these studies are; fasting insulin and post-load insulin in children is strongly positively correlated with current weight or ponderal index or BMI which are in turn positively correlated with birthweight.[45,49,51–53] An inverse relationship between birthweight and fasting and/or post-load insulin was found in several studies but only on adjustment for some measure of current size, either BMI or weight or ponderal index.[45,52–54] Neither birthweight nor ponderal index at birth are associated with fasting glucose but post-load glucose had either an inverse or U-shaped relationship with ponderal index[49] or birthweight[52–54] in some studies. This was not a consistent finding[45] and in one study the relationship with post-load glucose was only present on adjustment for current weight.[52] In Jamaican children glycated haemoglobin was inversely associated with hospital recorded birthweight and positively associated with current fatness as assessed by triceps thicknesss.[50] Most of the studies did not comment on any sex difference in the findings.

Thus the data are more consistent for relationships between size at birth and insulin levels than between size at birth and glucose levels and as noted above the meaning of insulin levels in childhood is unclear. Where examined, the effect is present in girls and boys and is most prominent in those who are also fat as children. Of themselves, these studies cannot indicate whether a policy of trying to increase average birthweights is advisable. In particular, we do not know whether having higher insulin levels from being big in childhood is innocuous whilst having higher insulin levels from being small at birth is detrimental. Nor do we know whether childhood blood glucose or insulin predicts adult diabetes risk better if adjustment for childhood body size is made. None the less these studies support the idea that reduced size at birth could be a marker of later deranged glucose metabolism. However, Lucas *et al.*[55] noted that the association of lower size at birth with higher insulin levels is only present when adjustment for current size or weight is made which is at least as consistent with a more rapid change in size postnatally being the determinant of higher insulin levels, rather than a lower size at birth *per se*.

6.4.1.4 Hypotheses on the pathophysiological mechanisms linking early life nutrition and size to adult risk of diabetes

There is emerging consensus that the association between reduced fetal size and diabetes risk is mediated through insulin resistance rather than beta cell failure.[56] The precise mechanisms are not well understood. The evidence is less consistent that birthweight is associated with the lipid disturbances usually found in the insulin resistance syndrome (elevated triglyceride, low high-density lipoprotein cholesterol (HDLc)) than with the other aspects of the insulin resistance syndrome suggesting that a distinct, less lipid related, pathway is involved. Studies suggest that the fetal response to undernutrition may involve alterations in the hormonal axes that control growth and fuel availability and utilization which are then disadvantageous in postnatal life. In particular, disordered function of the hypothalamic–pituitary–adrenal axis has been proposed with higher serum cortisol and lower growth hormone levels being found in men with lower birthweight.[57,58] Involvement of the sympathetic nervous system has been suggested by an independent association between lower birthweight and higher resting pulse rate.[59]

6.4.1.5 Does the relationship of size at birth to diabetes risk have a genetic or environmental explanation?

At least part of the size at birth relationship to diabetes risk may have a genetic explanation, particularly since insulin is a critical hormone in fetal growth.[60] About 30–40% of the variance in fetal growth is likely to have a genetic basis[61,62] with genes being equally important in females and males.[62] Infants with rare genetic defects in insulin secretion, for example the glucokinase gene[63] or insulin resistance,[64] are small at birth. In one study offspring of fathers with type 2 diabetes had lower birthweight.[65] Thus the same genes could cause reduced birthweight and later diabetes. That part of the size at birth relationship to diabetes risk is attributable to the intrauterine environment is indicated by the finding in 14 pairs of genetically identical twins discordant for type 2 diabetes that the affected twin had a birthweight 300 g less than the unaffected twin.[66] However, in the Birmingham twin study 44 identical and 91 non-identical twin pairs were studied and in neither type of twin was the difference in birthweight associated with a difference in adult glucose tolerance or insulin levels.[62] Perhaps the strongest evidence that intrauterine programming of glucose homeostasis in later life can occur is the extensive data demonstrating the effects of maternal diabetes during pregnancy on longer term diabetes risk in the offspring as discussed in the next section.

6.4.2 Maternal diabetes and diabetes risk in offspring

In addition to maternal history of diabetes at any time, there is a considerable body of evidence that maternal diabetes specifically during pregnancy leads to heavier birthweight, and later an increased risk of obesity and diabetes in the offspring.[67,68] Among the Pima Indians, offspring of a diabetic pregnancy had an incidence of diabetes 20 times that of the offspring of a non-diabetic pregnancy, higher BMI and a higher prevalence of impaired glucose tolerance (19% versus 2.5%) at age 10–30 years.[69] Higher rates of insulin resistance and obesity have also been confirmed in the offspring of European women with gestational diabetes and, importantly, with type 1 diabetes.[26,70,71] The higher incidence of type 2 diabetes in offspring of type 1 diabetic mothers strongly suggests an intrauterine effect of maternal diabetes rather than a genetic effect since type 1 diabetic mothers would pass genes for type 1 not type 2 diabetes to their offspring. Of course shared postnatal environment, or a greater genetic load in women who are diagnosed earlier in life with type 2 diabetes, might partly explain the data on diabetes risk in offspring of type 2 diabetic mothers. However, arguing against these explanations is that the offspring of the same diabetic mother are more at risk of type 2 diabetes if they were *in utero* when she had diabetes than their siblings who were *in utero* prior to the development of maternal diabetes. This excess risk is not explained by maternal age. Among the Pima Indians, offspring of diabetic pregnancies had a 3.7-fold odds of developing diabetes compared with siblings born prior to the development of maternal diabetes.[72] However replication of these data in other groups will be important for more definitive evidence of the role of intrauterine environment.

Diabetes associated with maternal diabetes occurs earlier in life and is an important factor in the growing epidemic of type 2 diabetes in children. The changes in prevalence of type 2 diabetes in Pima Indian children was reported for various time points between 1967 and 1996. In the most recent period 1987–96, the youngest age at diagnosis was just 3.5 years. The prevalence had increased substantially over time, doubling for those aged 15–19 years from 2.7% to 5.3%.[73] Exposure to diabetes *in utero* almost quadrupled from 2% to 7.5% during this period. In the 1987–96 examination, 35% of diabetes in Pima children was attributable to exposure to diabetes in pregnancy (an odds ratio of 10) and along with increasing BMI in childhood was the main factor explaining the increasing prevalence over time. This growing epidemic of type 2 diabetes in children is affecting girls more than boys. The age of diagnosis of type 2 diabetes in children is about a year earlier on average in girls than boys.[74] In case series where African American children have predominated, the female to male ratio among type 2 diabetic children is about 1.6:1.[74,75] In the Pima Indians this ratio is lower, but is still greater in girls than boys. Whether this reflects in part a greater susceptibility of female offspring to *in utero* exposure to maternal diabetes is not clear. The effect of maternal diabetes has potentially enormous implications for accelerating the incidence of diabetes. As the average BMI of women continues to increase (and as pregnancy is deferred to an older age) a greater proportion of fetuses will be exposed to maternal diabetes and glucose intolerance and later risk of diabetes. In many high risk societies this poses a much greater future public health challenge than the effects of maternal under-nutrition in pregnancy.

6.5 Catch-up growth hypothesis

The catch-up growth hypothesis attributes particular importance to the period of postnatal catch-up growth for the mediation of the effects of impaired fetal growth on diabetes risk. Under this hypothesis increased insulin-like growth factor (IGF) production in the postnatal period, whilst achieving catch-up growth, causes the development of insulin resistance in order to counteract the insulin-like effects of IGF.[76] As yet there is little definitive evidence to support this hypothesis. However an earlier adiposity rebound has been associated with a greater risk of adult obesity and through this mechanism may increase diabetes risk.[77] The term adiposity rebound refers to the age at which BMI reaches its lowest point in childhood (usually around five or six years) (see Chapter 14). An earlier adiposity rebound may in part reflect accelerated growth.

6.6 Physical activity

The impact of physical activity on obesity is dealt with in Chapter 14. However, physical activity may have an impact on diabetes risk that is independent of obesity. In the US Nurses' Health Study after adjusting for BMI, the relative risks from the lowest to highest fifths of physical activity were 1.0, 0.84, 0.87, 0.77, 0.74 (p for trend = .002).[78] This risk reduction was found whether physical activity was vigorous or moderate. The evolution of physical activity patterns across the life course is discussed in Chapter 13.

6.7 Alcohol consumption

There is a positive association between the level of alcohol consumption and insulin sensitivity in young adults, and this appears to be independent of physical activity and socioeconomic status. An interaction with current BMI has been reported, with those of low BMI benefiting the most from alcohol consumption in terms of insulin sensitivity.[79]

6.8 Menarche and menstrual cycle

A few studies have examined the association between age at menarche and menstrual pattern and risk of diabetes. Since a higher BMI is associated with earlier menarche an association between menarche and later risk of diabetes might be expected. However, Cooper *et al.* found no association with menarche in a cohort of 668 women that included 49 self reported cases of diabetes.[80] Neither were there any associations between cycle length or variability except that longer cycle length was associated with an 2.6 fold risk of diabetes of borderline significance (95% confidence interval 1.0–6.5). In an abstract publication from the US Nurses' Health Study, a long cycle length was associated with an increased risk of type 2 diabetes that was attenuated when adjusted for key confounders.[81] Age at menarche was not associated with diabetes risk. Of course, as discussed in Chapter 2, polycystic ovary syndrome, in which amenorrhoea or disordered cycle length are common, is also associated with insulin resistance.

6.9 Effect of parity on subsequent risk of diabetes

Observations that parity may be associated with an enhanced risk of subsequent type 2 diabetes were made several decades ago[82,83] and since then, there have been well over 20 studies attempting to determine the nature of such a relationship, and establish the causes of it. The results of these studies have been conflicting, with some indicating a positive relationship, others a negative[84] or U-shaped relationship[85,86] and yet others showing no relationship.[87–90] Each of these findings can be accounted for by biologically plausible hypotheses.

It is reasonable to suggest that parity should be associated with diabetes risk, as increasing parity is generally associated with obesity, and an increased risk of insulin resistance[91], which may occur independently of obesity, due to the insulin antagonizing effects of oestrogen, progesterone and corticosteroids.[92] Parity is also positively associated with age, and also with lower socioeconomic status, and these factors need to be accounted for in any analysis.

The largest study to explore this relationship is the US Nurses' Health Study, including 113 606 women with self report of both diabetes and parity.[86] Initially, there was a U-shaped relationship between parity and birthweight, with the crude relative risk of diabetes being 0.80 in those with two births compared to nulliparous women, rising to 1.56 with six or more births. This latter relative risk was attenuated to 0.95 when age and BMI were adjusted for, and the U-shaped association was broadly replaced by an inverse relationship.

Socioeconomic status was not included, as it was argued that these women were all nurses, but no account was taken of husband's social class. Increased surveillance for diabetes during pregnancy may account for a positive relationship, but the observed relationship persisted when the data were restricted only to those who demonstrated symptoms of diabetes before diagnosis. This suggests that although there is an association between parity and diabetes, this can be accounted for by age and obesity, and a specific diabetogenic effect of pregnancy need not be sought. This is in broad agreement with two previous studies which also adjusted for key confounders.[89,90] Those demonstrating a positive relationship have not generally adjusted for all these factors in a simultaneous model.

Others however have argued for a negative or U-shaped relationship, with a particularly enhanced risk in nulliparous women, even after accounting for confounders.[84,85] The explanation for such a relationship coud be the effects of hyperinsulinaemia on androgen metabolism, associated with both obesity and the polycystic ovary syndrome, a not unusual condition in women resulting in poor fertility. Certainly the study of Pima Indians did show that nulliparous women were more obese than their parous counterparts.[84] A U-shaped relationship could therefore be due to hyperinsulinaemia associated with the polycystic ovary syndrome in nulliparous women on the one hand, and increasing obesity associated with insulin resistance in grand multiparous women on the other.

6.10 Risk of diabetes associated with oral contraceptive pill use

Oral contraceptives are known to cause a transitory elevation of glucose and insulin levels, which could therefore lead to later diabetes. A small study of 593 high risk women[93] reported that there was an increased risk of diabetes in current users, but only in the subgroup with few other risks of diabetes (i.e. no family history and absence of obesity). A larger UK based study of 46 000 women found no increased risk of diabetes over a 21-year period in current or past users.[94] These previous studies did not adjust fully for potential confounders. The US Nurses' Health Study found that past users had a very marginal increase in risk (unadjusted relative risk, 1.04), whereas current users had a lower risk of diabetes (unadjusted relative risk, 0.56).[95] These risks were barely altered after adjustment for confounders and when restricted to cases which were symptomatic before diagnosis. Unfortunately, information on brands, composition and dosage were not available. More recent interest has focused on women with gestational diabetes, who already have a threefold increase in risk of developing diabetes with a subsequent pregnancy. Previous studies have produced inconclusive findings;[96–99] but these had relatively short follow-up, and numbers were generally small. In a study of 904 Latina women with gestational diabetes, 12% of oral contraceptive users developed diabetes over a 7.5-year follow-up period, compared with 9% in those who were using other forms of contraception.[100] The enhanced risk appeared to be confined to progestin-only preparations, with a 2.5-fold increase in risk compared to combination preparations. This enhanced risk persisted when confounders were adjusted for, and a dose–response relationship was also demonstrated. Previous studies have shown that progestin can increase the risk of insulin resistance,[101] whereas oestrogens are neutral,[102] or may in some cases have an insulin sensitizing role.[103] These previous studies must be interpreted with caution however, as they were not randomized trials, and between group differences may have an impact on the observed elevated risk in progestin-only users.

6.11 **Gestational diabetes**

Gestational diabetes (transient diabetes that comes on during pregnancy) is a strong risk factor or risk marker for diabetes risk in later life, with progression to type 2 diabetes estimates ranging from 13% to 62%.[104] The risk of gestational diabetes itself in a given population is difficult to estimate with certainty, as detection and screening rates vary, and the occurrence of diabetes before pregnancy cannot be excluded. The risk will also largely depend on the underlying risk of the majority ethnic group. Thus risks may vary from around 1% to 15% of all pregnancies.[105]

Gestational diabetes occurs more frequently in women whose mothers have a history of diabetes, and the risk increases with age and parity. A study of Norwegian women noted that those with both low (<2500 g) and high (>4500 g) birthweights had an increased risk of gestational diabetes, with odds ratios of 1.8 and 1.5 respectively.[106] This association persisted when adjusted for age, parity, and maternal diabetes status. Advanced maternal age, family history of diabetes mellitus, non-White ethnicity, higher BMI, weight gain in early adulthood, and cigarette smoking all predicted increased gestational diabetes risk in the US Nurses' Health Study.[107]

6.12 **Menopause**

Oestradiol-17 β has beneficial effects on the metabolic syndrome, so its decline at the menopause, in association with the increase in central adiposity, should result in an increased risk of impaired glucose tolerance.[108] However prospective epidemiological studies do not find an increase in plasma glucose or insulin levels with menopause.[109] Recent metabolic studies indicate that the menopause is associated with both lower insulin secretion and a reduced rate of insulin elimination, so that resulting insulin concentrations are similar to those in premenopausal women,[110] and also insulin resistance.[111]

6.13 **Conclusions**

The burden of diabetes is set to reach epidemic proportions worldwide and the emergence of childhood type 2 diabetes is a serious threat to public health. There is an excess maternal transmission of diabetes that may be partly attributable to genetic and genetic-related factors such as mitochondrial inheritance and genomic imprinting and may partly reflect an effect of intrauterine environment. The intrauterine environment is important in determining adult risk of diabetes both via undernutrition as manifest by reduced birth size and exposure to maternal diabetes *in utero*. As the age of onset of type 2 diabetes is falling and overnutrition is rising in women the latter is set to have increasing importance for diabetes risk. The role of accelerated *catch-up* growth in early life on glucose metabolism is not yet clear. Many life course risk factors for diabetes are similar for men and women. Factors specific to women such as parity largely operate through obesity. Sparse data suggest a possible association between menstrual abnormalities and risk. The role of exogenous sex hormones is not conclusive but may depend on the balance of oestrogen and progesterone. Gestational diabetes itself is a strong risk marker of type 2 diabetes in later life. Policy interventions designed to reduce the burden of obesity and to increase physical activity from early life offer the greatest likelihood of combating the expected rise of diabetes.

Commentary on 'A life course approach to diabetes'

Janet Rich-Edwards

Diabetes is undeniably one of the world's most destructive diseases. Its prevalence and cost is high and rising in both the developed and the developing world. Type 2 diabetes constitutes a present public health crisis in the developed world, and a coming crisis in the developing world. Yet type 2 diabetes is largely preventable. A life course approach offers a new appreciation of diabetes as the result of accumulated and interacting risks, many of which originate in childhood.

In their chapter, Colhoun and Chaturvedi correctly point out that the increasingly early onset of diabetes exposes the roots of the disease in early life. Diabetes is a paradigmatic example of interaction between a background risk set early in life and environmental risk factors met and set throughout childhood, adolescence, and adulthood. In fact, we may come to view diabetes aetiology as similar to the initiation and promotion stages of cancer. Their chapter outlines the ways in which diabetes susceptibility may be conferred before birth through several means: by genetic transmission (whether autosomal, mitochondrial, or imprinted), by a hyperglycaemic womb of a diabetic mother, or by other as yet unknown factors that are guilty by association with poor fetal growth. It is against this background risk, this metabolic setting for feast or famine, that childhood and adult environment plays out its effects.

In childhood and adulthood, obesity and overweight trump all other risk factors for diabetes. Few normal weight individuals develop type 2 diabetes. Insulin resistance and adiposity are so intertwined that adiposity may not be so much a cause of diabetes as it is an intermediate variable, the first manifestation of a general metabolic disturbance. If a joint susceptibility to weight gain and diabetes share early life antecedents, early interventions may be found that would simultaneously reduce the risk of obesity and the risk of diabetes. Although later interventions are important, they have met with only limited success.

There are several charges to researchers. First, we need to specify modifiable early life determinants of susceptibility to obesity and diabetes. These may include physiological 'programmers' operating in critical developmental windows. As examples, Colhoun and Chaturvedi refer to the possible impact of maternal glycaemia on fetal insulin receptors or the effect of high postnatal insulin-like growth factor on insulin resistance. Genes would also fall in this category. Secondly, we must identify sensitive developmental stages for diabetogenic behaviours: when, how, and to what extent are eating and exercise patterns set in childhood? Finally, as documented by the chapter, we now know that adult physical activity, diet composition, alcohol consumption, and use of medicines alters diabetes risk and prognosis. We may eventually see these adult lifestyle factors as modifers of background diabetes susceptibility set earlier in life. As we continue to enumerate the determinants of diabetes, we must question closely the strong social patterning of exposure to risk factors and incidence of diabetes. In industrialized nations, diabetes is predominantly a disease of ethnic minorities and the poor. In Asia, now negotiating the 'epidemiological transition', these factors are more prevalent among the affluent.

In particular, as we describe overweight as a gateway to diabetes, we must also investigate the social and economic context that underlies overweight. We need to abandon the short-sighted view that blames the individual for overweight. The individualistic approach ignores the likely early life determinants of obesity, appetite, and diabetes. It also overlooks the enormous social and corporate processes that bear on individuals' diet, exercise, stress, and access to medical care. Where girls attend schools that serve pizza for lunch and cut out physical education classes, we should not be surprised that teens become obese. Where women work all day and return home to care for children and elders, there is little time or support to prepare low glycaemic index meals or take a brisk walk in the park. Institutional change is needed in every sector: in the schools and workplaces, in the systems of transportation and recreation, in the food industry, in the distribution of workload, and in health care systems.

A life course perspective makes it abundantly clear that the most successful tactic against the diabetes epidemic is prevention, that prevention must start (but not end) in childhood, and that it must involve the entire community. We must identify the points in the life course which offer particular leverage for intervention. For example, promoting fitness among girls will help prevent gestational diabetes, thereby avoiding its consequences for the fetus. Gestational diabetes itself offers a leverage point: postpartum counselling and support may help the mother to avert diabetes for herself and for her next pregnancy. While further research will help target such leverage points, we already know enough to begin the enormous public health challenge to turn the tide of diabetes.

References

1 **WHO**. *Definition, Diagnosis and Classification of Diabetes Mellitus and its complications*. Geneva: World Health Organisation, 1999.

2 **Walker M, Fulcher G R, Alberti KGMM**. The assessment of insulin action *in vivo*. In Alberti KGMM, Zimmet P, DeFronzo RA, Keen H, eds. *International Textbook of Diabetes Mellitus*. Chichester: Wiley, 1997:595–610.

3 **Kenny SJ, Aubert RE, Geiss LS**. Prevalence and Incidence of Non-Insulin-Dependent Diabetes. In Harris MI, Cowie CC, Stern MP, Boyko EJ, Reiber GE, Bennett PH, eds. *Diabetes in America*. National Institutes of Health, 1995:47–67.

4 **Amos AF, McCarty DJ, Zimmet P**. The rising global burden of diabetes and its complications: estimates and projections to the year 2010. *Diabet Med* 1997;**14 Suppl 5**:S1–85.

5 **King H, Rewers M, WHO Ad Hoc Diabetes Reporting Group**. Global estimates for prevalence of diabetes mellitus and impaired glucose tolerance. *Diabetes Care* 1993;**16**:157–77.

6 **Harris MI, Flegal KM, Cowie CC, Eberhardt MS, Goldstein DE, Little RR** *et al*. Prevalence of Diabetes, Impaired Fasting Glucose, and Impaired Glucose Tolerance in US Adults. The Third National Health and Nutrition Examination Survey, 1988–1994. *Diabetes Care* 1998;**21**:518–24.

7 **Valle T, Eriksson J, Tuomilehto J**. Epidemiology of NIDDM in Europids. In Alberti KGMM, Zimmet P, DeFronzo RA, Keen H, eds. *International Textbook of Diabetes Mellitus*. Chichester: Wiley, 1997:125–42.

8 **De Courten M, Bennett PH, Tuomilehto J, Zimmet P**. Epidemiology of NIDDM in Non-Europids. In Alberti KGMM, Zimmet P, DeFronzo RA, Keen H, eds. *International Textbook of Diabetes Mellitus*. Chichester: Wiley, 1997:143–70.

9 **Rewers M, Hamman R F**. Risk Factors for Non-Insulin-Dependent Diabetes. In Harris MI, Cowie CC, Stern MP, Boylo EJ, Reiker GE, Bennett PH, eds. *Diabetes in America (2nd Edn)*. NIH Publication, 1995:179–220.

10 **West KM**. Factors Associated with Occurrence of Diabetes. *Epidemiology of Diabetes and Its Vascular Lesions*. New York: Elsevier, 1978:191–288.

11 **Kobberling J, Tillil H**. Empirical risk figures for first degree relatives of non-insulin dependent diabetics. *The genetics of diabetes mellitus*. London: Academic Press, 1982:201–9.

12 **Barnett AH, Eff C, Leslie RD, Pyke DA**. Diabetes in identical twins. A study of 200 pairs. *Diabetologia* 1981;**20**:87–93.

13 **Newman B, Selby JV, King MC, Slemenda C, Fabsitz R, Friedman GD**. Concordance for type 2 (non-insulin-dependent) diabetes mellitus in male twins. *Diabetologia* 1987;**30**:763–8.

14 **McKeigue PM, Marmot MG, Syndercombe Court YD, Cottier DE, Rahman S, Riemersma RA**. Diabetes, hyperinsulinaemia, and coronary risk factors in Bangladeshis in East London. *Br Heart J* 1988;**60**:390–6.

15 **Williams RC, Long JC, Hanson RL, Sievers ML, Knowler WC**. Individual estimates of European genetic admixture associated with lower body-mass index, plasma glucose, and prevalence of type 2 diabetes in Pima Indians. *Am J Hum Genet* 2000;**66**:527–38.

16 **McCarthy M, Menzel S**. The genetics of type 2 diabetes. *Br J Clin Pharmacol* 2001;**51**:195–9.

17 **Horikawa Y, Oda N, Cox NJ, Li X, Orho-Melander M, Hara M** *et al*. Genetic variation in the gene encoding calpain-10 is associated with type 2 diabetes mellitus. *Nat Genet* 2000;**26**:163–75.

18 **Ong KK, Phillips DI, Fall C, Poulton J, Bennett ST, Golding J** *et al*. The insulin gene VNTR, type 2 diabetes and birth weight. *Nat.Genet* 1999;**21**:262–3.

19 **Huxtable SJ, Saker PJ, Haddad L, Walker M, Frayling TM, Levy JC** *et al*. Analysis of parent-offspring trios provides evidence for linkage and association between the insulin gene and type 2 diabetes mediated exclusively through paternally transmitted class III variable number tandem repeat alleles. *Diabetes* 2000;**49**:126–30.

20 **Alcolado JC, Alcolado R**. Importance of maternal history of non-insulin dependent diabetic patients. *Br Med J* 1991;**302**:1178–80.

21 **Thomas F, Balkau B, Vauzelle-Kervroedan F, Papoz L**. Maternal effect and familial aggregation in NIDDM. The CODIAB Study. CODIAB-INSERM-ZENECA Study Group. *Diabetes* 1994;**43**:63–7.

22 **Klein BE, Klein R, Moss SE, Cruickshanks KJ**. Parental history of diabetes in a population-based study. *Diabetes Care* 1996;**19**:827–30.

23 **Karter AJ, Rowell SE, Ackerson LM, Mitchell BD, Ferrara A, Selby JV** *et al*. Excess maternal transmission of type 2 diabetes. The Northern California Kaiser Permanente Diabetes Registry. *Diabetes Care* 1999;**22**:938–43.

24 **Young CA, Kumar S, Young MJ, Boulton AJ**. Excess maternal history of diabetes in Caucasian and Afro-origin non- insulin-dependent diabetic patients suggests dominant maternal factors in disease transmission. *Diabetes Res Clin Pract* 1995;**28**:47–9.

25 **Knowler WC, Pettitt DJ, Savage PJ, Bennett PH**. Diabetes incidence in Pima Indians: Contributions of obesity and parental diabetes. *Am J Epidemiol* 1981;**113**:144–56.

26 **Harder T, Plagemann A**. A role for gestational diabetes in the excess maternal transmission of type 2 diabetes? *Diabetes Care* 2000;**23**:431–2.

27 **Ballinger SW, Shoffner JM, Hedaya EV, Trounce I, Polak MA, Koontz DA** *et al*. Maternally transmitted diabetes and deafness associated with a 10.4 kb mitochondrial DNA deletion. *Nat Genet* 1992;**1**:11–5.

28 **Poulton J, Brown MS, Cooper A, Marchington DR, Phillips DI**. A common mitochondrial DNA variant is associated with insulin resistance in adult life. *Diabetologia* 1998;**41**:54–8.

29 **Casteels K, Ong K, Phillips D, Bendall H, Pembrey M**. Mitochondrial 16189 variant, thinness at birth, and type-2 diabetes. ALSPAC study team. Avon Longitudinal Study of Pregnancy and Childhood. *Lancet* 1999;**353**:1499–500.

30 Pfeifer K. Mechanisms of genomic imprinting. *Am J Hum Genet* 2000;**67**:777–87.

31 Georgiades P, Watkins M, Burton GJ, Ferguson-Smith AC. Roles for genomic imprinting and the zygotic genome in placental development. *Proc Natl Acad Sci U.S.A* 2001;**98**:4522–7.

32 Moore T. Genetic conflict, genomic imprinting and establishment of the epigenotype in relation to growth. *Reproduction* 2001;**122**:185–93.

33 Moore GE, Abu-Amero SN, Bell G, Wakeling EL, Kingsnorth A, Stanier P *et al*. Evidence that insulin is imprinted in the human yolk sac. *Diabetes* 2001;**50**:199–203.

34 Hales CN, Barker DJP, Clark PMS, Cox LJ, Fall C, Osmond C *et al*. Fetal and infant growth and impaired glucose tolerance at age 64. *Br Med J* 1991;**303**:1019–22.

35 Lithell HO, McKeigue PM, Berglund L, Mohsen R, Lithell U-B, Leon DA. Relation of size at birth to non-insulin dependent diabetes and insulin concentrations in men aged 50–60 years. *Br Med J* 1996;**312**:406–10.

36 McCance DR, Pettitt DJ, Hanson RL, Jacobsson LTH, Knowler WC, Bennett PH. Birth weight and non-insulin dependent diabetes: thrifty genotype, thrifty phenotype, or surviving small baby genotype? *Br Med J* 1994;**308**:942–5.

37 Yarbrough DE, Barrett-Connor E, Kritz-Silverstein D, Wingard DL. Birth weight, adult weight, and girth as predictors of the metabolic syndrome in postmenopausal women: the Rancho Bernardo Study. *Diabetes Care* 1998;**21**:1652–8.

38 Fall CH, Osmond C, Barker DJ, Clark PM, Hales CN, Stirling Y *et al*. Fetal and infant growth and cardiovascular risk factors in women. *Br Med J* 1995;**310**:428–32.

39 Forsen T, Eriksson J, Tuomilehto J, Reunanen A, Osmond C, Barker D. The fetal and childhood growth of persons who develop type 2 diabetes. *Ann Intern Med* 2000;**133**:176–82.

40 Rich-Edwards JW, Colditz GA, Stampfer MJ, Willett WC, Gillman MW, Hennekens CH *et al*. Birthweight and the risk for type 2 diabetes mellitus in adult women. *Ann Intern Med* 1999;**130**:278–84.

41 Phipps K, Barker DJ, Hales CN, Fall CH, Osmond C, Clark PM. Fetal growth and impaired glucose tolerance in men and women. *Diabetologia* 1993;**36**:225–8.

42 Fall CH, Stein CE, Kumaran K, Cox V, Osmond C, Barker DJ *et al*. Size at birth, maternal weight, and type 2 diabetes in South India. *Diabet Med* 1998;**15**:220–7.

43 Valdez R, Athens AA, Thompson GH, Bradshaw BS, Stern MP. Birthweight and adult health outcomes in a biethnic population in the USA. *Diabetologia* 1994;**37**:624–31.

44 Flanagan DE, Moore VM, Godsland IF, Cockington RA, Robinson JS, Phillips DI. Fetal growth and the physiological control of glucose tolerance in adults: a minimal model analysis. *Am J Physiol Endocrinol Metab* 2000;**278**:E700–E706.

45 Whincup PH, Cook DG, Adshead F, Taylor SJ, Walker M, Papacosta O *et al*. Childhood size is more strongly related than size at birth to glucose and insulin levels in 10–11-year-old children. *Diabetologia* 1997;**40**:319–26.

46 Ronnemaa T, Knip M, Lautala P, Viikari J, Uhari M, Leino A *et al*. Serum insulin and other cardiovascular risk indicators in children, adolescents and young adults. *Ann Med* 1991;**23**:67–72.

47 Spyckerelle Y, Steinmetz J, Deschamps JP. Comparison of measurements of cholesterol, glucose and uric acid taken at 5-year intervals in children and adolescents. *Arch Fr Pediatr* 1992;**49**:875–81.

48 Burke GL, Webber LS, Srinivasan SR, Radhakrishnamurthy B, Freedman DS, Berenson GS. Fasting plasma glucose and insulin levels and their relationship to cardiovascular risk factors in children: Bogalusa heart study. *Metabolism* 1986;**35**:441–6.

49 Law CM, Gordon GS, Shiell AW, Barker DJ, Hales CN. Thinness at birth and glucose tolerance in seven-year-old children. *Diabet Med* 1995;**12**:24–9.

50 Forrester TE, Wilks RJ, Bennett FI, Simeon D, Osmond C, Allen M *et al*. Fetal growth and cardiovascular risk factors in Jamaican schoolchildren. *Br Med J* 1996;**312**:156–60.

51 Yajnik CS, Fall CH, Vaidya U, Pandit AN, Bavdekar A, Bhat DS *et al*. Fetal growth and glucose and insulin metabolism in four-year-old Indian children. *Diabet Med* 1995;**12**:330–6.

52 Bavdekar A, Yajnik CS, Fall CHD, Bapat S, Pandit AN, Deshpande V *et al*. Insulin Resistance Syndrome in 8-Year-Old Indian Children. Small at Birth, Big at 8 Years, or Both? *Diabetes* 1999;**48**:2422–9.

53 Crowther NJ, Cameron N, Trusler J, Gray IP. Association between poor glucose tolerance and rapid postnatal weight gain in seven-year-old children. *Diabetologia* 1998;**41**:1163–7.

54 Dabelea D, Pettitt DJ, Hanson RL, Imperatore G, Bennett PH, Knowler WC. Birth weight, type 2 diabetes, and insulin resistance in Pima Indian children and young adults. *Diabetes Care* 1999;**22**:944–50.

55 Lucas A, Fewtrell MS, Cole TJ. Fetal origins of adult disease – the hypothesis revisited. *Br Med J* 1999;**319**:245–9.

56 Phillips DI. Birth weight and the future development of diabetes. A review of the evidence. *Diabetes Care* 1998;**21 Suppl 2**:B150-B155.

57 Phillips DI, Barker DJ, Fall CH, Seckl JR, Whorwood CB, Wood PJ *et al*. Elevated plasma cortisol concentrations: a link between low birth weight and the insulin resistance syndrome? *J Clin Endocrinol Metab* 1998;**83**:757–60.

58 Flanagan DE, Moore VM, Godsland IF, Cockington RA, Robinson JS, Phillips DI. Reduced foetal growth and growth hormone secretion in adult life. *Clin Endocrinol (Oxf)* 1999;**50**:735–40.

59 Phillips DI,Barker DJ. Association between low birthweight and high resting pulse in adult life: is the sympathetic nervous system involved in programming the insulin resistance syndrome? *Diabet Med* 1997;**14**:673–7.

60 Hattersley AT, Tooke JE. The fetal insulin hypothesis: an alternative explanation of the association of low birthweight with diabetes and vascular disease. *Lancet* 1999;**353**:1789–92.

61 Penrose LS. Some recent trends in human genetics. *Caryolgia* 1954;**6**:521–9.

62 Baird J, Osmond C, MacGregor A, Snieder H, Hales CN, Phillips DI. Testing the fetal origins hypothesis in twins: the Birmingham twin study. *Diabetologia* 2001;**44**:33–9.

63 Hattersley AT, Beards F, Ballantyne E, Appleton M, Harvey R, Ellard S. Mutations in the glucokinase gene of the fetus result in reduced birth weight. *Nat Genet* 1998;**19**:268–70.

64 Gluckman PD. The role of pituitary hormones, growth factors and insulin in the regulation of fetal growth. *Oxford Revision Reproduction Biology* 1986;**1986**:1–60.

65 Lindsay RS, Dabelea D, Roumain JM, Hanson RL, Bennett PH, Knowler WC. Type 2 diabetes and low birth weight: the role of paternal inheritance in the association of low birth weight and diabetes. *Diabetes* 2000;**49**:445–9.

66 Poulsen P, Vaag AA, Kyvik KO, Moller JD, Beck-Nielsen H. Low birth weight is associated with NIDDM in discordant monozygotic and dizygotic twin pairs. *Diabetologia* 1997;**40**:439–46.

67 Freinkel N. Banting Lecture 1980. Of pregnancy and progeny. *Diabetes* 1980;**29**:1023–35.

68 Pettitt DJ, Aleck KA, Baird HR, Carraher MJ, Bennett PH, Knowler WC. Congenital susceptibility to NIDDM. Role of intrauterine environment. *Diabetes* 1988;**37**:622–8.

69 Lindsay RS, Hanson RL, Bennett PH, Knowler WC. Secular trends in birth weight, BMI, and diabetes in the offspring of diabetic mothers. *Diabetes Care* 2000;**23**:1249–54.

70 Silverman BL, Metzger BE, Cho NH, Loeb CA. Impaired glucose tolerance in adolescent offspring of diabetic mothers. Relationship to fetal hyperinsulinism. *Diabetes Care* 1995;**18**:611–7.

71 Plagemann A, Harder T, Kohlhoff R, Rohde W, Dorner G. Glucose tolerance and insulin secretion in children of mothers with pregestational IDDM or gestational diabetes. *Diabetologia* 1997;**40**:1094–100.

72 Dabelea D, Hanson RL, Lindsay RS, Pettitt DJ, Imperatore G, Gabir MM *et al*. Intrauterine exposure to diabetes conveys risks for type 2 diabetes and obesity: a study of discordant sibships. *Diabetes* 2000;**49**:2208–11.

73 Dabelea D, Hanson RL, Bennett PH, Roumain J, Knowler WC, Pettitt DJ. Increasing prevalence of Type II diabetes in American Indian children. *Diabetologia* 1998;**41**:904–10.

74 Pinhas-Hamiel O, Dolan LM, Daniels SR, Standiford D, Khoury PR, Zeitler P. Increased incidence of non-insulin-dependent diabetes mellitus among adolescents. *J Pediatr* 1996;**128**:608–15.

75 Scott CR, Smith JM, Cradock MM, Pihoker C. Characteristics of youth-onset noninsulin-dependent diabetes mellitus and insulin-dependent diabetes mellitus at diagnosis. *Pediatrics* 1997;**100**:84–91.

76 Cianfarani S, Germani D, Branca F. Low birthweight and adult insulin resistance: the 'catch-up growth' hypothesis. *Arch Dis Child Fetal Neonatal Ed* 1999;**81**:F71–F73.

77 Whitaker RC, Pepe MS, Wright JA, Seidel KD, Dietz WH. Early adiposity rebound and the risk of adult obesity. *Pediatrics* 1998;**101**:E5.

78 Hu FB, Sigal RJ, Rich-Edwards JW, Colditz GA, Solomon CG, Willett WC *et al*. Walking compared with vigorous physical activity and risk of type 2 diabetes in women: a prospective study. *J Am Med Assoc* 1999;**282**:1433–9.

79 Flanagan DE, Moore VM, Godsland IF, Cockington RA, Robinson JS, Phillips DI. Alcohol consumption and insulin resistance in young adults. *Eur J Clin Invest* 2000;**30**:297–301.

80 Cooper GS, Ephross SA, Sandler DP. Menstrual patterns and risk of adult-onset diabetes mellitus. *J Clin Epidemiol* 2000;**53**:1170–3.

81 Solomon CG, Rich-Edwards J, Dunaif A, Willett WC. Abnormal menstrual cycle length predicts subsequent non-insulin-dependent diabetes mellitus. *Am J Epidemiol* 1998;**147**:S60.

82 Mosenthal HO, Bolduan C. Diabetes Mellitus—problems of present day treatment. *Am J Med Science* 1933;**186**:605.

83 Joslin EP, Lombard HL. Diabetes epidemiology from death records. *N Engl J Med* 1936;**214**:7–9.

84 Charles MA, Pettitt DJ, McCance DR, Hanson RL, Bennett PH, Knowler WC. Gravidity, obesity, and non-insulin-dependent diabetes among Pima Indian women. *Am J Med* 1994;**97**:250–5.

85 Simmons D. Parity, ethnic group and the prevalence of type 2 diabetes: the Coventry Diabetes Study. *Diabet Med* 1992;**9**:706–9.

86 Manson JE, Rimm EB, Colditz GA, Stampfer MJ, Willett WC, Arky RA *et al*. Parity and incidence of non-insulin-dependent diabetes mellitus. *Am J Med* 1992;**93**:13–8.

87 Sicree RA, Hoet JJ, Zimmet P, King HO, Coventry JS. The association of non-insulin-dependent diabetes with parity and still- birth occurrence amongst five Pacific populations. *Diabetes Res Clin Pract* 1986;**2**:113–22.

88 Zimmet P, Seluka A, Collins J, Currie P, Wicking J, DeBoer W. Diabetes mellitus in an urbanized, isolated Polynesian population. The Funafuti survey. *Diabetes* 1977;**26**:1101–8.

89 Alderman BW, Marshall JA, Boyko EJ, Markham KA, Baxter J, Hamman RF. Reproductive history, glucose tolerance, and NIDDM in Hispanic and non- Hispanic white women. The San Luis Valley Diabetes Study. *Diabetes Care* 1993;**16**:1557–64.

90 Collins VR, Dowse GK, Zimmet PZ. Evidence against association between parity and NIDDM from five population groups. *Diabetes Care* 1991;**14**:975–81.

91 Kuhl C. Glucose metabolism during and after pregnancy in normal and gestational diabetic women. 1. Influence of normal pregnancy on serum glucose and insulin concentration during basal fasting conditions and after a challenge with glucose. *Acta Endocrinol (Copenh)* 1975;**79**:709–19.

92 Porte D, Halter JB. The endocrine pancreas and diabetes mellitus. *Textbook of endocrinology*. Philadelphia: WB Saunders, 1981:716–843.

93 Duffy TJ, Ray R. Oral contraceptive use: prospective follow-up of women with suspected glucose intolerance. *Contraception* 1984;**30**:197–208.

94 Hannaford PC, Kay CR. Oral contraceptives and diabetes mellitus. *Br Med J* 1989;**299**:1315–6.

95 Rimm EB, Manson JE, Stampfer MJ, Colditz GA, Willett WC, Rosner B *et al*. Oral contraceptive use and the risk of type 2 (non-insulin-dependent) diabetes mellitus in a large prospective study of women. *Diabetologia* 1992;**35**:967–72.

96 Kjos SL, Shoupe D, Douyan S, Friedman RL, Bernstein GS, Mestman JH *et al*. Effect of low-dose oral contraceptives on carbohydrate and lipid metabolism in women with recent gestational diabetes: results of a controlled, randomized, prospective study. *Am J Obstet Gynecol* 1990;**163**:1822–7.

97 Skouby SO, Andersen O, Saurbrey N, Kuhl C. Oral contraception and insulin sensitivity: in vivo assessment in normal women and women with previous gestational diabetes. *J Clin Endocrinol Metab* 1987;**64**:519–23.

98 Skouby SO, Kuhl C, Molsted-Pedersen L, Petersen K, Christensen MS. Triphasic oral contraception: metabolic effects in normal women and those with previous gestational diabetes. *Am J Obstet Gynecol* 1985;**153**:495–500.

99 Kung AW, Ma JT, Wong VC, Li DF, Ng MM, Wang CC *et al*. Glucose and lipid metabolism with triphasic oral contraceptives in women with history of gestational diabetes. *Contraception* 1987;**35**:257–69.

100 Kjos SL, Peters RK, Xiang A, Thomas D, Schaefer U, Buchanan TA. Contraception and the risk of type 2 diabetes mellitus in Latina women with prior gestational diabetes mellitus. *J Am Med Assoc* 1998;**280**:533–8.

101 Godsland IF, Crook D, Simpson R, Proudler T, Felton C, Lees B *et al*. The effects of different formulations of oral contraceptive agents on lipid and carbohydrate metabolism. *N Engl J Med* 1990;**323**:1375–81.

102 Spellacy WN, Buhi WC, Birk SA, McCreary SA. Studies of ethynodiol diacetate and mestranol on blood glucose and plasma insulin. I. Six month oral glucose tolerance test. *Int J Fertil* 1971;**16**:55–65.

103 Wilcox JG, Hwang J, Hodis HN, Sevanian A, Stanczyk FZ, Lobo RA. Cardioprotective effects of individual conjugated equine estrogens through their possible modulation of insulin resistance and oxidation of low-density lipoprotein. *Fertil Steril* 1997;**67**:57–62.

104 Ali Z, Alexis SD. Occurrence of diabetes mellitus after gestational diabetes mellitus in Trinidad. *Diabetes Care* 1990;**13**:527–9.

105 King H. Epidemiology of glucose intolerance and gestational diabetes in women of childbearing age. *Diabetes Care* 1998;**21 Suppl 2**:B9–13.

106 Egeland GM, Skjaerven R, Irgens LM. Birth characteristics of women who develop gestational diabetes: population based study. *Br Med J* 2000;**321**:546–7.

107 Solomon CG, Willett WC, Carey VJ, Rich-Edwards J, Hunter DJ, Colditz GA *et al*. A prospective study of pregravid determinants of gestational diabetes mellitus. *J Am Med Assoc* 1997;**278**:1078–83.

108 Kelleher C, Kingston SM, Barry DG, *et al*. Hypertension in diabetic clinic patients and their siblings. *Diabetologia* 1988;**31**:76–81.

109 Matthews KA, Meilahn E, Kuller LH, Kelsey SF, Caggiula AW, Wing RR. Menopause and risk factors for coronary heart disease. *N Engl J Med* 1989;**321**:641–6.

110 Walton C, Godsland IF, Proudler AJ, Wynn V, Stevenson JC. The effects of the menopause on insulin sensitivity, secretion and elimination in non-obese, healthy women. *Eur J Clin Invest* 1993;**23**:466–73.

111 Spencer CP, Godsland IF, Stevenson JC. Is there a menopausal metabolic syndrome? *Gynecol Endocrinol* 1997;**11**:341–55.

Chapter 7

A life course approach to musculoskeletal ageing: muscle strength, osteoporosis, and osteoarthritis

Joan Bassey, Avan Aihie Sayer, and Cyrus Cooper

Musculoskeletal disorders increase in frequency with age and are one of the most important causes of morbidity and mortality in women in western populations. We review the development and ageing of three key components of the musculoskeletal system (muscle, bone, and cartilage), as well as considering their consequences for adult disease. The clinical correlates of age-related decline in the function of these three components are muscle weakness and its associated functional impairments, osteoporosis and osteoarthritis. Genetic and environmental factors operating before birth and during childhood, adolescence and adult life can be identified as sources of risk of these disorders. A life course approach to minimizing age related decline in these three body components will enhance the musculoskeletal health of the female population in future decades.

7.1 Introduction

The ability to move, the protection of vital organs, and stable support for the body are the principal roles of the musculoskeletal system.[1] This system accounts for a large proportion of the body mass; for example, the muscle mass of a healthy 70 kg adult is about 20 kg.[2] The outlines of the musculoskeletal system are apparent from the first trimester. At this stage the fetus is only a few millimetres long. The growing fetus usually obtains nourishment at the expense of the mother, who tends to suffer in periods of adversity, but placental size and unrestricted blood flow through placental vessels to and from the fetus is important for optimal growth especially during the last trimester. Fetal nutrition and the uterine environment are likely to play a part in the transcription of the genomic blueprint acquired at conception into the phenotypic newborn. Some of these influences may have long-term effects and so are known as 'programming'. During early childhood, growth is rapid and there are opportunities for environmental or lifestyle factors to have long-term effects, especially on the skeleton.

Adolescence, which occurs much earlier in girls than boys, brings growth to an end and its timing will have long-term consequences for adult stature. Women are on average physically disadvantaged compared with men throughout adult life because they have smaller skeletons and about 30% less absolute strength. Women have an even poorer strength for weight ratio compared with men due to their extra body fat, and lower levels of physical activity, at least in the developed western countries, compound their inevitable disadvantage.

Human ageing is accompanied by marked changes in the quantity and composition of all three musculoskeletal components. These changes underlie the enormous public health problem attributable to muscle weakness and musculoskeletal disorders in later life. Thus, it has been estimated that around 40% of adult women suffer from pain in their joints, neck, or back.[3] The prevalence increases markedly with age, so that at age 75–84 years some 20% of women report current back pain, and 30% report current knee pain. The main contributor to this burden is osteoarthritis, a disorder characterized by the loss of articular cartilage.[4] The age related loss of bone which leads to osteoporosis (the most common skeletal disorder in western populations), is also a contributor to considerable morbidity, and even mortality. Thus, it is estimated that around 40% of all White women and 13% of White men in the United States aged over 50 years experience a clinically apparent fragility fracture during their lifetime,[5] as a result of age related bone loss. Women are at greater risk because of their smaller skeletons and their dependence on the protective effect of oestrogen which is lost at menopause.

7.2 Muscle strength

Skeletal muscle cells can convert chemical energy derived from food into mechanical energy for doing work and generating the power to move. Individual muscle fibres are bundled in connective tissue that transmits the force of muscle contraction through tendons to attachments on bone. Each fibre can do work only in the direction of its long axis; it is the great variety of arrangements of muscles attached to the levers of the skeleton, and the cooperation between them, that permits the full range of human activities. Muscle contraction would be ineffective unless it could produce directed motion through a skeletal lever.

Muscles are highly responsive to the use made of them, becoming stronger if they are used. Habitual activity throughout life is therefore an important influence on strength. It is useful in adult life to be strong, and in old age it can make the difference between the satisfactions of an independent lifestyle or the dwindling horizons of institutionalized care.[6] Muscle diseases are rare but any chronic disease which reduces activity levels will indirectly reduce muscle strength due to disuse.

7.2.1 Intrauterine and early postnatal life

Muscle strength depends to a large extent on body size. Individuals who are relatively large at birth often grow into large adults who are therefore strong; birth size tracks though childhood and adolescence into adult life.[7,8] For example, studies in which parental size has been controlled, show that babies born small for gestational age achieve less than expected adult stature.[7] Birthweight is influenced by the intrauterine environment; genetic influences on birth size are relatively modest.[9–11] The adult number of muscle fibres are all present at birth, no more can be added later, so any events *in utero* which limit the number of muscle fibres would have long-term consequences, setting potential ultimate limits on muscle size and strength. In piglet litters the smallest piglets, which have been relatively malnourished *in utero*, develop fewer muscle fibres compared with their largest litter mates.[12] The difference can be as much as 17%. As the piglets mature the muscle fibres grow larger to compensate but this leaves smaller safety margins and greater vulnerability to loss of fibres later in life.

Evidence from humans is beginning to accumulate which shows that adult muscle mass and strength might also be modified by environmental influences during critical periods of early development. Birthweight is positively associated with lean tissue in the upper arm of children at age 8 years,[13] and with thigh muscle-bone area at age 17–22 years.[8] In a cohort study of 102 men and 41 women aged 70–75 years who were born in Sheffield, UK, a strong association was found between birthweight and adult lean mass (which is 60–70% muscle) as assessed by dual energy X-ray absorptiometry.[14] In this study, around 25% of the variation in whole body lean mass among these men and women could be explained by birthweight. The relationship remained highly statistically significant after adjusting for age, adult height and adult weight.[14] Another British cohort study has evaluated the relationship between birthweight and muscle strength in late adulthood.[15,16] Grip strength was measured in 306 women and 411 men, aged 60–74 years. Strong positive associations were found between birthweight, weight at one year, and adult grip strength. Subjects in the lowest fifth of the distribution of birthweight had 12% lower grip strength than those in the highest fifth of the distribution, after adjusting for age, sex, socioeconomic status, and adult height (Fig. 7.1).[16] The association between birthweight and adult grip strength was confirmed in a study of 1365 men and 1381 women born in 1946 and followed to age 53 years and shown to be independent of body size in childhood as well as adult life.[17]

These findings show that the association between birth size and adult muscle mass and function is not simply a skeletal size effect because large individuals tend to have large muscles. They suggest additional programming influences *in utero* that may depend on nutrition, since strong associations remain after controlling for adult stature in women after middle-age.

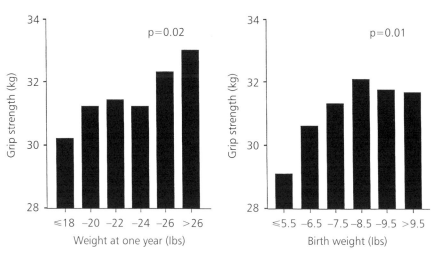

Fig. 7.1 Relationship between birthweight, weight at one-year and adult grip strength among 717 British men and women aged 60–74 years [derived from ref. 15].

7.2.2 **Childhood and adolescence**

As a child grows its muscles grow larger; this is partly under genetic control but the stretch imposed by growth of the skeleton also stimulates muscle to increase its length. Muscle mass and bone mass are related throughout life[18] and muscle in turn stimulates bone through the tension it imposes on the skeleton during physical activity. From 6 to 15 years of age, muscle strength and cross-sectional area increase steadily as more contractile protein is produced, unless the child is severely malnourished.

At around 15 years the rate of increase of muscle mass slows. The slow-down is under hormonal control and its timing has profound consequences for adult size and strength. The slow-down occurs much later in boys, who continue to gain muscle at a substantial rate into late adolescence.[19] During these years, sedentary lifestyles, which are common among girls in western societies (see Chapter 14), and may begin as young as five years, will result in loss of muscle strength[20] but there is no evidence that this has irrevocable effects on adult muscularity. However, patterns of physical activity and attitudes to active lifestyles take root in adolescence and may be formative for adult life (see Chapter 13). Menstrual periods, breast development, and sometimes a marked increase in the fat to lean ratio of the body (teenage puppy-fat) may all combine with psychological changes to prevent some adolescent girls from enjoying physical activity.

7.2.3 **Adulthood**

Physical activity drops off steadily throughout life and is associated with a steady loss of cardiorespiratory endurance.[21] However, perhaps because brief bouts of activity are enough to maintain muscle, strength remains on a plateau from young adulthood to late middle-age and then falls after the age of about 60 years.[22] Safety margins are usually adequate for the demands of daily life until old age.

The changes in the hormonal levels of oestrogen and progestogen at the menopause, which may have marked effects on the skeleton, do not appear to have direct implications for muscle strength. Cross-sectional data from representative surveys do not show a dip in strength at the time of menopause, as is found for bone.[23] There are no effects of hormone replacement therapy (HRT) status on muscle in elderly women, nor are there any effects of oestrogen status (natural or therapeutic) at age 45–54 years.[24] Randomized controlled trials of HRT in postmenopausal women show no effect on strength.[25–27] In younger women studies of changes through the natural cycle[28] or during hormone manipulation for *in vitro* fertilization,[29] in which hormone levels are confirmed by blood samples, show either no effect or a fall in strength associated with increased oestrogen levels.

7.2.4 **Old age**

In old age muscle strength declines slowly.[30] In common with the ageing of the human body as a whole, the intrinsic atrophy of skeletal muscle fibres appears to be controlled by many different genes. This loss is exacerbated by increasingly sedentary lifestyles which are part of the pattern of ageing, especially in developed countries.[6] With lack of use the remaining muscle becomes weaker. However, this loss remains potentially reversible by increased physical activity even in extreme old age.[31] Muscle mass forms up to a third of the body mass in adult life but in old age it falls back to about one fifth; the muscle is normal but there is too little of it.[31,32] It is important as a nutritional defence during illness, a source of metabolic heat, and for protection of vulnerable tissues such as osteoporotic bone. Mortality in old age as an outcome of serious illness is much more likely if nutritional stores of fat and muscle are low. The function of remaining muscle cells seems to be little affected by the inevitable insults that will occur in a lifetime and the accumulation of 'junk' within the cells. It is remarkable that these highly differentiated non-renewable cells continue to transmit electrical signals and to contract energetically for up to 100 years; a testimony to their remarkable powers of self-repair and adaptation.

7.2.5 Back pain and other over-use injuries

Back pain is the most common musculoskeletal problem, whether measured as a symptom in the general population, as a source of disability, as a reason for seeking health care, or as a cause of both short- and long-term work loss. In any one year, around 40% of women experience at least one day of low back pain—a figure which does not include menstrual pain or pain accompanying a feverish illness.[33] Back pain typically arises from injury to the muscles and ligaments that support the thoracolumbar spine. There are constitutional risk factors for back pain, the most well established is tall stature,[34] but narrow spinal canals may also increase susceptibility, an anatomical characteristic perhaps determined early in life.[35] A small proportion of cases of back pain can be attributed to specific problems such as infection, inflammation, vertebral fracture, or cancer. However, most back pain episodes are non-specific, and attributable to musculoligamentus strain. Back pain is common in those occupations that require heavy lifting, such as nursing.[36] Poor physical condition, muscle weakness, and poor psychological health increase susceptibility to back pain.[37]

Stiffness after a severe bout of exercise is a manifestation of repair of over-use damage. However, over-use can cause more intransigent problems, associated not just with heavy lifting but also with excessively prolonged use of the same muscles, as in repetitive strain injury. This is associated with a chronic inflammatory condition of the tendons and ligaments surrounding the muscle, for example sports injuries such as 'tennis elbow'. Once established, these over-use syndromes are difficult to cure and require permanent avoidance of the causal activity.

7.2.6 Summary: a life course model of muscle strength

Muscle strength depends upon muscle size. Limits to this are set *in utero*, since the number of muscle fibres does not increase after birth. Body size is partly inherited, but low levels of nutrition *in utero* may also determine the number of muscle fibres formed. Muscle fibres increase in size with growth during childhood, provided nutrition is adequate. Muscles respond to use increasing or decreasing in size according to activity levels; early lack of activity does not preclude improvements in later life even into old age. Adequate and appropriate patterns of habitual physical activity are therefore important to ensure freedom from back pain and other over-use injuries, to offset potentially debilitating effects of chronic diseases in middle-age and to maintain independence in old age when there is some inevitable loss of muscle fibres. Encouraging appropriate lifelong physical activity should be the focus of preventive strategies.

7.3 Bone strength and osteoporosis

Bone is formed from calcium mineral deposited in a collagen protein matrix that confers both rigidity and elasticity. The bone surfaces are covered with a population of bone cells that can remove bone and then deposit new bone in the resulting space. This linked process of bone turnover, which is under complex local and systemic hormonal control, ensures that microfractures are repaired and that bone can re-model in response to load. During adult life, the skeleton is completely renewed many times over, and it is therefore much 'younger' than other tissues in the body such as the muscles and nerves. However, from middle-age onwards, turnover becomes inadequate with less new bone replacing the old. This leads eventually to bone fragility and a greatly increased risk of fracture.

The bone mass of an individual is established early in adult life. It then remains on a plateau referred to as peak bone mass, and any variations due to lifestyle are small. In later adult life bone mass depends upon the peak attained during skeletal growth and the subsequent rate of bone loss.

Bone strength depends mainly on bone mineral density (BMD) which accounts for 75–90% of the variance. Other determinants are skeletal size and shape to which bone mineral content (BMC) is related. Thus, slight build is associated with increased fracture risk. Genetic factors,[9] especially maternal osteoporosis, have a significant influence on the skeleton.[38–40] Parental height, especially maternal height, influences the birth length of offspring that in turn tracks through to adult height.[7,41–45]

Osteoporosis is a skeletal disorder characterized by low BMD due to bone loss with the consequence of increasing the risk of fracture.[5] These fractures typically occur at the hip, spine, and wrist; the annual cost attributable for them in England and Wales is £1.7 billion, with over 90% of this figure ascribed to hip fracture. Prevalence is increasing world-wide, mainly due to the demographic shifts towards older populations, but the age-adjusted incidence of these fractures continues to rise and cohort effects are evident.[46] White Caucasian ethnic groups are at greater risk than Black African groups, with Asian groups intermediate.

7.3.1 Intrauterine and early postnatal life

The risk of osteoporosis may be programmed to some extent by environmental influences during early life. Both BMC and BMD in neonates and early childhood are related to birthweight and to various parental characteristics, including maternal smoking in pregnancy.[42,47–49] Premature babies followed up to later childhood have deficits in BMC and BMD.[50] Do these relationships continue into adult life? So far, a number of studies have looked at the associations between weight at birth or in infancy and adult BMC and BMD.

Weight at one year was related to BMC in a UK cohort of 153 women aged 21 years[41] and in an older UK cohort which included 201 women aged 60–75 years after adjustment for known genetic and adult environmental factors.[51] Reported birthweight was associated with BMC in a US cohort of 305 women aged 70 years after controlling for a number of adult factors.[52] These findings suggest that the trajectory of bone growth may be programmed in early life, an assertion previously supported only by inference from measurements of body height.[45] These data are compatible with the hypothesis that endocrine programming of growth hormone, perhaps interacting with the quality of the diet and exposure to infection in infancy,[53] affects adult stature and peak skeletal size. More importantly for fracture risk, a study of 41 women and 102 men from the Sheffield historical cohort showed that BMD (measured as bone mineral apparent density (BMAD)) as well as BMC was significantly related to birthweight (Fig. 7.2).[14]

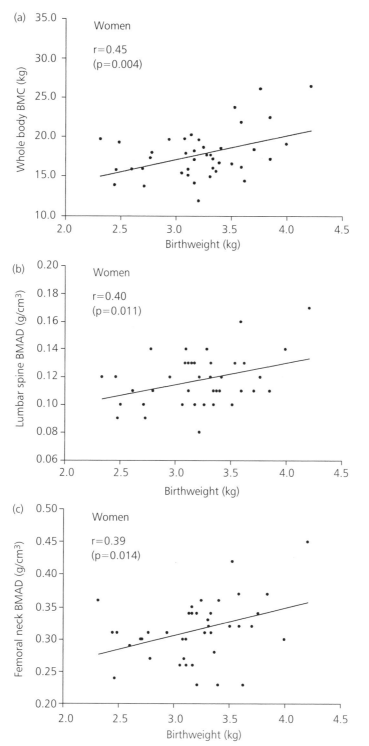

Fig. 7.2 Relation between birthweight and (a) whole body bone mineral content and (b) bone mineral apparent density (BMAD) at the lumbar spine and (c) BMAD at the femoral neck assessed by dual energy X-ray absorptiometry (DXA) among 41 women aged 70–75 years born in Sheffield, UK [derived from ref 14].

7.3.2 **Childhood and adolescence**

Skeletal growth is rapid during the first six months after birth and then proceeds slowly through childhood. Although young children of a given age vary considerably in their stature, there is no systematic gender difference. Bone mineral density changes little during these years; some studies find a gender difference in favour of boys but the difference is small (1–2%). The onset of puberty occurs in response to hormonal changes which control the skeletal growth spurt. During the two years of most rapid growth, 26% of adult bone mass is accrued so this is a critical period.[54] Girls reach puberty earlier than boys and also reach their adult stature sooner. In girls on average the growth spurt begins at 10 years of age, reaches its maximum rate at 12 years and subsides at 16 years. As the bone grows in size there are no major changes in density. However, compared with boys, adolescent girls develop smaller bones with less absolute bone strength, in keeping with their smaller adult stature and lower muscle strength.

Childhood growth has been linked to incidence of hip fracture many years later.[43] Records of body size at birth and measurements of height and weight throughout childhood were available for over 7000 adults (around half of them women) born in Helsinki during 1924–33 who still lived in Finland. Hospital discharge records showed that between 1971 and 1995, 57 of these women suffered a first hip fracture at a mean age of 64 years. After adjusting for age and socioeconomic status, poor growth between 7 and 15 years significantly increased fracture risk.

Chronic malnutrition or chronic disease will stunt growth and potential adult height may not be reached. Children who were fed from birth on a macrobiotic diet, which is low in calcium and vitamin D, had significantly lower BMC than their peers at 9–15 years even after adjustment for other significant factors.[55] Children growing up in severely deprived areas on such low dietary calcium intakes that their serum calcium was prejudiced had reduced BMAD at 6 and 20 years, after controlling for body size.[56] There are concerns that some girls have such low calcium intakes their long term skeletal health may be compromised.[57]

Physical activity needs to be optimal; there seems to be a critical window of opportunity during these childhood years, when the skeleton is most sensitive to the anabolic effects of bone loading. Studies in adults who took up racket sports competitively before menarche showed dramatic effects of the regular unilateral loading; they have differences of 25–30% in the arm bones which outlast the playing years whereas those who began to train as adolescents or in adult life showed much smaller differences.[58] In children aged under 10 years, regular brief bouts of jumping or skipping doubled the rate of increase of bone mass compared with a control group[59] but a similar exercise regime in young adult women achieved increases of a only few per cent.[60] Adolescent gymnasts have exceptionally high BMD, even compared with runners[61] but swimmers and cyclists do not differ in BMD from their sedentary peers because their chosen activity does not provide extra loading for the skeleton. These are exceptional groups but among more typical children aged 8–14 years, the more active girls had 17% higher bone mineral content in their skeletons after controlling for maturational age and size.[62] The low physical activity levels which are becoming prevalent among girls may result in their failure to achieve optimal bone strength.

There are adverse consequences of too much exercise. When excessive athletic activity is combined with poor diet, weight loss causes changes in the hypophyseal–gonadal hormonal axis which result in amennorhoea and bone loss (similar to what happens in anorexia nervosa). The effects on the skeleton may be serious despite the stimulating influence of bone loading exercise. The deficit is most marked at the spine; the femur is relatively protected by the exercise. When training routines are modified and diet and body weight improve, menses return but the BMD does not return to expected normal levels. Moreover, simple reversal of the oestrogen lack with oral administration of HRT has not been entirely successful.[63]

7.3.4 Adult life

The underlying patterns of maturation and ageing are different for the spine and femur. The vertebrae, which are more sensitive to oestrogen, continue to accumulate bone until the fourth decade, and then remain stable until the menopause. The femoral head, which is more affected by weight-bearing activity, begins to lose bone from the fourth decade onward and does not show an accelerated loss at the menopause.[38] Nutrition is important, particularly calcium intake; 700 mg daily is the recommended daily allowance (RDA) in Britain. Some studies show significant associations between BMD and dietary calcium at low levels of intake and a few show that supplementation increases BMD.[64] Absorption varies greatly so many women remain in good bone health on levels below the RDA but if absorption is compromised then the skeleton may suffer. Excessive weight loss, smoking,[65] alcohol abuse and some drug treatments, such as corticosteroids, have negative effects on bone.[39,40] Some of these may have long-term consequences.

Pregnancy imposes heavy demands on the mother's nutritional resources especially in the last trimester and also during lactation. In multiparous mothers who are severely malnourished skeletal damage may occur (such as osteomalacia). A drop in BMD is observed even in well-nourished mothers during pregnancy and lactation but this is reversed once the child is weaned and the mothers suffer no long-term disadvantage, unless they smoke.[66]

Active lifestyles that load the skeleton in a variety of ways will maintain bone mass.[67,68] Exercise interventions in controlled trials have improved bone mineral density at specific sites by modest amounts. Those that have been successful were based on high impact weight-bearing activity such as jogging or skipping,[27,60,69] or on strength training using heavy weights in slow lifts.[70] A small amount of activity appears to be sufficient to maintain the skeleton provided it is regular. Chronic disease, such as back pain, which restricts physical activity will have negative effects on bone, and prolonged bed rest causes substantial bone loss.[71]

During and after the menopause, as the ovaries fail, the withdrawal of circulating oestrogen causes bone loss due to increased bone resorption that is not matched by increased formation. Some women lose very little bone, others lose 5% per year over several postmenopausal years. Rapid loss combined with a low premenopausal bone mass leaves some women at a seriously increased risk of osteoporotic fracture. Women who have had an early menopause or oophorectomy or an early hysterectomy are at a disadvantage because of their premature loss of oestrogen. HRT appears to protect against bone loss while it is used, but this effect wanes rapidly on cessation of treatment. Some women are left with higher residual levels of oestrogen than others, and, since quite modest levels of oestrogen seem to be sufficient for bone maintenance, these women retain adequate bone strength.[72]

Slight build and low fat stores are known risk factors for osteoporosis. Adipose tissue produces small quantities of oestradiol, also body fat acts as a cushion to protect fragile bones from falls and body weight helps to load bones.[73] In women who weigh more than 70 kg osteoporotic fracture is rare, so the obsession with weight loss through dietary restriction, which is prevalent in western societies can have unfortunate consequences. Moderate amounts of fat may be more of a friend to postmenopausal women than is usually supposed.

7.3.5 Old age

Menopausal loss is followed by a decline in BMD of about 1% per year that continues into old age. This happens in both men and women and is part of normal ageing. Most body systems slow down in old age, but in the skeleton there is an increase in the rate of bone turnover. This should favour repair and response to loading but it is not adaptive because it is accompanied by an imbalance in favour of resorption that explains the bone loss. The increase in turnover has been attributed in part to increased levels of parathyroid hormone due to reduced serum calcium levels. Diets lacking adequate vitamin D and calcium may contribute to the high incidence of hip fractures in the institutionalized elderly.[74]

Physical activity helps to maintain the skeleton in old age; no formal interventions have been conducted beyond the eighth decade but sedentary lifestyles are known to be associated with increased osteoporotic fracture at this time of life.[68] Moreover, maintenance of muscle strength and balance contribute to reducing the risk of accidental falls[75] at an age when poor eyesight and sensory loss are prevalent.

7.3.6 Summary: a life course approach to osteoporosis

Individuals with small skeletons, low bone mineral density within the skeleton, and low body mass index are the most vulnerable to osteoporotic fracture in later life. Low birthweight and undernutrition *in utero* may contribute. Other life course factors that increase the risk of fracture include poor nutrition, especially with respect to calcium and vitamin D, and lack of bone-loading exercise. The years before puberty are the most vulnerable to lack of exercise. In middle-age, early menopause, low postmenopausal oestrogen levels, smoking and some drug treatments, can all increase the fracture risk substantially. In old age, poor physical condition, thinness and frequent falls are further risk factors. Osteoporotic fracture is a serious public health problem and it is a consequence of both genetic susceptibility and the cumulative effects of life course experience. Preventive approaches to osteoporotic fracture should be aimed at increasing the bone mass attained during intrauterine life, childhood and adolescence; reducing age-related rates of bone loss; and reducing the risk and severity of falling.

7.4 Joints and osteoarthritis

Osteoarthritis is the most common cause of joint disease and dysfunction and has a profound impact on women's health. In terms of disability adjusted life years, osteoarthritis is the fourth most frequent cause of health problems in women worldwide.[76] Despite this public health impact, understanding of the disease process remains incomplete and current interventions are directed at treatment rather than prevention.

The term osteoarthritis (OA) describes a complex disease process in which a combination of systemic and local mechanisms result in characteristic pathological and radiological changes. These include focal loss of articular cartilage in part of a synovial joint accompanied by a hypertrophic reaction in the subchondral bone and joint margin. X-rays show joint space narrowing, subchondral sclerosis, and cyst formation with marginal osteophytosis. These abnormalities are often, but not always, associated with the clinical features of joint pain, swelling, and tenderness.

Most currently available information on the epidemiology of OA comes from population-based radiographic surveys. The prevalence of radiographic OA rises steeply with age at all joint sites. Both hand and knee diseases appear to be more frequent in women than in men, particularly after the menopause but the reason for this gender difference is unclear. The female to male ratio varies among studies between 1.5 and over 4.0. Hip OA is less common than knee OA, and prevalence rates in men and women appear more similar.

The most recent data to characterize the incidence of symptomatic hand, hip, and knee OA were obtained from the Fallon Community Health Plan, a health maintenance organization located in the north-east United States.[77] In this study, the age- and sex-standardized incidence rate of hand OA was 100 per 100 000 person years, for hip OA, 88 per 100 000 person years, and for knee OA, 240 per 100 000 person years. The incidence of hand, hip, and knee disease increased with age, and women had higher rates than men, especially after the age of 50 years. A levelling off occurred for both groups at all joint sites around the age of 80 years. By the age of 70–89 years, the incidence of symptomatic knee OA among women approached 1% per year.

Osteoarthritis occurs worldwide and although some geographic differences in prevalence have been reported, these are often difficult to interpret because of different sampling procedures and lack of radiographic consistency. However, hip OA does appear to be more common in Caucasian populations.

Individual risk factors for OA appear to act through two main mechanisms: factors influencing or marking a generalized predisposition to the condition and factors resulting in abnormal biomechanical loading at a specific joint. Traditionally these risk factors have been divided into those acting through heredity and those occurring in later life. Twin and family studies suggest a hereditary component to the aetiology of early onset generalized OA.[78] However the importance of this in the general population remains unclear. There is growing evidence that OA is an age-related dynamic reaction of a joint in response to insult or injury.[79] Thus OA represents failure of the joint as an organ and the pathological observations in advance of the disease are as much a product of attempted repair as of the primary insult or damage which contributed to initiation of the process. In terms of risk factors for OA, it is therefore appropriate to consider influences acting throughout the life course rather than focusing on the events in later years.

7.4.1 Developmental influences

There has been little consideration of the effects of *in utero* influences on long-term joint function although it has been recognized that embryological events may provide insights into the study of 'mature' joints and their diseases.[80] There is rapid development and differentiation of the musculoskeletal system during the embryonic period and all bones and joints can be observed by the seventh week. Alteration in shape is clearly one of the critical events in embryological development and the shape of joints continues to be important in the occurrence of joint pathology in later life.

The change in cell phenotype during development probably arises as a result of a complex interaction of changes in extracellular matrix (ECM), peptide regulatory factors (PRFs) and changes in cell–cell interactions.[81,82] The recognition of the role that cell–cell and cell–ECM interactions play in determining both cell phenotype and spatial orientation may provide important clues into mechanisms that control the maintenance of normal joint structures.

The sites at which joint shape has been most closely linked with later development of OA are the hip and knee. Childhood hip disorders such as Perthes disease and congenital dislocation lead to premature OA.[79] It is also likely that more minor abnormalities in the shape of the hip joint account for a proportion of hip OA among younger people. These changes may alter the biomechanical stability of the knee joint and predispose to OA.

Movement is also important in the development of joints and in the maintenance of joint space throughout life.[83] Hypermobility (laxity of ligaments) can have adverse effects on joint function.[84] Joint laxity tends to diminish rapidly throughout childhood and then more slowly during later life due to wear and fibrosis in connective tissues. It is associated with overuse injuries as well as OA although the strength of this association and the precise mechanism remain unclear.

7.4.2 Obesity

Obesity is closely associated with OA at the knee, less strongly with hip OA, and probably not with hand OA. Population-based studies suggest that the increase in risk of knee OA between the highest and lowest fifths of the distribution of body mass index, lies between four and seven fold.[85] Until recently it was uncertain whether obesity preceded (and perhaps caused) OA, or whether obesity resulted from the sedentary lifestyle of patients with OA. There is now evidence that the former is correct. Analysis of the Framingham study in the US has revealed that obesity predicted knee OA up to 30 years later and more recent data from the Fallon Community Study showed that body weight was a predictor of incident OA of the hand, hip, and knee.[86] Also, analysis from a population-based American survey has shown that obesity is consistent in its association with both symptomatic and asymptomatic OA.[87]

The reason for the association between obesity and OA remains speculative. Although mechanical loading is an obvious mechanism, it does not explain differential effects of adiposity at the hip and knee. The association may be stronger in women than men, suggesting that metabolic, rather than mechanical factors may explain the link. The role of obesity in childhood on subsequent development of OA has been little considered but it is unlikely that the mechanical or metabolic effects are confined to adult life.

7.4.3 Nutrition

There is some evidence from animal models that early nutrition has long-term effects on joint function. A study on dogs showed that diet restriction instituted at eight weeks of age and continued through life resulted in reduced prevalence and severity of OA eight years later[88] but the influence of early growth and nutrition on the development of human OA is not known.

There has been some study of the role of specific nutritional factors in the adult diet.[89] Anecdotal evidence suggests that joint symptoms may be linked to the ingestion of certain types of food and immunological or inflammatory mechanisms may underlie this. Epidemiological studies have looked at the role of vitamin intake. Vitamins C and E are among the most potent of dietary antioxidants and it has been proposed that oxidative damage occurs in OA. There is some evidence that low levels of vitamin C are associated with disease progression although the evidence is less clear for vitamin E.[89] Reduced vitamin D has also been linked to progressive disease and its actions on bone remodelling and chondrocyte function may be important.[90]

7.4.4 Hormonal influences

The predominance of generalized OA in postmenopausal women has led to the suggestion that it may be hormonally mediated. Osteoarthritis has been associated with previous hysterectomy.[87] Oestrogen receptors have recently been identified on the osteoblast surface, and *in vitro* studies have suggested that female sex hormones modify chondrocytes in culture conditions.[85] Attempts to retard the development of OA using postmenopausal HRT, however, have had limited success. A recent study showed that HRT had a moderate but not statistically significant protective effect against worsening of radiographic knee OA among elderly White women.[91]

Osteoarthritis at particular sites also appears to have a negative association with osteoporosis. The strongest evidence for this lies at the hip joint, where studies consistently observe that elderly patients with hip OA are at lower risk of sustaining femoral neck fractures,[92] although in patients with generalized OA, studies of bone density have produced inconsistent results. This may be because excess body weight can damage weight-bearing joints leading to increased risk of OA, whereas load on the bones appears to be osteogenic and conversely, weight loss and low body mass index are associated with increased risk of osteoporosis. The OA–osteoporosis relationship supports the view that abnormal mechanical behaviour of subchondral bone underlies accelerated cartilage damage.

7.4.5 Trauma

Major injury is a common cause of knee OA. Two specific types of injury are associated: cruciate (ligament) damage and meniscal (cartilage) tears. Follow-up studies of patients with cruciate rupture have reported cartilage loss, even in young patients. For meniscectomy, most studies have reported an increased frequency of subsequent OA.[87] Major injury, particularly fracture, may alter mechanical function and predispose to OA at other sites. Most notable among these are fractures of the femoral shaft (hip OA), tibia (ankle OA), humerus (shoulder OA), and scaphoid (wrist OA). Sporting activity combines the risks of severe joint damage with those of repetitive use. The long-term effects of trauma sustained in childhood are less clear.

7.4.6 Adult risk factors

Occupational activity exemplifies stereotyped repetitive use of particular joint groups. The association of hand OA with handedness, and the relatively infrequent involvement of paralysed limbs by the condition, suggest a role for repetitive activity in the aetiology of OA. Several occupational groups have been shown at increased risk of developing OA. For example jobs involving repetitive knee bending are associated with increased risk of knee OA.

There is some evidence that cigarette smoking has a protective influence on the development of OA. This effect remains after adjustment for potential confounding variables such as body weight.[87] Other diseases have also been linked to OA including diabetes, hypertension, and hyperuricaemia.[87] These relationships are independent of obesity. The mechanisms are not known.

7.4.7 Summary: a life course model of osteoarthritis

Osteoarthritis may therefore be viewed as the result of exposures throughout life and the corresponding response in terms of regeneration and repair. Exposures may not be entirely independent and may form 'chains of risk'. This model is analogous to the lifelong exposure-response model of ageing which proposes that the ageing phenotype is determined by the response to intrinsic and extrinsic exposures starting at conception and occurring throughout life.[93] The close relationship between OA and ageing has been considered before.[94]

At present intervention in osteoarthritis is aimed primarily at treatment of established disease in adult life. The life course approach encourages consideration of wider preventive strategies. The use of postmenopausal HRT has shown limited benefit in secondary prevention but there is evidence that treatment of adult obesity reduces the risk of developing OA and may slow its progression. It is possible that intervention earlier in life may have additional benefit. This is an area for future research.

7.5 Conclusions

Musculoskeletal disorders are an important cause of morbidity and functional impairment in the general population. They are strongly age-related, and tend to occur more frequently among women than men. For the three important causes of musculoskeletal disability (age-related declines in muscle strength; osteoporosis; and osteoarthritis) evidence now exists to suggest aetiological factors acting throughout the life course. Although genetic influences are an important contributor to the risk of these three musculoskeletal disorders, modification of the environment to which an individual is exposed at different stages in their development, adult life, and later years, also determines risk. Many environmental risk factors, for example nutrition, physical activity, and occupational use, are modifiable both in the population as a whole, as well as among individuals at the greatest risk. A greater understanding of the health impact made by strategies aiming to intervene at different stages in the life course is urgently required.

Commentary on 'A life course approach to musculoskeletal ageing: muscle strength, osteoporosis, and osteoarthritis'

Jane Cauley

A life course approach to musculoskeletal ageing emphasizes that prevention of the losses in muscle mass and strength, bone mass and strength, and joint function must begin early in life. The chapter by Bassey, Aihie, Sayer, and Cooper provides persuasive evidence that, indeed, influences which occur early in life can have devastating consequences late in life. A life course approach emphasizes that 'prevention' must be a lifelong commitment that is integrated into an individual's lifestyle. It is, perhaps, a utopian ideal, mandating a lifelong commitment to practices which promote muscle, bone, and joint health throughout life.

On a population level, skeletal muscle and bone strength and joint function universally decline with age. On an individual basis, there is marked individual variability in the rate of decline. Identification of the risk factors which contribute to this marked individual variability could lead to identification of appropriate interventions to prevent, delay or attenuate these declines.

The aetiology of the decline in muscle, bone and joint function is complex. Multiple genes may contribute, each with modest effects. There are probably many gene-gene and gene-environmental interactions which have yet to be identified. Alterations in the neuronal and hormonal milieu are also likely to play a role. However, a central theme to the discussion of these changes in muscle, bone, and joints is the potential impact of our lifestyles, and environment, thus offering the promise of prevention. Indeed, a healthy diet, coupled with a lifelong persistence in engagement in physical activities may help us prevent their declines and their consequences.

A second central theme to the study of these age-related declines is that they are inter-related. For example, declines in muscle strength and muscle mass will lead to decreased mechanical stress on bone which in turn will lead to decreased bone mass. The implication of their inter-relatedness is that interventions aimed at increasing muscle strength, for example, resistance exercise, will also lead to improvements in bone strength and possibly joint function.

Cohorts of children and young adults today have had very different environmental exposures, consume different diets and are less physically active than previous cohorts. This could lead to secular increases in the rate of musculoskeletal ageing. A life course approach to prevention facilitates projections into the likely impact of these cohort differences on the secular increases in the consequences of these musculoskeletal changes.

Over the past several decades, we have made substantial improvement in our understanding of bone mass and strength and the risk factors that lead to the most important consequence, fractures. One of the most important advancements has been our ability to quantify bone mass and to identify a level of bone mass below which most fractures occur. Osteoporosis, the clinical consequence of the loss of bone strength is defined as a bone density 2.5 standard deviations below the normal mean.[95]

Sarcopenia, a term initially used by Rosenberg[96] in 1989, is used to describe the decline in muscle mass and strength that occurs with ageing. Much less is known about sarcopenia including the prevalence, incidence, aetiology, and consequences. The current chapter identifies many factors early in life which may contribute to sarcopenia and its related consequences. Nevertheless, a more systematic approach to sarcopenia is needed similar to that used to study osteoporosis several decades ago. Population-based normative data on lean mass across ages is needed. This could lead to the identification of an appropriate cut-off for sarcopenia similar to the approach used for osteoporosis.[95]

Finally, the prevalence of sarcopenia, osteoporosis or osteoarthritis in older women is substantial and increases markedly with age. It is estimated that 40% to 50% of women have osteoporosis or sarcopenia.[97,98] These conditions have a great impact on the quality of life, independence, disability of older persons. As described by Bassey, Aihie, Sayer, and Cooper, a life course research approach to determining their aetiology and prevention is likely to be the most effective public health approach.

References

1 **Simkin PA**. The musculoskeletal system. In: Klippel JH, Dieppe PA, eds. *Rheumatology*. London: Mosby; 1994:1.2.1–1.2.10.

2 **Kreisberg RA, Bowdoin B, Meador CK**. Measurement of muscle mass in humans by isotopic dilution of creatine 14C. *J Appl Physiol* 1970;**28**:264–7.

3 **Badley EM, Tennant A**. The changing profile of joint troubles with age: findings from a postal survey of the population. *Ann Rheum Dis* 1992;**51**:366–71.

4 **Cooper C, Dennison E**. The natural history and prognosis of osteoarthritis. In: Brandt K, Doherty M, Lohmander S, eds. *Textbook of osteoarthritis*. Oxford; Oxford University Press, 1998:237–49.

5 **Cooper C, Melton LJ**. Magnitude and impact of osteoporosis and fractures. In: Marcus R, Feldman D, Kelsey J, eds. *Osteoporosis*. Academic Press Inc, San Diego, 1996:419–34.

6 **Bassey EJ**. Physical capabilities, exercise and aging. *Rev Clin Geront* 1997;**7**:289–97.

7 **Leger J, Levy-Marchal C, Bloch J, Pinet A, Chevenne D, Porquet D**, *et al*. Reduced final height and indications for insulin resistance in 20 year olds born small for gestational age: regional cohort study. *Br Med J* 1997;**315**:341–7.

8 **Kahn H, Narayan K, Williamson D, Valdez R**. Relation of birthweight to lean and fat thigh tissue in young men. *Int J Obes Relat Metab Disord* 2000;**24**:667–72.

9 **Arden NK, Spector TD**. Genetic influences on muscle strength, lean body mass, and bone mineral density: a twin study. *J Bone Miner Res* 1997;**12**:2076–81.

10 **Penrose LS**. Some recent trends in human genetics. *Caryologia* 1954;**6**(**suppl**):521–30.

11 **Brooks AA, Johnson MR, Ster PJ, Pawson ME, Abdalla HI**. Birthweight: nature or nurture? *Early Hum Dev* 1999;**42**:29–35.

12 **Wigmore P, Stickland N**. Muscle development in large and small pig fetuses. *J Anatomy* 1983;**137**:235–45.

13 **Hediger M, Overpeck M, Kuczmarski R, McGlynn A, Maurer KR, Davis WW**, *et al*. Muscularity and fatness of infants and young children born small- or large-for-gestational age. *Paediatrics* 1998;**102**:E60.

14 **Gale CR, Martyn CN, Kellingray S, Eastell R, Cooper C**. Intrauterine programming of adult body composition. *J Clin Endocrinol Metab* 2001;**86**:267–72.

15 **Aihie Sayer A, Cooper C, Barker DJP**. Is lifespan determined *in utero*? *Arch Dis Child* 1997;**77**:162–4.

16 **Aihie Sayer A, Cooper C, Evans JR, Ralph A, Wormald RPL, Osmond C, Barker DJP**. Are rates of ageing determined *in utero*? *Age Ageing* 1998;**27**:579–83.

17 **Kuh D, Bassey, J, Hardy R, Aihie Sayer A, Wadsworth MEJ, Cooper C**. Birthweight, childhood size and muscle strength in adult life. *Am J Epidemiol*, in press.

18 **Doyle F, Brown J, Lachance C**. Relation between bone mass and muscle weight. *Lancet* 1970;**i**:391–3.

19 **Round J, Jones D, Honour J, Nevill A**. Hormonal factors in the development of differences in strength between boys and girls during adolescence: a longitudinal study. *Ann Human Biol* 1999;**26**:49–62.

20 **Eliakim A, Scheet T, Allmendiger N, Brasel JA, Cooper DM**. Training, muscle volume, and energy expenditure in non-obese American girls. *J Appl Physiol* 2001;**90**:35–44.

21 **Erens B, Primatesta P**. *Health Survey for England 1998. Cardiovascular disease. Volume 1*. Department of Health. The Stationery Office, London.

22 **Allied Dunbar National Fitness Survey**. *Main findings* 1992 (ISBN 1 872158 55 2) *and Technical Report* 1994 (ISBN 1 872158 48). The Sports Council and the Health Education Authority.

23 Taafe DR, Villa ML, Delay R, Marcus R. Maximal muscle strength of elderly women is not influenced by oestrogen status. *Age Ageing* 1995;**24**:329–33.

24 Bassey EJ, Mockett S, Fentem PH. Lack of variation in muscle strength with menstrual status in healthy women aged 45–54 years: data from a national survey. *Eur J Appl Physiol* 1996;**73**:382–6.

25 Armstrong AL, Osborne J, Coupland CAC, Macpherson MB, Bassey EJ, Wallace WA. Effects of hormone replacement therapy on muscle performance and balance in postmenopausal women. *Clin Sci* 1996;**91**:685–90.

26 Evans EM, Van Pelt RE, Binder EF, Williams DB, Ehsani AA, Kohrt WM. Effects of HRT and exercise training on insulin action, glucose tolerance and body composition in older women. *J Appl Physiol* 2001;**90**:2033–40.

27 Kohrt WM, Snead DB, Slatopolsky E, Birge S. Additive effects of weight-bearing exercise and estrogen on bone mineral density in older women. *J Bone Miner Res* 1995;**10**:1303–11.

28 Janse de Jonge XA, Boot CR, Thom JM, Ruell PA, Thompson MW. The influence of menstrual cycle phase on skeletal muscle contractile characteristics in humans. *J Physiol* 2001;**530**:161–6.

29 Greeves JP, Cable NT, Luckas MJM, Reilly T, Biljan MM. Effects of acute changes in oestrogen on muscle function of the first dorsal osseus muscle in humans. *J Physiol* 1997;**500**:265–70.

30 Bassey EJ. Longitudinal changes in selected physical capabilities: muscle strength, flexibility and body size. *Age Ageing* 1998;**27**:12–16.

31 Fiatarone MA, Marks EC, Ryan ND, Meredith CN, Lipsitz LA, Evans WJ. High intensity strength training in nonagenarians; effects on skeletal muscle. *J Am Med Assoc* 1990;**263**:3029–34.

32 Kallman D, Plato C, Tobin J. The role of muscle loss in the age-related decline of grip strength: cross-sectional and longitudinal perspectives. *J Gerontol A Biol Sci Med Sci* 1990;**45**:M82–8.

33 Waddell G, Feder G, McIntosh A, Lewis M, Hutchinson A. *Low back pain: evidence review*. Royal College of Practitioners, London, 1999.

34 Kuh DJL, Coggon D, Mann S, Cooper C, Yusuf E. Height, occupation and back pain in a national prospective study. *Br J Rheumatol* 1993;**32**:911–6.

35 Heliovaara M, Vanharanta H, Korpi J, Troup JDG. Herniated lumbar disc syndrome and vertebral canals. *Spine* 1986;**11**:433–5.

36 Smedley J, Egger P, Cooper C, Coggon D. Prospective cohort study of predictors of incident low back pain in nurses. *Br Med J* 1997;**314**:1225–8.

37 Harreby M, Hesseoe G, Kjer J, Neergaard K. Low back pain and physical exercise in leisure time in 38 year old women: a 25 year cohort study. *Eur Spine J* 1997;**6**:181–6.

38 Melton LJ, Atkinson EJ, O'Connor MK, O'Fallon WM, Riggs BL. Determinants of bone loss from the femoral neck in women of different ages. *J Bone Miner Res* 2000;**15**:24–31.

39 Hannan MT, Felson DT, Dawson-Hughes B, Tucker KL, Cupples LA, Wilson PW, *et al*. Risk factor for longitudinal bone loss in elderly men and women: the Framingham Osteoporosis Study. *J Bone Miner Res* 2000;**15**:710–20.

40 Cooper C, Barker DJP. Risk factors for hip fracture. *New Engl J Med* 1995;**332**:814–5.

41 Cooper C, Cawley MID, Bhalla A, Egger P, Ring F, Morton L, Barker DJP. Childhood growth, physical activity and peak bone mass in women. *J Bone Miner Res* 1995;**10**:940–7.

42 Godfrey K, Walker-Bone K, Robinson S, Taylor P, Shaw S, Wheeler T, Cooper C. Neonatal bone mass: influence of parental birthweight, maternal smoking, body composition and activity during pregnancy. *J Bone Miner Res* 2001;**16**:1694–1703.

43 Cooper C, Eriksson JF, Forsén T, Osmond C, Tuomilehto AJ, Barker DJP. Maternal height, childhood growth and risk of hip fracture in later life: a longitudinal study. *Osteoporosis Int* 2001;**12**:623–9.

44 Walker-Bone K, Dennison E, Cooper C. *Epidemiology of osteoporosis*. Rheumatic Disease Clinics of North America 2001;**27**:1–18.

45 Cooper C, Walker-Bone K, Arden N, Dennison E. Novel insights into the pathogenesis of osteoporosis: the role of intrauterine programming. *Rheumatology* 2000;**39**:1312–15.

46 Evans JG, Seagroatt V, Goldacre MJ. Secular trends in proximal femur fracture, Oxford record linkage study: area and England, 1968–1986. *J Epidemiol Comm Health* 1997;**51**:424–9.

47 Koo WW, Walters J, Bush AJ, Chesney RW, Carlson SE. Dual-energy X-ray absorptiometry studies of bone mineral status in new-born infants. *J Bone Miner Res* 1996;**11**:997–1102.

48 Jones G, Riley M, Dwyer T. Maternal smoking during pregnancy, growth, and bone mass in prepubertal children. *J Bone Miner Res* 1999;**14**:146–51.

49 Hamed HM, Purdie DW, Ramsden CS, Carmichael B, Steele SA, Howey S. Influence of birthweight on adult bone mineral density. *Osteoporosis Int* 1993;**3**:1–2.

50 Fewtrell MS, Prentice A, Jones SC, Bishop NJ, Stirling D, Buffenstein R, *et al.* Bone mineralization and turnover in preterm infants at 8–12 years of age: the effect of early diet. *J Bone Miner Res* 1999;**14**:810–20.

51 Cooper C, Fall C, Egger P, Hobbs R, Eastell R, Barker DJP. Growth in infancy and bone mass in later life. *Ann Rheum Dis* 1997;**56**:17–21.

52 Yarborough D, Barrett-Connor E, Morton D. Birthweight as a predictor of adult bone mass in postmenopausal women: the Rancho Bernardo Study. *Osteoporosis Int* 2000;**11**:626–30.

53 Cole T. Secular trends in growth. *Proc Nutr Soc* 2000;**59**:317–24.

54 Bailey DA, McKay HA, Mirwald RL, Crocker PR, Faulkner RA. A six-year longitudinal study of the relationship of physical activity to bone mineral accrual in growing children: the university of Saskatchewan bone mineral accrual study. *J Bone Miner Res* 1999;**14**:1672–9.

55 Parsons TJ, van Dusseldorp M, van der Vliet M, van der Werken K, Schaafama G, van Staveren WA. Reduced bone mass in Dutch adolescents fed a macrobiotic diet in early life. *J Bone Miner Res* 1997;**12**:1486–94.

56 Pettifor JM, Moodley GP. Appendicular bone mass in children with a high prevalence of low dietary calcium intakes. *J Bone Miner Res* 1997;**12**:1824–32.

57 Kardinaal AF, Ando S, Charles P, Charzewska J, Rotily M, Vaananen K, *et al.* Dietary calcium and bone density in adolescent girls and young women in Europe. *J Bone Miner Res* 1999;**14**:583–92.

58 Kannus P, Haapasalo H, Sankelo M, Sievanen H, Pasanen M, Heinonen A, *et al.* Effect of starting age of physical activity on bone mass in the dominant arm of tennis and squash players. *Ann Intern Med* 1995;**123**:27–31.

59 Fuchs R, Bauer J, Snow C. Jumping improves hip and lumbar spine bone mass in prepubescent childern: a randomized controlled trial. *J Bone Miner Res* 2001;**16**:148–56.

60 Bassey EJ, Ramsdale SJ. Increase in femoral bone density in young women following high impact exercise. *Osteoporosis Int* 1994;**4**:72–5.

61 Taaffe DR, Robinson TL, Snow CM, Marcus R. High-impact exercise promotes bone gain in well-trained female athletes. *J Bone Miner Res* 1997;**12**:255–60.

62 Kemper H, Twisk J, Van Mechelin W, *et al.* A fifteen-year longitudinal study in young adults on the relation of physical activity and fitness with the development of the bone mass: the Amsterdam Growth and Health Longitudinal Study. *Bone* 2000;**27**:847–53.

63 Keen A, Drinkwater B. Irreversible bone loss in former amenorrheic athletes. *Osteoporosis Int* 1997;**7**:311–5.

64 Welten DC, Kemper H, Post G, Van Staveren W. A meta-analysis of the effect of calcium intake on bone mass in young and middle-aged females and males. *J Nutr* 1995;**125**:2802–13.

65 Slemenda CW. Cigarettes and the Skeleton. *N Engl J Med* 1994;**330**:430–1.

66 Jones G, Scott FS. A cross-sectional study of smoking and bone mineral density in premenopausal parous women: effect of body mass index, breastfeeding, and sports participation. *J Bone Miner Res* 1999;**14**:1628–33.

67 Cooper C, Wickham C, Coggon D. Sedentary work in middle life and fracture of the proximal femur. *Br J Ind Med* 1990;**47**:69–70.

68 Jaglal SB, Kreiger N, Darlington G. Past and recent physical activity and risk of hip fracture. *Am J Epidemiol* 1993;**138**:107–18.

69 Kohrt WM, Ehsani AA, Birge SJ, Jr. Effects of exercise involving predominantly either joint-reaction or ground-reaction forces on bone mineral density in older women. *J Bone Miner Res* 1997;**12**:1253–61.

70 Kerr D, Morton A, Dick I, Prince R. Exercise effects on bone mass in postmenopausal women are site-specific and load-dependent. *J Bone Miner Res* 1996;**11**:218–25.

71 Krolner B, Toft B. Vertebral bone loss: an unheeded side effect of therapeutic bedrest. *Clin Sci* 1983;**64**:537–540.

72 Stone K, Bauer DC, Black DM, *et al.* Hormonal predictors of bone loss in elderly women: a prospective study. The Study of Osteoporotic Fractures Research Group. *J Bone Miner Res* 1998;**13**:1167–74.

73 Henderson NK, Price RI, Cole JH, Gutteridge DH, Bhagat CI. Bone density in young women is associated with body weight and muscle strength but not dietary intakes. *J Bone Miner Res* 1995;**10**:384–93.

74 Chapuy MC, Arlot ME, Duboeuf F, Brun J, Crouzet B, Arnaud S, *et al.* Vitamin D3 and calcium to prevent hip fractures in elderly women. *N Engl J Med* 1992;**327**:1637–42.

75 Buchner DM, Cress ME, de Lateur BJ, Esselman PC, Margherita AJ, Price R, *et al.* The effect of strength and endurance training on gait, balance, fall risk, and health services use in community-living older adults. *J Gerontol A Biol Sci Med Sci* 1997;**52**:M218–24.

76 Murray CJL, Lopez AD eds. The global burden of disease: a comprehensive assessment of mortality and disability from diseases, injuries and risk factors in 1990 and projected to 2020. Cambridge, MA: Harvard University Press, 1996.

77 Oliveria SA, Felson DT, Reed JI, Cirillo PA, Walker AM. Incidence of symptomatic hand, hip, and knee osteoarthritis among patients in a health maintenance organization. *Arthritis Rheum* 1995;**38**:1134–41.

78 Spector TD, Cicuttini F, Baker J, Loughlain J, Hart D. Genetic influences on osteoarthritis in women: a twin study. *Br Med J* 1996;**312**:940–44.

79 Hutton CW. Osteoarthritis: the cause not result of joint failure? *Ann Rheum Dis* 1989;**48**:958–61.

80 van den Berg R. The embryology of the musculoskeletal system. In Klippel JH, Dieppe PA, eds. *Rheumatology*. St Louis: Mosby, 1994:1.5.1–1.5.4.

81 Hay ED. Extracellular matrix, cell skeletons, and embryonic development. *Am J Med Genet* 1989;**34**:14–29.

82 Slack JM. Peptide regulatory factors in embryonic development. *Lancet* 1989;**i**:1312–5.

83 Drachman DB. Normal development and congenital malformation of joints. *Bull Rheum Dis* 1969;**19**:1.

84 Grahame R. Time to take hypermobility seriously (in adults and children). *Rheumatology* 2001;**40**:485–7.

85 Felson DT, Nevitt MC. The effects of oestrogen on osteoarthritis. *Curr Opin Rheumatol* 1998;**10**:269–72.

86 Oliveria SA, Felson DT, Cirillo PA, Reed JI, Walker AM. Body weight, body mass index, and incident symptomatic osteoarthritis of the hand, hip, and knee. *Epidemiology* 1999;**10**:161–6.

87 Cooper C. Osteoarthritis epidemiology. In Klippel JH, Dieppe PA, eds. *Rheumatology*. St Louis: Mosby, 1994:7.3.1–7.3.4.

88 Kealy RD, Lawler DF, Ballam JM, Lust G, Biery DN, Smith GK, Mantz SL. Evaluation of the effect of limited food consumption on radiographic evidence of osteoarthritis in dogs. *J Am Vet Med Assoc* 2000;**217**:1678–80.

89 McAlindon T, Felson DT. Nutrition: risk factors for osteoarthritis. *Ann Rheum Dis* 1997;**56**:397–402.

90 McAlindon TE, Felson DT, Zhang Y, Hannan MT, Aliabadi P, Weissman B, *et al*. Relation of dietary intake and serum levels of vitamin D to progression of osteoarthritis of the knee among participants in the Framingham Study. *Ann Intern Med* 1996;**25**:353–9.

91 Zhang Y, McAlindon TE, Hannan MT, Chaisson CE, Klein R, Wilson PW, Felson DT. Estrogen replacement therapy and worsening of radiographic knee osteoarthritis: the Framingham Study. *Arthritis Rheum* 1998;**41**:1867–73.

92 Dequeker J, Johnell O. Osteoarthritis protects against femoral neck fracture: the MEDOS study experience. *Bone* 1993;**14**:S51–S56.

93 Aihie Sayer A , Cooper C. Early undernutrition: good or bad for longevity? In Watson RR, ed. *Handbook of nutrition in the aged*. CRC Press Inc, 2000:97–114.

94 Kirkwood TB. What is the relationship between osteoarthritis and ageing? *Baillieres Clin Rheumatol* 1997;**11**:638–94.

95 Kanis JA, Melton LJ,III, Christiansen C, Johnston CC, Khaltaev N. The diagnosis of osteoporosis. *J Bone Miner Res* 1994;**9**:1137–41

96 Rosenberg IH. Summary comments. *Am J Clin Nutr* 1989;**50**:1231–33.

97 Looker AC, Orwoll ES, Johnston CC, *et al*. prevalence of low femoral bone density in older US adults from NHANES III. *J Bone Miner Res* 1997;**12**:1761–8.

98 Baumgartner RN, Koehler KM, Gallagher D, Romero L, Heymsfield SB, Ross RR, *et al*. Epidemiology of sarcopenia among the elderly in New Mexico. *Am J Epidemiol* 1998:**147**:755–63.

Chapter 8

Depression and psychological distress: a life course perspective

Barbara Maughan

Throughout the reproductive years, women are roughly twice as likely to experience clinically significant depression as men. The reasons for this increased vulnerability are not well understood, but a number of pointers are beginning to emerge. Depression is a complex disorder, reflecting influences of predisposing individual characteristics, early experiences and more immediately precipitating stressors; as a result, a number of different developmental pathways may be involved. Childhood adversities—including both lack of adequate parental care and exposure to abusive experiences—may predispose to depression in a variety of ways, affecting neurobiological, psychological, and social development. In addition, women's greater risk of exposure to sexual abuse may also contribute to their increased vulnerability. Childhood anxiety is more common in girls than boys, and often precedes depression, providing a further route for early sex-linked predispositions, while later in the life course women may be more susceptible than men to the depressogenic effects of some types of stressors, and use coping styles that reinforce rather than reduce an initial lowering of mood. Genetic factors also play a role in susceptibility to depression. Recent evidence suggests the possibility of sex differences in both the extent of heritability and the genetic risk factors involved. These variations may emerge after puberty, when women's increased risk of depression first becomes marked; as yet, however, the role of gonadal hormones is not well understood.

8.1 **Introduction**

Depression is a common, recurrent disorder, associated with both concurrent impairment and excess mortality.[1] In 1990, unipolar major depression was the fourth leading cause of disease burden in the world; by 2020, it is projected to be the second most important cause.[2] These findings are especially salient for women's health because throughout the reproductive years, women are roughly twice as likely to experience depression as men.[3] This gender difference in risk for depressive disorders is among the best replicated findings in psychiatric epidemiology; paradoxically, it also remains one of the least well understood.[4]

A complex array of factors—biological, psychological, and social—are now known to contribute to risk for depressive disorders. Understanding how they combine, their relative salience at different stages in the life course, and why women are at such markedly increased risk, constitute significant challenges for research. This chapter provides an overview of recent evidence on these three related themes. It begins by sketching in epidemiological findings on changing rates and gender ratios in depressive disorders from childhood to older age, highlighting the periods when women's increased vulnerability first emerges, and when it appears to decline. It then examines the main domains of risk for depressive conditions, exploring how far men and women differ in exposure or susceptibility to risks that affect both sexes, or whether some gender-specific risks may be involved. Throughout, it highlights the differing pathways through which individual vulnerabilities, childhood adversities and later stressors have been argued to combine in the genesis of depression.

8.2 Depression across the life course

Depressive phenomena—depressed mood, loss of interest and pleasure in life, and the negative cognitions and physiological disturbances that often accompany them—can be construed as both categories and dimensions. Debates continue over how best to sub-type severe depressions, and there is growing recognition that diagnostic criteria for depressive disorders impose somewhat arbitrary cut-points on what may well be a continuum of symptomatology.[5] Accepting that arbitrariness, epidemiological studies in the US,[6,7] Canada,[8] and the UK[9] converge in suggesting that in early and middle adulthood the point prevalence of the acute, two-week concurrence of symptoms required for a diagnosis of major depressive disorder (MDD) lies in the region of 2–5%. Estimates of lifetime prevalence are more varied; plausible estimates probably lie between 10% and 20%. In almost all studies women have been found to be about twice as likely to report unipolar depression as men. Adult women are also at increased risk of dysthymia (a less severe but more chronic lowering of mood) and of seasonal winter depression, though not of bipolar disorders (less common conditions involving both manic and depressive episodes). Historical trends in depression are difficult to determine, because both diagnostic criteria and assessment methods have changed with time; many commentators now agree, however, that overall rates of depression may have risen somewhat in recent decades, possibly accompanied by some slight narrowing of gender ratios.[10]

These findings relate to the main years of adulthood—broadly the period from the early 20s to the mid-50s. Data from childhood and adolescence qualify the epidemiological picture in important ways. Rates of depression are low in pre-pubertal children, and show few sex differences; where variations are reported, rates tend if anything to be higher in boys than in girls.[11,12] Two key changes then take place in the early teens. First, levels of depression begin to rise in both sexes; second, that rise is stronger in girls, so that by late adolescence the female preponderance typical of the adult years is clearly established. Figure 8.1 illustrates these trends with data from the Dunedin Multidisciplinary Study of Health and Development, a longitudinal study assessing the one-year prevalence of depression in the same age-cohort of young people at repeated points from ages 9 to 26 years.[13,14]

The precise timing of the increase amongst girls has been a matter of debate; evidence from a number of studies now converges, however, to suggest that the trend begins at or around age 13.[11] The Dunedin data suggest that gender ratios are at their most marked in the late teens and early twenties, and narrow a little thereafter. Figure 8.2 confirms this pattern, using data from the US National Comorbidity Survey—based on the same assessment protocol as the

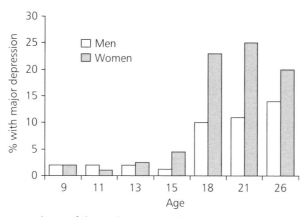

Fig. 8.1 One-year prevalence of depression, ages 9–26 years: Dunedin Multidisciplinary Health and Development Study.[13,14]

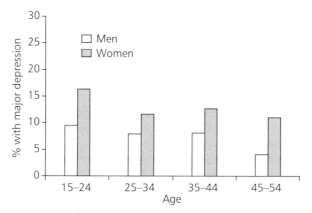

Fig. 8.2 One-year prevalence of depression, ages 15–54 years: National Comorbidity Survey.[15]

New Zealand study—showing cross-sectional findings on one-year prevalence rates for age-groups from the mid-teens to the mid-50s.[15] Surveys in older age often use somewhat different assessment tools, making it difficult to link trends at midlife with those later in the life course. Some studies have now, however, begun to bridge this epidemiological 'gap'. A large-scale Australian study, for example, found that rates of depression showed a slight decline between the mid-40s and the mid-60s in women, but a more marked drop thereafter.[16] For men, rates fell from the mid-50s, supporting the trends found in most studies of older adults[17] that levels of depression decline in older age, and that sex ratios narrow somewhat—or may even be reversed[18]—in the later adult years.

These striking gender differences in prevalence seem unlikely to be attributable to artefacts of measurement or diagnostic thresholds.[4] Although women do, for example, tend to report more depressive symptoms than men, a female preponderance is found even at sub-threshold symptom levels, and men and women who meet diagnostic criteria for depression show similar levels of associated impairment. One area where findings are less clear is in relation to risk of recurrence. Major depression is commonly a recurrent disorder, so that one possible basis for gender differences might lie in variations in vulnerability to second or subsequent episodes following an initial period of illness. At present, evidence is unclear on this issue. In the late teens and early 20s—when, as we have seen, gender differences are at their most marked—the Dunedin study found that the female excess was very largely explicable in terms of higher rates of new onsets among young women.[14] Studies in adulthood have produced less consistent findings. Some of the differences in point prevalence later in the life course might thus reflect variations in risk of recurrence; this could not, however, account for women's elevated rates of lifetime risk.

The sections that follow outline the core risks for adolescent and adult depression identified in the aetiological literature to date. Depression in childhood raises particular issues, beyond the scope of this chapter; these are discussed in several recent reviews.[11,19] Depression in older adults also raises specific concerns, and is associated with some specific patterns of risk. These are noted briefly here, and examined more fully elsewhere.[20]

8.3 Vulnerability and risk for depression in adolescence and adult life

Extensive evidence has now confirmed that depression is a complex disorder, showing influences of predisposing individual characteristics, prior experience, and more immediately precipitating stressors. Individual vulnerabilities appear to function in a variety of ways, influencing individual differences in responsivity to stress, in perceptions of the severity of stressful experiences, and also in the likelihood that individuals will follow life pathways that elevate risks of exposure to adversity. Many theoretical models postulate cumulating chains of risk reaching back to childhood; at this stage, however, most empirical evidence still rests on retrospective data collected in adult life. As prospective longitudinal studies mature, retrospective and short-term longitudinal findings are increasingly being tested in more appropriate designs. Wherever possible, prospective evidence of this kind is highlighted in the sections that follow.

8.3.1 Life events and difficulties

The pioneering studies of Brown and Harris in the 1970s[21] showed that acute stressful life events and longer term difficulties play an important role in the precipitation of many first episodes of depression. Experiences involving loss, humiliation or 'entrapment'—being caught, for example, in a poor job or a poor marriage—seem central to these effects in adult life. Exposure to stressful events markedly increases risk of a depressive episode in the immediately succeeding weeks or months; in one recent study, for example, 35% of women without prior histories of depression developed an episode within one month of experiencing a stressful event.[22] Acute events—especially those centring on relationship difficulties and personal disappointments—also function as risks for depression in adolescence, often developing in the context of more chronic stressors such as parental discord, bullying, and exposure to physical, sexual or emotional abuse.[23] In older age the nature of life stressors changes; health related disability and loss of close social contacts are among the most common precursors of first onsets of depression, but ongoing difficulties account for most episodes.[24]

There is now considerable evidence that the strength of the association between life events and onset declines progressively with the number of previous episodes; although adverse events are central in many first episodes, over the course of illness, risk of subsequent onsets becomes increasingly autonomous from environmental precipitants.[22] These findings are consistent with the view (often described as the 'kindling' hypothesis), that the experience of an initial episode sensitizes individuals to future depression through changes in cognitions or neurobiological processes associated with response to stress.[25]

Do men and women differ in exposure or response to life stresses? Findings on exposure vary, but a number of studies have now reported that women seem more likely to develop depression in response to particular types of stress. Losses or interpersonal problems involving immediate loved ones seem equally likely to provoke depression in both sexes. Where differences have been noted is in relation to 'network' events that affect a broader circle of kin and friends (perhaps reflecting the 'cost of caring' arising from women's greater involvement in the lives of those around them),[26] or in role domains where women typically have greatest investment.[27] In addition, there is some evidence that women are more likely to become depressed following other types of events such as moving house, physical attack, and life-threatening illness or injury.[28] These findings are less easily understood in terms of differential role involvement. If replicated, they suggest that sex differences in stress responsivity—whether genetically, biologically, psychologically, or socially determined—may contribute in important ways to women's increased risk for depression. We turn now to explore some of those possibilities.

8.3.2 Genetic influences

Numerous family and twin studies have now shown that depression is a familial disorder, and that a substantial part of that familiality reflects heritable risks. A recent meta-analysis of results from twin studies in early and middle adulthood produced a point estimate of heritability of the liability to MDD of 37%, 95% confidence interval (CI)=31–42%.[29] Corrected for unreliability in diagnostic assessments, the true figure could be considerably higher. Evidence for environmental influences shared within the family was minimal; the remaining variance in these twin studies—estimated at just over 60%—was thus attributable to individual-specific environmental risks. Twin studies in adolescence (currently based on depression scale scores, rather than on measures of diagnostic categories) suggest a similar picture. Although findings vary somewhat by reporter, adolescent depressive symptomatology also appears to involve a clear heritable component.[11] At this stage, evidence from genetically sensitive designs is not available in older age. In one cross-sectional study of older adults, however, family history was less strongly predictive of depression than in younger age-groups, and a past history of depression declined in predictive power with age.[30] In part, these findings may reflect failure of recall of past episodes with increasing age. In addition, the selective early death of individuals with prior histories of depression may mean that the heritability of late-life depression is indeed lower than in younger age-groups.

Genetic risks are likely to act through multiple mechanisms, direct and indirect. Indirect influences include effects on previous episodes of disorder, on personality characteristics such as neuroticism that show strong links with depression,[31] and on the interplay between genetic and environmental risks. Two mechanisms have attracted particular attention here: first, genetic control of *sensitivity* to the environment—whereby genetic predisposition affects vulnerability to environmental stressors—and second, genetic control of *exposure* to the environment, whereby genetic factors influence the probability that individuals select themselves into environments carrying different degrees of risk.[32] This second model—supported by evidence, for example, that exposure to stressful life events also shows genetic influence, overlapping with risk for MDD[33]—is especially salient from a life course perspective.

For many years it was thought unlikely that genetic factors could contribute to sex differences in depression. One recent large-scale study has, however, reported a significantly greater heritability of the liability to lifetime risk of broadly-defined MDD in women, with similar but non-significant trends on more stringent definitions of disorder.[34] This study also found that although positively correlated, genetic risk factors were not identical in the two sexes. Possible bases for such genetic variations are not known, but the authors raise a number of speculative suggestions. Variations in biological factors—especially perhaps exposure to gonadal hormones—might elicit genetic variations in men and women; differences in social experiences might function in a similar way. Alternatively, the 'psychopathological pathways' to depression might differ between the sexes, with precursors in men centring on externalizing traits, those in women depending more heavily on internalizing syndromes such as anxiety.

Findings in adolescence add to this picture. As outlined above, rates of depression rise sharply around the time of puberty, especially in girls. One study of pre- and post-pubertal twins[35] found that the impact of life events was significantly increased in post-pubertal girls, and that heritability for depression was also higher in this older group. Part of the liability to both depression and to life events could be linked to a common set of genes, and the data reflected a clear developmental increase in genetic variance for life events in post-pubertal girls. If replicated, these findings raise the intriguing possibility that new genes for depression may be 'switched on' at puberty in girls.

8.3.3 Childhood adversities

In addition to adult stressors, an extensive body of evidence has now documented links between adverse childhood experiences and vulnerability to depression in adult life.[36–38] Lack of adequate parental care,[39] along with potentially traumatic experiences such as exposure to physical or sexual abuse[40] seem central to these effects. Other factors often associated with poor parenting such as discord or violence between parents, parental divorce, or a family history of mental health or alcohol problems, also show links with increased risk of depression.[41]

How might early experiences affect vulnerability to later psychiatric disturbance? Two different issues are involved: first, how early adversity affects development in childhood, and second, how effects are carried forward to adult life.[42] Studies of the short-term impact of abusive experiences in childhood suggest effects on multiple developmental systems including emotion regulation, attachment security, quality of peer relationships and the development of the self-system.[43] Each of these might plausibly contribute to long-term risk. In addition, neurobiological processes may also be involved. Recent years have seen an expansion in pre-clinical studies of the effects of early stress, providing clear evidence that adverse rearing conditions can promote long-term changes in many of the neurotransmitter systems and brain structures implicated in vulnerability to depression.[44] In animal studies these effects are moderated both by subsequent caregiving and by genetic factors: species with more intrinsic reactivity show greater response to environmental manipulations, and environmental change has greater impact on some neurobiological systems than others. Although caution is clearly needed in extrapolating from these findings, early evidence suggests that women with retrospectively reported histories of child abuse do show increased pituitary-adrenal and autonomic responses to stress.[45]

Mechanisms mediating the long-term impact of these effects are likely to be complex. At the most general level commentators have distinguished between *latency* or *trauma* models (also referred to as 'programming')—whereby early experience has a direct effect on later functioning—and *pathways* models, whereby effects cumulate across development, mediated and moderated by individual characteristics and intervening events. In the psychosocial domain, for example, Brown and his colleagues[46] have developed a two-route model, with early adversity functioning to elevate risks through both 'external' environmental and 'internal' psychological pathways. Figure 8.3 provides a simplified version of key elements of this model. On the external, 'outer world' path, lack of childhood care is seen as increasing risks of a cumulating chain of environmental adversities in childhood and early adulthood, each contributing to increased social vulnerability later in life. Early or unplanned pregnancy, often followed by single parenthood, low social status and poor emotional support in adulthood, have emerged as central themes in this path. On the internal, psychological pathway lack of childhood care is argued to contribute to emotional vulnerability through effects on the self-system and on coping skills. Prospective evidence from the MRC National Survey of Health and Development (NSHD) has now extended this picture, highlighting the role of interpersonal competence in mediating effects of early parental style,[47] consonant with formulations from attachment theory that the key sequelae of disrupted or inadequate parent–child relationships may lie in effects on later relationship capacities. The first study of monozygotic (MZ) twins discordant for depression[48] provides further echoes of this pattern. It highlighted three distinct clusterings of risk, one centring on childhood anxiety and overprotective parenting, a second on adolescent rebelliousness and stress-prone adult life pathways, and a third on lack of warmth in parenting, disturbed interpersonal relationships, and poor social support.

These findings provide a rich basis for the development of life course models of vulnerability to depression, with the potential to integrate findings across many established domains of risk. However, they suggest a complex interweaving of effects, and raise as many questions as they answer. For many years, debates centred on the extent to which early adversity conveyed a general susceptibility to psychological distress or a more latent vulnerability, only activated in the face of later stressors. More recent concerns have centred on the specificity of the effects involved, both in terms of developmental pathways and psychopathological outcomes;[49] how findings on early experience can best be integrated with

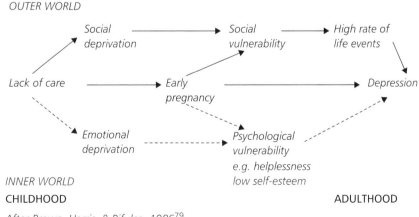

After Brown, Harris, & Bifulco, 1986[79]

Fig. 8.3 Hypothesized life course pathways for effects of childhood adversity.

knowledge of genetic risks; how far adverse effects of early experience persist or attenuate with age;[41,50] and, especially pertinent from the perspective of gender differences, the extent to which childhood adversities function more strongly as predisposing factors in women than in men.[51] Although there is little reason to think that boys and girls will be differentially exposed to many types of early adversity, one—sexual abuse—is clearly more common among girls. Numerous retrospective studies have now documented the much increased risks of depression (and other psychiatric disorders) faced by women who report sexual abuse in childhood. Prospective data in this area are still limited, and may suggest more modest effects; at this stage, however, it seems likely that early abusive experiences may play a more significant role in contributing to women's increased vulnerability than has previously been appreciated.

8.3.4 Reproductive age, gonadal hormones, and depression

The sharp rise in depression in the teens has inevitably highlighted this period as a key developmental 'window' for investigating risk. In addition to the biological changes of puberty, the early adolescent years are typically marked by changes in young people's social roles, in relationships with parents, peers and romantic partners, and often in the school environment. Each might plausibly be implicated in risk for depression. Particular interest has focused on the social/psychological effects of the timing of puberty, following evidence that disruptive behaviour problems increase in adolescence among girls who mature earlier than their peers, mediated via their increased likelihood of associating with older friends.[52] In relation to depression, however, current findings suggest that pubertal status *per se* may be more influential. One recent epidemiological study has reported, for example, that rates of unipolar depression rose sharply in girls at Tanner stage III.[53] Examination of associated hormonal changes showed no effects of the trophic hormones (follicle-stimulating hormone and luteinizing hormone), but high levels of testosterone and oestrogen were strongly implicated, accounting for all of the effects of Tanner stage in multivariate analyses.[54]

These findings suggest that rather than simply acting as a marker for the morphological changes of puberty, gonadal hormones may be more directly involved in susceptibility to depression. Oestrogens are known to influence a broad range of central nervous system (CNS) sub-systems putatively involved in the regulation of mood, behaviour, and cognition, generally functioning in protective and homeostatic ways.[55] The literature on links between oestrogen levels and mood changes during the course of women's reproductive years is, however, far from straightforward. Low oestrogen levels have been implicated in the mood changes of the late-luteal premenstrual period, and there is some evidence both that follicular phase oestrogen levels are lower in depressed women than controls,[56] and that transdermal oestrogen replacement is effective in the treatment of depression in perimenopausal women.[57] The rise in oestrogen levels in pregnancy is not, however, accompanied by any marked decrease in depression, and falling oestrogen levels at the menopause—although clearly associated with vasomotor symptoms, accelerated decrease in bone mineral density, and with a decrease in some cognitive functions—do not appear to be associated with any increase in depression. Indeed, though it has long been assumed that the menopause constitutes a period of increased risk for low mood for many women, both the broader epidemiological literature and studies specific to the menopausal years[58] have now shown that this view may be misplaced. In the NSHD, for example, repeated assessments between ages 47 and 52 showed no association between menopausal status and levels of psychological symptoms, though hormone replacement therapy (HRT) users did show higher levels of symptomatology.[59] Instead, pre-existing vulnerabilities, poor physical health and exposure to stressors constituted the key risks for anxiety and low mood over the menopausal transition.

How can these varying findings be reconciled? One proposal[54] is that rather than reflecting absolute oestrogen levels (high or low), vulnerability to depression may be associated with *cyclicity* in gonadal hormones. Throughout the reproductive years, women are exposed to repeated fluctuations in hormone levels, and so also to associated increases and decreases in the CNS and other processes influenced by them. These repeated fluctuations may function as an instability factor contributing—probably in interaction with heritable characteristics and environmental stressors—to risk for depression in vulnerable individuals.

8.3.5 Personality, psychological vulnerability, and prior disorder

A variety of personality characteristics, cognitive styles and coping strategies are also strongly associated with depression. Among personality features, neuroticism shows the most consistent links, and shares genetic variance with MDD.[31] Personality characteristics might affect risk for depression in a variety of ways; adult studies have shown, for example, that neuroticism is associated with differential risk of exposure to life events, with variations in the perceived severity of events, and also with variations in vulnerability to event-related psychological distress. Longer term prospective studies are now beginning to clarify that picture. In the NSHD, neuroticism assessed in the teens predicted exposure to life events some twenty years later, and also increased sensitivity to the depressogenic effects of adult stress.[60] It is unclear at this stage how far early personality factors function primarily as markers for adult characteristics that constitute the key moderators, or whether more complex developmental processes are involved, with effects cumulating across the life course.

Cognitive theories of depression highlight the negative attributional styles and cognitive biases seen in many depressed individuals, whereby the self, the future and the world are viewed in negative, dysfunctional ways.[61,62] Depressed people regard themselves as unworthy and undesirable, expect failure and rejection, and often interpret their experiences as confirming those expectations. These cognitive schemas are argued to be acquired from early experience, and to be activated by exposure to experiences of rejection or deprivation later in life. Low self-esteem may also mediate the difficulties in establishing and sustaining close interpersonal relationships found in many individuals with depression. From an aetiological perspective, however, there are problems in determining the direction of effects involved here, as low self-esteem may be an outcome of, as much as a contributor to, depression.[63] From the perspective of gender differences, there is also little clear evidence that men and women in non-depressed samples differ in their attributional styles. Clearer gender differences have emerged in relation to coping styles—the ways in which individuals respond to an initial lowering of mood.[64] Here, evidence suggests that men tend to use more active coping strategies, distracting themselves through involvement in activity, while women have a more ruminative style, likely to prolong depressed mood. Neurocognitive studies suggest that variations of this kind may indeed have implications for differential activation of brain regions associated with depression.[65]

One further set of precursor conditions lies in the realm of early onset psychiatric disorders. Depression is frequently comorbid with anxiety disorders in adulthood, and there has been considerable interest in the developmental patterning of these conditions earlier in life. As we have seen, diagnoses of depression are rare before puberty, but pre-pubertal anxiety is much more common, and shows a clear female excess.[66] First onset of anxiety disorders typically occurs in childhood and early adolescence—well before the main rise in rates of depression—and prospective studies have now confirmed that pre-existing anxiety disorders function as strong risks for onset of depression in adolescence and early adulthood, with odds ratios in one study ranging from 1.7 for specific phobias to 3.9 for generalized anxiety disorder.[67] How far these associations reflect shared risk factors or other aetiological mechanisms remains to be clarified. In addition, girls who show conduct problems may also be at increased risk of depression later in life. Though little highlighted in the depression literature to date, this pattern has been noted in a number of prospective follow-up studies,[68,69] and is reminiscent of the 'rebellious' cluster identified among discordant MZ twins.[48] Adolescent girls with conduct problems often follow stress-prone life pathways likely to increase exposure to adverse life events.[69] It is unclear at this stage how far these alone account for their increased risk, or whether prior comorbidity with depression or other vulnerability factors are also involved.

8.3.6 Social and cultural influences

In addition to these individually-based influences, epidemiological findings suggest that broader social factors are also implicated in risk for depression. Low socioeconomic status is associated with a higher prevalence of affective disorders,[70] and though part of this association may reflect selection effects, some causal influences also seem likely to be involved.[71] Quite how these are mediated is far from certain; most commentators conclude, however, that the effects of low social status and financial hardship are likely to be indirect, operating to increase exposure to more proximal personal and interpersonal risks.[72]

Rates of depression also vary by marital status. In general, marriage shows 'protective' effects against low mood, while higher rates of distress are found among the separated, widowed, and divorced. Importantly, these marital status effects also vary by gender: the excess of depression in women is most marked among the married, less notable among the widowed and divorced, and least evident of all among adults who remain single.[3,73] Young married women looking after small children seem especially at risk, as do single mothers.[72] This suggests that aspects of social roles may contribute to risk for depression, whether through role overload or underload, through overinvestment in a limited number of roles, or through the value (or lack of it) that individuals attach to the social categories they occupy. This last possibility is underscored by findings that gender differences are much less marked in cultural groups where a high value is typically placed on caring and homemaker roles.[74,75]

Increasingly women combine childcare with work outside the home. In general, employment has been found to be beneficial for psychological health, providing interest, fulfilment, and social contacts as well as access to financial rewards. Not unexpectedly, however, these benefits vary between men and women, and also among women in different social circumstances: the advantages of work are less marked for married than for single women, weaker if they have children, and weakest of all for those with children of pre-school age.[3] Once again, role strain and role overload have been argued to be key contributors to these effects.

8.4 Conclusions

The female preponderance in adult depression has been evident for many years. Perhaps surprisingly, the developmental 'profile' of these effects at different stages in the life course has only been established quite recently, and evidence on possible contributory factors is evolving even more rapidly, often overturning previously held views. As we have seen, it is now plausible to assume that heritable, biological, psychological, and experiential influences all contribute to women's increased vulnerability to depression, and that a variety of distinct developmental pathways may be involved. New research strategies continue to contribute new insights. The advent of molecular genetic studies, along with fuller exploration of neurobiological effects, promise especially important advances here. Integrating findings from these diverse areas of enquiry will undoubtedly present significant challenges; the heavy burden of psychological distress faced by many women across the life course underscores the urgency of this task.

Commentary on 'Depression and psychological distress: a life course perspective'

Bryan Rodgers

Barbara Maughan has provided a very thorough account of the current research evidence on life course influences on depression and psychological distress, with an emphasis on processes that differ between men and women. It is a puzzle that an apparently simple and well-replicated finding, that women have roughly double the rates of disorder of men over the adult years, has no ready explanation. We are still pursuing answers through research strategies involving a wide range of genetic, biological and psychosocial mechanisms. What is clear from this chapter, however, is the fundamentally developmental nature of the aetiology of these disorders. The first onset of depression most often occurs in the teenage years or early adulthood, a pattern not unlike that for many other adult psychiatric disorders (dementia being the notable exception), and often follows a chronic or recurrent course. Risk factors include genetic predisposition, environmental exposures in early life, and triggering events and circumstances at the time of onset of episodes. Unlike many chronic physical disorders, the prevalence of depression appears substantially lower in late adulthood compared to midlife.

Even in regard to basic findings on age differences, our existing knowledge has limitations. The results from the Dunedin Multidisciplinary Health and Development Study (Fig. 8.1) are one of the few examples of such data from longitudinal investigation and most evidence comes from cross-sectional studies. Consequently, there is no certainty that the lower prevalence of depression found in older adults represents a true developmental age change rather than a difference between cohorts born in different circumstances.[10] The answers to more subtle questions as to whether age changes follow a steady linear gradient, an accelerating decrease with age[76] or a plateau followed by a more precipitous fall in prevalence must await further prospective studies.

The emergence of gender differences in depression around puberty does have the support of longitudinal evidence and there is growing evidence of links with the timing of menarche[77] and associated hormonal changes in adolescent girls. However, research on pregnancy and the menopause does not fit neatly with a model of hormonal-mediated changes. There are several possible explanations. One is that pubertal change could be a marker or mediator of emerging differences in social roles, especially those relating to affiliative and caring behaviour in women.[26,78] Another is that biological changes may only influence the first onset of disorder. The significance of first onset is a recurring theme in relation to gender differences in depression at puberty,[14] for gender differences later in the life course,[15] and for the significance of childhood adversity for adult disorder.[49] Studies of the menopause may fail to detect any changes comparable to those associated with puberty because of their focus on the prevalence rather than the incidence of depression.

One further theme to emerge from studies to date is that research has moved away from delineating simple differences in rates of disorder between men and women towards addressing more complex interactions, in both the statistical and developmental senses. As a minimum, our explanatory models now need to consider how gender differences in depression vary across different environmental exposures. In some instances, these models are moving towards the description of processes that are gender-specific. This does not imply that depression has different consequences for men and women, in terms of personal distress or disability, nor deny that there are common aetiological factors, but it emphasizes that there are gender differences in mechanisms and not just outcomes. There is a potential for further consideration of more complex interactions, not only involving gender but other combinations of risk factors, including factors from the different domains covered by this review (genetic, biological and psychosocial). The magnitude of this task appears daunting but drawing on relevant theoretical models provides a guide to the prioritizing of research questions.

Although a considerable amount of research has been conducted in this area over several decades, there are clear gaps in our knowledge. There is a need for more prospective longitudinal research, for studies that encompass the incidence as well as prevalence of depression, and for an interdisciplinary approach that brings together data on genetic, biological, and psychosocial factors. Such research may not only improve explanations of gender differences in depression but can also identify better the underlying processes that apply separately to women and men.

References

1 Harris EC, Barraclough BB. Excess mortality of mental disorder. *Br J Psychiatry* 1998;**173**:11–53.

2 Murray CJL, Lopez AD. Evidence-based health policy: lessons from the Global Burden of Disease Study. *Science* 1996;**274**:740–3.

3 Bebbington PE. Sex and depression. *Psychol Med* 1998;**28**:1–8.

4 Piccinnelli M, Wilkinson G. Gender differences in depression: critical review. *Br J Psychiatry* 2000;**177**:486–92.

5 Kendler KS, Gardner CO. Boundaries of major depression: an evaluation of DSM-IV criteria. *Am J Psychiatry* 1998;**155**:172–77.

6 Weissman MM, Leaf PJ, Tishchler GL, Blazer DG, Karno M, Bruce ML, Florio LP. Affective disorders in five United States communities. *Psychol Med* 1988;**18**:141–53.

7 Blazer DG, Kessler RC, McGonagle KA, Swartz MS. The prevalence and distribution of major depression in a national community sample: the National Comorbidity Survey. *Am J Psychiatry* 1994;**151**:979–86.

8 **Bland RC, Orn H, Newman SC**. Epidemiology of psychiatric disorders in Edmonton. *Acta Psychiatr Scand* 1988;(**Suppl 1–80**).

9 **Jenkins R, Lewis G, Bebbington P, Brugha T, Farrell M, Gill B, Meltzer**. The National Psychiatric Morbidity Surveys of Great Britain—initial findings from the household survey. *Psychol Med* 1997;**27**:775–89.

10 **Fombonne E**. Time trends in affective disorders. In Cohen P, Slomkowski C, Robins LN, eds. *Historical and geographical influences on psychopathology*. New Jersey: Lawrence Erlbaum; 1999:115–39.

11 **Angold A, Costello EJ**. The epidemiology of depression in children and adolescents. In: Goodyer IM ed. *The Depressed Child and Adolescent*. 2nd ed Cambridge: Cambridge University Press; 2001:143–78.

12 **Harrington R**. Affective disorders. In: Rutter M, Taylor E, eds. *Child and Adolescent Psychiatry: Modern Approaches, Fourth Edition*, in press.

13 **Moffitt TE, Caspi A**. Personal communication 2001.

14 **Hankin BL, Abramson LY, Moffitt TE, Silva PA, McGee R, Angell K**. Development of depression from preadolescence to young adulthood: emerging gender differences in a 10-year longitudinal study. *J Abnorm Psychol* 1998;**107**:128–40.

15 **Kessler RC, McGonagle KA, Swartz M, Blazer DG, Nelson CB**. Sex and depression in the National Comorbidity Survey I: Lifetime prevalence, chronicity and recurrence. *J Affective Disord* 1993;**29**:85–96.

16 **Henderson S, Andrews G, Hall W**. Australia's mental health: an overview of the general population survey. *Aus NZ J Psychiatry* 2000;**34**:197–205.

17 **Beekman ATF, Copeland JRM and Prince MJ**. Review of community prevalence of depression in later life. *Br J Psychiatry* 1999;**174**:307–11.

18 **Bebbington PE, Dunn G, Jenkins R, Lewis G, Brugha T, Farrell M, Meltzer H**. The influence of age and sex on the prevalence of depressive conditions: report from the National Survey of Psychiatric Morbidity. *Psychol Med* 1998;**28**:9–19.

19 **Goodyer IM**. *The Depressed Child and Adolescent*. 2nd ed. Cambridge: Cambridge University Press; 2001.

20 **Prince MJ, Beekman AJF**. The aetiology of late-life depression. In: Copeland J, Abou-Saleh M, Blazer D, eds. *Principles & Practice of Geriatric Psychiatry*. Second edition. Chichester: Wiley;2001:

21 **Brown GW, Harris T**. *Social origins of depression*. London: Tavistock; 1978.

22 **Kendler KS, Thornton LM, Gardner CO**. Stressful life events and previous episodes in the etiology of major depression in women: an evaluation of the 'kindling' hypothesis. *Am J Psychiatry* 2000;**157**:1243–51.

23 **Goodyer IM**. Life events: their nature and effects. In: Goodyer IM, ed. *The Depressed Child and Adolescent*. 2nd ed. Cambridge: Cambridge University Press, 2001, pp. 204–32.

24 **Brilman EI, Ormel J**. Life events, difficulties and onset of depressive episodes in later life. *Psychol Med* 2001;**31**:859–69.

25 **Post RM**. Transduction of psychosocial stress into the neurobiology of recurrent affective disorder. *Am J Psychiatry* 1992;**149**:999–1010.

26 **Kessler RC, McLeod JD**. Sex differences in vulnerability to undesirable life events. *American Sociological Review* 1984;**49**:620–31.

27 **Nazroo JY, Edwards AC, Brown GW**. Gender differences in onset of depression following a shared life event: a study of couples. *Psychol Med* 1997;**27**:9–19.

28 **Maciejewski PK, Prigerson HG, Mazure CM**. Sex differences in event-related risk for major depression. *Psychol Med* 2001;**31**:593–604.

29 **Sullivan PF, Neale MC, Kendler KS**. Genetic epidemiology of major depression: review and meta-analysis. *Am J Psychiatry* 2000;**157**:1552–62.

30 **van Ojen R, Hooijer C, Bezemer D, Jonker C, Lindeboom J, van Tilburg W**. The relationship between psychiatric history, MMSE and family history. *Br J Psychiatry* 1995;**166**:316–9.

31 **Roberts SB, Kendler KS**. Neuroticism and self-esteem as indices of the vulnerability to major depression in women. *Psychol Med* 1999;**29**:1101–9.

32 **Kendler KS**. Major depression and the environment: a psychiatric genetic perspective. *Pharmacopsychiatry* 1998;**31**:5–9.

33 **Kendler KS, Karkowski-Shuman L**. Stressful life events and genetic liability to major depression: genetic control of exposure to the environment? *Psychol Med* 1997;**27**:539–47.

34 **Kendler KS, Gardner CO, Neale MC, Prescott CA**. Genetic risk factors for major depression in men and women: similar or different heritabilities and same or partly distinct genes? *Psychol Med* 2001;**31**:605–16.

35 **Silberg J, Pickles A, Rutter M, Hewitt J, Simonoff E, Maes H, Carbonneau R, Murrelle L, Foley D, Eaves L**. The influence of genetic factors and life stress on depression among adolescent girls. *Arch Gen Psychiatry* 1999;**56**:225–32.

36 **Maughan B, McCarthy G**. Childhood adversities and psychosocial disorders. *Br Med Bull* 1997;**53**:156–69.

37 **Rodgers B**. Adult affective disorder and early environment. *Br J Psychiatry* 1990;**157**:539–550.

38 **Sadowski H, Ugarte B, Kolvin I, Kaplan C, Barnes J**. Early life family disadvantages and major depression in adulthood. *Br J Psychiatry* 1999;**174**:112–20.

39 **Parker G**. Early environment. In Paykel ES, ed. *Handbook of affective disorders*. 2nd ed. New York: Guilford; 1992:171–83.

40 **Mullen PE, Martin JL, Anderson JC, Romans SE, Herbison GP**. Childhood sexual abuse and mental health in adult life. *Br J Psychiatry* 1993;**163**:721–32.

41 **Kessler RC, Magee WJ**. Childhood adversities and adult depression: basic patterns of association in a US national survey. *Psychol Med* 1993;**23**:679–90.

42 **Rutter M, Maughan B**. Psychosocial adversities in childhood and adult psychopathology. *J Personal Disord* 1997;**11**:4–18.

43 **Cicchetti D, Toth SL**. A developmental psychopathology perspective on child abuse and neglect. *J Am Acad Child Adolesc Psychiatry* 1995;**34**:541–65.

44 **Kaufman J, Plotsky PM, Nemeroff CB, Charney DS**. Effects of early adverse experience on brain structure and function: clinical implications. *Biol Psychiatry* 2000;**48**:778–90.

45 **Heim C, Newport DJ, Heit S, Graham YP, Wilcox M, Bonsall R, Miller AH, Nemeroff C**. Pituitary-adrenal and autonomic responses to stress in women after sexual and physical abuse in childhood. *J Am Med Assoc* 2000;**284**:592–7.

46 **Harris T, Brown GW, Bifulco A**. Loss of parent in childhood and adult psychiatric disorder: a tentative overall model. *Dev Psychopathol* 1990;**2**:311–28.

47 **Rodgers B**. Reported parental behaviour and adult affective symptoms. 2. Mediating factors. *Psychol Med* 1996;**26**:63–77.

48 **Kendler KS, Gardner CO**. Monozygotic twins discordant for major depression: a preliminary exploration of the role of environmental experiences in the aetiology and course of illness. *Psychol Med* 2001;**31**:411–23.

49 **Kessler RC, Davis CG, Kendler KS**. Childhood adversity and adult psychiatric disorder in the US National Comorbidity Survey. *Psychol Med* 1997;**27**:1101–19.

50 **Bifulco A, Brown GW, Moran P, Ball C, Campbell C**. Predicting depression in women: the role of past and present vulnerability. *Psychol Med* 1998;**28**:39–50.

51 Veijola J, Puukka P, Lehtinen V, Moring J, Lingholm T, Väisänen E. Sex differences in the association between childhood experiences and adult depression. *Psychol Med* 1998;**28**:21–7.

52 Stattin H, Magnusson D. *Paths Through Life: Pubertal Maturation in Female Development.* Hillsdale, NJ: Lawrence Erlbaum, 1990.

53 Angold A, Costello EJ, Worthman CM. Puberty and depression: the roles of age, pubertal status and pubertal timing. *Psychol Med* 1998;**28**:51–61.

54 Angold A, Costello EJ, Erkanli A, Worthman CM. Pubertal changes in hormone levels and depression in girls. *Psychol Med* 1999;**29**:1043–53.

55 Halbreich U. Gonadal hormones, reproductive age, and women with depression. *Arch Gen Psychiatry* 2000;**57**:1163–4.

56 Young EA, Midgley AR, Carlson NE, Brown MB. Alteration in the hypothalamic-pituitary-ovarian axis in depressed women. *Arch Gen Psychiatry* 2000;**57**:1157–62.

57 de Novaes Soares C, Almeida OP, Joffe H, Cohen LS. Efficacy of estradiol for the treatment of depressive disorders in perimenopausal women. *Arch Gen Psychiatry* 2001;**58**:529–34.

58 Dennerstein L, Lehert P, Burger H, Dudley E. Mood and menopausal transition. *J Nerv Ment Dis* 1999;**187**:685–91.

59 Kuh D, Hardy R, Rodgers B, Wadsworth MEJ. Lifetime risk factors for women's psychological distress at midlife, *Soc Sci Med*, in press.

60 van Os J, Jones P. Early risk factors and adult person-environment relationships in affective disorder. *Psychol Med* 1999;**29**:1055–67.

61 Abramson LY, Metalsky GI, Alloy LB. Hopelessness: a theory-based subtype of depression. *Psychol Rev* 1989;**96**:358–72.

62 Beck AT, Rush AJ, Shaw BF, Emery G. *Cognitive Therapy of Depression.* London: John Wiley, 1980.

63 Haaga DAF, Dyck MJ, Ernst D. Empirical status of cognitive theory of depression. *Psychol Bull* 1991;**110**:215–36.

64 Nolen-Hoeksma S, Parker LE, Larson J. Ruminative coping with depressesd mood following loss. *J Pers Soc Psychol* 1994;**67**:92–104.

65 Heller W. Gender differences in depression: perspectives from neuropsychology. *J Affective Disord* 1993;**29**:129–43.

66 Meltzer H, Gatwood R, Goodman R, Ford T. *Mental Health of Children and Adolescents in Great Britain.* London: The Stationery Office, 2000.

67 Wittchen H-U, Kessler RC, Pfister H, Lieb M. Why do people with anxiety disorders become depressed? *Acta Psychiatr Scand* 2000;**102** (**Suppl 406**):14–23.

68 Bardone AM, Moffitt TE, Caspi A, Dickson N, Silva P. Adult mental health and social outcomes of adolescent girls with depression and conduct disorder. *Dev Psychopathol* 1996;**8**:811–29.

69 Fergusson DM, Woodward LJ. Educational, psychosocial, and sexual outcomes of girls with conduct problems in early adolescence. *J Child Psychol Psychiatr* 2000;**41**:779–92.

70 Weich S, Lewis G. Material standard of living, social class, and the prevalence of the common mental disorders in Great Britain. *J Epidemiol Community Health* 1998;**52**:8–14.

71 Dohrenwend BP, Levav I, Shrout PE, Schwartz S, Naveh G, Link BG, Skodol AE, Steuve A. Socioeconomic status and psychiatric disorder: the causation-selection issue. *Science* 1992;**255**:946–52.

72 Brown GW, Moran PM. Single mothers, poverty and depression. *Psychol Med* 1997;**27**:21–33.

73 Bebbington P. The origin of sex differences in depressive disorder: bridging the gap. *Int Rev Psychiat* 1996;**8**:295–332.

74 Vásquez-Barquero JL, Diez-Manrique JF, Pena C, Aldana J, Samaniego-Rodriguez C, Menedez-Arango J, Mirapiex C. A community mental health survey in Cantabria: a general description of morbidity. *Psychol Med* 1987;**17**:227–42.

75 Lowenthal K, Goldblatt V, Gorton T, Lubitsch G, Bicknell H, Fellowes D, Sowden A. Gender and depression in Anglo-Jewry. *Psychol Med* 1995;**25**:1051–64.

76 Jorm AF. Sex and age differences in depression: a quantitative synthesis of published research. *Aust N Z J Psychiatry* 1987;**21**:46–53.

77 Patton GC, Hibbert ME, Carlin J, *et al.* Menarche and the onset of depression and anxiety in Victoria, Australia. *J Epidemiol Community Health* 1996;**50**:661–6.

78 Cyranowski JM, Frank E, Young E, Shear K. Adolescent onset of the gender difference in lifetime rates of major depression. *Arch Gen Psychiatry* 2000;**57**:21–7.

79 Harris T, Brown GW, Bifulco A. Loss of parent in childhood and adult psychiatric disorder: the role of lack of adequate parental care. *Psychol Med* 1986;**16**:641–59.

Chapter 9

Body image: a life course perspective

Lindsay McLaren and Jane Wardle

Interest in women's body image has focused primarily on the life stages of adolescence and young adulthood since it is during these periods that peak prevalence of clinical eating disorders is observed. However it is increasingly clear that body dissatisfaction is reported by women at midlife and beyond, and can adversely impact women's health and well-being throughout the life span. Although current cultural standards for women's bodily attractiveness constitute an important backdrop for dissatisfaction, such contextual factors do not easily explain variation in dissatisfaction within and across age-groups. Body dissatisfaction can emerge for the first time at midlife, or may reflect a continuation of dissatisfaction experienced at earlier periods. Retrospective research indicates that particular risk factors in early life (for example overweight body size, body-related teasing) may contribute to body dissatisfaction later on. These predictors, in turn, probably interact with developmental events (puberty, pregnancy, and menopause) which can facilitate fat storage and bring women's bodies further from the thin 'ideal' with increasing age. These pathways appear to differ for women of different racial and social class groups. In this chapter, with the goal of explaining body dissatisfaction at midlife, we review the literature on body dissatisfaction across the life span, highlighting enduring, cumulative, or interactive effects of early predictors where research exists to support such pathways.

9.1 Introduction

While 'body image' encompasses any affective, cognitive, or perceptual beliefs individuals hold about their bodies,[1] 'body dissatisfaction' is a narrower, evaluative term that involves the feeling or belief that one's current body is discrepant from an ideal, coupled with a negative affective evaluation of this discrepancy. Dissatisfaction is assessed in a variety of ways, including ratings of self-reported dissatisfaction, or based on the endorsement of some related concept such as 'feeling fat' or wishing to lose weight, or is inferred from a current–ideal discrepancy. The contribution of body dissatisfaction to the occurrence of eating disorders underlies a substantial proportion of the literature on this topic; however, the focus here is body dissatisfaction in its own right.

We aim to integrate existing literature on body dissatisfaction in a way that highlights possible pathways or trajectories that explain variation in body dissatisfaction at midlife. To this end, we focus on three main questions: first, what is the extent or prevalence of body dissatisfaction in women beyond young adulthood, and what trends have there been over time? Second, what are the consequences of body dissatisfaction for health and well-being among older women? Third, what are the determinants of dissatisfaction at different stages of the life span that may be relevant in explaining midlife dissatisfaction? A life course perspective will be considered in this third goal, and since this perspective is a new framework for the study of body image, identification of gaps in the literature is inevitable.

9.2 **Prevalence and time trends**

Body dissatisfaction is often described as 'normative' among women in contemporary western society.[2] This position has emerged primarily from research with adolescent and young adult samples, which invariably reports that a large proportion, if not a majority, of these girls are dissatisfied.[3–5] Furthermore, dissatisfaction is increasingly documented among female children,[6,7] attesting to the early emergence of this discontent. Research on body image beyond young adulthood is more limited, and its conclusions are less consistent. Several studies indicate less body dissatisfaction among older women relative to younger women.[8–11] However, other research has found an increase in body dissatisfaction with increasing age among females aged 7 to 65,[12] and 17 to 40.[13] A further study[14] found that 62% of a sample of women over 65 wanted to lose weight, a value comparable with that obtained in younger samples.[5]

Widespread body dissatisfaction is inextricably tied to what type of body is considered 'attractive' at a given time, and insight into body dissatisfaction among middle-aged and older women can be gained from looking at changes in the 'standards' of beauty over time. It is widely accepted that the ubiquitous images of ultra-thin women in western media, by conveying the message that beauty is equated with thinness, serve as the primary source of dissatisfaction felt by most women about their bodies. Today's cultural 'ideal' defined by these images is very thin, and researchers have attempted to quantify changes in this 'ideal' by tracking the body dimensions of female fashion models over time. Classic research in the eating disorder literature documented a steady decline in body size and curvaceousness of the 'ideal' over the course of the 1960s and 1970s, a trend which paralleled a steady increase in the population weight norms for young women.[15] Thus the gap between 'actual' and 'ideal' was widening over this period, a trend believed to underline the 'normative discontent' described in the 1980s.[2] During the 1980s and 1990s, the body size of models was essentially constant;[16] however, the prevalence of obesity has risen and continues to rise strongly.[17,18] Thus, although the 'ideal' may not be changing, the actual–ideal gap may well continue to increase. Furthermore, this 'ideal' remains underweight by normative guidelines (i.e. body mass index below 18.5 kg/m^2), and is therefore an unrealistic pursuit for most women. Among American women, for example, less than 4% have a body size that is comparable to these models.[19] The 'thin ideal' is widely believed to have emerged in the mid-1960s with media images of 'Twiggy', and therefore it is important to emphasize that the cohort of women currently entering middle-age has been exposed to these unrealistic images for much of their lifetime (i.e. since adolescence).

Studies comparing body dissatisfaction in women of different age groups are typically cross-sectional in nature. Thus it is difficult to determine whether findings reflect cohort effects (i.e. impact of values and attitudes unique to one's generational group), period effects (i.e. impact of time-specific sociocultural context), or maturational effects (i.e. impact of age-related changes in attitudes and values). Women of different age groups may resemble one another in contemporaneous cross-sectional surveys of body dissatisfaction simply because they are all living in an environment that emphasizes a slim body. They may differ from one another due to cohort-specific values, attitudes, and experiences, or due to maturational changes that are independent of one's birth cohort.

In terms of a cohort effect, a qualitative study found that older women (aged 61 to 92 years) expressed a preference for women's bodies that were larger and more rounded than the cultural model of beauty espoused today.[20] The author suggested that older women hold standards of beauty that are more in keeping with standards that existed when they were growing up (i.e. that are unique to their birth cohort), than with contemporary standards. Alternatively, this could reflect a shifting ideal in response to one's own changing body shape. Age differences in body dissatisfaction have also been attributed to cohort effects in other studies;[21] however, convincing empirical support for this type of effect is limited due to the lack of research following different age groups of women over a lengthy period of time. The Women's Health Australia project[22] looks promising in this regard.

Evidence for an age-independent period effect is strong. First, in contrast to qualitative research cited above, another study found different generations of women to espouse similar 'ideals' for body size.[4] This suggests that, regardless of age, women are aware of and perhaps aspire to today's standard of beauty. Furthermore, results from two studies indicate that when older women are asked about their current and past diet and weight loss behaviours, they indicate higher use of these tactics currently (i.e. when social pressures for thinness are high) than when they were adolescents (i.e. when thinness was less strongly valued). Rosenzweig and Spruill[23] studied a sample of 159 women (mean age 38 years) in the mid to late 1980s, when social pressures for thinness were quite strong. They found women were more likely to report current and more frequent use of diet pills, diuretics, and laxatives at this time than when they were at school or college during the early 1960s, just prior to the emergence of 'Twiggy'. Similarly, Hetherington and Burnett[24] found that among an elderly sample of 65 women who reported dieting, most had started between the ages of 40 and 50, which corresponded to the late 1960s, the time period when a thin body first became popular. Very few women had dieted in their teens or twenties during the pre-Twiggy era. Since weight loss behaviours in these women emerged—having been absent before—in a social climate characterized by a slim ideal and social sanction of dieting, these studies suggest an influence of the sociocultural climate in the onset of behaviours related to body dissatisfaction, which is independent of age.

Evidence for maturational changes in body dissatisfaction is also compelling. Cross-sectional research across a sample of 334 women and 305 men aged 10–79 documented a decrease in the self-reported importance of appearance with increasing age.[8] In addition, weight concern was found to be inversely correlated with self-esteem among 30–49-year-old women, but uncorrelated with self-esteem among women over 50[10] suggesting that even if women over 50 report weight concern, it may be less central to their self-esteem and therefore less distressing. Another study[25] found that the range of body sizes chosen as 'acceptable' increased with age, such that middle-aged adults were the most tolerant of bodies that did not resemble the cultural ideal. Finally, qualitative research indicates that some women adopt more relaxed attitudes towards their body during middle and late adulthood. For example, they view weight gain as an inevitable part of ageing, or something that is no longer their responsibility,[20,26] or feel that at their age they deserve to be free to eat what they like and to ignore appearance-related pressures imposed by spouses and others.[26]

Distinguishing the relative impact of age and current context is difficult because of the virtual absence of research which allows for the teasing apart of such effects, such as comparable longitudinal studies of women from different birth cohorts during different eras. However, in an interesting pair of studies, Heatherton and colleagues[27,28] attempted to tease apart these effects by comparing eating disorder symptoms across a 10-year period in both a cross-sectional and longitudinal manner. Specifically, these authors examined self-reported symptoms among samples of (a) women and men in 1982 when they were in college, (b) those women and men from 1982 who agreed to participate again in 1992 (now approximately 30 years old), and (c) college-aged women and men in 1992, comparable to sample (a). Body dissatisfaction was expressed as a desire for weight loss. There was both a cross-sectional decrease (i.e. fewer college-aged women desiring to lose weight in 1992 relative to 1982), and a longitudinal decrease (i.e. women who desired to lose weight in 1982 were less likely to report this ten years later in 1992). The magnitude of the longitudinal decrease was larger than that of the cross-sectional decrease. Coupled with evidence that the 'ideal' has not changed appreciably over this time period,[16] this provides some evidence for an independent age-related decline in this behaviour.

In summary, research generally suggests that middle-aged and older women are slightly less likely to report body dissatisfaction than younger women. This appears to reflect maturational changes in attitudes toward the body and thinness, coupled with some 'protection' offered among older women (i.e. age 65 and older) by having grown up in an era when standards of beauty were larger and more womanly. However, the prevalence of dissatisfaction among middle-aged and older women is still high, and in general women from these earlier born cohorts are acutely aware of contemporary standards of attractiveness and means of attaining them. Furthermore, the cohort of women now entering middle-age have experienced a thin ideal since adolescence, and therefore we may well expect a constant or even increasing prevalence of body dissatisfaction among women of this age group, since such lifelong exposure may overwhelm any protective maturational effect.

9.3 Health consequences

Body dissatisfaction in middle-aged women has effects on health and well-being. Body dissatisfaction has been linked with greater depressive affect, lower overall quality of life, fewer pleasant feelings (e.g. energetic, happy, upbeat), and more unpleasant feelings (e.g. fatigued, tired, worn-out) among a sample of women aged 35–75.[11] It has also been associated with diminished sexual interest and sexual activity, and less enjoyment of sex.[29] Body dissatisfaction has been associated with marital dissatisfaction, independent of the woman's body size.[30] Importantly, the direction of causality in these latter relationships is not clear: if a woman who is dissatisfied with her body is reluctant to engage in physical intimacy, it is easy to see how this could place strain on the sexual/marital relationship. Alternatively, in the case of a relationship that is already strained, a woman may begin to feel undesirable and consequently develop dissatisfaction with her body or appearance.

Also, body dissatisfaction may adversely influence health behaviour. The related construct of social physique anxiety[31]—anxiety about having one's body evaluated by others—has been linked with lesser involvement in physical activity among postmenopausal women, independent of percentage body fat.[32] The explanation is that a woman who is dissatisfied with her body may be reluctant to exercise in public or in circumstances where she must wear revealing clothing (such as a swimsuit). As smoking cessation is linked with weight gain, body dissatisfaction has been cited as one reason why women are reluctant to stop cigarette smoking,[33] notwithstanding the far more negative health consequences of failure to quit. Body dissatisfaction is also linked with unhealthy weight loss tactics and disordered eating among older women just as in younger ones.[14] Finally, body dissatisfaction may influence women's medical decisions at menopause. Women have cited perceived cosmetic benefits and anti-ageing effects of hormone replacement therapy as important reasons for choosing or not choosing this therapeutic option at menopause.[34,35] Thus there are several reasons to consider body dissatisfaction an important health issue for women across the life span.

9.4 Determinants of body dissatisfaction across the life span

This section considers the correlates of body dissatisfaction and how they might be involved in dissatisfaction at midlife. Following a discussion of 'age-independent' factors (i.e. factors whose influence is not restricted to a particular age period), the developmental spectrum and correlates of body dissatisfaction that are associated with particular periods in the life course are considered. Enduring, cumulative, or interactive effects will be highlighted where research exists to support such pathways.

9.4.1 Age-independent risk factors

9.4.1.1 Gender

Particularly when expressed as a desire to lose weight, body dissatisfaction is more prevalent among women than men. This female preponderance becomes apparent at about eight to ten years of age[7] and remains evident across a wide age span. Women have also been shown to accord greater importance to appearance and weight control than men regardless of age.[8] Using cross-sectional data, one study found that the gender gap in body dissatisfaction was smaller among older adults (mean age 74 years) than among young adults (mean age 19 years).[9] However, another study reported that the gender difference remained constant across a 10–74-year-old sample[8] with women consistently feeling less satisfied with their appearance. Longitudinal research suggests that women gain more weight with age than men across 11 years[36] and 25 years[37] in adulthood (based on individuals who were in their thirties at baseline). Since higher weight is associated with greater body dissatisfaction in women (see below), it is perhaps most likely that the female preponderance of body dissatisfaction will remain constant or even increase with increasing age. In any case, it seems clear that being female places one at a disadvantage in terms of body dissatisfaction from childhood onwards, and this disadvantage does not subside with age.

9.4.1.2 Body size

Among women, perhaps the strongest predictor of body dissatisfaction is body size. In general, a higher body mass index is associated with greater body dissatisfaction, and this relationship has been consistently demonstrated from childhood through late adulthood.[5,11,14,38,39] Although overweight women are perhaps at greatest risk for body dissatisfaction at any age, a substantial number of normal weight women are dissatisfied, although within the normal weight range, a heavier woman is likely to be more dissatisfied than a lighter woman.[24] Notably, the small percentage of women who report being satisfied with their bodies are typically underweight (body mass index less than 20 kg/m²), and even among these underweight women, several (up to 10%) report a desire to lose weight.[17,40]

This negative consequence of being or feeling 'overweight' appears to accumulate over time, such that the longer an individual has been overweight, the worse her body dissatisfaction will be. Research indicates that women whose overweight or obese status emerged in childhood have more body dissatisfaction in adulthood than those whose overweight or obese status emerged in adulthood.[41,42] And, the earlier the onset of obesity, the worse the adult body image, even controlling for adult body mass index.[43] Thus, overweight status during childhood appears to be one early predictor of adult body dissatisfaction.

9.4.1.3 Social and cultural context

Highlighted earlier in this chapter, the contemporary western sociocultural climate is characterized by strong pressure for women to be thin. Ubiquitous media images of very thin women convey this message. Studies have demonstrated that greater exposure to media representations of the thin ideal—whether through experimentally manipulated exposure to slides of thin, versus average or oversize, models[44] or through high self-reported frequency of reading fashion magazines[45]—is linked with increased body dissatisfaction. Furthermore, coupled with the pressure for women to be thin is the societal aversion to fatness. Studies using primarily young samples have shown that fat people are judged more negatively and attributed more negative character traits than thin people.[46,47] In addition to thinness being equated with beauty for women in western cultures, research shows that physically attractive people are judged as possessing more positive qualities[48] and are treated more positively[49] than unattractive people. In such a context, 'normative' body dissatisfaction, typically in the direction of wanting to become thinner, is hardly surprising.

9.4.1.4 Individual characteristics

Individual attributes can help explain which individuals are more or less vulnerable to ubiquitous sociocultural factors. Body dissatisfaction is associated with high neuroticism in young samples,[50] and with low self-esteem, in both young and middle-aged women.[5,51] Young women who endorse feminine gender roles have shown more negative appearance evaluation,[50] and endorsement of non-traditional or feminist values has been associated with less weight concern among young samples[52] and among 30–49-year-old women.[10] To the extent that individual characteristics remain stable across the life span, they may provide baseline protection from, or vulnerability to, the impact of other stressors. For example, women with high neuroticism or low self-esteem may be more likely to experience body dissatisfaction at periods of rapid weight gain such as puberty or pregnancy.

9.4.1.5 Race

'Race' is a difficult variable to consider. Increasingly, social science research recognizes that 'race' has little biological foundation, and typically a great deal of variation is detected within racial groups; issues that underline the question of what 'race' is really tapping. None the less, some patterns have emerged from the work that has examined racial differences in body dissatisfaction, mostly pertaining to the differences between White and Black or African American women.

Comparisons of Black and White women within western societies generally indicate that for any given weight, Black women report less body dissatisfaction than White women. This finding has been demonstrated in women ranging from adolescence[53] through middle-age and beyond.[11,54] Furthermore, Black women are less likely than White women to diet during puberty, after pregnancy, and during menopause, periods which are considered 'high-risk' for body dissatisfaction among White women due to their potential for weight gain.[55] Among Black women, this lower prevalence of body dissatisfaction coupled with higher prevalence of overweight[56] has led to the suggestion that these women experience cultural norms that are more permissive of larger body sizes and that place less importance on thinness in women.[56,57] In line with this hypothesis, White women express more negative social pressure about their weight than Black women,[55] White women express more negative attitudes toward overweight than Black women,[58] and Black girls perceive less concern about weight from their family and friends than White girls.[59] This suggests that the more relaxed attitudes towards weight seen in Black girls emerge early on and are maintained throughout adulthood. Research on body dissatisfaction in other racial groups is limited, particularly from a life course perspective, and will not be discussed here.

9.4.1.6 Social class

Body size is socially stratified for women in developed countries, with a larger average body mass index and a higher prevalence of obesity found in lower than in higher social class groups.[60] In general, body dissatisfaction is positively associated with social class, with girls and women of higher social class more likely to report body dissatisfaction, weight concern, and attempts at weight loss.[61–64] Exceptions to this pattern exist but appear to be few.[53,65] A positive relationship between social class and body dissatisfaction is consistent with the epidemiological transition in the social distribution of body weight: as overweight and obesity become common among the lower class, a thin body becomes a mark of affluence or social distinction.[66] From this theoretical perspective, it is the wealthy in developed countries who will aspire to be thin, and in turn be most distressed by a discrepancy between their own body and that of the ideal (i.e. experience the most body dissatisfaction).

Low income women have been found to be both less attentive to their weight and more tolerant of weight gain than high income women, independent of body mass index.[62] Also, higher social class individuals appear to be more interested in their weight as indicated by more regular weight monitoring than lower social class individuals, controlling for body mass index.[64] In terms of negative attitudes toward fatness, one study found these attitudes to be more prevalent among girls from higher-class schools;[46] however, another study found negative attitudes to be more prevalent among adolescents from a lower-class school,[63] controlling for participants' body size. Thus, low social class women may be less interested in their weight, but they do not necessarily hold more positive attitudes toward larger body sizes than high income women. Alternatively, it may be that attitudes toward fatness are being diffused down the social hierarchy and thus relationships between social class and attitudes are going through a transition, accounting for the mixed findings. A 'cultural' explanation for social class differences in obesity[62] asserts that lower social class women hold different standards of physical attractiveness; however, research has found that high and low social class women do not differ in their 'ideal' body size.[62,64] This suggests that women acknowledge the same standard for female attractiveness regardless of social class. All of these studies implicitly consider social class to be a stable attribute, and research on social mobility and body image is lacking.

An emerging hypothesis is that the social or material–physical climate in which low income women live is less conducive to body dissatisfaction. Research has documented a relationship between the affluence of one's local living environment (i.e. neighbourhood) and body dissatisfaction: for a given body mass index, high affluence neighbourhoods have a higher proportion of women reporting body dissatisfaction than low affluence neighbourhoods, independent of women's individual income.[67] This contextual effect suggests that affluent neighbourhoods have certain features that promote body dissatisfaction; examples might include easy availability of fashion magazines, weight-loss centres or gyms that emphasize physical appearance and diet food products. It also suggests that the impact of these environmental features are independent of individual-level 'risk factors' including social class and body size.

9.4.1.7 Summary—age independent factors

Against the backdrop of a society that values thinness in women, it is generally true that regardless of age, larger women are more likely to be dissatisfied with their bodies, and the negative impact of overweight appears to endure, or even to accumulate, over time. For women of any weight, the likelihood of dissatisfaction is greater for Caucasian women, and for women from higher social classes. Particular personality characteristics, as well as the amount of exposure to sociocultural ideals through western media channels, may further modify vulnerability to dissatisfaction.

9.4.2 Determinants across the life span

Against the backdrop of factors operating at all life stages discussed above, we will now consider determinants of body dissatisfaction that exert their effects during particular developmental periods as well as, where applicable, their enduring effects for dissatisfaction later in life.

9.4.2.1 Childhood

Throughout the early years, the parents are a primary influence on children's developing body image. Parents' own weight-related concerns may influence their child's body image; for example, one study found that mother's investment in her own thinness, father's complaints about his own weight, and father's own dieting all predicted more negative body esteem in their children.[68] In addition, daughters have been found to resemble their mothers in terms of body dissatisfaction,[69] suggesting that some modelling of dissatisfaction may occur. Girls who believe that their parents think they are overweight have been found to experience reduced satisfaction with their appearance.[70] Girls who believe that it is important to their parents that they are thin were found to be more likely to become weight-concerned over a one-year period of study.[71] Importantly, mothers may also be a source of positive body image development in their daughters,[72] for instance by modelling body acceptance and positive appearance evaluation. The enduring impact of early parent variables (positive or negative) on later body dissatisfaction is not known, but a lasting effect of these important early influences is certainly plausible.

An increasing amount of research—typically retrospective in nature—has documented the adverse impact of body-related comments or teasing on children's body esteem. Mothers' comments, positive or negative, about their child's weight have been found to be associated with negative body esteem in the child, particularly for daughters.[68] A self-reported history of teasing has been associated with greater body dissatisfaction among children,[73] and a history of weight/size-related teasing appears to be more damaging to body esteem than general appearance teasing.[74] One study reported that teasing from family members (particularly brothers) was more damaging than teasing from peers,[75] although teasing from both sources undoubtedly carries very negative consequences for some women. Among adult women, retrospective research indicates a potentially long-term adverse impact of teasing: women with poor body esteem in adulthood are more likely to recall criticism of their appearance and weight-related teasing in childhood than women with positive body esteem.[58,72,76]

Children may be involved in extra-curricular activities that are more or less conducive to body dissatisfaction. Competitive environments emphasizing weight and appearance are believed to be particularly detrimental; ballet class has perhaps been most widely studied and has consistently been associated with heightened prevalence of eating disturbance.[77–79] On the other hand, a meta-analysis found that involvement in some sport contexts may be protective against the development of eating problems. Specifically, girls and women involved at the non-elite level in sports that do not emphasize a thin body type (for example, basketball or volleyball as opposed to gymnastics or long-distance running) appear to be at less risk than non-athletes of developing eating problems including body dissatisfaction.[80] Since parents may determine their child's activities, the nature of these extra-familial activities will in turn reflect attitudes and values of the parents, and family circumstances such as social class will dictate the accessibility of various activities.

9.4.2.2 Adolescence

With its dramatic physical, psychological, and social sequelae, the event of puberty is perhaps the most plausible trigger for body dissatisfaction, and is certainly the developmental period most often studied. Girls gain a substantial amount of weight at puberty, much of which is fat,[81] and this weight gain inevitably represents a movement away from the androgynous body shape of childhood which societal messages indicate is attractive. Thus it is not surprising that 'normal development' is generally a negative experience for girls, a comment substantiated by the dramatic increase in prevalence of body dissatisfaction from pre-pubescence (e.g. 34%) to post-pubescence (e.g. 76%).[82] Some studies indicate that the experience of a puberty that is early relative to one's peers is associated with worse body esteem and more disordered eating,[83] however not all studies have found this association.[84] A link between early maturation and body dissatisfaction may be due to body size differences, since girls who experience an early menarche are, on average, larger before puberty than girls who experience an on-time or late puberty.[75]

Changes in the nature of social interaction at adolescence are an important precursor to body dissatisfaction. Peers have been found to influence eating disorder symptoms both by modelling particular behaviours and by discussing body concerns,[85] although one study found that the importance of thinness to peers was not related to girls' development of weight concern.[71] Heterosexual interaction may be a particularly important type of peer influence. Girls who believe that boys will like them more if they are thin showed poorer body image in one study.[86] Also, adolescent girls identified as being at increased risk for disordered eating were more likely to be involved in social situations where boys were present, and were more likely to report being physically involved with a boyfriend.[87] The impact on body concern may be particularly negative among those girls for whom onset of dating and puberty occur synchronously, based on a significant interaction effect found by Levine and colleagues.[85]

In the absence of research indicating whether events at adolescence affect later body dissatisfaction, two observations can be made. First, since individual differences in physical and emotional maturity are particularly salient during adolescence, events during this period may have an acute impact on body dissatisfaction that diminishes when differences even out (for example, when other girls have 'caught up'). From this perspective, determinants of adolescent body image would not be expected to have any enduring effect. Second, given that adolescence marks the initiation of the 'adult' body, it is possible that one's body image and events that precipitated its development are important indicators of dissatisfaction later in the life span. In this latter context, a longitudinal examination of the lasting impact of these factors at adolescence is an important task for future research.

9.4.2.3 Early adulthood

A woman's spouse or partner may become a primary source of body-related and appearance-related social feedback in early adulthood and beyond. The physical appearance of a wife has been hypothesized to be more important to a relationship—in terms of husband commitment and quality and quantity of sexual relations—than the physical appearance of the husband.[88] Further, research has found that men but not women exposed to photographs of physically attractive, versus average-looking, members of the opposite sex rated their current partner as less attractive and reported less love for them.[89] This supports the position that physical appearance in a partner is more important to men than to women. Another study[90] found that within heterosexual couples, the men were more dissatisfied with their partners' body than the women were with the man's body. This suggests that men do not only value physical appearance in relationships more so than do women, but they are also more likely to evaluate this aspect of their partner negatively. Giesen[91] found that single women were more likely than married women to believe they were becoming more attractive with age. On the other hand, women who are satisfied with their marriage are also likely to report satisfaction with their body,[30] indicating that the partner can also be a source of positive social feedback. The extent to which a romantic partner instils dissatisfaction (or satisfaction) where it previously did not exist, or simply reinforces existing satisfaction or dissatisfaction, is not known. Furthermore, to our knowledge, research examining the role of lesbian partners on women's body dissatisfaction is non-existent.

Pregnancy, with its concomitant changes in body size and shape, carries much potential to influence body dissatisfaction. Research results on body image in pregnancy and the postpartum have been mixed, with the use of both quantitative and qualitative methods contributing to the complexity of findings. Some studies document increased body satisfaction in pregnant women, as though pregnancy 'legitimizes' a large body and weight gain.[92,93] Other research has found decreased body satisfaction during pregnancy,[94] and postpartum.[95] Changes in body image during pregnancy have also been found to depend on prepregnancy weight status, with overweight women reporting an increase in satisfaction and normal weight women reporting a decrease in satisfaction during pregnancy.[94] Still other research has demonstrated considerable stability in women's orientations to their body weight across pregnancy and the postpartum.[96] A possible explanation for dissatisfaction during pregnancy is offered by Davies and Wardle[93] who found that women maintained their view of what constituted an 'ideal' body throughout the pregnancy transition, despite a significant change in their 'actual' body size. Negative attitudes by men regarding their partners' pregnancy weight were found to be rare in one study,[93] suggesting that women's potential body image concerns during this event are not unduly influenced by negative social feedback from their intimate partners.

9.4.2.4 The middle years

As women age, their body becomes further removed from the 'ideal' in many respects—size, shape, composition, colouring, and texture. In the light of the thin, youthful standard of beauty, these normal changes may be among the most important determinants of body dissatisfaction in middle-aged and older women. The impact of this developmental period on women is likely to be more detrimental than for men as indicated by the widely cited 'double standard of ageing' whereby physical ageing is believed to be judged more harshly in women than in men.[97] There may be an acute effect of the menopause on women's body dissatisfaction: one study found substantially higher social physique anxiety among perimenopausal women (i.e. age 45–54 years) than among older women.[98] Body-related comments from husbands may still be important contributors to dissatisfaction, although qualitative research suggests that some women feel less distressed by such comments as they get older.[26] One study found that middle-aged women who felt less in control of their lives were less satisfied with their bodies.[51]

In general, research on the determinants of body dissatisfaction at midlife is limited. As mentioned earlier, women who are now entering middle-age were teenagers when the 'thin ideal' first became popular (the mid-1960s), and these women have thus been exposed to a lifetime of unreasonably thin beauty ideals. Against the backdrop of this sociocultural trend, it is reasonable to hypothesize that body dissatisfaction will become more common among women in their middle years.

9.5 Conclusions

Body dissatisfaction arises from a confluence of factors. The biological (e.g. body size), psychosocial (e.g. self-esteem), and social/interpersonal (e.g. parental influence, ongoing social feedback, body-related teasing) operate in interaction with developmental events (puberty, pregnancy, menopause) and developmental trends (e.g. increase in weight with age) within a particular context (sociocultural standards for attractiveness). Although empirical evidence for long-term pathways is lacking, particular events and characteristics evident at earlier life stages may contribute to dissatisfaction at midlife.

It was shown, retrospectively, that a large body size and body-related teasing during childhood predicted body dissatisfaction in adulthood. It is possible that these early influences have an enduring impact on body dissatisfaction; for example, a woman who is overweight during early life and then loses weight may retain a poor body image from her earlier overweight period. Alternatively, the pathway underlying midlife dissatisfaction may show less continuity: for example, the aforementioned woman who loses weight may experience an improvement in body image following weight loss. Two studies indicate reasonable continuity in body image across adulthood,[99,100] although these studies are limited to six and ten years' duration, respectively. Extent of continuity or change assessed prospectively over a longer time period is not known.

Any life span pathway is likely to show evidence of social patterning. Body dissatisfaction is less common among lower social class and non-White women, and these social groups appear to value thinness less. A young White girl from a higher social class background is likely to grow up in an environment characterized by social pressure for thinness, with parents who diet or who are concerned about their weight. This social environment is probably maintained throughout development within peer groups and romantic relationships, emphasizing a lifelong social environment in which risk factors for body dissatisfaction are both more prevalent and more powerful among White, middle and upper class girls and women. This social class patterning is likely to be continued in an intergenerational manner, although it may change as a function of social mobility.

As is evident from the speculative nature of these pathways, research that directly examines the influence on longer term trajectories is lacking. Presently, within the context of the Medical Research Council National Survey of Health and Development,[101,102] we are working towards the development of a coherent life course model of body dissatisfaction. Being a long-term, prospective cohort study of a nationally representative sample of British individuals, this survey provides the unique opportunity to examine midlife health outcomes as a function of lifelong developmental trajectories. Data on body dissatisfaction and its functional consequences are being collected among the female survey members, currently in their mid-fifties. With these data, we plan to evaluate the viability of the life course framework that shaped this chapter.

Commentary on 'Body image: a life course perspective'

J. Kevin Thompson

The field of body image has experienced a rapid growth over the past 10–15 years.[103] Once a topic of interest primarily of researchers and clinicians interested in the study of eating disorders, body image issues are now examined routinely in men and women of diverse ethnicities, ages, avocations (gymnasts, dancers, runners, weightlifters, etc.), and sexual orientation. Indeed, appearance concerns once confined supposedly to adult White women in western societies now appear in much younger ages and across a variety of individuals regardless of ethnic or cultural background.[104] The time could not be more appropriate for a new theoretical perspective to guide future research in the area of body image.

Such a formulation is provided by McLaren and Wardle. In this excellent review and synthesis of the confusing field of body image research, these researchers succinctly review the essentials related to prevalence and health consequences, then provide an integration of research using the life course perspective. This reformulation of a vast array of studies into sections on age-independent risk factors and determinants across the life span forms the framework and analysis that may guide much future research. Factors that appear to produce or perpetuate body image problems at all life stages include: social class, ethnicity, individual dispositional variables (i.e. self-esteem), social/cultural context, body size, and gender. Some factors or 'determinants' appear to operate uniquely to affect body image at a certain developmental period. For instance, appearance-related feedback (i.e. teasing) may operate selectively or predominantly during the childhood years. Peers and menarcheal development may have unique effects on adolescents. Partners, spouses, and the role of pregnancy on body image may play a large role for young adults. Menopause may affect women of the middle years.

This chapter identifies particular factors associated with body image problems at unique age periods and reviews some of the few findings indicative of a prospective prediction from one epoch to another (such as body size and teasing). It speculates on additional pathways, such as social patterning (i.e. some individuals of a higher social class may encounter and experience familial and peer group appearance pressures throughout life). Although there is actually very little prospective work currently available to draw on, the authors manage to articulate clear cut ideas for future such investigations. Importantly, they also review two ongoing studies—the Medical Research Council National Survey of Health and Development[101,102] and the Women's Health Australia project[22]—that should reveal relevant data in the near future.

Additional studies might consider evaluation of theoretical models for body image and eating disturbance (applied to the prediction of body image problems) tailored for females, or perhaps males, of various life stages. Some of these multivariate models were reviewed by Stice[105] and include Levine and Smolak's cumulative stress model, Heatherton and Polivy's spiral model, Stice's dual pathway approach, and Thompson *et al.*'s tripartite influence (peers, parents, media) and two-part mediational (internalization of the 'thin ideal' and appearance comparison) model of body image development. Such models might be tested cross-sectionally using regression or covariance structure modelling, yielding information regarding unique predictors of body image for different life stages.

Future reviews will probably view this chapter as the primary impetus for an examination of body image from a life course perspective. The authors present the theory, examine the quantitative and qualitative data, explain the methods, and offer a heuristic guide for the work. Body image researchers take note: the next stage of body image research is the life course perspective.

References

1 **Thompson JK**. Assessment of body image. In: Allison DB, ed. *Handbook of assessment methods for eating behaviors and weight-related problems*. New York: Sage, 1995, pp. 119–48.

2 **Rodin J, Silberstein L, Striegel-Moore R**. Women and weight: a normative discontent. In: Sonderegger TB, ed. *Nebraska symposium on motivation: vol 32. Psychology and gender*. Lincoln, NE: University of Nebraska Press, 1985, pp. 267–307.

3 **Wardle J, Beales S**. Restraint, body image and food attitudes in children from 12 to 18 years. *Appetite* 1986;7:209–17.

4 **Tiggemann M**. Body-size dissatisfaction: individual differences in age and gender, and relationship with self-esteem. *Pers Ind Diff* 1992;**13**:39–43.

5 **Kostanski M, Gullone E**. Adolescent body image dissatisfaction: relationships with self-esteem, anxiety, and depression controlling for body mass. *J Child Psychol Psychiatry* 1998;**39**:255–62.

6 **Ambrosi-Randic N**. Perception of current and ideal body size in preschool age children. *Percept Mot Skills* 2000;**90**:885–9.

7 **Ricciardelli LA, McCabe MP**. Children's body image concerns and eating disturbance: a review of the literature. *Clin Psychol Rev* 2001;**21**:325–44.

8 **Pliner P, Chaiken S, Flett GL**. Gender differences in concern with body weight and physical appearance over the life span. *Pers Soc Psychol Bull* 1990;**16**:263–73.

9 Franzoi SL, Koehler V. Age and gender differences in body attitudes: a comparison of young and elderly adults. *Int J Aging Hum Dev* 1998;**47**:1–10.

10 Tiggemann M, Stevens C. Weight concern across the life-span: relationship to self-esteem and feminist identity. *Int J Eat Disord* 1999;**26**:103–6.

11 Reboussin BA, Rejeski WJ, Martin KA, Callahan K, Dunn AL, King AC, Sallis JF. Correlates of satisfaction with body function and body appearance in middle- and older aged adults: the Activity Counseling Trial (ACT). *Psychol Health* 2000;**15**:239–54.

12 Guaraldi GP, Orlandi E, Boselli P, Tartoni PL. Body size perception and dissatisfaction of female subjects of different ages. *Psychother Psychosom* 1995;**64**:149–55.

13 Altabe M, Thompson JK. Body image changes during early adulthood. *Int J Eat Disord* 1993;**13**:323–8.

14 Allaz AF, Bernstein M, Rouget P, Archinard M, Morabia A. Body weight preoccupation in middle-age and ageing women: a general population survey. *Int J Eat Disord* 1998;**23**:287–94.

15 Garner DM, Garfinkel PE, Schwartz D, Thompson M. Cultural expectations of thinness in women. *Psychol Rep* 1980;**47**:483–91.

16 Katzmarzyk PT, Davis C. Thinness and body shape of playboy centerfolds from 1978 to 1998. *Int J Obes Relat Metab Disord* 2001;**25**:590–2.

17 Ledoux M, Rivard M. Poids corporel. *Collection la santé et le bien-être: enquête sociale et de santé 1998*. Institut de la statistique du Québec, 2001:185–99.

18 World Health Organisation. Controlling the global obesity epidemic 2001 [online]. Available from: URL: http://www.who.int/nut/obs.htm

19 Kuczmarski RJ, Carroll MD, Flegal KM, Troiano RP. Varying body mass index cutoff points to describe overweight prevalence among US adults: NHANES III (1988 to 1994). *Obes Res* 1997;**5**:542–8.

20 Hurd LC. Older women's body image and embodied experience: an exploration. *J Women Aging* 2000;**12**:77–97.

21 Lamb CS, Jackson LE, Cassiday PB, Priest DJ. Body figure preferences of men and women: a comparison of two generations. *Sex Roles* 1993;**28**:345–58.

22 Brown WJ, Dobson AJ, Bryson L, Byles JE. Women's Health Australia: on the progress of the main cohort studies. *J Womens Health Gend Based Med* 1999;**8**:681–8.

23 Rosenzweig M, Spruill J. Twenty years after Twiggy: a retrospective investigation of bulimic-like behaviors. *Int J Eat Disord* 1987;**16**:59–65.

24 Hetherington MM, Burnett L. Ageing and the pursuit of slimness: dietary restraint and weight satisfaction in elderly women. *Br J Clin Psychol* 1994;**33**:391–400.

25 Rand CSW, Wright BA. Continuity and change in the evaluation of ideal and acceptable body sizes across a wide age span. *Int J Eat Dis* 2000;**28**:90–100.

26 Tunaley JR, Walsh S, Nicolson P. 'I'm not bad for my age': The meaning of body size and eating in the lives of older women. *Ageing Society* 1999;**19**:741–59.

27 Heatherton TF, Nichols P, Mahamedi F, Keel P. Body weight, dieting, and eating disorder symptoms among college students, 1982 to 1992. *Am J Psychiatry* 1995;**152**:1623–9.

28 Heatherton TF, Mahamedi F, Striepe M, Field AE, Keel P. A 10-year longitudinal study of body weight, dieting, and eating disorder symptoms. *J Abnorm Psychol* 1997;**106**:117–25.

29 Fooken I. Sexuality in the later years-the impact of health and body-image in a sample of older women. *Patient Educ Couns* 1994;**23**:227–33.

30 Friedman MA, Dixon AE, Brownell KD, Whisman MA, Wilfley DE. Marital status, marital satisfaction, and body image dissatisfaction. *Int J Eat Disord* 1999;**26**:81–85.

31 **Hart EA, Leary MR, Rejeski WJ.** The measurement of social physique anxiety. *J Sport Exerc Psychol* 1989;**11**:94–104.

32 **Ransdell LB, Wells CL, Manore MM, Swan PD, Corbin CB.** Social physique anxiety in postmenopausal women. *J Women Ageing* 1998;**10**:19–39.

33 **King TK, Matacin M, Marcus BH, Bock BC, Tripolone J.** Body image evaluations in women smokers. *Addict Behav* 2000;**25**:613–8.

34 **Hunter MS, O'Dea I, Britten N.** Decision-making and hormone replacement therapy: a qualitative analysis. *Soc Sci Med* 1997;**45**:1541–8.

35 **Fauconnier A, Ringa V, Delanoë D, Falissard B, Bréart G.** Use of hormone replacement therapy: women's representations of menopause and beauty care practices. *Maturitas* 2000;**35**:215–28.

36 **Heitmann BL, Garby L.** Patterns of long-term weight changes in overweight developing Danish men and women aged between 30 and 60 years. *Int J Obes* 1999;**23**:1074–8.

37 **Stevens J, Knapp RG, Keil JE, Verdugo RR.** Changes in body weight and girths in black and white adults studied over a 25 year interval. *Int J Obes* 1991;**15**:803–8.

38 **Mendelson BK, White DR, Mendelson MJ.** Children's global self-esteem predicted by body-esteem but not by weight. *Percept Mot Skills* 1995;**80**:97–8.

39 **Pingitore R, Spring B, Garfield D.** Gender differences in body satisfaction. *Obes Res* 1997;**5**:402–9.

40 **Green KL, Cameron R, Polivy J, Cooper K, Liu L, Leiter L, Heatherton T.** Weight dissatisfaction and weight loss attempts among Canadian adults. *Can Med Assoc J* 1997;**157** (**Suppl 1**):S17–25.

41 **Grilo CM, Wilfley DE, Brownell KD, Rodin J.** Teasing, body image, and self-esteem in a clinical sample of obese women. *Addict Behav* 1994;**19**:443–50.

42 **McLaren L, Gauvin L.** The cumulative impact of overweight status on women's body esteem. *Eat Weight Disord,* in press.

43 **Wardle J, Waller J, Fox E.** Age of onset and body dissatisfaction in obesity. *Addict Behav,* in press.

44 **Irving LM.** Mirror images: effects of the standard of beauty on the self- and body-esteem of women exhibiting varying levels of bulimic symptoms. *J Soc Clin Psychol* 1990;**9**:230–42.

45 **Field AE, Cheung L, Wolf AM, Herzog DB, Gortmaker SL, Colditz GA.** Exposure to mass media and weight concerns among girls. *Pediatrics* 1999;**103**:E36.

46 **Wardle J, Volz C, Golding C.** Social variation in attitudes to obesity in children. *Int J Obes* 1995;**19**:562–9.

47 **Shapiro S, Newcomb M, Burns Loeb T.** Fear of fat, disregulated-restrained eating, and body-esteem: prevalence and gender differences among eight- to ten-year-old children. *J Clin Child Psychol* 1997;**26**:358–65.

48 **Cash TF.** The psychology of physical appearance: aesthetics, attributes, and images. In: Cash TF, Pruzinsky T, eds. *Body images: development, deviance, and change*. New York: The Guilford Press, 1990, pp. 51–79.

49 **Langlois JH, Kalakanis L, Rubenstein AJ, Larson A, Hallam M, Smoot M.** Maxims or myths of beauty? a meta-analytic and theoretical review. *Psychol Bull* 2000;**126**:390–423.

50 **Davis C, Dionne M, Lazarus L.** Gender-role orientation and body image in women and men: the moderating influence of neuroticism. *Sex Roles* 1996;**34**:493–505.

51 **Rackley JV, Warren SA, Bird GW.** Determinants of body image in women at midlife. *Psychol Rep* 1988;**62**:9–10.

52 **Dionne M, Davis C, Fox J, Gurevich M.** Feminist ideology as a predictor of body dissatisfaction in women. *Sex Roles* 1995;**33**:277–87.

53 **Story M, French SA, Resnick MD, Blum RW.** Ethnic/racial and socioeconomic differences in dieting behaviors and body image perceptions in adolescents. *Int J Eat Disord* 1995;**18**:173–9.

54 Stevens J, Kumanyika SK, Keil JE. Attitudes toward body size and dieting: differences between elderly black and white women. *Am J Public Health* 1994;**84**:1322–5.

55 Striegel-Moore RH, Wilfley DE, Caldwell MB, Needham ML, Brownell KD. Weight-related attitudes and behaviors of women who diet to lose weight: a comparison of black dieters and white dieters. *Obes Res* 1996;**4**:109–16.

56 Flynn KJ, Fitzgibbon M. Body images and obesity risk among black females: a review of the literature. *Ann Behav Med* 1998;**20**:13–24.

57 Kumanyika S, Wilson JF, Guilford-Davenport M. Weight-related attitudes and behaviors of black women. *J Am Diet Assoc* 1993;**93**:416–22.

58 Thompson SH, Sargent RG. Black and white women's weight-related attitudes and parental criticism of their childhood appearance. *Women Health* 2000;**30**:77–92.

59 Adams K, Sargent RG, Thompson SH, Richter D, Corwin SJ, Rogan TJ. A study of body weight concerns and weight control practices of 4th and 7th grade adolescents. *Ethn Health* 2000;**5**:79–94.

60 Sobal J, Stunkard AJ. Socioeconomic status and obesity: a review of the literature. *Psychol Bull* 1989;**105**:260–75.

61 Drewnowski A, Kurth CL, Krahn DD. Body weight and dieting in adolescence: impact of socioeconomic status. *Int J Eat Disord* 1994;**16**:61–5.

62 Jeffery RW, French SA. Socioeconomic status and weight control practices among 20- to 45- year old women. *Am J Public Health* 1996;**86**:1005–10.

63 Ogden J, Thomas D. The role of familial values in understanding the impact of social class on weight concern. *Int J Eat Disord* 1999;**25**:273–9.

64 Wardle J, Griffith J. Socioeconomic status and weight control practices in British adults. *J Epidemiol Community Health* 2001;**55**:185–90.

65 Stevens C, Tiggemann M. Women's body figure preferences across the life span. *J Genet Psychol* 1998;**159**:94–102.

66 Wilkinson RG. Unhealthy societies: the afflictions of inequality. London: Routledge, 1996.

67 McLaren L, Gauvin L. Neighborhood- vs. individual-level correlates of women's body dissatisfaction: toward a multilevel understanding of the role of affluence. *J Epidemiol Community Health* 2002;**56**:193–9.

68 Smolak L, Levine MP, Schermer F. Parental input and weight concerns among elementary school children. *Int J Eat Disord* 1999;**25**:263–71.

69 Rozin P, Fallon A. Body image, attitudes to weight, and misperceptions of figure preferences of the opposite sex: a comparison of men and women in two generations. *J Abnorm Psychol* 1988;**97**:342–5.

70 Walsh Pierce J, Wardle J. Self-esteem, parental appraisal and body size in children. *J Child Psychol Psychiat* 1993;**34**:1125–36.

71 Field AE, Camargo CA, Taylor CB, Berkey CS, Roberts SB, Colditz GA. Peer, parent, and media influences on the development of weight concerns and frequent dieting among preadolescent and adolescent girls and boys. *Pediatrics* 2001;**107**:54–60.

72 Rieves L, Cash TF. Social developmental factors and women's body-image attitudes. *J Soc Behav Pers* 1996;**11**:63–78.

73 Gardner RM, Sorter RG, Friedman BN. Developmental changes in children's body image. *J Soc Behav Pers* 1997;**12**:1019–36.

74 Thompson JK, Heinberg LJ. Preliminary test of two hypotheses of body image disturbance. *Int J Eat Disord* 1993;**14**:59–63.

75 Collins E. Body dissatisfaction—social and emotional influences in adolescent girls. M. Phil thesis. University of London, 1996.

76 **Schwartz DJ, Phares V, Tantleff-Dunn S, Thompson JK**. Body image, psychological functioning, and parental feedback regarding physical appearance. *Int J Eat Disord* 1999;**25**:339–43.

77 **Garner DM, Garfinkel PE, Rockert W, Olmsted, MP**. A prospective study of eating disturbance in the ballet. *Psychother Psychosom* 1987;**48**:170–5.

78 **Abraham S**. Characteristics of eating disorders among young ballet dancers. *Psychopathology* 1996;**29**:223–9.

79 **Bettle N, Bettle O, Neumarker U, Neumarker KJ**. Adolescent ballet school students: their quest for body weight change. *Psychopathology* 1998;**31**:153–9.

80 **Smolak L, Murnen SK, Ruble AE**. Female athletes and eating problems: a meta-analysis. *Int J Eat Disord* 2000;**27**:371–80.

81 **Graber JA, Brooks-Gunn J, Warren MP**. The vulnerable transition: puberty and the development of eating pathology and negative mood. *Women's Health Issues* 1999;**9**:107–14.

82 **Thompson AM, Chad KE**. The relationship of pubertal status to body image, social physique anxiety, preoccupation with weight and nutritional status in young females. *Can J Public Health* 2000;**91**:207–11.

83 **Swarr AE, Richards MH**. Longitudinal effects of adolescent girls' pubertal development, perceptions of pubertal timing, and parental relations on eating problems. *Dev Psychol* 1996;**32**:636–46.

84 **Stormer SM, Thompson JK**. Explanations of body image disturbance: a test of maturational status, negative verbal commentary, social comparison, and sociocultural hypotheses. *Int J Eat Disord* 1996;**19**:193–202.

85 **Levine MP, Smolak L, Moodey AF, Shuman MD, Hessen LD**. Normative developmental challenges and dieting and eating disturbances in middle school girls. *Int J Eat Disord* 1994;**15**:11–20.

86 **Oliver KK, Thelen MH**. Children's perceptions of peer influence on eating concerns. *Behav Ther* 1996;**27**:25–39.

87 **Cauffman E, Steinberg L**. Interactive effects of menarcheal status and dating on dieting and disordered eating among adolescent girls. *Dev Psychol* 1996;**32**:631–5.

88 **Blumstein P, Schwartz P**. *American couples: money, work, sex*. New York: William Morrow and Company, 1983.

89 **Kenrick DT, Gutierres SE, Goldberg LL**. Influence of popular erotica on judgments of strangers and mates. *J Exp Soc Psychol* 1989;**25**:159–67.

90 **Ogden J, Taylor C**. Body dissatisfaction within couples. *J Health Psychol* 2000;**5**:25–32.

91 **Giesen CB**. Aging and attractiveness: marriage makes a difference. *Int J Aging Hum Dev* 1989;**29**:83–94.

92 **Clark M, Ogden J**. The impact of pregnancy on eating behaviour and aspects of weight concern. *Int J Obes Rel Metab Disord* 1999;**23**:18–24.

93 **Davies K, Wardle J**. Body image and dieting in pregnancy. *J Psychosom Res* 1994;**38**:787–99.

94 **Fox P, Yamaguchi C**. Body image change in pregnancy: a comparison of normal weight and overweight primigravidas. *Birth* 1997;**24**:35–40.

95 **Jenkin W, Tiggemann M**. Psychological effects of weight retained after pregnancy. *Women Health* 1997;**25**:89–98.

96 **Devine CM, Bove CF, Olson CM**. Continuity and change in women's weight orientations and lifestyle practices through pregnancy and the postpartum period: the influence of life course trajectories and transitional events. *Soc Sci Med* 2000;**50**:567–82.

97 **Berman PW, O'Nan BA, Floyd W**. The double standard of aging and the social situation: judgments of attractiveness of the middle-aged woman. *Sex Roles* 1981;**7**:87–96.

98 **McAuley E, Bane SM, Rudolph DL, Lox CL**. Physique anxiety and exercise in middle-aged adults. *J Gerontol B Psychol Sci Soc Sci* 1995;**50B**:P229–35.

99 **Rizvi SL, Stice E, Agras WS**. Natural history of disordered eating attitudes and behaviors over a 6-year period. *Int J Eat Disord* 1999;**26**:406–13.

100 **Joiner TE, Heatherton TF, Keel PK**. Ten-year stability and predictive validity of five bulimia-related indicators. *Am J Psychiatry* 1997;**154**:1133–8.

101 **Wadsworth MEJ**. *The imprint of time: childhood, history and adult life*. Oxford: Oxford University Press, 1991.

102 **Wadsworth MEJ, Kuh DJL**. Childhood influences on adult health: a review of recent work in the British 1946 national birth cohort study, the MRC National Survey of Health and Development. *Paediatr Perinat Epidemiol* 1997;**11**:2–20.

103 **Thompson JK, Heinberg LH, Altabe MN, Tantleff-Dunn S**. *Exacting beauty: theory, assessment and treatment of body image disturbance*. Washington, DC: American Psychological Association, 2001.

104 **Thompson JK, Smolak L, eds**. *Body image, eating disorders and obesity in youth: assessment, prevention and treatment*. Washington, DC: American Psychological Association, 2001.

105 **Stice E**. Risk factors for eating pathology: Recent advances and future directions. In: Striegel-Moore R, Smolak L, eds. *Eating disorders: innovative directions in research and practice*. Washington, DC: American Psychological Association, 2001, pp. 51–74.

Part III

Biological, social, and psychosocial pathways

Chapter 10

Endocrine pathways in differential well-being across the life course

Carol M. Worthman

Current challenges in population health require better specification of the pathways to differential health outcomes, and such pathways are often gender specific. In this chapter, considerations of organic design from evolutionary biology are combined with physiological data, to suggest the importance of endocrine pathways in health across the life course. Endocrine bases of function and health risk are surveyed, and life course action and trajectories for a set of four exemplary endocrine axes (reproductive, adrenal, thyroid, and adiposal) are described, to illustrate the role of neuroendocrine-endocrine action in well-being. Reviews of acute and organizational impacts of ecological and behavioural factors on each of these axes demonstrate that hormones translate variation in behaviour, experience, and environmental quality into differential health outcomes over the long- and short-term. This analysis suggests the value to epidemiology of considering endocrine mediation in pathways to health, particularly women's health.

10.1 Introduction

The formidable task of meeting new or, until recently, intractable challenges to human well-being has prompted resurgent evaluation of and debate over the relative roles of population versus individual level interventions in social and public health policy. On the population side, social policy is confronting the need to expand from resource management, to include inequality *per se*,[1–4] while public health is evolving toward population health as it stretches to incorporate cultural, behavioural, and developmental factors that imply new targets for prevention.[5–8] These literatures share a common theme, namely the absence of well-specified pathways underlying the associations of context with health. Biomedical treatments and prophylaxis are challenged by emerging diseases fostered by structural and ecological conditions, and likewise from changing health risk related to demographic ageing and lifestyle changes.[9] Our extensive knowledge of how things work needs to be integrated into design principles that support predictions or hypotheses about life course impact of changing behaviours or circumstances.

A pathway-oriented, developmental life history approach may help to track the root causes of health outcomes. Attention to pathways between context and health is particularly salient for women, and has been a rationale for women's health initiatives during the last fifteen years.[10–12] Variation in the treatment and status of women and in their reproductive and productive roles and life histories, along with gender-specific physiology and health risks, set up distinctive ecologies, biologies, and pathways to health for women.[13] Furthermore, women's well-being affects that of their offspring, thereby accruing a multiplier effect into the future.[14–18]

This chapter provides a survey of endocrine axes (gonadal, adrenal, thyroid, adiposal) to show how mediating pathways operate. Hormones are central agents in the pathways to differential well-being: they regulate virtually every aspect of function, from gestation onwards. Integrated endocrine action also allocates limited resources (energy, materials, time) between the competing demands of living. Such demands range from the immediate necessities for survival, to the life course projects of growing up, reproducing, producing, and being social. This last demand strongly engages the physiological systems responsible for health maintenance because for humans, social context and human relationships are crucial to well-being.[6] By such physiological routes, many of the linkages between context and individual well-being are forged.

10.2 Endocrine architecture of the life course

Contemporary biological views of the life course build on life history theory, which proposes that biological design of the life course for any species is constrained by limited resources. Limited resources include time as well as energy, information, and relationships, and must be apportioned among the crucial enterprises of growth, reproduction, and survival/maintenance.[19,20] Schedules for deployment of resources among these enterprises with accompanying trade-offs among competing demands (live fast, die young versus live slowly, die old; offspring quality versus offspring quantity) form the macroarchitecture of life history. Distinctive features of the human life course include single relatively immature births, prolonged provisioning of young, slow growth with delayed maturation, low mortality, menopause, and long life span. These features apparently co-evolved with a singular cognitive-behavioural complex, including obligate sociality, use of language, pair bonding, and culture.[21] Evolutionary biology explains sex differences in life history, including biology and behaviour, as consequent to their different roles in reproduction.[22,23]

How the macroarchitecture of life history relates to the microarchitecture of physiology has scarcely interested biologists, but hormones are prime candidates.[24] Hormones establish the short- and long-term balance of resource allocation between growth, reproduction, and maintenance. Hormones juggle net energy availability by modulating metabolism and setting internal regulatory parameters, they regulate the rate of growth and the timing of developmental transitions such as puberty, and they dynamically manage the interface between the individual and environment by orchestrating responses to everything from stress to workload. Hormones establish an individual's sex and drive the reproductive life course, including for women the processes of pregnancy, parturition, lactation, and menopause. Endocrine regulation also determines timing of life history events (e.g. puberty, ageing), with physiological consequences that shape health risks.

A vivid example comes from the concept of fetal programming, which Barker and colleagues proposed to explain associations of neonatal outcomes (e.g. birthweight, body proportions, placental size) with risk for adult cardiovascular and metabolic disorders.[25–28] Neonatal outcomes, they proposed, reflect the impact of early environments on fetal development that, in turn, set parameters for function and further development over the life course and thereby affects risk for chronic disease. Endocrine factors mediate many of these phenomena.[27–30] This burgeoning literature on fetal programming not only has raised the importance of early environments for health risk[31–33] (see also special section, *International Journal of Epidemiology* **30**: 15–23, 50–98) and emphasized the importance of maternal conditions in pregnancy for long-term well-being of offspring,[34] but also it has yielded evidence for impact on life history. Specifically, neonatal size and maturity have been linked to age at menarche: among females thin at birth, those who are long reach menarche six months before those who are short.[35] This effect is most pronounced among those with above-average postnatal growth, and postnatal growth is known to be a sensitive indicator of environmental quality. Incidentally, this literature illustrates the value of specifying proximal bases for epidemiological findings.

Another instance is puberty, in which neuroendocrine mechanisms establish the childhood phase and initiate the process leading to reproductive competence.[36,37] Humans delay maturation and extend the pre-adult period to an extent unusual even for primates. Gonadal quiescence, and possibly adrenal androgen damping, are required to establish and maintain immaturity. Although the mechanisms responsible for sustained gonadal quiescence and triggering the onset of puberty remain uncertain, they operate via regulatory pathways through the hypothalamus. The brain acts as the pacemaker for puberty once it commences, and regulates ovarian cyclicity and reproductive ageing thereafter.

Hormones, then, are pivotal for guiding the life course through day-to-day prioritization of resource allocation, as well as the long-term scheduling of growth, reproductive effort, and ageing (Fig. 10.1). Knowledge of hormone action explains ongoing function, adaptation, and differential well-being, while consideration of life history offers a view of adaptive goals and trade-offs subserved by hormones.

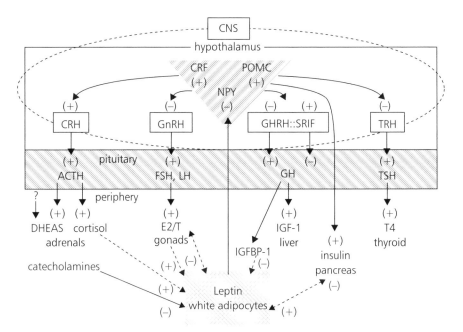

Fig. 10.1 Overview of exemplar endocrine systems.

10.3 Endocrine trajectories across the life course

We lack an integrated theory of physiological development that proceeds from life history through design to function. Emphasizing the roles hormones play in the physiological architecture of human adaptation and life course requires a rather different view of endocrinology than is prevalent in the endocrine, clinical, and epidemiological literature. Such literature has focused on the identification, characterization, regulation, and molecular biology of hormones and hormone action, on establishing normative ranges for expectable values, and on identifying correlates of risk. Comparative endocrine research has gradually established that, although the endocrine actors and main functional pathways are nearly universal, endocrine function can vary for specific axes and their interrelationships and thus play adaptive roles.[38]

Some of this cross-population variation may be based on genetic diversity, but much of it is influenced by the specific ecologies in which humans grow up and function.[39] The present discussion concerns the endocrine architecture of the life course with respect to differential health outcomes for women. Portions of that architecture are summarized in Fig. 10.1. Subsequent sections provide life course overviews of the following endocrine axes: hypothalamo–pituitary–gonadal (HPG), hypothalamo–pituitary–adrenal (HPA), hypothalamo–pituitary–thyroid (HPT), and weight regulation (lipostatic). For brevity, the somatotropic axis regulating growth, metabolic regulation, and energy partitioning is excluded. Data are drawn mainly from work on North Americans and, where that is unavailable, on western Europeans, to construct a functional picture for populations with roughly similar (though still diverse) cultural and physical ecologies. Sources have been selected on the basis of assay quality and comparability to other sources, of sample size, and of appropriateness or representativeness of the sampling strategy. Where possible, 95% confidence intervals are shown.

Understanding endocrine action and regulation entails more than the key peripheral hormone/s of a given endocrine axis, such as oestradiol or cortisol. The biological impact of circulating hormones involves several factors that moderate the relationships of hormones to health outcomes. These include:

1. Regulators of hormone production, such as the pituitary hormones that stimulate target gland activity (e.g. pituitary gonadotropins that control ovarian activity and thus, oestradiol levels) or blood sugar levels that drive insulin production. Altered ratios of stimulus to endocrine response indicate developmental transitions (puberty, menopause) or pathogenesis (diabetes, obesity).

2. Temporal patterns of endocrine release, produced both by endogenous rhythms and by exposure to stimuli. Circadian and pulsatile release patterns often convey information for endocrine action. Disruption of these patterns may contribute to pathogenesis, as in the case of dysregulated gonadotropin pulsatility in amenorrhoea[40] or of trauma-induced changes in circadian HPA activity.[41]

3. Binding proteins and soluble receptors significantly moderate the bioavailability of hormones and thus their biological impact. Although individual differences in carrier protein concentrations have been linked to endocrinopathies such as hirsutism in women, little research has explored the potential contributions of varying concentrations

of binding protein, soluble receptors, or immunoglobulins to individual or population variation in endocrine function and health.

4. Cross-talk among endocrine axes modulates the activity of any one axis in relation to others, and regulates partitioning of the body's resources between competing physiological and adaptive demands. Endocrine mediation of short- and long-term trade-offs in the allocation of scarce biological resources represents a rich vein for future research, but lies outside the scope of this survey.

This analysis provides a platform for future research by not only presenting what is known about function and regulation, but also indicating the scope of variation and suggesting its bases in sensitive organizational periods revealed by intervals of change or reorganization. It points, where possible, to potential epigenetic-ecological sources of variation, and draws attention to areas of potential investigation by clarifying the temporal and regulatory dynamics of several hormonal axes.

10.4 Hypothalamo–pituitary–gonadal (HPG) axis

The HPG axis exemplifies centrally regulated endocrine function, controlled via pulsatile secretion by the hypothalamus of gonadotropin-releasing hormone (GnRH) that, in turn, stimulates pulsatile release by the anterior pituitary of the gonadotropins follicle-stimulating hormone (FSH) and luteinizing hormone (LH). The amount and pattern of FSH and LH release drive ovarian activity, including ovarian steroid production, of which the principal form in females is oestradiol (E2), along with substantial progesterone (P) output in the latter half (luteal phase) of an ovulatory ovarian cycle. The regulatory loop is closed by feedback effects of circulating ovarian steroids on release of hypothalamic GnRH and anterior pituitary gonadotropins. The axis performs two key tasks: it controls reproductive maturation and closure, and maintains and regulates adult reproductive function. These tasks are central to women's reproductive health, and bear on health through the direct and indirect impact of ovarian steroids on central and peripheral function.

10.4.1 Age-related change

HPG activity in women changes markedly across the life course (Fig. 10.2), in this sequence: a brief postnatal burst of activity, followed by centrally-mediated early gonadal quiescence, a centrally-organized reactivation at puberty, a period of mature reproductive function supported by ongoing hypothalamic stimulation (represented here by LH), and menopausal closure of reproductive function following a process of reproductive senescence. A neuroendocrine 'switch' is required to break the HPG quiescence of childhood and initiate puberty, although the precise trigger for this centrally-mediated mechanism remains uncertain.[42] Thereafter, the axis requires several years to attain mature rates of ovulation and luteinization, a maturational period characterized by menarcheal subfecundity.[43] At the other end of the reproductive lifespan, menopause is a process comprising several years' altered HPG activity before and after the last menstrual bleed. Reproductive closure occurs mainly through follicle depletion despite accelerated central stimulation compounded by diminishing central sensitivity to ovarian feedback. As described in Chapter 4, menopause occurs on average in the fifth or sixth decade and is generally followed by massive gonadotropin output which gradually declines with age. Life course HPG activity exemplifies the neuroendocrine underpinnings of women's life history, including a prolonged juvenile period

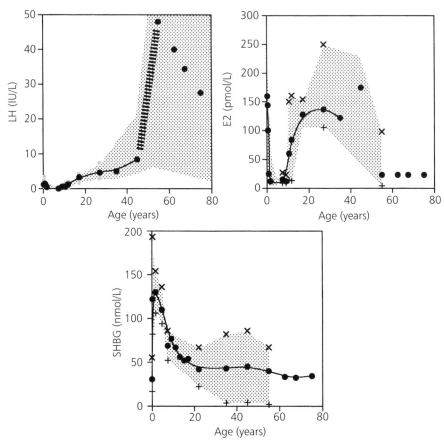

Fig. 10.2 Activity of women's reproductive axis across the life span. Top left panel: circulating concentrations of LH from birth through senescence (heavy dashed line indicates period of highly individually variable HPG dysregulation that accompanies the menopausal transition). Top right panel: E2 at all ages; line discontinued at age 40 years, due to high individual variability and conflicting reports, some suggesting that LH increases despite sustained or increasing E2 in this period. Bottom panel: circulating concentrations of SHBG, the gonadal steroid carrier protein. On all panels, values for postmenarcheal women are based on mid-follicular measures. (mean, solid circle; 95% confidence interval, stippled area). Data sources: LH: [191–195]. E2: [191, 193, 196, 197]. SHBG: [116, 198–203].

of reproductive immaturity, late onset of puberty and first birth, and early reproductive senescence.

A commonly overlooked moderator of bioavailable oestrogen is the blood-borne carrier protein, sex hormone binding globulin (SHBG), which binds circulating oestradiol and other steroids.[44,45] The lifespan profile of SHBG is distinct from that of its target hormones (Fig. 10.2). Levels of SHBG in women notably exceed those in men, despite the absolutely greater molar amounts of gonadal output in men than women, pregnancy excepted. This suggests a larger role for SHBG in modulating gonadal steroid action in women than men.

10.4.2 Ecological and behavioural factors

Unlike men, in whom gonadal activity is continuous and high after puberty, women produce varying levels of ovarian hormones depending on follicular activity. Behavioural and ecological factors heavily influence ovarian activity.[46] First, timing of puberty and onset of menses varies widely within and between populations: such variation is partly attributable to genetic effects but principally to environmental conditions such as gestational factors, nutrition, and infection (see Chapter 2).[47] Similarly strong environmental effects on reproductive ageing, or menopause in particular, have not been observed (see Chapter 4).[48] Second, timing of marriage, patterns of sexual activity, and contraceptive practices influence timing and numbers of pregnancies, during which follicular activity is suppressed.[43] Third, intensive sustained breastfeeding suppresses ovarian activity, maintaining postpartum amenorrhoea for months and damping ovarian activity once menses resume.[49] Moreover, women's nutritional status and workload are known to affect steroid output over the ovarian cycle, and hence also modulate exposure. Unfavourable energetic status from marginal nutrition, heavy workload, or illness, is accompanied by increased menstrual irregularity, increased anovulation, and reduced ovarian steroid output overall.[50] Other moderators of ovarian steroid levels include smoking, psychological stress, diet composition, and steroid contraceptive use.

Dietary sources of and environmental exposures to oestrogen agonists and antagonists (phytooestrogens, PCBs) have recently been implicated as modulators of steroid exposure that influence both reproductive function and health risk.[51] For instance, the very low prevalence of menopausal symptoms among Japanese has been attributed to habitual phytooestrogen consumption.[52] By contrast, decades of high steroid levels may contribute to symptom prevalence and severity at menopause in western populations.

Social, cultural, and individual factors that affect women's well-being (health, nutritional status, workload, stress) and reproductive life histories also affect amount and degree of ovarian activity across the life course. Such factors, as well as the gene-environment interactions they catalyse, produce inter- and intra-population variation in life course pattern and amount of ovarian activity and degree of ovarian output. For instance, Ellison and colleagues' comparative studies have shown population differences in luteal progesterone levels that persist across the reproductive life course and correspond to their degrees of behavioural and ecological stress (Fig. 10.3).[53]

10.4.3 Ovarian steroid exposure and risk

Steroids act on target tissues via receptors and other intracellular mechanisms; the nature and intensity of their action depends on receptor distribution, type, and density. The nuclear-level role of steroid activation also mediates their carcinogenic effects in target tissues. Considerable evidence links amount of steroid exposure to degree of cancer risk (see Chapter 3), and implicates culturally- and behaviourally-mediated variation of women's reproductive life course, health and nutrition, and workloads in cancer risk by moderating exposure to ovarian steroids.[54] Therefore, with early age at menarche, late age at first birth, few births, little or no breastfeeding, excellent nutrition, low physical activity, and high ovarian output per cycle, women in western postindustrial societies experience substantially increased ovarian steroid exposure and hence increased risk of reproductive cancer.[55] Chronic exposure to high levels of ovarian steroids may also exacerbate the risk of adverse

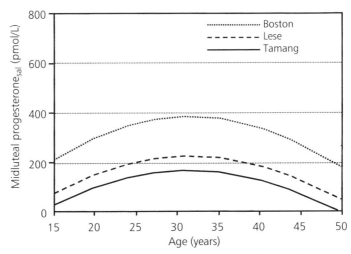

Fig. 10.3 Population differences in luteal function. Ellison and colleagues have assessed luteal function in several populations living in divergent societies and ecologies, including Lese horticulturalists of Zaire (dashed line), Tamang agriculturalists of Nepal (solid line), and postindustrial Americans in Boston (dotted line). Curves are fitted to mean for age of maximum salivary progesterone in saliva collected every two days from samples of women of each group[53].

symptoms in menopause: although a minority of western women experience the core symptoms of menopause (hot flushes, night sweats), a much smaller proportion report such symptoms in populations as diverse as Japan or Guatemala.[13,56] Population differences in HPG activity, as illustrated in Fig. 10.3, suggest a possible need for population-adjusted formulations of steroid contraceptives to reduce side-effects.[57]

Ovarian steroid exposure and its moderators influence risk for other morbidities.[58] Patterns of exposure in western postindustrial societies, combined with sedentary lifestyles and prolonged life span, contribute to dramatic increases in rates of osteoporosis in these populations (see Chapter 7). Ovarian steroid effects on metabolism promote fat deposition, which results in a visible change in body contours at puberty and contributes to the large sex difference in adult body composition.[59] Such energy storing action has adaptive value in settings of uncertain food supply, but among overnourished populations, contributes to risk for obesity. Additionally, where lean body image is valued in women, the adiposity-promoting action of ovarian steroids both sets up women for a conflict between social values and biology, and may promote vulnerability to eating disorders that address both problems (body image and ovarian activity) (see Chapter 9).

Where reproductive risk is low, women outlive men, which implies the existence of protective factors in women, risk factors in men, or both. Changes in relative risk for diverse chronic diseases (cardiovascular, mood disorder) after menopause imply endocrine involvement (see Chapters 5 and 8).[60] Ovarian steroids moderate risk for hypertension and cardiovascular events, through direct action on serum lipid profiles and plaque formation.[61]

Turning from physical to mental health, ovarian steroids exert multiple effects on the central nervous system (CNS)[62] and have been implicated in risk for mood disorders, specifically for depression (reviewed in Chapter 8). Oestrogens also act as neurogenic agents that promote dendrite and synapse formation, blunt neurotoxicity from glucocorticoids and free radicals, and acutely enhance mood and cognitive performance,[63–66] whereas progesterone acts neuroprotectively by reducing secondary neural damage in cerebral trauma or stroke.[67,68]

10.5 Hypothalamo–pituitary–adrenal (HPA) axis

The adrenal gland secretes a range of hormones with diverse physiological roles across the life course, but which spread resources among competing physiological demands. Such adaptive adjustments are essential but costly, and carry a cost-benefit trade-off: adrenal hormones mobilize resources to accommodate small and large physiological and psychological challenges, but continual or prolonged activation leads to functional impairment.[97] The adrenal comprises two functionally distinct compartments, cortex and medulla. The former produces mineralocorticoids, glucocorticoids, and adrenal androgens that regulate basic functions, from electrolyte balance to glucose metabolism and stress response. The medulla acts as a neuroendocrine structure by releasing the adrenergic neurotransmitters epinephrine and norepinephrine into the bloodstream.

Both compartments operate synergistically to promote short- to long-term adjustments to physiological and environmental load (Fig.10.1, left). The sympatheto–adrenal–medullary (SAM) axis organizes swift (in milliseconds) endocrine responses that rapidly initiate physiological (e.g. heart rate) and cognitive (e.g. heightened arousal, vigilance) adjustments and, in turn, facilitate behavioural reactions. This axis has been implicated in the aetiology of hypertension under conditions of chronic stress or arousal. A rather slower (15–30 minutes to peak response) HPA cascade involves corticotropin releasing hormone (CRH), adrenocorticotropic hormone (ACTH), and cortisol, and mediates adjustments in physiological priorities from long-term (e.g. growth, reproduction, digestion) to short-term (vigorous activity, alertness) functions.

Two kinds of adrenocortical hormones, the glucocorticoid cortisol and the adrenal androgen dehydroepiandrosterone-sulfate (DHEAS), are discussed below. The contrast in functional roles illustrates two aspects of endocrine action, for cortisol mediates acute, rapid responses to arousal or stress, whereas the adrenal androgen DHEAS shows little episodic or diurnal variability, but undergoes distinctively patterned changes across the life course that reflect pacemakers of life history.

10.5.1 Cortisol

This portion of the HPA axis is regulated by episodic and circadian hypothalamic output of CRH, that consequently stimulates the anterior pituitary to release ACTH. In turn, ACTH stimulates adrenocortical release of cortisol. Commonly viewed as a stress hormone, cortisol might be better imagined as an activational hormone that facilitates or mobilizes responses to psychobiological load.[69,70] Release is pulsatile and episodic, exhibits strong diurnal variation, and responds acutely to psychobehavioural conditions including sleep-wake patterns, eating, vigorous physical activity, and psychological challenge (worry, excitement, performance anxiety, new situations).[71,72] Hence, at any given moment, circulating levels reflect impact of experience and behaviour within the last hour, although physiological and affective load drive cortisol release by different pathways.[73,74] HPA reactivity—threshold, latency, magnitude, and duration of cortisol release—has been identified as a factor in well-being, including cardiovascular,[75] infectious,[76] and psycho-behavioural[77] risk.

Cortisol acts to promote immediate survival needs at the expense of long-term processes by stimulating catabolic and inhibiting anabolic pathways.[70] It increases blood glucose, vigilance, and attention focusing, reduces food intake, HPG activity, gut motility, growth, and memory formation, and alters immune activity. Cortisol exerts non-linear (inverted U-shaped) effects on memory, arousal, sensory integration, and emotion regulation, due to the concentration dependent differential activation of two glucocorticoid receptors.[78]

10.5.1.1 Age-related change

The adrenal gland undergoes a brief period of postnatal reorganization, and achieves diurnal periodicity by 6 months of age.[79–81] Thereafter, little age-related change occurs until a trend of gradually increasing cortisol emerges from the third decade (Fig. 10.4).[82,83] No early sex differences in circulating cortisol have been reported, but sex differences in HPA regulation obtain from birth, whereby a lower level of circulating cortisol accompanies a given level of the trophic hormone, ACTH, in males than females. ACTH exhibits both

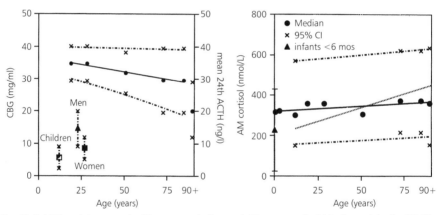

Fig. 10.4 HPA activity over the life course. Left panel: Plasma cortisol binding globulin (CBG) concentrations (left axis; solid circle, solid line) by age and mean 24-hour serum ACTH values in children (mean age 11.3 years; hatched box) and adults (mean age 25 years) of both sexes (with 95% confidence interval; X, dashed line). Slope by age for CBG insignificant and age-specific variance is large. Note apparent large drop in advanced age, possibly implying increased free, bioactive cortisol. Age and sex differences in ACTH (children, hatched box; women, solid box; men, solid triangle), and absent concomitant cortisol correlates, indicate regulatory differences. Right panel: Morning cortisol in circulation. Median (closed circle, solid line) and 95% confidence interval (X, dash-dot line) shown for all age groups, except infants, shown separately because their HPA axes undergo substantial reorganization in the first six months (solid triangle, AM circulating cortisol values by age, both sexes with 95% confidence interval). Lines represent slope by age (solid for male, dotted for female) (71) applied to this value range. Age trend significant in both sexes; infants under 6 months show differences in cortisol output that indicate a developmental period. CBG, ACTH: [85, 87, 204, 205]. Cortisol: [95, 205].

lower levels and lack of sex differences in childhood, and sex differences in adulthood with small or absent cortisol differences.[84,85] Both age and sex discrepancies suggest differences in ACTH delivery to the adrenal, or in adrenocortical sensitivity or responsiveness to ACTH stimulation.

Indeed, sex differences in responsivity of the HPA emerge with age.[71] In a psychosocial challenge test, young men were both more likely to have raised cortisol levels (75%, 6 times more than women), and showed larger cortisol increments than female responders (no sex difference in non-responders). Conversely, cortisol responses in older female responders greatly exceeded that in male responders, aged or young.[84,86] Age-related shifts in sex differences in HPA response to such challenge may reflect real differences in vulnerability to psychosomatic stressors over the life course. Concurrently declining cortisol-binding protein (CBP) leaves more free, bioavailable cortisol and magnifies such differences. Age-related enzymatic shifts in adrenal function may contribute to changing neurological risk: increased ratios of cortisol to adrenal androgens have been observed in the cerebrospinal fluid of children (aged 3–8 years) and elderly (over 60 years), who may be more vulnerable to neurolytic effects of stress.[70,87] Greater increases in ratios of glucocorticoids to adrenal androgens in women may compound neurological risk.[88,89] Finally, circadian cortisol variation increases markedly with age in women (Fig. 10.5), such that the early adult sex difference (greater variation in men) reverses with ageing.

10.5.1.2 Ecological and behavioural factors

Since cortisol operates through its responsivity to ecological and behavioural conditions, virtually all literature on cortisol could be relevant. Initially, cortisol was viewed as acutely driven by 'stress', and neither summed nor habituated; hence, increasing cortisol must reflect escalating stimulus, and previous activity of the axis should not affect its current

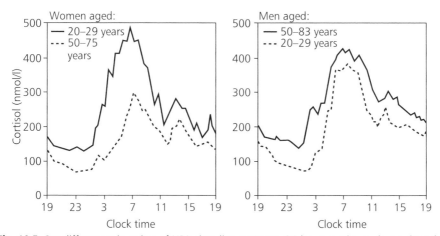

Fig. 10.5 Sex differences in aging of HPA circadian patterns. 24 hour continuously monitored plasma cortisol, by sex and age. Left panel: women 20–29 years (dashed line) versus 50–75 years (solid line). Right panel: men 20–29 (dashed line) versus 50–83 years (solid line). Women show greater acrophase and phase shift with age than do men. Data source: [71].

activity. Lately, a body of animal literature has established the importance of experience and begun to unpack the epigenetic bases of variation in HPA function.[90–92] This and human clinical work has shown that HPA function is affected by gestational conditions, postnatal care, and other early experiences, acute trauma, and chronic deprivation.[17,41,93]

Cortisol exhibits wide individual variation that can persist over time and represent stable individual characteristics.[94] For instance, a large cross-sectional study of circadian cortisol levels in Swedish children showed over five-fold variation in individual mean diurnal values.[95] Diurnal measures repeated over 0.5 to 8 years on a subset of pubertal children, showed high longitudinal stability of cortisol output. The broad, stable individual variation in cortisol was not associated with anthropometric correlates, which suggests little effect on lypolysis and glucose homeostasis, although cortisol is related to their regulation. Such findings may be due to differences in target tissue sensitivity, but they may also be due to organizational effects on metabolic regulation. Reports of a U-shaped relationship between birthweight and glucocorticoid excretion in childhood,[28] as well as of persistently higher adrenocortical activity in rhesus exposed to prenatal stress,[96] support the latter possibility.

10.5.1.3 Cortisol and health risk

As a component of stress response, cortisol has been implicated in an extensive range of health risks, including cardiovascular, metabolic, gastrointestinal, reproductive, immunological, neurological and related cognitive and psychiatric disorders.[70,75,97] Target tissue variation in sensitivity to glucocorticoids contributes to individual differences in cortisol effects.[98] Glucocorticoids have been found to impede memory formation and mediate selective neuronal loss in the brain.[70,99] Socioculturally mediated gender differences in exposure to and coping with stressors may thereby contribute to differential health risk. Additionally, increased stress responsivity and central resistance to glucocorticoid feedback is thought to exacerbate risk for depression in women, and contribute to the paradox that adult women have greater rates of physical morbidity than men but lower risk of mortality.[100]

10.5.2 Adrenal androgens

The role of the adrenal androgens in life history merits attention, for humans and few other primates possess qualitatively and quantitatively distinctive adrenal activity patterns. Adrenal androgens—androstenedione, dehydroepiandrosterone (DHEA) and its sulfate (DHEAS)—are weak androgens produced by the zona reticularis of the adrenal cortex in abundant quantities that, from puberty, exceed those of all other steroids. Circulating adrenal androgens exhibit progressive changes across the life course[101,102] that are most evident for DHEAS, the quantitatively predominant steroid hormone.(Fig. 10.6). Changes in adrenal androgen output after birth, at adrenarche and puberty, and with ageing reflect adrenal reorganizations that dismantle or elaborate zones having enzyme activity favouring their production.[103] Although adrenal steroidogenesis is well understood, regulation of adrenal androgen production is not: ACTH stimulates episodic, pulsatile and circadian DHEA release in parallel with cortisol (DHEAS does not), but these hormones run contrary under other circumstances. Under stress or physical trauma, cortisol may be elevated or flat while adrenal androgens are reduced. Moreover, ACTH does not account for the lifetime pattern of change. Alternatively, insulin-like growth factors (IGFs) stimulate adrenal androgen

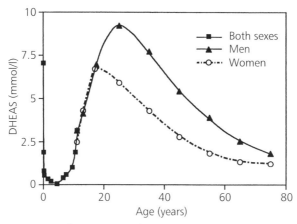

Fig. 10.6 Lifespan trajectory of DHEAS. Data for circulating DHEAS are combined for both sexes until differences emerge in puberty. Data source: [206].

production, and insulin-like growth factor-I (IGF-I) correlates with DHEA/S production from adrenarche into old age.[104]

Functions of adrenal androgens remain perplexing, for their massive production begs an explanation.[105] DHEA(S) provide substrates for substantial peripheral intracrine production of oestrogens and androgens that exert significant steroid target tissue bioactivity.[106] Where synthesized in brain, they exhibit neurosteroid activity with mood-, sleep-, and memory-enhancing effects. Multiple suggested carcinoprotective, immunoenhancing, neurogenic, antiobesity, antidiabetic, and antiageing effects scarcely explain the unusual DHEAS production of humans.[104]

10.5.2.1 Age-related change

Circulating concentrations of DHEAS (Fig. 10.6) are high at birth, decline rapidly over the first year of life to the low and slightly rising levels in early childhood, and show an increase in slope between six and eight years of age. This shift, adrenarche, occurs somewhat earlier in girls than boys. Increased adrenal androgen output in mid-childhood is probably unrelated to timing of puberty; adrenarche occurs at similar ages in very late as in early maturing populations.[107,108] At puberty, adrenal androgen output escalates sharply and climbs steadily to reach peak values in the early-mid 20s, and thereafter declines with age.[109] These age-related changes in DHEAS may either have functional implications on their own, related to direct effects of DHEAS, or they may indirectly index ageing processes reflected in DHEAS. Otherwise, DHEAS may serve a background or buffering role that moderates the impact of variation in other steroid hormones, such as glucocorticoids. Marked sex differences in adrenal androgens emerge with adrenarche and puberty: adrenals generate the great preponderance of DHEAS and gonads a minor fraction, yet circulating levels in men exceed those in women.[103] Consequent to divergent age-related change, the ratio of cortisol to DHEAS follows a U-shaped curve with age[104] that is particularly pronounced for women, in whom age- and body mass index (BMI)-adjusted cortisol is 10% higher and DHEAS 40% lower than in men.[83]

10.5.2.2 Ecological and behavioural factors

Because interest in life course patterns of adrenal androgens has been so recent, and largely focused on ageing, data concerning their sensitivity to ecological and developmental factors remain sketchy. Initial reports document large population differences in DHEAS output across the life course that track maturational timing and show that western populations have chronically elevated values from puberty onwards.[39,110] Reduced DHEAS and hence reduction of its anticarcinogenic, chemoprotective, and endocrinological buffering activities may reflect action of life history trade-offs to prioritize immediate needs over long-term maintenance in populations confronting lower environmental quality and greater health risks. More acutely, DHEA(S) is reduced by severe illness or chronic stress.[103] For instance, by contrast with cortisol, DHEAS is reduced in depression.[111]

10.5.2.3 DHEAS and health risk

DHEA(S) may offer sex-differentiated protective effects against cardiovascular disease (CVD), cancer, immune-based diseases, mood and memory disorders, and ageing.[104,112,113] Lower DHEAS characterizes Alzheimer's disease and diabetes, and is associated with reduced bone density in middle-aged women (not men), depressed mood in older women (not men), and prospectively with risk for premenopausal breast cancer and for CVD mortality in elderly men (not women).[111,114] A direct aetiological role is difficult to infer even from prospective studies, because DHEA(S) may simply reflect differential ageing and its associated morbidities or index other physiological processes that influence health status. Relationships of adrenal androgens to life expectancy seem complex. Follow-up of populations showing short-term associations of DHEAS with cardiovascular mortality risk has diminished the estimate of their effect on survival risk for men, and shown no effect on women.[115–117] Nevertheless, enthusiasm for DHEA replacement therapy focuses on its putative role in ageing[114,118] and possible direct protective actions including buffering neurolytic effects of glucocorticoids.[119]

10.6 Thyrotropic axis and central metabolic regulation

The hypothalamo–pituitary–thyroid axis (HPT) comprises a primary endocrine pathway regulating energy homeostasis. Central regulation originates in the hypothalamus, proceeds through secretion of thyrotropin-releasing hormone (TRH) to stimulate anterior pituitary release of thyroid stimulating hormone (TSH), and thence prompt thyroid hormone (thyroxine (T4) and triiodothyronine (T3)) production. Thyroid activity responds to energy expenditure, increases metabolic rate, and hence serves an important adaptive function.[120]

10.6.1 Age-related change

The formulation of reference ranges for normal thyroid (euthyroid) functioning are of considerable public health importance in determining the widespread risk for and functional impact of hypothyroidism.[121] Yet reference values remain elusive for lack of a definitive marker of euthyroid status.[122,123] The pituitary hormone, TSH, represents actual thyroid function indirectly, while 92–94% of the principal thyroid hormone, thyroxine (T4), is tied up by circulating binding proteins that themselves undergo developmental change.[123,124] As the bioactive form, free T4 is considered an optimal marker of thyroid activity. T4 exhibits a

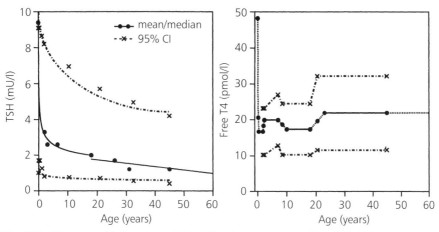

Fig. 10.7 Lifespan activity patterns of the HPT axis. Means or medians (solid circle, solid line) with 95% confidence intervals (X, dot-dash line) for plasma TSH (left panel) and free T4 (right panel), for the first six decades, both sexes combined. Data sources: TSH: [126, 129, 207, 208]; free T4: [124, 126, 129].

complex pattern of age-related change over a narrow range of variation across the lifespan (Fig. 10.7) that is thought to indicate maturational shifts in pituitary and thyroid regulation.[124] But, following a neonatal TSH and T4 surge, little[125] or no[126] age-related change in T4 has been observed, although TSH declines through childhood and adolescence.[127] Sex differences have not been seen systematically at any age. Reports of elevated TSH with age[128] are based on populations unscreened for health status. Studies of well-screened healthy aged populations, by contrast, indicate TSH does decline steadily from late infancy throughout adulthood, reflecting diminishing pituitary response to hypothalamic releasing hormone.[129–131]

10.6.2 Ecological and behavioural factors

Of the endocrine axes discussed here, the HPT is most overtly influenced by ecology and behaviour. Thyroid dysfunction arises principally from iodine deficiency or overnutrition; iodine bioavailability depends on diet, soil and water content, and is antagonized by goitrogens.[132] Overall, one billion people are considered at risk for iodine deficient disorders (IDD).[132] Consequently, most postindustrial countries run national neonatal screening programs to detect congenital hypothyroidism, and international salt iodization campaigns in the last decade have decreased IDD rates.[133] Deficiencies of cofactors essential for thyroid action (selenium, zinc, copper, iron) also compromise HPT function.[134,135]

10.6.3 Thyroid function and health risk

Thyroid dysfunction related to iodine malnutrition is readily prevented by iodine prophylaxis but persists widely, even in Europe,[136] despite massive international campaigns. Juvenile hypothyroidism (congenital or iodine deficient, characterized by elevated TSH, above 10 IU/ml) galvanizes concern because it impairs brain development and is the main preventable cause of mental retardation.[137–139] If congenital or severe and chronic, hypothyroidism results in cretinism or goitre, respectively. Within a broad zone of subclinical hypothyroidism, inadequate thyroid function at any age associates with poor cognitive functioning and motor performance (learning, memory, attention, reaction time), and depression.[140] Distractability, insomnia, anxiety, and emotional instability accompany hyperthyroidism.[137] But the most significant long-term consequence of mild-to-moderate iodine insufficiency is hyperthyroidism in ageing, associated with osteoporosis, muscle atrophy, and cardiac dysfunction.[141,142] Conversely, high iodine intake increases risk of autoimmune hypothyroidism, which increases consistently with age.[143] Indeed, iodine supplementation must be monitored and moderated to maintain intakes within a range that avoids hypo- and hyperthyroidism.[125,144]

HPT function particularly affects women's health: women experience much more thyroid disorder than men, having 3–6, 2–5, and 2.5–5 times the population prevalence of hypothyroidism, hyperthyroidism, and thyroid autoimmunity than men, respectively.[125,145,146] The gender disparity increases with ageing. Autoimmune hypothyroidism disrupts reproductive health, associating with ovarian dysfunction and infertility, increased pregnancy failure, and autoimmune postpartum rebound from immunosuppression of pregnancy.[147] Increased risk for goitre in women has been attributed to goitrogenic effects of pregnancy;[148] thyroid volume increases with parity, so that adequate iodine supply is crucial to avert even moderate iodine deficiency.[149] Hypothyroidism further contributes to risk for chronic depression, more prevalent in women.[150,151] Hence, much of the burden of dietary and autoimmune thyroid disease is borne by women, and the gender disparity of that burden increases with age.

10.7 Leptin and distributed metabolic regulation

Although it had long been thought that the brain must monitor energy status (energy stores minus expenditure) in order to regulate physiological and behavioural determinants of such status, the bases for signalling energy (net from energy intake and expenditure) remained uncertain until leptin was reported in late 1994.[152,153] Subsequent research has expanded the view of its role as 'lipostat' in weight regulation, to include an array of central and peripheral actions in metabolic, reproductive, affective, and even haemopoeitic activity.[154–157] It has also widened our views of endocrine function. Leptin is a cytokine-related hormone produced principally by white adipocytes and shows pulsatility as well as diurnal rhythmicity (nadir [range] ~1030 h [0800–1740 h]; peak [range]~0120 h [2200–0300 h]).[158] Receptors for leptin are not only found in fat, muscle, pancreas, and liver, but also richly represented in the CNS, particularly at its principal site of action and the seat of energetics regulation, the hypothalamus.[159] A host of neuropeptides (most importantly, neuropeptide Y, proopiomelanocortin, and agouti-related peptide) moderate or transduce the central actions of leptin on thermogenesis, energy metabolism, and food intake, as well as hypothalamically-mediated impact on other axes, including the gonadal, adrenal, and thyroid. The soluble form of its receptor circulates as a carrier protein for leptin, regulates its bioavailability, and increases markedly at puberty.[160]

Circulating levels of leptin acts as a trait (energy stores, weight maintenance, long-term energy balance) and a state (acute energy imbalance) marker. Leptin correlates exponentially with body fat stores and provides a metabolic signal to the hypothalamic regions regulating satiety, energy expenditure, and multiple related endocrine axes. But it also preemptively signals acute energy imbalance by shifting during weight loss or gain, such that fasting decreases and overfeeding increases leptin, even though meal ingestion has no acute effect. The modulatory impact of leptin on other endocrine domains contributes to its actions over different time horizons: from acute effects on food intake, to effects over hours on glucose metabolism, to changes in CNS gene expression over days, to impacts on weight and body composition over days or weeks, and permissive effects on puberty onset and reproductive function over years.[154]

Body composition, specifically per cent body fat versus lean body mass, is the most sexually dimorphic feature in humans, whereby per cent body fat in young women is nearly 50% greater than in young men.[161] Accordingly, shortly after birth onwards, leptin concentrations in females exceed those in males of the same body weight among lean as well as obese individuals (Fig. 10.8).[154,162–165] Reasons for this difference include effects of sex hormones, the difference in body composition itself, and greater output of leptin by adipocytes in women from mid-puberty.[166–171] The strong negative relationship of leptin to testosterone in males and the less robust positive one to oestradiol in females has been observed in studies of endocrine change in puberty.[172,173] Grounds for manifest differences not only in body composition but also in eating disorders and overall weight regulation have been sought in such distinctive leptin patterns, but actions of leptin are not so direct. Given the importance of energy status to reproduction, particularly the high energy outlays required of women for pregnancy and lactation, relationships of leptin and reproductive function are necessarily complex. Gonadal steroids may alter sensitivity of the CNS to leptin-mediated signals; reciprocally, leptin output is altered by direct and indirect effects of gonadal steroids, and leptin permissively influences HPG function.[59,174]

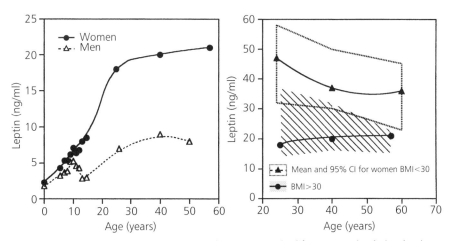

Fig. 10.8 Relationship of gender and BMI to leptin across the life course. Circulating leptin concentrations over the first six decades. Left panel: Sex differences in leptin (women: closed circle, solid line; men: open triangle, dotted line), commence from birth, becoming pronounced at puberty and remaining so in adulthood. [163, 177, 180]. Right panel: Relationship between leptin and BMI, largely mediated by fat mass. Mean and 95% confidence interval for women with BMI <30 (solid circle, solid line; hatched area) versus those with BMI > 30 (solid triangle, solid line; dot-outlined area) [180].

10.7.1 Age-related change

Age-related changes in leptin are difficult to disentangle from changes in body composition due to developmental (growth, puberty) or behavioural (activity) factors. As noted above, girls have higher leptin than boys before, during, and after puberty even discounting girls' greater adiposity,[175] though not all reports confirm this pattern (Fig. 10.8).[59] Because it signals energy stores, leptin was also expected to play a permissive role in puberty onset.[176] Consistent with this expectation, leptin increases markedly at puberty,[177] but animal data do not support a causal role.[42] During the years of ovarian cyclicity, leptin varies with the ovarian cycle in conjunction with progesterone and peaks in the luteal phase. Leptin increases in pregnancy and declines sharply postpartum, which changes correspond to those in oestradiol and (human chorionic gonadotropin (hCG).[178,179] Thereafter, BMI-adjusted levels decline progressively with age, including after menopause. In contrast to the relationship of oestradiol and leptin over the ovarian cycle, such decline appears independent of diminishing oestradiol and other endocrine changes, although these make some contribution.[180]

10.7.2 Ecological and behavioural factors

Adjustments in leptin production and regulation could provide powerful means for facultative adjustment of energy management. For instance, early energy restriction might influence the organization of metabolic regulation reflected in alterations of leptin output by adipocytes, autonomic regulation of fat cells, or of hypothalamic and thus behavioural responses to leptin signals.[181] Relevant data are as yet unavailable, but support for one such effect comes from a report that lower birth or infant weight is associated with greater adult leptin, controlling for adult weight.[182] A small literature on specific ethnicities[170,183] or non-western populations[184,185] is complicated by complexities of controlling for body fat and does not support generalities, though it indicates potential population variation in correlates of leptin.

10.7.3 Leptin and health risk

Initially, it was hoped that leptin might provide a pharmacological or even genetic 'magic bullet' for weight regulation, particularly prevention and treatment of obesity and eating disorders, through effects on eating behaviour, on metabolism, or both. That hope swiftly faded. Hopefully further research will be able to address worldwide patterns of both undernutrition and pandemic overnutrition and its attendant disorders (diabetes, CVD).[156,157] For instance, leptin apparently plays a key role in adaptation to sustained nutritional deprivation by maintaining elevated cortisol and GH to ensure fat mobilization. These effects, with concurrent suppression of IGF-1, divert energy from growth to metabolic demands.[186] Genetic defects account for a minor fraction of obesity cases; obesity is usually accompanied by leptin resistance, and receptor and post-receptor mechanisms for such resistance are under scrutiny. The roles of adrenal, and less so of gonadal, steroids in modulating leptin regulation and action may be particularly pertinent to unravelling the physiological, psychobehavioural, and ecological bases of increased vulnerability of women for eating disorders and obesity. Additionally, patterns of leptin production (Fig. 10.8) emphasize that the biology of women reflects adaptation to the heavy energetic demands of reproduction.[46,187,188] At puberty, changes in oestradiol and leptin drive the accumulation of body fat in anticipation of reproductive needs, but in low fertility, overnourished populations, this capacity becomes a potential health liability. Further, where leanness denotes beauty and virtue, the potential for distress and eating disorders is exacerbated.[189]

10.8 Pathways to women's health

Historically, attribution of women's health issues to women's biology or behaviour led to targeting women themselves for prevention and treatment.[190] Recognition that such issues are the life course product of women's specific needs and capacities, with the context in which they develop, function, and age, points to societal-structural targets for health promotion. This survey has integrated the epidemiological and biomedical literatures concerning women's health by sketching pathways to differential well-being from macro-architectual (life history) through microarchitectural (endocrinology) levels. Figure 10.9 outlines a framework for pathway analysis. The upper tier depicts an evolutionary view of life history and its endocrine architecture in relation to life course analysis on the level of the individual. It shows relationships of life history parameters (life history box at top) to

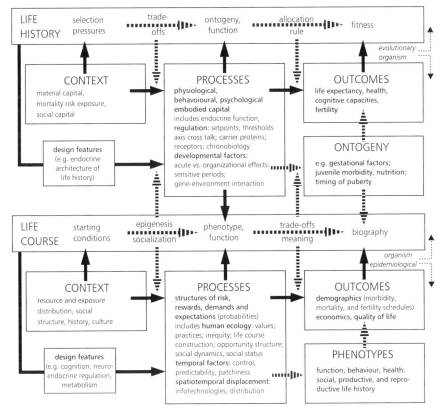

Fig. 10.9 Framework for pathways analysis, from the evolutionary through the individual-organismic, to the population-epidemiologic levels.

individual ontogeny and function, focusing on mediating endocrine factors, that determine adult outcomes in health, survival, and competence (at organism level; 'ontogeny' and 'outcomes' boxes, upper right), as well as fitness (on the evolutionary level; top right) and gene frequencies. The lower tier concerns relationships of individual life course processes ('life course' box at centre) to population-level epidemiology ('phenotypes' and 'outcome' boxes, lower right), focusing on interactions of social conditions with organism design features to determine population-level outcomes, including quality of life, productivity, and demographics, as well as individual life courses ('biography', centre right).

This framework relates design features from evolutionary processes to the population outcomes that concern epidemiologists, through the individual level of the organism. Phenotype emerges from the individualized intersection of evolutionary history with human ecology (political economy, economics, culture) that through time, makes the life course. In aggregate, on the population level, the combined probabilities for exposure and vulnerability established by population ecology and biology produce the array of phenotypes counted in demography as morbidity, mortality, and fertility, and in epidemiology as differential outcomes. We use breast cancer risk in contemporary postindustrial societies as an example. Changes in practices (decreased breastfeeding), life course construction (delayed reproduction), and values (reduced fertility goals; education and employment for women) increase lifetime exposure to steroids (summed in the phenotype). Concurrent changes in practices (child care, public sanitation, vaccination), values (gender equality), and life course construction (education rather than labour for children) result both in increased life expectancy, and in biological changes (accelerated maturation, upregulated ovarian activity) mediated by organic design features associated with life history trade-offs. Together, increased life expectancy and increased steroid exposure converge at the individual level with constitutional-genetic conditions and epigenetic processes (moderators of steroid action [receptors, enzymes, exogenous steroids], of breast tissue development, and of immune function [stress, exposures]) that determine probability of carcinogenesis and progression.

Tracking pathways to health risk (and prevention) brings epidemiology to life, because proximal pathways effect lifespan development and function, and hence the health of all members of society. Pathway analysis integrates existing epidemiological with biomedical-physiological data to both explain recognized trends (increased breast cancer) and suggest new hypotheses concerning cause (e.g. compromised immune function) or intervention (e.g. increase breastfeeding). Identification of mediating pathways facilitates recognition of trade-offs such as those between lifestyle choice and health, of early versus later patterns of morbidity, or among diverse dimensions of well-being. Individual processes emerge as central, highlighting the value of rich individual level data for epidemiology.

A life course approach constrains health research to follow the problem rather than vice versa, mandates pursuit of the problem through multiple levels and time frames, suggests routes for intervention, and predicts consequences of social change and lifestyle variation. This is particularly true for certain areas such as women's health. Social change or structural reforms can cause broad spectrum improvements in well-being, but need to be accompanied by processes at the individual level that operate synergistically to produce specific health trade-offs. The pathways approach should help all concerned with the present complex challenges to health, to meet those challenges through new ideas, research, and policy.

Commentary on 'Endocrine pathways in differential well-being across the life course'

Elizabeth Barrett-Connor

> Biology is the study of complicated things that give the appearance of having been designed for a purpose.[209]

This chapter, with its impressively broad sweep, is a grand effort to pull together data from diverse sources and disciplines. Many ideas and challenges are presented. I expect that readers who have not considered hormones in the context of anthropology will find the first few pages hard reading. Soldier on, for there are numerous provocative ideas and observations that follow, despite the limitations of the available data.

The study of hormones throughout the human life span, never mind their relation to adult health and longevity, is incredibly complex for several reasons, beginning with the spotty data drawn from different sources. Figure 10.10 describes the large variation over the

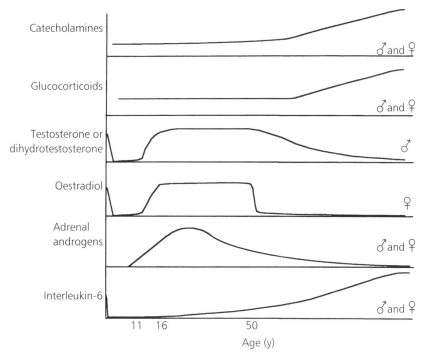

Fig. 10.10 Changes in circulating hormones and interleukin-6 with ageing in men and women[210].

adult life course in circulating levels of four hormone groups, catecholamines, and inter-leukin-6,[210] but some of these lines 'connect the dots' over large or important periods of life for which there is little intervening data, and the data do not come from the same people or even the same laboratory.

The number of hormones and the number of outcomes is overwhelming; this topic could have been the subject of an entire book, rather than the limited number of pages permitted in a book chapter. As a consequence of enforced brevity, it may be difficult for the reader to evaluate the studies cited (although there is an impressive bibliography), or whether the reported hormone patterns were derived from studies with only a few subjects (as is often the case), or whether the source of subjects was patients or populations. (When the sample is too small or the study subjects are not representative of a population, results may be misleading.) Other details important to the interpretation of results are also lacking, such as laboratory methods, and hour of day and follicular phase when blood for hormone assays was obtained. (The paucity of large studies in premenopausal women undoubtedly reflects the problems of the timing of blood samples to measure sex hormones in cycling women.) Few studies have repeated hormone levels in the same individuals, and none for more than a few years out of a lifetime. Thus, the life course graph shown in Fig. 10.10 does not repre-sent cohorts followed over time, but separate studies in different people and places.

The challenges become more complex when attempting to link women's hormone levels to health outcomes at some remote time in their lives. Most studies reporting the relation of endogenous sex hormones to subsequent disease are recent, reflecting the relatively new availability of sensitive, reliable, and affordable hormone assays suitable for large popula-tion samples. Although animal studies and epidemiological data leave little doubt that oestrogen promotes breast cancer, the first pooled analysis of nine studies of baseline oestrogen levels and subsequent breast cancer to confirm this thesis was not completed until 2001.[211] Animal and epidemiological data also support a role for oestrogen deficiency and osteoporosis in women, but the first prospective study showing that lower endogenous oestrogen levels predict spine fracture risk in men was published in 2000.[212]

Originally, interest in sex hormones was related to their critical role in gender dimor-phism and reproduction. Now it is recognized that sex steroids also are responsible for developmental and metabolic effects in many other tissues and organs. One of the earliest interests in sex hormones and later disease was an attempt to explain the striking and uni-versal gender difference in coronary heart disease. This gender difference is classically attributed to a protective effect of endogenous oestrogen, although at least three prospective studies have failed to show that high endogenous oestrogen levels are cardioprotective in postmenopausal women or in men.[213–215] Nevertheless, the oestrogen-heart disease hypothesis is not dead. No prospective studies have examined the possibility that the higher premenopausal oestrogen levels are cardioprotective. There are no adequately sized hormone studies of healthy premenopausal women who have been followed long enough to have cardiovascular events in sufficient numbers for analysis.

One reason for weak or absent associations may be that circulating sex steroids vary too much during a day or week or month to be characterized by a single assay. The most informative blood levels may be samples obtained in the afternoon or at night (particularly during puberty), times when blood samples are rarely obtainable for studies of large populations. Another reason for weak or absent associations is that circulating hormone levels do not necessarily parallel concentrations in the target tissues of interest; this may be particularly true for postmenopausal women (who form the bulk of the hormone-disease studies in populations). After the menopause, oestrogen is mainly synthesized from circulating C19 steroids in sites remote from the ovary, including bone, breast, and brain; these locally produced hormones are thought to be locally active in a paracrine or intracrine fashion.[216] Much of the action of locally produced oestrogen appears to be mediated by the classic oestrogen receptors, and very little oestradiol is needed for an effect. The expression of oestrogen and androgen receptors in nonreproductive tissues is at least 10-fold lower than the expression of these receptors in reproductive sites.[217] In fact, the concentration of oestrogen receptors in cells of the cardiovascular system is about 50-fold less than the concentration in cells of the reproductive system.[218]

Another difficulty is that oestrogen receptor expression may change over the life course. A particularly striking example is the transient expression of oestrogen receptor alpha in the cerebral cortex during neonatal development, a period of impressive neurogenesis and differentiation, and its disappearance thereafter.[219] Considering lifelong changes in sex hormone synthesis and receptor expression, it is surprising that important oestrogen or androgen effects are ever detected by studies of plasma hormones!

Two adrenal hormones, cortisol and dehydroepiandrosterone sulfate (DHEAS), are currently attracting considerable attention in relation to life course theories of adult disease. DHEAS is present in the human circulation in higher concentrations than any other hormone and easily measured in plasma. It shows little intra-individual variation over a few years, and changes dramatically over the life course as shown in Fig. 10.11.[220] DHEAS levels fall after very high levels during fetal growth, and rise again in adolescence—only to show a progressive fall after age 30 to about 10% of young adult levels by age 80. The reasons for these age-related changes are only partially understood.[221]

DHEAS is an androgen and oestrogen precursor, but its principal function is uncertain. Initially DHEAS attracted attention as a hormone with remarkable anti-ageing, anti-obesity,

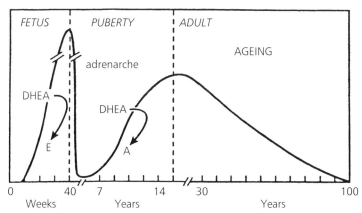

Fig. 10.11 Diagrammatic representation of circulating DHEA (also DHEA-S) over the life span in humans[220]. (Note that the fetal adrenal is most active in the production of DHEA, which is the key precursor for aromatization with the formation of estrogen by the placenta during pregnancy. The second wave of accelerated secretion occurs at the time of adrenarche when DHEA serves as a precursor for the formation of androgen independent of ACTH on gonadotropin.)

anti-cancer, and anti-diabetic effects. These early reports were from animal experiments, largely conducted in rodents. The relevance of these studies to humans is uncertain, because only humans and a few primates synthesize and secrete DHEA and DHEAS.

Although the first isolation of DHEAS from human blood was reported by Baulieu in 1960,[222] it was not until 1986 that the first prospective study of DHEAS blood levels and heart disease was published.[223] In this cohort study, high DHEAS levels were cardioprotective in men[223] but not in women.[224] Subsequent enthusiasm for DHEAS as a cardioprotective, anti-ageing hormone was only slightly dimmed when less impressive benefits after longer follow-up were published from the same cohort eight years later.[225]

It is unclear whether DHEAS-developmental or -disease associations reflect the role of DHEAS as a sex hormone precursor or its interaction with other proteins, cytokines, or hormones. Ebeling and Koivisto have suggested that DHEA may act as an androgen in premenopausal women and as an oestrogen in postmenopausal women,[226] but this hypothesis contradicts the clinical and epidemiological observations that DHEAS levels are inversely related to heart disease in men and show no protective association in women, although older men have higher circulating oestrogen levels than postmenopausal women of similar age.

DHEAS secretion increases in parallel with a pre-pubertal increase in insulin-like growth factor 1 (IGF-1).[227] With ageing, there is a parallel decline in serum DHEAS and IGF-1.[228] Several small clinical trials reviewed elsewhere[220] have shown that DHEA treatment increases IGF-1 levels. DHEAS may modify the inflammatory response. Serum levels of the cytokine interleukin 6 (IL-6) increase with age in both sexes and are inversely correlated with DHEAS levels.[229] This age associated increase in the cytokine IL-6 may be returned to normal by DHEAS. Physiological levels of DHEA inhibit the production of IL-6 by human peripheral blood mononuclear cells[230] and unstimulated spleen cells.[231]

Much of current interest in DHEAS relates to its interface with cortisol. Cortisol levels increase by 20–50% in both men and women between the ages of 20 and 80 years, in direct contrast with DHEAS.[228] A greater age-related increase in 24-hour cortisol excretion is reported for women than men, including a higher evening nadir and a shorter quiescent period.[231] This pattern is unexplained but is characteristic of depression. Cortisol levels are higher in older women than older men,[232] an observation that has led more than one female investigator to postulate that men usually come home from work to a beer and newspaper, while women usually cook dinner, wash up, fold laundry, write the grocery list, and so on. In the Rancho Bernardo Study we found a higher molar ratio of cortisol to DHEAS in women than men.[232] An antiglucocorticoid effect of DHEAS has been proposed, based primarily on animal studies,[233] and is thought to mediate the putative neuroprotective effects of DHEA.[234]

Cortisol levels increase in response to stress; such elevated levels are thought to be useful (for adaptation and survival) when transient, and noxious when sustained. What are the presumably adaptive reasons for the relatively sustained high levels of cortisol in infancy, pregnancy, and old age?

McEwen and Stellar introduced the concept of allostatic load as a multi-system measure of the physiological burden exacted on the body through attempts to adapt to life's demands.[235] Current interest in the combined effects of cortisol and DHEAS relate to this theory, which suggests that biological factors such as cortisol reflect cumulative stress and result in impaired mental and physical function,[236,237] and that DHEAS serves as a 'buffer' to cortisol's stress-induced effects.[233] In one small study, healthy older men and women who had both high cortisol levels and low DHEAS levels at baseline experienced a fourfold increased risk of cognitive impairment after a two-year follow-up.[238] The MacArthur Study of Successful Aging data calculated baseline allostatic load scores based in part on DHEAS and cortisol levels and reported an increased 2–3 year risk for new coronary heart disease (CHD) events;[236] these associations were less evident at 7 years.[237]

The increase in cortisol relative to DHEA(S) may also play a role in the metabolic shift to a catabolic state during ageing[239] and has been speculated to be causally linked to several physical diseases and psychiatric disorders.[240,241]

As provocative as these findings are, many future studies of health outcomes in relation to hormones over the life course will not be based on blood or tissue hormone levels, but on surrogates for lifetime hormone exposure. For example, good bone mineral density is, in part, a surrogate for lifetime oestrogen exposure, and studies showing higher breast cancer rates in women with better bone mineral density are compatible with the thesis that lifetime oestrogen exposure is a risk factor for breast cancer.[242] Similarly, fractures in postmenopausal women, a surrogate measure of bone density reflecting long-term lower oestrogen levels, appear to be inversely associated with endometrial cancer.[243] The observation that women with polycystic ovary syndrome, who have high levels of endogenous testosterone and insulin, have no increased risk of cardiovascular disease suggests that testosterone is not atherogenic in women.[244] The problem with the surrogate methods is that other explanations for these associations (or lack thereof) can only rarely be excluded.

What next? The surface of life course endocrinology and its consequences has barely been scratched, with advances made in separate age groups (newborns, infants, children, adolescents, young adults, and middle-aged and older adults), and little coordination of the overall life course. Most of the studies of adult disease have their baseline observations made in adults when they were usually only a few years (out of the total lifespan) younger. The field of hormone-related research in this adult age range is expanding rapidly with improved methodology and insights, but future research needs to address how to link up age-specific or phase specific (e.g. premenopause, menopause transition, and early and late postmenopause) hormone patterns in large enough samples to examine possible predictors of current and future health and well-being. The challenge of linking fetal, infant, childhood, and adolescent endocrinology to late life health will be great, and requires a commitment to the archiving and future analyses of today's data. Reading this chapter by Carol Worthman serves to illustrate many possible associations and the importance of their further study.

References

1 Dasgupta P. *An inquiry into well-being and destitution*. Oxford: Clarendon Press; 1993.

2 Farmer P. *Infections and inequalities*: The modern plagues. Berkeley: University of California Press, 1999.

3 Sen A. *Inequality reexamined*. Cambridge, MA: Harvard University Press, 1992.

4 Wilkinson RG. *Unhealthy societies: The afflictions of inequality*. London: Routledge, 1996.

5 Kaufman JS, Cooper RS. Seeking causal explanations in social epidemiology. *Am J Epidemiol* 1999;**150**:113–20.

6 Krieger M. Commentary: Society, biology and the logic of social epidemiology. *Int J Epidemiol* 2001;**30**:44–6.

7 Macinko J, Starfield B. The utility of social capital in research on health determinants. *Milbank Q* 2001;**79**:387–427.

8 Murray CJ, J.A. S, Mathers C. A critical examination of summary measures of population health. *Bull WHO 2000*;**78**:981–94.

9 **Callahan D**. Ageing, death, and population health. *J Am Med Assoc* 1999;**282**:2077.

10 **Anonymous**. Design of the Women's Health Initiative clinical trial and observational study. The Women's Health Initiative Study Group. *Control Clin Trials* 1998;**19**:61–109.

11 **Matthews KA, Shumaker SA, Bowen DJ, R.D. L, Hunt JR, Kaplan RM, et al**. Women's Health Initiative. Why now? What is it? What's new? *Am Psychol* 1997;**52**:101–16.

12 **Pinn VW**. The role of the NIH's Office of Research on Women's Health. *Acad Med* 1994;**69**:698–702.

13 **Lock MM**. *Encounters with ageing*: Mythologies of menopause in Japan and North America. Berkeley: University of California Press, 1993.

14 **Champagne F, Meaney MJ**. Like mother, like daughter: Evidence for non-genomic transmission of parental behavior and stress responsivity. *Prog Brain Res* 2001;**133**:287–302.

15 **Chung TK, Lau TK, Yip AS, Chiu HF, Lee DT**. Antepartum depressive symptomatology is associated with adverse obstetric and neonatal outcomes. *Psychosom Med* 2001;**63**:830–4.

16 **Dubowitz H, Black MM, Kerr MA, Hussey JM, Morrel TM, Everson MD, et al**. Type and timing of mothers' victimization: Effects on mothers and children. *Pediatrics* 2001;**107**:728–35.

17 **Heim C, Nemeroff CB**. The role of childhood trauma in the neurobiology of mood and anxiety disorders: Preclinical and clinical studies. *Biol Psychiatry* 2001;**49**:1023–39.

18 **Martorell R, Ramakrishnan U, Schroeder DG, Ruel M**. Reproductive performance and nutrition during childhood. *Nutr Rev* 1996;**54**:S15–21.

19 **Charnov E**. *Life history invariants: Some explorations of symmetry in evolutionary ecology*. Oxford: Oxford University Press, 1993.

20 **Stearns S**. *The evolution of life histories*. New York: Oxford, 1992.

21 **Kaplan H, Hill KR, Lancaster J, Hurtado AM**. A theory of human life history evolution: Diet, intelligence, and longevity. *Evolutionary Anthropol* 2000;**9**:156–85.

22 **Hill K, Hurtado A**. *Ache life history: The ecology and demography of a forageing people*. New York: Aldine de Gruyter; 1995.

23 **Hill KR, Kaplan H**. Life history traits in humans: Theory and empirical studies. *Annu Rev Anthropol* 1999;**28**:397–430.

24 **Finch C, Rose M**. Hormones and the physiological architecture of life history evolution. *Quart Rev Biol* 1995;**70**:1–52.

25 **Barker DJP**. *Fetal and infant origins of adult disease*. London: British Medical Journal Publishing; 1992.

26 **Barker D**. Intra-uterine programming of the adult cardiovascular system. *Curr Opin Nephrol Hypertens* 1997;**6**:106–10.

27 **Fall C, Pandit A, Law C, Yajnik C, Clark P, Breier B, et al**. Size at birth and plasma insulin-like growth factor-1 concentrations. *Arch Dis Child* 1995;**73**:287–93.

28 **Clark P, Hindmarsh P, Shiell A, Law C, Honour J, Barker D**. Size at birth and adrenocortical function in childhood. *Clin Endocrinol (Oxf)* 1996;**45**:721–6.

29 **Law C, Gordon G, Shiell A, Barker D, Hales C**. Thinness at birth and glucose tolerance in seven-year-old children. *Diabet Med* 1995;**12**24–9.

30 **Seckl JR, Cleasby M, Nyirenda MJ**. Glucocorticoids, 11[beta]-hydroxysteroid dehydrogenase, and fetal programming. *Kidney Int* 2000;**57**1412–17.

31. **McDade TW, Beck MA, Kuzawa CW, Adair LS**. Prenatal undernutrition and postnatal growth are associated with adolescent thymic function. *J Nutr* 2001;**131**:1225–1231.

32 **Susser M, Levin B**. Ordeals for the fetal programming hypothesis: The hypothesis largely survives one ordeal but not another. *Br Med J* 1999;**318**:885–6.

33 **Williams S, Poulton R**. Twins and maternal smoking: Ordeals for the fetal origins hypothesis? A cohort study. *Br Med J* 1999;**318**:897–900.

34 Godfrey KM. Maternal regulation of fetal development and health in adult life. *Eur J Obstet Gynecol Reprod Biol* 1998;**78**:141–50.

35 Adair LS. Size at birth predicts age at menarche. *Pediatrics* 2001;**107**:E59.

36 Worthman C. Evolutionary perspectives on the onset of puberty. In: Trevathan W, McKenna J, Smith E, eds. *Evolutionary medicine*. New York: Oxford University Press, 1999:135–63.

37 Worthman C. Bio-cultural interactions in human development. In: Pereira M, Fairbanks L, eds. *Juvenile primates: Life history, development and behavior*. Oxford: Oxford University Press, 1993:339–58.

38 Ellison PT. Developmental influences on adult ovarian hormonal function. *Am J Hum Biol* 1996;**8**:725–34.

39 Worthman CM. The epidemiology of human development. In: Panter-Brick C, Worthman CM, eds. *Hormones, health and behavior*. Cambridge: Cambridge University Press, 1999:47–104.

40 Marshall J, Griffen M. The role of changing pulse frequency in the regulation of ovulation. *Hum Reprod* 1993;**8**:57–61.

41 Yehuda R, Teicher MH, Trestman RL, Levengood RA, Siever LJ. Cortisol relguation in posttraumatic stress disorder and major depression: A chronological analysis. *Biol Psychiatry* 1996;**40**:79–88.

42 Plant TM. Neurobiological bases underlying the control of the onset of puberty in the rhesus monkey: A representative higher primate. *Front Neuroendocrinol* 2001;**22**:107–39.

43 Wood JW. *Dynamics of human reproduction*. New York: Aldine de Gruter, 1994.

44 Rosner W. Plasma steroid-binding proteins. *Endocrinol Metab Clin North Am* 1991;**20**:697–20.

45 Rosner W, Hryb DJ, Khan MS, Nakhla AM, Romas NA. Sex hormone-binding globulin mediates steroid hormone signal transduction at the plasma membrane. *J Ster Biochem Mol Biol* 1999;**69**:481–5.

46 Ellison PT. *On fertile ground*. Cambridge, MA. Harvard University Press, 2001.

47 Eveleth P, Tanner J. *Worldwide variation in human growth*. New York: Cambridge University Press, 1990.

48 Thomas F, Renaud F, Benefice E, de Meeus T, Guegan JF. International variability of ages at menarche and menopause: Patterns and main determinants. *Hum Biol* 2001;**73**:271–90.

49 Worthman CM, Jenkins CL, Stallings JF, Lai D. Attenuation of nursing-related ovarian suppression and high fertility in well-nourished, intensively breast-feeding Amele women of lowland Papua New Guinea. *J Biosoc Sci* 1994;**25**:425–43.

50 Ellison PT. Advances in human reproductive ecology. *Annu Rev Anthropol* 1994;**23**:255–75.

51 Whitten PL, Naftolin F. Reproductive actions of phytoestrogen s. *Bailliere Clin Endoc* 1998;**12**:667–90.

52 Lock M, Kaufert P. Menopause, local biologies, and cultures of ageing. *Am J Hum Biol* 2001;**13**:494–504.

53 Ellison P, Panter-Brick C, Lipson S, O'Rourke M. The ecological context of human ovarian function. *Hum Reprod* 1993;**8**:2248–58.

54 Eaton SB, Pike MC, Short RV, Lee NC, Trussell J, Hatcher RA, *et al*. Women's reproductive cancers in evolutionary context. *Q Rev Biol* 1994;**69**:353–67.

55 Jasienska G, Thune I, Ellison PT. Energetic factors, ovarian steroids and the risk of breast cancer. *Eur J Cancer Prev* 2000;**9**:231–9.

56 Beyene Y, Martin MC. Menopausal experiences and bone density of Mayan women in yucatan, Mexico. *Am J Hum Biol* 2001;**13**:505–11.

57 Bentley GR. Ranging hormones—do hormonal contraceptives ignore human biological variation and evolution. *Ann NY Acad Sci* 1994;**709**:201–3.

58 Kuller LH, Matthews K, Meilahn EN. Oestrogens and women's health: Interrelation of coronary heart disease, breast cancer and osteoporosis. *J Ster Biochem Mol Biol* 2000;**74**:297–309.

59 Rosenbaum M, Leibel RL. Role of gonadal steroids in the sexual dimorphisms in body composition and circulating concentrations of leptin. *J Clin Endocrinol Metab* 1999;**84**:1784–9.

60 Greendale G, Lee N, Arriola E. The menopause. *Lancet* 1999;**353**:571–80.

61 Haynes MP, Russell KS, Bender JR. Molecular mechanisms of oestrogen actions on the vasculature. *J Nucl Cardiol* 2000;**7**:500–8.

62 McEwen B. Multiple ovarian hormone effects on brain structure and function. *J Gender-Specific Med* 1998;**1**:33–41.

63 Mooradian A. Antioxidant properties of steroids. *J Ster Biochem Mol Biol* 1993;**45**:509–11.

64 Wong M, Thompson T, Moss R. Nongenomic actions of oestrogen in the brain l physiological significance and cellular mechanisms. *Crit Rev Neurobiol* 1996;**10**:189–203.

65 Wise PM, Dubal DB, Wilson ME, Rau SW, Böttner M. Neuroprotective effects of oestrogen-new insights into mechanisms of action. *Endocrinology* 2001;**143**:969–73.

66 Wolf OT, Kudielka BM, Hellhammer DH, Törber S, McEwen BS, Kirschbaum C. Two weeks of transdermal estradiol treatment in postmenopaussal elderly women and its effects on memory and mood: Verbal memory changes are associated with the treatment induced estradiol levels. *Psychoneuroendocrinol* 1999;**24**:727–41.

67 Roof R, Duvdevani R, Heyburn J, Stein D. Progesterone rapidly decreases brain edema: Treatment delayed up to 24 hours is still effective. *Exp Neurol* 1996;**138**:246–51.

68 Roof R, Hoffman S, Stein D. Progesterone protects against lipid peroxidation following traumatic brain injury in rats. *Mol Chem Neuropathol* 1997;**31**:1–11.

69 McEwen B. Hormones as regulators of brain development: Life-long effects related to health and disease. *Acta Paediatrica* 1997;**422 (Suppl)**:41–4.

70 Sapolsky RM. *Why zebras don't get ulcers: An updated guide to stress, stress-related diseases, and coping.* 2nd ed. New York: W.F. Freeman, 1998.

71 Van Cauter E, Leproult R, Kupfer D. Effects of gender and age on the levels and circadian rhythmicity of plasma cortisol. *J Clin Endocrinol Metab* 1996;**81**:2468–73.

72 van Eck M, Berkhof H, Nicolson N, Sulon J. The effects of perceived stress, traits, mood states, and stressful daily events on salivary cortisol. *Psychosom Med* 1996;**58**:447–58.

73 Herman J, Cullinan W. Neurocircuitry of stress: Central control of the hypothalamo-pituitary-adrenocortical axis. *Trends Neurosci* 1997;**20**:78–84.

74 Singh A, Petrides JS, Gold PW, Chrousos GP, Deuster PA. Differential hypothalmic-pituitary-adrenal axis reactivity to psychological and physical stress. *J Clin Endocrinol Metab* 1999;**84**:1944–8.

75 Rosmond R, Bjørntørp P. The hypothalamic-pituitary-adrenal axis activity as a predictor of cardiovascular disease, type 2 diabetes and stroke. *J Intern Med* 2000;**247**:188–197.

76 Boyce W, Chesney M, Alkon A, Tschann J, Adams S, Chesterman B, *et al.* Psychobiological reactivity to stress and childhood respiratory illnesses: Results of two prospective studies. *Psychosom Med* 1995;**57**:411–22.

77 Young E, Midgley A, Carlson N, Brown M. Alteration in the hypothalamic-pituitary-ovarian axis in depressed women. *Arch Gen Psychiatry* 2000;**57**:1157–62.

78 Lupien SJ, McEwen BS. The acute effects of corticosteroids on cognition: Integration of animal and human model studies. *Brain Res Rev* 1997;**24**:1–27.

79 de Zegher F, Vanhole C, Van den Berghe G, Devlieger H, Eggermont E, Veldhuis J. Properties of thyroid-stimulating hormone and cortisol secretion by the human newborn on the day of birth. *J Clin Endocrinol Metab* 1994;**79**:576–81.

80 Onishi S, Miyazawa G, Nishimura Y, Sugiyama S, Yamakawa T, Inagaki H, *et al.* Postanatal development of circadian rhythm in serum cortisol levels in children. *Pediatrics* 1983;**72**:399–404.

81 Ramsay D, Lewis M. The effects of birth condition on infants' cortisol response to stress. *Pediatrics* 1995;**95**:546–9.

82 Deuschle M, Gotthardt U, Schweiger U, Weber B, Korner A, Schmider J, *et al.* With ageing in humans the activity of the hypothalamus-pituitary-adrenal system increases and its diurnal amplitude flattens. *Life Sci* 1997;**61**:2239–46.

83 Laughlin GA, Barrett-Connor E. Sexual dimorphism in the influence of advanced on adrenal hormone levels: The Rancho Bernardo study. *J Clin Endocrinol Metab* 2000;**85**:3561–8.

84 Kudielka BM, Hellhammer J, Hellhammer DH, Wolf OT, Pirke K-M, Varadi E, *et al.* Sex differences in endocrine and psychological responses to psychosocial stress in healthy elderly subjects and the impact of a 2-week dehydroepiandrosterone treatment. *J Clin Endocrinol Metab* 1998;**83**:1756–61.

85 Wallace W, Crowne E, Shalet S, Moore C, Gibson S, Littley M, *et al.* Episodic acth and cortisol secretion in normal children. *Clin Endocrinol (Oxf)* 1991;**34**:215–21.

86 Seeman T, Singer B, Wilkinson C, BcEwen B. Gender differences in age-related changes in HPA axis reactivity. *Psychoneuroendocrinol* 2001;**26**:225–40.

87 Guazzo E, Kirkpatrick P, Goodyer I, Shiers H, Herbert J. Cortisol, dehydroepiandrosterone (DHEA), and DHEA sulfate in the cerebrospinal fluid of man: Relation to blood levels and the effects of age. *J Clin Endocrinol Metab* 1996;**81**:3951–60.

88 Ferrari E, Arcaini A, Gornati R, Pelanconi L, Cravello L, Fioravanti M, *et al.* Pineal and pituitary-adrenocortical function in physiological ageing and in senile dementia. *Exp Gerontol* 2000;**35**:1239–50.

89 Ferrari E, Cravello L, Muzzoni B, Casarotti D, Paltro M, Solerte SB, *et al.* Age-related changes in the hypothalamic-pituitary-adrenal axis: Pathophysiological correlates. *Eur J Endocrinol* 2001;**144**:319–29.

90 Ladd CO, RLH, Thrivikraman KV, CBN, Meaney MJ, Plotsky PM. Long-term behavioral and neuroendocrine adaptations to adverse early experience. *Prog Brain Res* 2000;**122**:81–103.

91 Meaney MJ. Maternal care, gene expression, and the transmission of individual differences in stress reactivity across generations. *Annu Rev Neurosci* 2001;**24**:1161–92.

92 Suomi S. Early stress and adult emotional reactivity in rhesus monkeys. In: Bock G, Whelan J, eds. *The childhood environment and adult disease*. Chichester, NY: Wiley; 1991:171–88.

93 Young EA, Vazquez D. Hypercortisolemia, hippocampal glucocorticoid receptors, and fast feedback. *Mol Psychiatry* 1996;**1**:149–59.

94 Young EA, Aggen SH, Prescott CA, Kendler KS. Similarity in saliva cortisol measures in monozygotic twins and the influence of past major depression. *Biol Psychiatry* 2000;**48**:70–4.

95 Knutsson U, Dahlgren J, Marcus C, Rosberg S, Bronnegard M, Stierna P, *et al.* Circadian cortisol rhythms in healthy boys and girls: Relationship with age, growth, body composition, and pubertal development. *J Clin Endocrinol Metab* 1997;**82**:536–40.

96 Clarke A, Wittwer D, Abbott D, Schneider M. Long-term effects of prenatal stress on HPA axis activity in juvenile rhesus monkeys. *Dev Psychobiol* 1994;**27**:257–69.

97 McEwen BS. The neurobiology of stress: From serendipity to clinical relevance. *Brain Res* 2000;**886**:172–89.

98 Ebrecht M, Buske-Kirschbaum A, Hellhammer D, Kern S, Rohleder M, Walker B, *et al.* Tissue specificity of glucocorticoid sensitivity in healthy adults. *J Clin Endocrinol Metab* 2000;**85**:3733–9.

99 McEwen BS. Effects of adverse experiences for brain structure and function. *Biol Psychiatry* 2000;**48**:721–31.

100 Young EA. Sex differences and the HPA axis: Implications for psychiatric disease. *J Gender-Specific Med* 1998;**1**:21–7.

101 Parker L. Control of adrenal androgen secretion. *Endocrinol Metab Clin North Am* 1991;**20**:401–21.

102 Phillips G. Relationship between serum dehydroepiandrosterone sulfate, androstenedione, and sex hormones in men and women. *Eur J Endocrinol* 1996;**134**:201–6.

103 Parker CR. Dehydroepiandrosterone and dehydroepiandrosterone sulfate production in the human adrenal during development and ageing. *Steroids* 1999;**64**:640–7.

104 Yen SSC, Laughlin GA. Ageing and the adrenal cortex. *Exp Gerontol* 1998;**7/8**:897–910.

105 Ebeling P, Koivisto V. Physiological importance of dehydroepiandrosterone. *Lancet* 1994;**343**:1479–81.

106 LaBrie F, Belanger A, Cusan L, Candas B. Physiological changes in dehydroepiandrosterone are not reflected by serum levels of active androgens and oestrogens but of their metabolites: Intracrinology. *J Clin Endocrinol Metab* 1997;**82**:2403–9.

107 Parker L. Adrenarche. *Endocrinol Metab Clin North Am* 1991;**20**:71–83.

108 Palmert MR, Hayden DL, Mansfield MJ, Crigler JF, Crowley WF, Chandler DW, *et al*. The longitudinal study of adrenal maturation during gonadal suppression: Evidence that adrenarche is a gradual process. *J Clin Endocrinol Metab* 2001;**86**:4536–42.

109 LaBrie F, Belanger A, Cusan L, Gomez J-L, Candas B. Marked decline in serum concentrations of adrenal C19 sex steroid precursors and conjugated androgen metabolites during ageing. *J Clin Endocrinol Metab* 1997;**82**:2397–402.

110 Zemel B, Worthman C, Jenkins C. Differences in endocrine status associated with urban-rural patterns of growth and maturation in Bundi (Gende-speaking) adolescents of Papua New Guinea. In: Schell L, Smith N, Bilsborough A, eds. *Urban health and ecology in the third world*. Cambridge: Cambridge University Press, 1993:38–60.

111 Michael A, Jenaway A, Paykel ES, Herbert J. Altered salivary dehydroepiandrosterone levels in major depression in adults. *Biol Psychiatry* 2000;**48**:989–95.

112 Khaw KT. Dehydroepiandrosterone, dehydroepiandrosterone sulphate and cardiovascular disease. *J Endocrinol* 1996;**150 Suppl**:S149–53.

113 Young EA. DHEA: Mood, memory, and ageing. *Biol Psychiatry* 1999;**45**:1531–2.

114 Gurnell EM, Chatterjee KK. Dehydroepiandrosterone replacement therapy. *Eur J Endocrinol* 2001;**145**:103–6.

115 Barrett-Connor E, Khaw K, Yen S. A prospective study of dehydroepieandrosterone sulfate, mortality, and cardiovascular disease. *N Engl J Med* 1986;**315**:1519–24.

116 Goodman-Gruen D, Barrett-Connor E. A prospective study of sex hormone-binding globulin and fatal cardiovascular disease in Rancho Bernardo men and women. *J Clin Endocrinol Metab* 1996;**81**:2999–3003.

117 Trivedi DP, Khaw KT. Dehydroepiandrosterone sulfate and mortality in elderly men and women. *J Clin Endocrinol Metab* 2001;**86**:4171–7.

118 Harper AJ, Buster JE, Casson PR. Changes in adrenocortical function with ageing and therapeutic implications. *Sem Reprod Endocrinol* 1999;**17**:327–38.

119 Leblhuber F, Neubauer C, Peichl M, Reisecker F, Steinparz F, Windhager E, *et al*. Age and sex differences of dehydroepiandrosterone sulfate (DHEAS) and cortisol (CRT) plasma levels in normal controls and Alzheimer's disease (AD). *Psychopharmacology (Berl)* 1993;**111**:23–6.

120 Geelhoed GW. Metabolic maladaptation: Individual and social consequences of medical intervention in correcting endemic hypothyroidism. *Nutrition* 1999;**11/12**:908–32.

121 WHO, UNICEF, ICCIDD. *Progress towards the elimination of iodine deficiency disorders (IDD)*. Geneva: WHO, 1999.

122 **WHO, UNICEF, ICCIDD.** *Indicators for assessing iodine deficincy disorders and their control through salt iodinization.* Geneva: WHO, 1994.

123 **Smallridge RC.** Disclosing subclinical thyroid disease. An approach to mild laboratory abnormalities and vague of absent symptoms. *Postgrad Med* 2000;**107**:143–6.

124 **Nelson J, Clark S, Borut D, Tomei R, Carlton E.** Age-related changes in serum free thyroxine during childhood and adolescence. *J Pediatr* 1993;**123**:899–905.

125 **Knudsen N, Jorgensen T, Rasmussen S, Christiansen E, Perrild H.** The prevalence of thyroid dysfunction in a popualtion with borderline iodine deficiency. *Clin Endocrinol* 1999;51:361–7.

126 **Wiedemann G, Jonetz-Mentzel L, Panse R.** Establishment of reference ranges for thyrotropin, triiodothyronine, thyroxine and free thyroxine in neonates, infants, children and adolescents. *Eur J Clin Chem Clin Biochem* 1993;**31**:277–8.

127 **Fisher DA, Nelson JC, Carlton EI, Wilcox RB.** Maturation of human hypothalamic-pituitary-thyroid function and control. *Thyroid* 2000;**10**:229–34.

128 **Hesse V, Jahreis G, Schambach H, Vogel H, Vilser C, Seewald H, et al.** Insulin-like growth factor I correlations to changes of the hormonal status in puberty and age. *Exp Clin Endocrinol* 1994;**102**:289–98.

129 **Mariotti S, Barbesino G, Caturegli P, Bartalena L, Sansoni P, Fagnoni F, et al.** Complex alteration of thyroid function in healthy centenarians. *J Clin Endocrinol Metab* 1993;**77**:1130–34.

130 **Runnels B, Garry P, Hunt W, Standefer J.** Thyroid function in a healthy elderly population: Implications for clinical evaluation. *J Gerontol: Biological Sciences* 1991;**46**:B39–44.

131 **Van Coevorden A, Laurent E, Decoster C, Kerkhofs M, Neve P, Van Cauter E, et al.** Decreased basal and stimulated thyrotropin secretion in healthy elderly men. *J Clin Endocrinol Metab* 1989;**69**:177–185.

132 **Delange F.** The disorders induced by iodine deficiency. *Thyroid* 1994;**4**:107–128.

133 **Delange FdBB, Pretell E, Dunne JT.** Iodine deficiency in the world: Where do we stand at the turn of the century? Thyroid 2001;**11**:437–47.

134 **Larsen PR, Berry MJ.** Nutritional and hormonal regulation of thyroid hormone deiodinases. *Ann Rev Nutr* 1995;**15**:323–52.

135 **Köhrle J.** The trace element selenium and the thyroid gland. *Biochimie* 1999;**81**:527–33.

136 **Delange F, Van Onderbergen A, Shabana W, Vandemeuleboucke E, Vertongen F, Gnat D, et al.** Silent iodine prophylaxis in Western Europe only partly corrects deficiency; the case of Belgium. *Eur J Endocrinol* 2000;**143**:189–96.

137 **Anderson GW.** Thyroid hormones and the brain. *Front Neruoendocrinol* 2001;**22**:1–17.

138 **Hetzel B, Potter B, Dulberg E.** The iodine deficiency disorders: Nature, pathogenesis, and epidemiology. In: Bourne G, ed. *Aspects of some vitamins, minerals, and enzymes in health and disease.* Basel: Karger, 1990:59–112.

139 **Thompson C, Potter G.** Thyroid hormone action in neural development. *Cerebral Cortex* 2000;**10**:939–45.

140 **Tiwari B, Godbole M, Chattopadhyay N, Mandal A, Mithal A.** Learning disabilities and poor motivation to achieve due to prolonged iodine deficiency. *Am J Clin Nutr* 1996;**63**:782–6.

141 **Laurberg P, Nohr SB, Pedersen KM, Hreidarsson AB, Andersen S, Bulow Pedersen I, et al.** Thyroid disorders in mild iodine deficiency. *Thyroid* 2000;**10**:951–63.

142 **Bakker SJ, ter Maaten JC, Popp-Slaets JP, Heine RJ, Gans RO.** The relationship between thyrotropin and low density lipoprotein cholesterol is modified by insulin sensitivity in healthy euthyroid subjects. *J Clin Endocrinol Metab* 2001;**86**:1206–11.

143 **Bonar BD, McColgan B, Smith DF, Darke C, Guttridge MG, Williams H, et al.** Hypothyroidism and ageing: The Rosses' survey. *Thyroid* 2000;**10**:821–7.

144 Stanbury JB, Ermans AE, Bourdoux P, Todd C, Oken E, Tonglet R, *et al*. Iodine-induced hyperthyroidism: Occurrence and eidemiology. *Thyroid* 1998;**8**:83–100.

145 Bjoro T, Holmen J, Kruger O, Midthjell K, Hunstad K, Schreiner T, *et al*. Prevalence of thyroid disease, thyroid dysfunciton and thyroid peroxidase antibodies in a large, unselected population. The health study of Nord-Trondelag (HUNT). *Eur J Endocrinol* 2000;**143**:639–47.

146 Laurberg P, Bulow Pedersen I, Pedersen KM, Vestergaard H. Low incidence rate of overt hypothyroidism compared with hyperthyroidism in an area with moderately low iodine intake. *Thyroid* 1999;**9**:33–8.

147 Chiovato L, Lapi P, Fiore E, Tonacchera M, Pinchera A. Thyroid autoimmunity and female gender. *J Endocrinol Invest* 1993;**16**:384–91.

148 Schulte KM, Jonas C, Krebs R, Roher HD. Activin A and activin receptors in the human thyroid: A link to the female predominance of goitre? *Horm Metab Res* 2000;**32**:390–400.

149 Rotondi M, Amato G, Biondi B, Mazziotti G, Del Buono A, Rotonda Nicchio M, *et al*. Parity as a thyroid size-determining factor in areas with moderate iodine deficiency. *J Clin Endocrinol Metab* 2000;**85**:4534–7.

150 Hickie I, Bennett B, Mitchell P, Wilhelm K, Orlay W. Clinical and subclinical hypothyroidism in patients with chronic and treatment-resistant depression. *Aust New Zealand J Psychiat* 1996;**30**:246–52.

151 Fardella C, Gloger SG, Figueroa R, Santis R, Gajardo C, Salgado, *et al*. High prevalence of thyroid abnormalities in a Chilean psychiatric outpatient population. *J Endocrinol Invest* 2000;**23**:102–6.

152 Caro J, Sinha M, Kolaczynski J, Zhang P, Considine R. Leptin: The tale of an obesity gene. *Diabetes* 1996;**45**:1455–62.

153 Zhang Y, Proenca R, Maffei, Barone M, Leopold L, Friedman JM. Positional cloning of the mouse *obese* gene and its human homologue. *Nature* 1994;**372**:425–31.

154 Wauters M, Considine RV, Van Gaal LF. Human leptin: From an adipocyte hormone to an endocrine mediator. *Eur J Endocrinol* 2000;**143**:293–311.

155 Mohamed-Ali V, Pinkney JH, Coppack SW. Adipose tissue as an endocrine and paracrine organ. *Int J Obes Relat Metab Disord* 1998;**22**:1145–58.

156 Mantzoros CS, Moschos SJ. Leptin: In search of role(s) in human physiology and pathophysiology. *Clin Endocrinol (Oxf)* 1998;**49**:551–67.

157 Mantzoros CS. The role of lepin in human obesity and disease: A review of current evidence. *Ann Intern Med* 1999;**130**:671–80.

158 Saad MF, Riad-Gabriel MG, Khan A, Sharma A, Michael R, Jinagouda SD, *et al*. Diurnal and ultradian rhythmicity of plasma leptin: Effects of gender and adiposity. *J Clin Endocrinol Metab* 1998;**83**:453–9.

159 Baskin DG, Hahn TM, Schwartz MW. Leptin sensitive neurons in the hypothalamus. *Horm Metab Res* 1999;**31**:345–50.

160 Quinton ND, Smith RF, Clayton PE, Gill MS, Shalet S, Justice SK, *et al*. Leptin binding activity changes with age: The link between leptin and puberty. *J Clin Endocrinol Metab* 1999;**84**:2336–41.

161 Ogle GD, Allen JR, Humphries I, Lu PW, Briody J, Morley K, *et al*. Body-composition assessment by dual-energy x-ray absorptiometry in subjects aged 4–26 y. *Am J Clin Nutr* 1995;**61**:746–53.

162 Ostlund R, Yang J, Klein S, Gingerich R. Relation between plasma leptin concentration and body fat, gender, diet, age, and metabolic covariates. *J Clin Endocrinol Metab* 1996;**81**:3909–13.

163 Hytinantti T, Koistinen HA, Koivisto V, Karonen S-L, Andersson S. Changes in leptin concentration during the early postnatal period: Adjustment to extrauterine life? *Pediatr Res* 1999;**45**:197–201.

164 Hassink S, Sheslow D, de Lancey E, Opentanova I, Considine R, Caro J. Serum leptin in children with obesity: Relationship to gender and development. *Pediatrics* 1996;**98**:201–3.

165 Ruige JB, Dekker JM, Blum WF, Stehouwer CD, Nijpels G, Mooy J, *et al*. Leptin and variables of body adiposity, energy balance, and insulin resistance in a population-based study: The Hoorn study. *Diabetes Care* 1999;**22**:1097–104.

166 Anderson LA, P.G. M, Barnett AH, Kumar S. The effects of androgens and oestrogens on preadipocyte proliferation in human adipose tissue: Influence of gender and site. *J Clin Endocrinol Metab* 2001;**86**:4951–5956.

167 Ahmed ML, Ong KK, Morrell DJ, Cox L, Drayer M, Perry L, *et al*. Longitudinal study of leptin concentrations during puberty: Sex differences and relationships to changes in body composition. *J Clin Endocrinol Metab* 1999;**84**:899–905.

168 Kennedy A, Gettys TW, Watson P, Wallace P, Ganaway E, Pan O, *et al*. The metabolic significance of leptin in humans: Gender-based differences in relationship to adiposity, insulin sensitivity, and energy expenditure. *J Clin Endocrinol Metab* 1997;**82**:1293–1300.

169 Hellstrom L, Wahrenberg H, Hruska K, Reynisdottir S, Arner P. Mechanisms behind gender differences in circulating leptin levels. *J Intern Med* 2000;**247**:457–62.

170 Marshall JA, Grunwald GK, Donahoo WT, Scarbro S, Shetterly SM. Percent body fat and lean mass explain the gender difference in leptin: Analysis and interpretation of leptin in hispanic and non-hispanic white adults. *Obes Res* 2000;**8**:543–52.

171 Roemmich JN, Clark PA, Berr SS, Mai V, Mantzoros CS, Flier JS, *et al*. Gender differences in leptin levels during puberty are related to the subcutaneous fat depot and sex steroids. *Am J Physiol* 1998;**275**:E543–51.

172 Blum WF, Englaro P, Hanitsch S, Juul A, Hertel MT, Muller J, *et al*. Plasma leptin levels in healthy children and adolescents: Dependence on body mass index, body fat mass, gender, pubertal stage, and testosterone. *J Clin Endocrinol Metab* 1997;**82**:2904–10.

173 Horlick MB, Rosenbaum M, Nicolson M, Levine LS, Fedun B, Wang J, *et al*. Effect of puberty on the relationship between circulating leptin and body composition. *J Clin Endocrinol Metab* 2000;**85**:2509–18.

174 Mystkowski P, Schwartz MW. Gonadal steroids and energy homeostasis in the leptin era. *Nutrition* 2000;**16**:937–46.

175 Demerath EW, Towne B, Wisemandle W, Blangero J, Chumlea WC, Siervogel RM. Serum leptin concentration, body composition, and gonadal hormones during puberty. *Int J Obesity Relat Metab Disord* 1999;**23**:678–85.

176 Vogel G. Leptin: A trigger for puberty. *Science* 1996;**274**:1466–7.

177 Garcia-Mayor RV, Andrade MA, Rios M, Lage M, Dieguez C, Casanueva FF. Serum leptin levels in normal children: Relationship to age, gender, body mass index, pituitary-gonadal hormones, and pubertal stage. *J Clin Endocrinol Metab* 1997;**82**:2849–55.

178 Hardie L, Trayhurn P, Abramowich D, Fowler P. Circulating leptin in women: A longitudinal study in the menstrual cycle and during pregnancy. *Clin Endocrinol (Oxf)* 1997;**47**:101–6.

179 Riad-Gabriel MG, Jinagouda SD, Sharma A, Boyadjian R, Saad MF. Changes in plasma leptin during the menstrual cycle. *Eur J Endocrinol* 1998;**139**:528–31.

180 Isidori A, Strollo F, More M, Caprio M, Aversa A, Moretti C, *et al*. Leptin and ageing: Correlation with endocrine changes in male and female healthy adult populations of different body weights. *J Clin Endocrinol Metab* 2000;**85**:1954–62.

181 Pénicaud L, Cousin B, Leloup C, Lorsignol A, Casteilla L. The autonomic nervous system, adipose tisssue plasticity, and energy balance. *Nutrition* 2000;**16**:903–8.

182 Phillips DI, Fall CH, Cooper C, Norman RJ, Robinson JS, Owens PC. Size at birth and plasma leptin concentrations in adult life. *Int J Obesity Relat Metab Disord* 1999;**23**:1025–9.

183 Sumner AE, Flakner B, Kushner H, Considine RV. Relationship of leptin concentration to gender, menopause, age, diabetes, and fat mass in African Americans. *Obes Res* 1998;**6**: 128–33.

184 Snehalatha C, Ramachandran A, Satyavani K, Sivasankari S, Vijay V. Difference in body fat percentage does not explain the gender dimorphism in leptin in Asian Indians. *J Assoc Physicians India* 1999;**47**:1164–7.

185 Zimmer P, Hodge A, Nicolson MS, de Courten M, Moore J, Morawiecki A, *et al.* Serum leptin concentration, obesity, and insulin resistance in Western Samoans: Cross sectional study. *Br Med J* 1996;**313**:965–9.

186 Soliman AT, ElZalabany MM, Salama M, Ansari BM. Serum leptin concentrations during severe progein-energy malnutrition: Correlation with growth parameters and endocrine function. *Metabolism* 2000;**49**:819–25.

187 Lancaster J. Sex and gender in evolutionary perspective. In: Katchadourian HA, ed. *Human sexuality: a comparative and developmental perspective*. Berkeley, CA: U California Press, 1979:51–80.

188 Lancaster JB. Human reproduction, the evolution of the brain, and fat storage. *Am J Phys Anthropol* 2000;**30 Suppl**:205.

189 Brown PJ. An anthropological perspective on obesity. *Ann NY Acad Sci* 1987;**499**:29–46.

190 Martin E. The woman in the body: A cultural analysis of reproduction. 2nd ed. Boston: Beacon Press, 2001.

191 Burger H, Yamada Y, Bangah M, McCloud P, Warne G. Serum gonadotropin, sex steroid, and immunoreactive inhibin levels in the first two years of life. *J Clin Endocrinol Metab* 1991;**72**:682–5.

192 Genazzani A, Petraglia F, Sgarbi L, Montanini V, Hartmann B, Surico N, *et al.* Difference of LH and FSH secretory characteristics and degree of concordance between postmenopausal and ageing women. *Maturitas* 1997;**26**:133–8.

193 Kwekkeboom D, deJong F, van Hemert A, Vandenbroucke J, Valkenburg H, Lamberts S. Serum gonadotropins and α-subunit decline in ageing normal postmenopausal women. *J Clin Endocrinol Metab* 1990;**70**:944–50.

194 Veldhuis J. Neuroendocrine mechanisms mediating awakening of the human gonadotropic axis in puberty. *Pediatr Nephrol* 1996;**10**:304–17.

195 Wu F, Butler G, Kelnar C, Huhtaniemi I, Veldhuis J. Ontogeny of pulsatile gonadotropin releasing hormone secretion from midchildhood, through puberty, to adulthood in the human male: A study using deconvolution analysis and an ultrasensitive immunofluorometric assay. *J Clin Endocrinol Metab* 1996;**81**:1798–1805.

196 Apter D, Cacciatore B, Alfthan H, Stenman H. Serum luteinizing hormone concentrations increase 100-fold in females from 7 years of age to adulthood, as measured by time-resolved immunoflourometric assay. *J Clin Endocrinol Metab* 1989;**68**:53–7.

197 Reame N, Kelch R, Beitins I, Yu M-Y, Zawacki C, Padmanabhan V. Age effects on follicle-stimulating hormone and pulsatile luteinizing hormone secretion across the menstrual cycle of premenopausal women. *J Clin Endocrinol Metab* 1996;**81**:1512–8.

198 Belgorosky A, Rivarola M. Progressive decrease in serum sex hormone-binding globulin from infancy to late prepuberty in boys. *J Clin Endocrinol Metab* 1986;**63**:510–2.

199 Belgorosky A, Rivarola M. Changes in serum sex hormone-binding globulin and in serum non-sex hormone-binding globulin-bound testosterone during prepuberty in boys. *J Steroid Biochem* 1987;**27**:291–5.

200 Belgorosky A, Rivarola M. Progressive increase in nonsex hormone-binding globulin-bound testosterone and estradiol from infancy to late prepuberty in girls. *J Clin Endocrinol Metab* 1988;**67**:234–7.

201 Bolton N, Tapanainen J, Koiviston M, Vihko R. Circulating sex hormone-binding globulin and testosterone in newborns and infants. *Clin Endocrinol (Oxf)* 1989;**31**:201–7.

202 Cunningham S, Loughlin T, Culliton M, McKenna T. The relationship between sex steroids and sex-hormone-binding globulin in plasma in physiological and pathological conditions. *Ann Clin Biochem* 1985;**22**:489–97.

203 Field A, Colditz G, Willett W, Longcope C, McKinlay J. The relation of smoking, age, relative weight, and dietary intake to serum adrenal steroids, sex hormones, and sex hormone-binding globulin in middle-aged men. *J Clin Endocrinol Metab* 1994;**79**:1310–6.

204 Horrocks P, Jones A, Ratcliffe W, Holder G, White A, Holder R, *et al.* Patterns of ACTH and cortisol pulsatility over twenty-four hours in normal males and females. *Clin Endocrinol (Oxf)* 1990;**32**:127–34.

205 Tietz N, Shuey D, Wekstein D. Laboratory values in fit ageing individuals—sexagenarians through centenarians. *Clin Chem* 1992;**38**:1167–85.

206 Orentreich N, Brind J, Rizer R, Vogelman J. Age changes and sex differences in serum dehydroepiandrosterone sulfate concentrations throughout adulthood. *J Clin Endocrinol Metab* 1984;**59**:551–5.

207 Brabant G, Prank K, Ranft U, Schuermeyer T, Wagner T, Hauser H, *et al.* Physiological regulation of circadian and pulsatile thyrotropin secretion in normal man and woman. *J Clin Endocrinol Metab* 1990;**70**:403–9.

208 van Coevorden A, Mockel A, Laurent E, Kerkhofs M, L'Hermite-Baleriaux M, Decoster C, *et al.* Neuroendocrine rhythms and sleep in ageing men. *Am J Physiol* 1991;**260**:E651–61.

209 Bateson P. Fetal experience and good adult design. *Int J Epidemiol* 2001;**30**:928–34.

210 Chrousos GP. Integration of the immune and endocrine systems by interleukin-6, pp. 133–134. In: Papanicolaou DA. Moderator. The pathophysiological roles of interleukin-6 in human disease. *Ann Intern Med* 1998;**128**:127–37.

211 The Endogenous Hormones and Breast Cancer Collaborative Group. Endogenous sex hormones and breast cancer in postmenopausal women: re-analysis of nine prospective studies. *J Natl Cancer Inst* 2002;**94**:606–16.

212 Barrett-Connor E, Mueller JE, von Mühlen DG, Laughlin GA, Schneider DL, Sartoris DJ. Low levels of estradiol are associated with vertebral fractures in older men, but not women: the Rancho Bernardo Study. *J Clin Endocrinol Metab* 2000;**85**:219–23.

213 Cauley JA, Gutai JP, Kuller LH, Dai WS. Usefulness of sex steroid hormone levels in predicting coronary artery disease in men. *Am J Cardiol* 1987;**60**:771–7.

214 Barrett-Connor E, Khaw KT. Endogenous sex hormones and cardiovascular disease in men. A prospective population-based study. *Circulation* 1988;**78**:539–45.

215 Barrett-Connor E, Goodman-Gruen D. Prospective study of endogenous sex hormones and fatal cardiovascular disease in postmenopausal women. *Br Med J* 1995;**311**:1193–1196.

216 Simpson E, Rubin G, Clyne C, Robertson K, O'Donnell, Jones M, *et al.* The role of local oestrogen biosynthesis in males and females. *Trends Endocrinol Metabol* 2000;**11**:184–8.

217 Manolagas SC, Kousteni S. Perspective: nonreproductive sites of action of reproductive hormones. *Endocrinology* 2001;**142**:2200–4.

218 Karas RH, Patterson BL, Mendelsohn ME. Human vascular smooth muscle cells contain functional oestrogen receptor. *Circulation*. 1994;**89**:1943–50.

219 Wise PM, Dubal DB, Wilson ME, Rau SW, Bottner M, Rosewell KL. Estradiol is a protective factor in the adult and ageing brain: understanding of mechanisms derived from in vivo and in vitro studies. *Brain Res Rev* 2001;**37**:313–9.

220 Yen SSC. Adrenal andropause and ageing. *J Anti-Ageing Med* 2000;**3**:315–28.

221 Parker Jr, CR. Adrenal function in ageing. *Curr Opin Endocrinol Diabetes* 1999;**3**:210–5.

222 Baulieu EE. Three sulfate esters of 17-ketosteroids in the plasma of human subjects and after the administration of ACTH. *J Clin Endocrinol Metab* 1960;**20**:900–4.

223 Barrett-Connor E, Khaw KT, Yen SS. A prospective study of dehydroepiandrosterone sulfate, mortality, and cardiovascular disease. *N Eng J Med* 1986;**315**:1519–24.

224 Barrett-Connor E, Khaw KT. Absence of an inverse relation of dehydroepiandrosterone sulfate with cardiovascular mortality in postmenopausal women. *N Engl J Med* 1987;**317**:711.

225 **Barrett-Connor E, Goodman-Gruen D**. The epidemiology of DHEAS and cardiovascular disease. *Ann N Y Acad Sci* 1995;**774**:259–70.

226 **Ebeling P, Koivisto VA**. Physiological importance of dehydroepiandrosterone. *Lancet* 1994;**343**:1479–81.

227 **Hesse V, Jahreis G, Schambach H, Vogel H, Vilser C, Seewald HJ, Borner A, Deichl A**. Insulin-like growth factor I correlations to changes of the hormonal status in puberty and age. *Exp Clin Endocrinol* 1994;**102**:289–98.

228 **Yen SS, Laughlin GA**. Ageing and the adrenal cortex. *Exp Gerontol* 1998;**33**:897–910.

229 **Straub RH, Konecna L, Hrach S, Rothe G, Kreutz M, Scholmerich J, Falk W, Lang B**. Serum dehydroepiandrosterone (DHEA) and DHEA sulfate are negatively correlated with serum interleukin-6 (IL-6), and DHEA inhibits IL-6 secretion from mononuclear cells in man in vitro: possible link between endocrinosenescence and immunosenescence. *J Clin Endocrinol Metab* 1998;**83**:2012–7.

230 **James K, Premchand N, Skibinska A, Skibinski G, Nicol M, Mason JI**. IL-6, DHEA and the ageing process. *Mech Ageing Dev* 1997;**93**:15–24.

231 **Van Cauter E, Leproult R, Kupfer DJ**. Effects of gender and age on the levels and circadian rhythmicity of plasma cortisol. *J Clin Endocrinol Metab* 1996;**81**:2468–73.

232 **Laughlin GA, Barrett-Connor E**. Sexual dimorphism in the influence of advanced ageing on adrenal hormone levels: The Rancho Bernardo Study. *J Clin Endocrinol Metab* 2000; **85**:3561–8.

233 **Kalimi M, Shafagoj Y, Loria R, Padgett D, Regelson W**. Anti-glucocorticoid effects of dehydroepiandrosterone (DHEA). *Mol Cell Biochem* 1994;**131**:99–104.

234 **Wolf OT, Kirschbaum C**. Actions of dehydroepiandrosterone and its sulfate in the central nervous system: effects on cognition and emotion in animals and humans. *Brain Res Rev* 1999;**30**:264–88.

235 **McEwen BS, Stellar E**. Stress and the individual: mechanisms leading to disease. *Arch Intern Med* 1993;153:2093–2101.

236 **Seeman TE, Singer Bh, Rowe JW, Horwitz RI, McEwen BS**. Price of adaptation—allostatic load and its health consequences. MacArthur studies of successful ageing. *Arch Intern Med* 1997;**157**:2259–68.

237 **Seeman TE, McEwen BS, Rowe JW, Singer BH**. Allostatic load as a marker of cumulative biological risk: MacArthur studies of successful ageing. *Proc Natl Acad Sci* 2001;**98**:4770–5.

238 **Kalmijn S, Launer LJ, Stolk RP, de Jong FH, Pols HA, Hofman A, Breteler MM, Lamberts SW**. A prospective study on cortisol, dehydroepiandrosterone sulfate, and cognitive function in the elderly. *J Clin Endocrinol Metab* 1998;**83**:3487–92.

239 **Baulieu EE**. Dehydroepiandrosterone (DHEA): a fountain of youth? *J Clin Endocrinol Metab* 1996;**81**:3147–51.

240 **Hechter O, Grossman A, Chatterton Jr, RT**. Relationship of dehydroepiandrosterone and cortisol in disease. *Med Hypotheses* 1997;**49**:85–91.

241 **Dubrovsky B**. Natural steroids counteracting some actions of putative depressogenic steroids on the central nervous system: potential therapeutic benefits. *Med Hypotheses* 1997;**49**:51–5.

242 **Cauley JA, Lucas FL, Kuller LH, Vogt MT, Browner WS, Cummings SR**, Bone mineral density and risk of breast cancer in older women: the study of osteoporotic fractures. Study of Osteoporotic Fractures Research Group. *J Am Med Assoc* 1996;**276**:1404–8.

243 **Newcomb PA, Trentham-Dietz A, Egan KM, Titus-Ernstoff L, Baron JA, Storer BE,Willett WC, Stampfer MJ**. Fracture history and risk of breast and endometrial cancer. *Am J Epidemiol* 2001;**153**:1071–8.

244 **Wild S, Pierpoint T, McKeigue P, Jacobs H**. Cardiovascular disease in women with polycystic ovary syndrome at long-term follow-up: a retrospective cohort study. *Clin Endocrinol (Oxf)* 2000;**52**:595–600.

Chapter 11

Social and economic trajectories and women's health

Mel Bartley, Amanda Sacker, and Ingrid Schoon

In this chapter we describe some of the complexity and change in
women's lives, and propose an approach to the study of socioeconomic
and psychosocial pathways through the life course, as precursors of physical
and mental health outcomes. The first section outlines what is known about
women's socioeconomic life trajectories: the relationship between social
origins and destinations, labour force participation, and their relationship
to marriage and child rearing. The second section of the paper describes a
theoretical and methodological approach to the analysis of the life course
that takes account of social structure and changing individual
characteristics over time.

11.1 Socioeconomic pathways in women and men

There are strong continuities of social, cultural[1] and economic[2] advantage between generations and across the life course of individuals, whether they are male or female. In study
after study, in most industrialized nations, children of families with greater economic
resources and higher social status are far more likely to acquire and keep these characteristics during their own lifetimes than children from less privileged family backgrounds.
These findings are now being linked by many researchers to studies from epidemiology
showing the relationships of education, social position based on occupation, prestige, and
income to risk factors for major diseases.[3–6] The implication of these studies is that the
aetiological processes of major diseases of adult life involve intricate combinations of
biological and social processes.[7]

   Although complex, the payoff for the understanding of these processes would be very
great. Large differences between people in more and less advantaged social and economic
circumstances in disabling disease and quality of life make an important contribution to the
demands for social and health care in modern societies.[8,9] To these should be added the
socioeconomic component in the development of cardiovascular,[10,11] respiratory,[12] and
malignant disease.[13] Clearly the scope for improvement of population health and quality of
life that could follow greater understanding of socioeconomic trajectories is considerable.

11.2 **From parents to children**

One of the most important ways in which continuity and change in socioeconomic circumstances take place over the life course is social mobility. Social mobility is of two types: intergenerational and intragenerational. The former refers to the movement between socioeconomic positions that takes place as the young person leaves their family of origin and establishes their own occupational and social trajectory. Intragenerational social mobility is that which takes place within the period of adult working life. Most research on social mobility has concentrated on men, with the result that intragenerational mobility is usually thought of in terms of movement between occupations with their associated prestige and income. However, changes in prestige and income may also take place as a result of marriage; traditionally this type of social mobility has been regarded as more relevant to women than to men.

There is found to be a large degree of continuity of class and income from father to son, which is well documented elsewhere.[14,15] The causes of this inheritance are far more controversial.[16,17] There is disagreement about the extent to which it is due to higher intelligence and better motivation at school in sons of more advantaged families, or whether these families are able to make sure that their sons achieve similarly favoured social position regardless of their own abilities. Research on this topic invariably finds that children from more economically privileged backgrounds perform better in school.

The ways in which these processes of social reproduction differ between men and women has been subject to rather less research effort. The understanding of social reproduction is complicated in the case of women by the different role played by marriage in social mobility. As well as asking whether the daughters of socially advantaged families are more likely to acquire advantaged occupations, it is also necessary to ask the question: are daughters likely to marry men in similar social positions to their own fathers?

The largest international study of social mobility from which data are available for both men and women is the CASMIN study, which examined patterns of intergenerational inheritance of social class in the 1970s in 12 nations, only 5 of which included data on women.[15] Young men and women entered widely differing occupations. In all five nations for which data were available, women were over-represented in routine non manual and non-skilled manual employment, and under-represented in skilled manual and technical work. The mobility path from unskilled parents into skilled manual, supervisory and lower technical occupations was therefore far less available to women than men. Women were also found to be more likely to be downwardly mobile in their own occupational careers than men, regardless of their class of origin. This was due to the more limited range of jobs open to women: different patterns of mobility in women could not be attributed to differences in attitudes or aspirations.[15]

The CASMIN study contained data on class by marriage. Patterns of social mobility by marriage in women were found to be not greatly different (though there were some differences) to patterns of occupational mobility in men. 'If we know how men of a given class origin have themselves become distributed within the class structure in the course of their employment, we can predict, with no great inaccuracy, how their 'sisters' will have been distributed through marriage'.[15] The overall outcome of these patterns of mobility is that, in the sample of industrial nations chosen for the CASMIN study, women tend to be concentrated in less advantaged occupations, resulting in lower rates of upward and higher rates of downward mobility. However, a large number of these women (particularly those with more advantaged parents) were married to men in the more privileged occupations, so that in terms of living standards and status, patterns of social reproduction were little different in men and women. Although this is one of the more recent studies of social mobility in women, its results accord with other earlier ones to a great extent.[18,19] Studies agree that mobility that takes place through a woman's own occupation is different to that which takes place as a result of marriage. Women are more likely to experience mobility over greater social distances, and with a pattern more similar to that found in men, by marriage than by work.

Of course, the CASMIN data are now 30 years old, and were collected at a time when 'over the lifetime of a marriage a woman's living standards most significantly derive from the status and conditions of her husband's employment, and from the level of his earnings'.[20,15] There are now many young women whose careers resemble those of men far more closely than at the time when most of the social mobility studies were carried out. At the present time, continuities of social advantage and disadvantage of women may become more and more a result of their own progress within the structure of employment rather than the result of marriage.

11.3 Intergenerational and intragenerational mobility in the 1980s and 1990s

Continuities in social advantage and disadvantage in women, and how these differ from those in men, were brought somewhat more up to date in the 1980s and 1990s in Great Britain using information taken from two British birth cohort studies: (the National Child Development Study (NCDS) and the 1970 British Birth Cohort (BCS70)), and the British Household Panel Survey. Data from these studies have been extensively used in research on social reproduction[21–24] and health.[25–27] The two British Birth Cohort Studies include all births in the first week of March 1958 and April 1970. The British Household Panel Survey is a representative, geographically clustered sample of private households in England, Wales, and Scotland, identified in 1991 and followed up every subsequent year.

Table 11.1 shows social mobility between the social class of the father and the daughters' and sons' own occupations at ages 26 or 33 in the two birth cohorts. Down the left hand side of the table is the social class, according to the UK Registrar-General's schema, of the parents of the cohort members. Along the top is the Registrar-General's social class of the cohort member in young adult life. Each of the rows (which sum to 100% for men and for women separately) represents the proportion of all men or women from a given class of origin who were themselves found in each class of destination. Thus, while 20% of men born to fathers in the professional class I in 1958 were themselves in social class I by age 33, only 10% of women born to class I fathers in this age cohort were found in class I according to their own occupation at age 33. The same pattern of mobility between parental and own class was seen in 25% of men and 15.8% of women born in 1970. The table allows us to see how similar or different are the trajectories from the family of origin to the occupation of the young adult women. The table illustrates a number of important aspects of social mobility. The first of these is the shift in the distribution of occupations over time. In the parental generation, class III manual (IIIM), the skilled manual occupations, made up by far the largest single group. This is no longer true for the generation of sons, where class IIIM has been narrowly overtaken by class II, the managerial occupations. In the daughters' class distribution, class III non manual (IIINM), clerical and sales occupations, is the largest, though closely followed by managerial class II. The second notable thing is the different distribution of men and women into classes IIIM and IIINM. Very few women are found in skilled manual occupations; the proportion of women in class IIINM is very similar to the proportion of men in IIIM.

Table 11.1 Intergenerational mobility of women and men born in 1958 and 1970 at ages 30 and 33

Class of father	Women: Own social class at age 33 (1958 cohort) and 30 (1970 cohort)												N in paternal class =100 % of paternal class	
	I		II		IIInm		IIIm		IV		V			
	1958	1970	1958	1970	1958	1970	1958	1970	1958	1970	1958	1970	1958	1970
I	10.0	15.8	50.6	52.0	25.9	21.4	3.2	4.1	9.6	6.6	0.8	0	251 (5.5)	196 (6.3)
II	5.6	7.9	42.2	43.8	31.2	34.4	6.4	5.7	12.0	7.7	2.7	0.4	702 (15.4)	454 (14.5)
IIInm	3.9	5.5	34.8	40.8	38.0	38.1	6.5	6.1	13.1	8.5	3.7	1.1	489 (10.7)	473 (15.1)
IIIM	1.8	2.6	27.7	31.9	34.7	41.1	8.6	8.7	20.3	13.5	6.9	2.1	2065 (45.3)	1490 (47.6)
IV	1.4	0.5	26.5	28.6	32.8	37.3	7.6	9.0	23.7	20.5	8.0	4.1	786 (17.2)	391 (12.5)
V	0.8	0	21.4	21.8	29.7	41.1	11.7	10.5	25.7	21.8	10.5	4.8	266 (5.8)	124 (4.0)
All	2.9	4.3	31.4	35.5	33.4	38.0	7.7	7.7	18.6	12.7	6.0	1.9		

Men: Own social class at age 33 (1958 cohort) and 30 (1970 cohort)

Social class	I		II		IIInm		IIIM		IV		V		N (%)	
	1958	1970	1958	1970	1958	1970	1958	1970	1958	1970	1958	1970	1958	1970
I	19.9	25.0	52.4	45.0	10.7	15.0	11.1	10.0	4.4	39.0	1.5	1.1	271 (6.0)	180 (6.5)
II	10.5	12.8	50.1	42.9	12.9	13.9	17.3	16.6	8.1	10.2	1.1	1.6	713 (15.7)	382 (13.8)
IIInm	6.9	12.1	47.0	36.5	17.1	21.3	19.5	18.1	7.4	10.1	2.2	1.9	462 (10.2)	414 (14.9)
IIIM	5.3	7.2	27.2	25.6	11.7	12.7	37.1	34.5	15.6	16.2	3.1	3.9	2026 (44.7)	1291 (46.5)
IV	5.6	4.4	21.5	23.2	11.0	12.8	37.6	32.6	20.3	23.5	3.9	3.4	817 (18.0)	383 (13.8)
V	2.9	0.8	19.5	20.3	6.6	13.3	39.0	33.6	22.8	22.7	9.1	9.4	241 (5.3)	126 (4.6)
All	7.1	9.2	32.9	30.3	12.0	14.3	30.8	28.0	14.2	15.0	3.0	3.3		

Source: National Child Development Study and 1970 British Birth Cohort study.

The main purpose of Table 11.1, however, is to throw some light on whether there are still substantial differences in intergenerational social mobility between men and women. The dark squares represent social stability: where a young woman or man is found in the same class as their father. Social stability between generations in social class I is clearly greater in men than women. There are two social classes where the male and female distributions are very different in the parental generation, that is, class IIINM which contains secretaries and clerical workers and class IIIM which contains the skilled manual occupations. In these cases, there is a matching tendency of daughters to move from parental class IIIM to own class IIINM. But apart from this, in the other classes where the marginal gender distributions are not very different, the differences between sons and daughters in social stability are not very great. Men are more likely than women to move upwards into class I from other classes. Women originating from classes I and II are more likely than men to be found in clerical or sales occupations (class IIINM) and to experience 'long range' downward social mobility into class IV. These differences are in accord with the larger size of class I in men and of classes IIINM and IV in women.

Did intergenerational social trajectories of women change between the two cohorts? The likelihood of a daughter of a man in class I having an occupation in those same classes when she was aged 33 increased, by over 50% (from 10% to 15.8%) between the two time periods, and the risk of downward mobility from class I into a clerical occupation (class IIINM) or semi-skilled or unskilled manual occupations (classes IV or V) decreased by around 20% (from 36.3% to 28.0%). Upward mobility of women with fathers in semi-skilled occupations (class IV) also increased. Very few moved into the shrinking social class V in either year: the most common destination for daughters of men in this class being semi-skilled rather than unskilled manual work.

Table 11.2 shows social mobility in men and women during their own adult lives (ages 18 to 60), for an eight-year period between 1991 and 1998 using British Household Panel Survey data. This table allows us to see a different aspect of women's social trajectories: movements between occupationally defined social classes over an eight-year period of adult life. Here the measure of social class is different to that used in Table 11.1. The National Statistics Socioeconomic Classes (NS-SEC) are used in the 2001 census of England and Wales. The schema organizes occupations according to employment relations and conditions such as the amount of job security, autonomy at work, and the presence of a career structure. It also distinguishes the self-employed (SEC 4) from employees. This allows us to see that within their own working lives, the class trajectories of men and women do differ in important respects. Women in SEC 1 are more likely to leave this class and to enter SEC 2 and 3 in particular. Women are also far more likely than men to remain in SEC 3 rather than moving upwards into SEC 1 or 2. Women are also less likely to become self-employed or owners of small firms by 1998, regardless of their class in 1991.

11.4 **Marriage and social trajectories**

Because studies have shown the importance of the income and status of the marital partner for women's living standards and status in adult life, tracing pathways from childhood context to women's own occupational attainment is not sufficient. We also need to understand what influences both the likelihood of marriage and the choice of marital partner. As in occupational mobility, educational level seems to be related to the income and education of the marital partner, but so are certain measures of health and health risk factors. A study by Garn

Table 11.2 Intra-generational mobility: comparison of adult women and men in Great Britain 1991–1998

SEC 1991	Socio-economic class (SEC) 1998												
	1		2		3		4		5		6		7	
	m	f	m	f	m	f	m	f	m	f	m	f	m	f
1 Higher managerial and professional	70.3	58.6	18.7	28.0	4.0	9.9	3.9	0.9	2.1	0.9	0.3	1.8	0.8	0
2 Lower managerial and professional	14.9	5.7	65.8	74.0	4.8	7.8	5.6	3.5	2.6	2.9	3.7	4.2	2.6	1.7
3 Intermediate	14.6	2.0	12.4	8.6	57.5	69.9	5.6	4.1	3.7	1.9	3.4	10.3	2.8	3.2
4 Small employers and self employed	1.3	1.2	7.9	6.0	1.8	10.1	71.2	66.3	6.3	1.5	2.9	7.0	8.4	7.0
5 Lower supervisory and technical	3.9	1.0	8.8	12.7	3.3	10.7	7.2	2.0	57.1	50.0	8.0	13.1	11.9	10.2
6 Semi-routine occupations	3.6	0.3	5.7	5.5	6.2	10.6	5.7	3.3	13.0	5.9	52.6	64.1	13.2	9.5
7 Routine occupations	1.8	0.3	4.0	2.9	2.2	6.2	6.5	3.3	12.5	5.2	8.3	18.1	64.7	63.9
All	15.0	3.9	18.4	19.0	9.7	25.6	14.5	7.1	15.4	6.9	11.1	21.8	15.9	15.7

Source: British Household Panel Study.

reported that women marrying men of higher educational levels than themselves tended to have lower body weight than women marrying men of similar education to their own.[28] In the 1958 British Birth cohort at age 33, women who were in the highest 10% of weight for height were 7% less likely to have married than those in the normal range, and their partners earned less than the husbands of slimmer women. Tall women in this study were also less likely to have married (tall men were more likely to do so), and the wives of tall men earned around 15 per cent more than the wives of men of average height.[29] Many[30–34], though not all[35,36] studies show that married men and women are in better health than their non-married peers. Because longitudinal studies are rare, it is harder to tell whether this is because marriage itself protects health or whether healthier people are more likely to marry. Studies have considered both 'direct' and 'indirect' health selection into marriage.[37,38] The concept of 'direct selection' proposes that those with significant illness may be less likely to marry; the notion of 'indirect selection' considers the possibility that there may be third factors such as psychological ill health that produce both a lower chance of marriage and a higher risk of illness.[36] Mastekaasa[39] found that having a limiting illness reduced the chances of marriage in men but not women. Joung et al.[38] investigated whether perceived general health, number of health complaints, or number of chronic conditions affected the chances of never-married, or divorced men and women marrying over a 4.5 year period in the Netherlands. Whereas social variables such as educational attainment, religion, and employment status were significantly related to marriage chances, the health variables in themselves were not.

The evidence in favour of health as a selective factor for marriage is fragmentary and as far as it goes not strongly supportive.[28,29] Thus to understand how the social trajectories of women may influence their health by affecting their experience of social advantage and disadvantage, we need to concentrate on social rather than biological continuities. However, few studies have examined the determinants of the social class of the marital partner. Prandy has shown that even within social classes, women's specific occupations had a significant influence on whom they were likely to marry. Secretaries, for example, were far more likely to marry men in social classes I and II than routine clerks or typists.[40] It has been more common to study the precursors of marriage itself, regardless of the partner's social or economic status. In most of these the focus has been on social factors such as educational attainment and employment status. These are often found to have some effect: both men and women with better education and who are active in the labour market appear to have more opportunity to form partnerships. Yet the better educated, particularly women, are also more likely to postpone partnerships and parenthood and remain single, and eventually childless.[41,42]

11.5 Parenthood and careers

Education is the primary route to social mobility, in both men and women, but the payoff of education in terms of employment, income, and promotion is found in most studies to be considerably less for women than it is for men. Several studies have compared the occupational attainments of women and men with similar ability levels, and most find that men gain more social and economic advantage than women for the same level of achievement.[43–45]

The extent to which women are engaged in paid work at all has varied sharply over time, and is still highly variable between countries. Table 11.3 shows that the rate of economic activity (being in work or looking for work) in women in Europe varies from under 50%

Table 11.3 Economic patterns in women in European nations 2001

						Country			
	Belgium	Denmark	Germany	Spain	France	Netherlands	Sweden	USA*	UK
% economically active	56.0	76.1	62.9	48.5	62.2	64.4	74.0	61.2	67.3
% employed part time	33.3	33.9	37.2	17.6	31.7	68.6	40.0	25.0	44.4
% unemployed	10.2	5.9	9.2	23.0	14.0	4.9	6.9	4.2	5.2
% of unemployed seeking part time work	22.1	27.5	23.7	8.9	22.5	76.5	17.7	not available	42.0
% with higher education	28.9	28.2	18.9	21.1	22.5	20.7	31.2	24.0	25.5

Source: Eurostat Statistics in Focus Theme 3, 5/2000.

*Source: US Bureau of Labor Statistics www.dol.gov and http://usgovinfo.about.com/newsissues/usgovinfo/library/weekly/aa031601a.htm?terms=women.

(in Spain) to over 70% (in Sweden and Denmark). This means that between 50% and 30% are not looking for work, most of the time due to family and caring responsibilities. Among those who are in work, between 18% (in Spain) and 69% (in the Netherlands) are working part-time. Among the unemployed (those without a job who are looking for one) anything between 9% (in Spain) and 76% (in the Netherlands) hope to find part-time rather than full-time employment.

The late 1970s saw the implementation of equal opportunity legislation and programmes aimed at overcoming inequalities in pay and opportunities for women. Educational levels have been constantly rising for women; by the early 1980s women's average educational attainment was the same as men's, and more women were moving into managerial and professional occupations.[46,47]

Women are having fewer children, or have their children later than they used to,[48,49] which gives them more freedom to enter the labour market and to pursue careers. However, formal equal opportunity policies have not completely overcome the problems entailed by women's family responsibilities. Women's pathways through the labour market and up the career ladders of organizations are still very different to men's. Joshi and colleagues show that women in the British 1958 Birth Cohort Study at age 33 were still worse paid than men with the same educational qualifications.[46] Much of this difference was because those who had children were working part-time, although even childless women earned less than their male peers. There is considerable debate as to the extent to which childcare affects women's career achievements: one estimate is that the average women loses £250 000 from her lifetime earnings for each child. Among women in their mid-30s in 1990s Great Britain, the lower pay of women with children relative to those without was entirely a result of the time they spent away from work due to home responsibilities.[50]

There are still far greater barriers for women wishing to combine career and parenthood than for men. A recent Dutch study showed that women's occupational success, in terms of the position they reached in their workplace or organization, was strongly influenced by their marital and parenthood histories. Never married, single, childless women, and divorcees as well as women in second marriages achieved relatively advantaged positions in the labour force. Among those who were married or formerly married, the childless also had greater success than mothers, suggesting that 'the absence rather than the presence of family ties seemed to foster women's occupational success'.[51] This illustrates one of the reasons for the continuation of a 'glass ceiling' in most organizations. With or without any effect of overt prejudice on promotion chances, and even in the presence of anti-discrimination legislation, the pressures of parenthood affect the choices women may regard as open to them in the labour market.

11.6 Pathways between childhood and adult social circumstances and health

Women's social trajectories can be seen to be complex and diverse. Even within a single nation changes in the past few decades make generalization difficult, and to this must be added the large variations between nations. These difficulties in modelling the complexity and diversity of women's trajectories are large even when confining oneself to an examination of adult life. They become even more challenging when, as any true life course approach must do, we attempt to consider the relationship of girls' earlier experiences to their pathways through adult life. Recent longitudinal research on health has combined a contextual-systems approach[52] with a 'life course view of human development'.[53–57] Research on the life course is concerned with the description, explanation, and modification of constancy and changes of behaviour throughout life, emphasizing the link between contextual change and individual development. The contextual systems approach regards the individual as embedded in multiple settings and multiple contexts. Those which have a direct impact, are termed 'proximal systems', whereas 'distal systems' have a more indirect impact which is often mediated by the more proximal contexts. Proximal systems include the immediate social and material setting in which the individual is situated: the home, family, and workplace. Distal systems include indicators of social position such as social class, and cultural or societal norms and customs.

At present we lack any detailed understanding of the ways by which social and economic circumstances affect the development of resources during childhood.[58] Figure 11.1 shows a contextual systems model that can be used to understand (and test) some of the pathways whereby childhood social class affects resources in girls.[59] This model aims to move beyond the simple quantification of the relationship between social class of origin and patterns of advantage and disadvantage in youth and early adulthood to a fuller understanding of how the relationships come about. The model begins with the child; specifically, her resources for successfully interacting with the current social environment and for social attainment and good health in adult life. At the first level are the proximal contextual systems, which are by definition directly related to the child. At the second level is the distal system that was under investigation: social class. In this model, inequalities in children's resources were hypothesized to be a result of differences in the proximal factors between children of different social classes. These proximal systems are defined and measured in terms of the social composition of the school, material deprivation at home, parental involvement with and parental aspirations for the child.

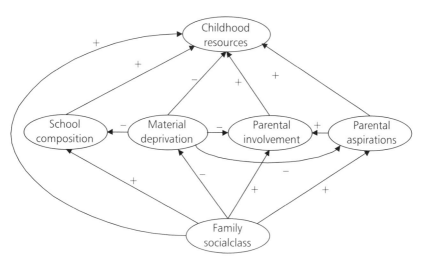

Fig. 11.1 Hypothesized path diagram for the contextual systems model of the relationship between family social class, material deprivation, school composition, parental involvement and aspirations, and children's resources.

The model predicts that attending a school with a more advantaged catchment population and having involved parents with high aspirations for their offspring are associated with higher resource levels in young girls. Relationships between the proximal systems of family and school are also included in the model. It is suggested that material deprivation will affect parental involvement and aspirations in the child because those living in financial and material hardship may have fewer resources of their own for interacting with and investing in their children. Parental involvement and aspirations are predicted to be related to each other. Parental social class is conceptualized as a 'distal' system, at one level removed from the child, which operates mainly through the proximal contexts of family, home, and school. Thus, there are pathways in the diagram from family social class to school social composition, material deprivation, parental involvement, and parental aspirations. The direct path from family social class to the child's resources represents any additional relationships between family social class and children's resources that are not taken account of in the theoretical model.

11.7 Influence of family circumstances and relationships to girls' resources

Two fully representative population samples of British children born 12 years apart, the 1958 NCDS and the 1970 BCS70, have made it possible to test this kind of model. A contextual systems model similar to that shown in Fig. 11.1 has been applied to the NCDS and BCS70 data when the cohort members were aged 11 and 10, respectively. The theoretical entities shown in Fig. 11.1 are modelled as latent or unobserved variables in a structural equation model (SEM). Latent variables represent hypothetical concepts that cannot be observed or measured directly. Instead, a set of observed variables are hypothesized to be imperfect indicators of the latent variable. For example, childhood resources were represented in terms of educational resources and measured by age-appropriate reading and mathematics comprehension tests. The estimated standardized coefficients for the 14 500 girls in the two surveys are shown in Table 11.4. They are interpreted in the same way as a standardized coefficient between a dependent variable and an independent variable in a linear regression analysis, but in the SEM the dependent and independent variables are latent or unobserved variables. The table shows that the relationship of social class to material deprivation was equally strong in 1969 and 1980. However changes in social and economic policies between 1960 and 1980 resulted in girls growing up in very different environments. By 1980, society had become more segregated with very poor families increasingly likely to be concentrated in urban 'areas of social exclusion'.[60,61] The effects of these policies can be seen in the changes in the relationship between class and school social composition in the 11-year period. In 1980, the relationship of their parents' social class to the social composition of the schools that 11-year-old girls attended was far more strongly mediated by material deprivation than it had been in 1969. This pattern of change was replicated in the pathways from social class and material deprivation to parental involvement.

In 1969, pathways from social class to girls' educational resources were mediated to a large extent through school social composition, parental involvement and to a lesser extent, through parental aspirations. In 1980, parental involvement and aspirations were again the main conduits for social inequalities in educational resources with material deprivation

Table 11.4 Standardized estimates of pathways in the contextual systems model for educational resources for girls in middle childhood from the National Child Development Study and the 1970 British Birth Cohort

	NCDS	BCS70	Difference	p-value
Family social class → Material deprivation	0.82	0.78	−0.03	0.63
Family social class → Parental aspirations	0.36	0.74	0.38	< 0.001
Material deprivation → Parental aspirations	0.11	−0.09	−0.19	0.02
Family social class → School social composition	0.72	0.32	−0.39	0.001
Family social class → Parental involvement	0.31	0.00	−0.31	< 0.001
Material deprivation → Parental involvement	0.25	0.48	0.23	0.004
Material deprivation → School social composition	0.04	0.33	0.29	0.002
Parental aspirations → Parental involvement	0.19	0.26	0.06	0.12
School social composition → Educational resources	0.31	0.07	−0.24	< 0.001
Parental involvement → Educational resources	0.31	0.24	−0.07	0.03
Family social class → Educational resources	0.06	0.07	0.00	0.99
Material deprivation → Educational resources	0.06	0.10	0.03	0.62
Parental aspirations → Educational resources	0.16	0.35	0.19	< 0.001

playing a greater role. But school environment now had little effect on girls' resources. In 1965, a change from selective secondary education to a comprehensive system in Great Britain began which was completed by the time children born in 1970 moved on to secondary school. BCS70 children in 1980 were equally likely to achieve educationally whether or not they were in a school with many disadvantaged peers. Given the strong transmission of parents' educational goals to their children[62,63] and the changes in occupational aspirations which took place across all social classes but primarily amongst women during the 1970s,[64] our results suggest that class affects children's educational resources in part through the internalization of their parents' educational aspirations. The stronger pathway from parental aspirations to girls' resources in the later born cohort suggests that higher aspirations have had positive effects on girls' achievements.

This example, adopting a contextual systems approach, makes it possible to move beyond a simple quantification of social inequalities in children's educational resources to a fuller understanding of the dynamics between home, child and the school which maintain these inequalities, and how this may be altered when macro-social conditions change.

11.8 Life course influences on adult psychosocial well-being

In order to analyse the social trajectories of women further, we need to consider how social class effects operating early in life have long-term effects on inequalities later in life including social destinations[2,27,65] and qualifications.[27,65] These are known to be related in women (and men) to mortality,[66] and physical and mental health.[67]

The two most consistent childhood determinants of social inequalities in adult psychoso-cial well-being, measured at the individual level, have been educational achievement and psychosocial adjustment,[5,68,69] both of which are socially patterned.[70,71] Figure 11.1 has shown the ways in which these are influenced by the material circumstances and relation-ships in the home during the school years. Schoon[72,73] has produced a developmental-contextual model examining the pathways linking childhood circumstances to adult outcomes. Figure 11.2 represents a developmental-contextual model for the study of adult health and well-being.[74]

The importance of the developmental-contextual perspective for the study of social inequality in adult adjustment lies in its scope to integrate process and structure and to link individual time with historical time. Repeated measures of social risk (such as parental class and material deprivation) and children's resources such as educational and behavioural adjustment in the face of that risk are assessed throughout childhood.

The model can provide estimates of the stability of social risk over time and the mainte-nance of adequate resources in the face of adversity. It also gives information on the timing and the accumulating effects of social risk on the development of individual resources, by estimating the additional incremental effects of social risk at subsequent time points over the life course (seen as the vertical paths from social risk to resources in Fig. 11.2). Finally, the model also examines intergenerational social mobility, and shows whether social desti-nations are determined solely by social origins or are mediated by individual resources. The model also enables us to quantify the contribution of early life circumstances to social inequalities in adult women's health and well-being.

Figures 11.3 and 11.4 show two examples of this model for women. In one example, individual resources in the domain of education are examined and in the other example, psychosocial resources are measured. Academic achievement is taken to identify educa-tional resources and behavioural adjustment identifies psychosocial resources. In both examples, the adult outcome is psychosocial well-being. The theoretical entities shown in Figs 11.3 and 11.4 are again modelled as latent or unobserved variables using SEM. Table 11.5 gives a description of the indicator variables of these latent variables at each measurement point.

Behavioural adjustment and academic achievement in childhood are related to own social class and psychological well-being in young adulthood in the BCS70 cohort. The

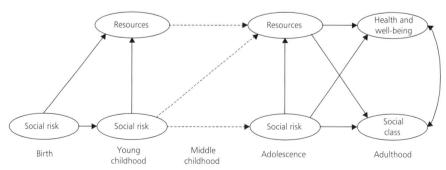

Fig. 11.2 Hypothesized path diagram for the developmental contextual model of adult health and well-being.

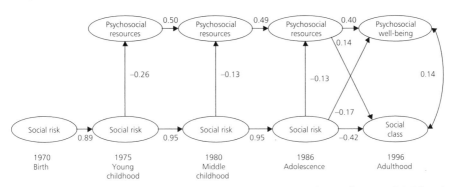

Fig. 11.3 Path diagram for the developmental contextual model of the influence of childhood psychosocial resources on adult psychosocial well-being at 26 years for women in the 1970 British Birth Cohort.

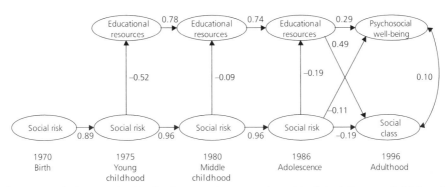

Fig. 11.4 Path diagram for the developmental contextual model of the influence of childhood educational resources on adult psychosocial well-being at 26 years for women in the 1970 British Birth Cohort.

positive correlation between cross-sectional measures of social class and educational and psychosocial resources throughout childhood (not shown here) indicate that pervasive social inequalities exist during childhood. The figures show the cumulative effect of social risk in childhood, which is consequently reflected in adult social destinations and psychosocial well-being. The experience of social risk at one time point can be seen to be a strong predictor of risk experienced at a subsequent time point. Over 90% of the variance in social risk at one time point can be predicted by knowing the extent of social risk experienced at the previous time point. Being born into a relatively disadvantaged family increases the probability of accumulating risks associated with that disadvantage. Even though there was much upward mobility for parents of the cohort between 1970 and 1986, the relative degree of social disadvantage experienced by the cohort was remarkably stable over the same time period. We can also see the relative stability of individual resources, with academic achievement (Fig. 11.4) being more stable than behavioural adjustment (Fig. 11.3), as indicated in the greater pathway coefficients. Young girls are not just influenced by the environment they experience, but are also shapers or producers of their own development. This is not to deny the impact of adversity on individual development. The experience of social risk weakens individual resources, and this detrimental effect is carried forward into the future through the maintenance of these lowered resources. Subsequent experiences of adversity add to this process of deterioration. A general premise of life course study postulates that adaptations to change are influenced by what people bring to the new situation. If individual resources are already weakened at a very early age, it becomes more and more difficult for the young person to develop their resources fully. This negative chain effect undermines the educational and psychosocial adjustment of the young person, and ultimately the individual attainments in adulthood.

Differences between the models in Figs 11.3 and 11.4 suggest that social risk has incremental detrimental effects on girls' behavioural adjustment throughout all of childhood. There was less consistency in the way that social risk lowered girls' academic achievements throughout childhood (Fig. 11.4). Adversity experienced early in the life course (before age five) had the strongest impact on the formation of both psychosocial and educational resources. Figure 11.4 shows that academic achievement is affected most at the key transitional stage of home to school (age 5) with an additional impact at the transition from school to work or further education (age 16). From Fig. 11.3, it appears that social inequalities in adult women's psychosocial well-being are maintained in roughly equal measure by the upward social mobility of behaviourally adjusted women, counter-balanced by the detrimental effects of adolescent social risk on well-being in early adult life. However, the academic achievements model (Fig. 11.4) indicates that individual educational resources mediate the maintenance of social inequality in well-being.

11.9 **Conclusion**

Developmental pathways do not exist in a social vacuum and cannot be isolated from the social contexts in which these attributes are encouraged to flourish. Educational achievement in adolescence may indeed be the strongest influence on the occupational destinations of young women but not all women can overcome the social risk experienced throughout their formative years to become educationally resilient. The models show that young girls who continue to be at risk throughout childhood face an uphill struggle to negotiate early adult life transitions successfully. The effects of socioeconomic disadvantage are cumulative.

Both the timing and duration of risk experiences play a crucial role in shaping the development of individual resources, and for a better understanding of successful adaptation we have to consider the dynamic interaction between a changing individual and a changing context. The whole life path is important in shaping individual development, not just the early years. Research on women's health in the life course poses a number of important challenges to contemporary researchers. Not least of these is the need to take account of social, economic, and demographic trajectories. In this chapter we have suggested some methodological approaches and presented some data from recent studies, in order to fill some gaps in the literature. There remains, however, a great deal to be done within this promising new field of study.

Commentary on 'Social and economic trajectories and women's health'

Kate Hunt

This chapter by Mel Bartley and her colleagues elegantly raises a number of important issues, central to them the immense complexity of understanding change and continuity in social position, resources and health over a woman's lifetime. Their empirical analysis of the trajectories of two generations of British women, from birth to relatively early adulthood, demonstrates the importance of a life course approach and the immense value of carefully conducted prospective studies such as the two birth cohorts that they draw on here. As the cohorts grow older and move into life stages which are characterized by a higher burden of chronic ill-health, it will be of great interest to see how these relationships are modified or amplified by later life experiences.

For many years, as Bartley and colleagues point out, the study of social mobility both inter- and intragenerationally was dominated by the study of men. At a time when the prevailing ideology about gender was more fixed, with its emphasis on the primacy of work for men and the domestic sphere for women, when fewer women were in the paid labour market and there were clearer divisions between 'working' and 'non-working' women in relation to other areas of life (such as marriage and parenting), there was an assumption that non-occupational routes to mobility predominated for women, whilst occupational routes were of primary importance to men. Changes in the last few decades in patterns of employment have rendered this increasingly problematic, and make the intergenerational shifts in occupational mobility difficult to interpret. Furthermore, we can see historically that, although the gender composition of different specific occupations continues to change over time with wider economic changes, gendered segregation of the labour market remains pervasive, albeit with some redefinitions of what constitutes 'men's' and 'women's' work.[75]

These changes in employment are rendered yet more complex by changes in patterns of marriage and parenting, and in the broader structure of society.[76] For example, fewer people marry and more of those that do dissolve their partnerships through separation and divorce. It is increasingly common to treat cohabiting partnerships not formalized by marriage as equivalent to marital relationships (e.g. in their assumed psychosocial benefits), despite variation in the way in which such relationships are seen institutionally (for example, in employers' policies for the transfer of pensions and other assets following death of a partner). As the prevalence of marriage has changed, this raises questions at all levels about the equivalence of being married in different generations.

Similarly, there have been shifts in patterns of parenting; these include the trend towards decreased fertility rates, dramatic changes in the prevalence of single parent families, and changes in the age at which people embark on parenting. For example, the mean age of women at the birth of a first child rose in Britain towards the end of the twentieth century to 26.8 in 1997. Such trends are likely to be both socially driven and differentially patterned by socioeconomic circumstances. However, factors such as parity and age at first birth continue to be understood in epidemiology predominantly as relatively unproblematized biological mediators of subsequent risk of disease (e.g. of breast cancer). But the social context and consequences of having a first child at an older age, or having no children, or a large family is likely to be different depending on whether a woman is challenging prevailing gender norms or reflecting them. Although life course epidemiology is looking more to biological pathways to explain the link between social influences or exposures and health, as yet there has been less attention on how the broader social context might challenge our understanding of more traditional biological risk factors.

There is greater recognition of the importance of place and context (historically and geographically) within more recent sociological and epidemiological research on the genesis of (inequalities in) health over the life course, but as yet we have made less progress in incorporating the wider socioeconomic context, and less still in understanding how changes within this may reinforce or disrupt current sociological or epidemiological interpretations of pathogenesis or salutogenesis over the life course. The social and economic rewards and penalties, and the experience, of combining various roles will differ according to the prevailing social milieu. The experiences and health consequences for women who were in paid work, with small children without a partner at home during the Second World War (when many women were perceived as 'doing the right thing' by responding to the war effort whilst their husbands were away at war), during the 1950s (when gender role ideology reasserted and reinforced the nuclear family with a non-working mother), and the 1990s (when patterns of work, marriage, and motherhood were all more fluid), for example. A dilemma for all life course research based on cohorts is that their participants are inevitably locked, to a degree at least, in historical time and space, and that the very data that exist on cohort members reflects, in part at least, ideas about causality which were prevalent at the time of data collection. All of this points to the importance of doing more of the kind of work presented here by Bartley and colleagues: comparisons of models based on careful thought about detailed pathways between exposures and later outcomes constructed for different generations may provide important leads to bringing in the wider and changing social context prevailing at different times in their lives.

References

1 Bourdieu P. *Distinction*. London: Routledge, 1984.

2 Kuh D, Wadsworth M. Childhood influences on adult male earnings: a longitudinal study. *Br J Sociol* 1991;**42**:537–55.

3 Brunner E. Socioeconomic determinants of health—stress and the biology of inequality. *Br Med J* 1997;**314**:1472–6.

4 Lynch J, Kaplan GA, Salonen R, Salonen JT. Socioeconomic status and progression of carotid atherosclerosis-Prospective evidence from the Kuopio Ischemic Heart Disease Risk Factor Study. *Arterioscler Thromb Vasc Biol* 1997;**17**:513–9.

5 Wadsworth MEJ. Health inequalities in a life course perspective. *Soc Sci Med* 1997;**44**:859–70.

6 McCarron P, Smith GD, Okasha M, McEwen J. Life course exposure and later disease: a follow-up study based on medical examinations carried out in Glasgow University (1948–68). *Public Health* 1999;**113**:265–71.

7 Eriksson JG, Forsen T, Tuomilehto J, Osmond C, Barker DJ. Early growth, adult income, and risk of stroke. *Stroke* 2000;**31**:869–74.

8 Kuh DJ, Wadsworth ME, Yusuf EJ. Burden of disability in a post war birth cohort in the UK. *J Epidemiol Community Health* 1994;**48**:262–9.

9 Sundquist J, Bajekal M, Jarman B, Johansson SE. Underprivileged area score, ethnicity, social factors and general mortality in district health authorities in England and Wales. *Scand J Prim Health Care* 1996;**14**:79–85.

10 Marmot M. Psychosocial factors and cardiovascular-disease—epidemiological approaches. *Eur Heart J* 1988;**9**:690–7.

11 Greenwood DC, Muir KR, Packham CJ, Madeley RJ. Coronary heart disease: a review of the role of psychosocial stress and social support. *J Public Health Med* 1996;**18**:221–31.

12 Malveaux FJ, Fletchervincent SA. Environmental risk-factors of childhood asthma in urban centers. *Environ Health Perspect* 1995;**103**:59–62.

13 Geyer S. Social factors in the development and course of cancer. *Cancer J* 1996;**9**:8–12.

14 Goldthorpe JH, Llewellyn C, Payne C. *Social mobility and class structure in modern Britain.* Oxford: Clarendon, 1980.

15 Erikson R, Goldthorpe JH. *The Constant Flux.* Oxford: Clarendon, 1992.

16 Bond R, Saunders P. Routes to success: influences on occupational attainment of young British males. *Br J Sociol* 1999;**50**:217–49.

17 Breen R, Goldthorpe JH. Class inequality and meritocracy. *Br J Sociol* 1999;**50**:1–27.

18 Chase ID. A comparison of men's and women's intergenerational mobility in the United States. *Am Sociol Rev* 1975;**40**:485–505.

19 Tyree A, Treas J. The occupational and marital mobility of women. *Am Sociol Rev* 1974;**39**:293–302.

20 Finch J. *Married to the Job: Wives' Incorporation into Men's Work.* London: Allen and Unwin, 1992.

21 Power C, Fogelman K, Fox AJ. Health and social-mobility during the early years of life. *Quarterly J Social Affairs* 1986;**2**:397–413.

22 Power C, Manor O, Fox AJ, Fogelman K. Health in childhood and social inequalities in health in young-adults. *J R Stat Soc Series A-Statistics in Society* 1990;**153**:17–28.

23 Montgomery SM, Bartley MJ, Cook DG, Wadsworth MEJ. Health and social precursors of unemployment in young men in Great Britain. *J Epidemiol Community Health* 1996;**50**:415–22.

24 Bynner J, Ferri E, Shepherd P. *Twenty-something in the 1990s: getting on, getting by, getting nowhere.* Aldershot: Ashgate, 1997.

25 Bartley M, Power C, Blane D, Smith GD, Shipley M. Birth weight and later socioeconomic disadvantage: evidence from the 1958 British cohort study. *Br Med J* 1994;**309**:1475–8.

26 Power C, Hertzman C, Matthews S, Manor O. Social differences in health: Life-cycle effects between ages 23 and 33 in the 1958 British birth cohort. *Am J Public Health* 1997;**87**:1499–503.

27 Power C, Matthews S. Origins of health inequalities in a national population sample. *Lancet* 1997;**350**:1584–9.

28 Garn SM, Sullivan TV, Hawthorne VM. Educational level, fatness, and fatness differences between husbands and wives. *Am J Clin Nutr* 1989;**50**:740–5.

29 Harper B. Beauty, stature and the labour market: a British cohort study. *Oxford Bull Econ Stat* 2000;**62**:771–800.

30 Waldron I, Hughes ME, Brooks TL. Marriage protection and marriage selection– prospective evidence for reciprocal effects of marital status and health. *Soc Sci Med* 1996;**43**:113–23.

31 Joung IM, van de Mheen H, Stronks K, van Poppel FW, Mackenbach JP. Differences in self-reported morbidity by marital status and by living arrangement. *Int J Epidemiol* 1994;**23**:91–7.

32 Sorlie PD, Backlund E, Keller JB. US mortality by economic, demographic, and social characteristics: the National Longitudinal Mortality Study see comments. *Am J Public Health* 1995;**85**:949–56.

33 Voges W. Unequal requirements for longevity—social determinants of mortality in longitudinal perspective. *Z Gerontol Geriatr* 1996;**29**:18–22.

34 Cheung YB. Marital status and mortality in British women: a longitudinal study. *Int J Epidemiol* 2000;**29**:93–9.

35 Ladwig KH, Marten Mittag B, Formanek B, Dammann G. Gender differences of symptom reporting and medical health care utilization in the German population. *Eur J Epidemiol* 2000;**16**:511–8.

36 Hope S, Rodgers B, Power C. Marital status transitions and psychological distress: longitudinal evidence from a national population sample. *Psychol Med* 1999;**29**:381–9.

37 Joung I. *Marital status and health*. Den Haag: CIP-DATA Koninklijke Bibliotheek; 1996.

38 Joung IM, van de Mheen HD, Stronks K, van Poppel FW, Mackenbach JP. A longitudinal study of health selection in marital transitions. *Soc Sci Med* 1998;**46**:425–35.

39 Mastekaasa A. Marriage and psychological well-being: some evidence on selection into marriage. *J Marriage Fam* 1992;**54**:901–11.

40 Prandy K. Similarities of life-style and the occupations of women. In: *Gender and Stratification*. Crompton R, Mann M, eds. Cambridge: Polity Press, 1986:137–53.

41 Han SK, Moen P. Work and family over time: A life course approach. *Ann Am Acad Pol Soc Sci* 1999;**562**:98–110.

42 Brewster KL, Rindfuss RR. Fertility and women's employment in industrialised nations. *Annu Rev Sociol* 2000;**26**:271–96.

43 Terman LM, Oden MH. *Genetic studies of genius: Vol. 5. The gifted group at mid-life*. Stanford CA: Stanford University Press, 1959.

44 Feldman DH. A follow-up of subjects scoring above 180 IQ in Terman's 'Genetic studies of genius'. *Except Child* 1984;**50**:518–23.

45 Subotnik RF, Arnold KD. *Beyond Terman: Longitudinal studies: Contemporary longitudinal studies of giftedness and talent*. Norwood, NJ: Ablex; 1993.

46 Joshi H, Paci P, Waldvogel J. The wages of motherhood: better or worse? *Cambridge J Econ* 1999;**23**:543–64.

47 Crompton R. *Class and Stratification*. Cambridge: Polity, 1993.

48 Haskey J. Families and households in Great Britain. *Popul Trends* 1996;**86**:12–20.

49 Haskey J. Families: Their historical context, and recent trends in the factors influencing their formation and dissolution. In: David ME,ed. *The Fragmenting Family: Does it matter?* Bury St. Edmunds: St Edmundsbury Press, IEA Health and Welfare Unit 1998:9–47.

50 Joshi H. The cash opportunity cost of childbearing: an approach to estimation using British evidence. *Popul Stud (Camb)* 1990;**44**:41–60.

51 Dykstra PA, Fokkema T. Partner and children: burden or asset for occupational attainment? Occupational mobility of men and women with different marriage and parenthood careers. *Mens en maatschappij* 2000;**75**:110–28.

52 **Bronfenbrenner U**. *The Ecology of Human Development: experiments by Nature and Design*. Cambridge, MA: Harvard University Press, 1979.

53 **Elder GH**. *Life course dynamics*. Ithaca, NY: Cornell University Press, 1985.

54 **Giele JZ, Elder GH**. Life course research: development of a field. In: *Methods of Life Course Research. Qualitative and Quantitative Approaches*. NY: Sage 1998:5–27.

55 **Lerner RM**. *On the nature of human plasticity*. NY: Cambridge University Press, 1984.

56 **Featherman DL, Lerner RM**. Ontogenesis and sociogenesis. Problematics for theory about development across the life-span. *Am Sociol Rev* 1985;**50**:659–76.

57 **Lerner RM**. Relative plasticity, integration, temporality, and diversity in human development: A developmental contextual perspective about theory, process, and method. *Dev Psychol* 1996;**32**:781–6.

58 **Brooks-Gunn J, Duncan GJ, Britto PR**. Are socioeconomic gradients for children similar to those for adults? In: *Developmental health and the wealth of nations*. Keating DP, Hertzman C, eds. NY: The Guildford Press 1999:94–124.

59 **Sacker A, Schoon I, Bartley M**. Social inequality in educational achievement and psychosocial adjustment throughout childhood: magnitude and mechanisms. *Soc Sci Med* 2001, in press.

60 **Bradshaw A**. Child welfare in the United Kingdom: Rising poverty, falling priorities for children. In: *Child poverty and deprivation in the industrialized countries, 1945–1995*. Cornia GA, Danziger S, eds. Oxford: Clarendon Press, 1997:210–32.

61 **Cornia GA**. Child poverty and deprivation in the industrialized countries: from the end of World War II to the end of the Cold War era. In: *Child poverty and deprivation in the industrialized countries, 1945–1995*. Cornia GA, Danziger S, eds. Oxford: Clarendon Press, 1997:25–63.

62 **Dekkers HPMJ, Bosker RJ, Driessen GWJM**. Complex inequalities of educational opportunities. A large-scale longitudinal study on the relation between gender, social class, ethnicity and school success. *Educat Res Evaluation* 2000;**6**:59–82.

63 **Schoon I, Parsons S**. Teenage aspirations for future careers and occupational outcomes. *J Vocat Behav* 2002;**60**:262–88.

64 **Shu X, Marini MM**. Gender-related change in occupational aspirations. *Sociol Educ* 1998;**71**:234–40.

65 **Lauder H, Hughes D**. Social origins, destinations and educational inequality. Political Issues in New Zealand Education. 2nd edition. Palmerston North, NZ: Dunmore Press Ltd, 1990:43–60.

66 **Smith GD, Hart C, Blane D, Gillis C, Hawthorne V**. Lifetime socioeconomic position and mortality: prospective observational study. *Br Med J* 1997;**314**:547–52.

67 **Power C, Hertzman C**. Health, well-being and coping skills. In: *Developmental health and the wealth of nations*. Keating DP, Hertzman C, eds. NY: The Guildford Press, 1999:41–54.

68 **Roberts H**. Children, inequalities and health. *Br Med J* 1997;**314**:1122–5.

69 **Montgomery SM, Bartley MJ, Wilkinson RG**. Family conflict and slow growth. *Arch Dis Child* 1997;**77**:326–30.

70 **Marmot M, Ryff CD, Bumpass LL, Shipley M, Marks NF**. Social inequalities in health: next questions and converging evidence. *Soc Sci Med* 1997;**44**:901–10.

71 **Wadsworth MEJ**. Family and education as determinants of health. In: *Health and Social Organisation*. Blane D, Brunner E, Wilkinson R, eds. London: Routledge, 1996:56–75.

72 **Schoon I**. Towards a dynamic-interactive model of talent development: A life-span perspective. In: *International handbook of giftedness and talent*. Heller KA, Mönks FJ, Sternberg R, Subotnik R, eds. Oxford: Pergamon Press 2000:213–25.

73 **Schoon I**. Risiko, Ressourcen und sozialer Status im frühen Erwachsenenalter. *Zeitschrift für Soziologie der Erziehung und Sozialisation* 2001;**21**:60–79.

74 **Schoon I, Sacker A, Bartley M**. Modelling the accumulation of risk in the life course. Paper to Society for Psychotherapy Research (SPR) Congress, Leiden. Leiden: SPR; 2001.

75 **Alvesson M, Billing YD**. *Understanding gender and organizations*. London: Sage, 1997.

76 **Walby S**. *Gender transformations*. London: Routledge, 1997.

Chapter 12

Life course influences on women's social relationships at midlife

Nadine F. Marks and Kristy Ashleman

Social relationships are an important factor influencing health. Existing research linking social relationships with health gives inadequate attention to differential quality of social relationships, potential gender differences in processes linking social relationships and health, and the multiplicity of factors that influence the trajectory of women's social relationships across the life course. This chapter reviews evidence documenting how the structure and quality of women's social relationships with mothers, fathers, siblings, partners, other kin, and friends change from childhood to middle adulthood. It considers how biological, psychological, and social factors uniquely, cumulatively, and interactively influence the quantity and quality of women's social relationships over time. The relative importance of early life course factors for helping to determine later life relationships and relationship quality is discussed. Life course differences between women and men and differences among women of varying socioeconomic status are noted. The chapter concludes with suggestions for future research and implications for policy.

12.1 Introduction

The importance of social relationships for health has become increasingly recognized.[1–5] Several prospective studies of mortality from the United States and Europe provide evidence that the existence of social ties predicts lower mortality rates.[6–9] Social support has also been linked to factors implicated in the aetiology of physical disease and morbidity, although evidence for these outcomes is less consistent.[1,3–5,10–12] The inconsistency in results linking social relationships and morbidity may be due to lack of differentiation of health outcomes as well as lack of sufficient differentiation of social relationship *quality* in much existing research. Not all social relations are equally beneficial for mental and physical health. Considering the demands, burden, and strain as well as the beneficial support involved in social relationships is critical to discerning whether and how social ties will influence health,[13] particularly since evidence suggests that negative aspects of people's social networks are more highly associated with well-being than positive aspects.[13–16]

The 'ties that bind', therefore, have the potential to provide both health-promoting solidarity and health-deterring demands, sometimes at the same time. Social relationships that incur strains as well as gains, or even mainly strains, may be more common among women than men, because women internalize and enact more responsibility for maintaining and providing support in social relationships, especially kin relationships, than men.[17–19] Women may thus be more vulnerable to the costs of caring and maintaining their commitments to social relations.[20,21] These considerations suggest that potential gender differences must be more systematically evaluated when considering linkages between social relationships and health. The mortality advantage of social ties, in fact, has been noted to be somewhat smaller (and sometimes non-existent, or even reversed) for women in contrast to men when the genders are considered separately,[4,22] and a qualitatively different meaning of social ties and processes linking social relationships with health for women may play a part in this.[22,23]

There has been inadequate attention to relationship quality and gender differences in much previous epidemiological research linking social relationships to health across the life course. This chapter aims to review evidence documenting how the structure and quality of women's social relationships change from childhood to middle adulthood; considering how biological, psychological, and social factors uniquely, cumulatively, and interactively influence the quantity and quality of women's social relationships over time, which might, in turn, be expected to influence women's health. Several types of relationships comprising the 'convoy' of social ties[24] shaping women's lives are considered—with mothers, with fathers, with siblings, with partners, with children, and with friends. The relative importance of early life course factors for helping to determine later life relationships and relationship quality is examined. Wherever possible, life course differences between women and men, and differences between persons of varying socioeconomic status (SES) are addressed. It concludes with suggestions for future research and implications for policy.

12.2 Women's relationships with their mothers

The first significant relationship in a woman's life is most typically with her mother, who is usually her primary caregiver. Attachment theory gives the primary caregiver relationship significant primacy and suggests that this tie is the prototypical social tie, that it has significant organic underpinnings, and lifelong consequences for the formation and development of other social relationships.[25–27] Not all early ties with mothers are of similar quality. Attachment researchers have differentiated three main styles of early attachment—secure, anxious-avoidant, and anxious-ambivalent.[28] Attachment style results from the degree to which mothers are sensitive, responsive, and accessible to the cues of need provided by infants. Securely attached infants (about 67%) evidence successful use of the caregiver as a secure base when distressed; anxious-avoidant infants (about 21%) show avoidance of the caregiver and exhibit signs of detachment when distressed; anxious-ambivalent infants (about 12%) display a mixture of attached behaviours with overt expressions of protest and anger toward the primary caregiver when distressed.[29] A fourth attachment type—disorganized—has been added in recent years to accommodate the incoherent attachment patterns of seriously maltreated children, and is characterized by an anomalous mixture of clinging, avoiding, ambivalent, stilling, freezing, and fear reactions in response to the caregiver.[30,31]

Attachment style is assumed to result in internal 'working models' both of self and of typical patterns of interaction with significant others.[26,28,32] These internal schemas, in turn, guide social behaviour and the development of social relationships. Securely attached persons view themselves as likable and friendly and view significant others as trustworthy and reliable. People with an anxious-ambivalent attachment style consider themselves unconfident and misunderstood, and view significant others as being unreliable and either unwilling or unable to commit to permanent relationships. Those with an anxious-avoidant attachment style view themselves as suspicious and aloof, and view significant others as generally unreliable or overly eager to commit to unreliable relationships. People with a disorganized attachment style consider themselves 'bad' and unworthy of care and display hypervigilance to threat of harm in relationships. Some theorists have also emphasized the importance of attachment style for managing negative affect, which is critical for making and maintaining satisfying and harmonious social relationships.[33]

Continuity in attachment style has been observed during preschool ages, particularly among middle class, relatively stable families.[32,34,35] However, research with economically disadvantaged families who report more life stress and life change has also suggested much less stable early attachment patterns,[36,37] which is consistent with the life course paradigm's emphasis on ongoing person–environment interaction and plasticity. Insecure attachment styles are also more typically reported among children reared in poverty in every culture, families with a history of abuse, and families where the mother has been diagnosed as seriously depressed.[38] Depression among mothers, more typical in lower socioeconomic groups,[39,40] is associated with less ability to respond effectively to infants and children, resulting in poorer attachment style outcomes in infancy, and problematic developmental outcomes.

Considerable empirical research has now confirmed that different mental models regarding attachment exist in adults as well as children,[41–43] and that they are associated with retrospective accounts of childhood relationships with mothers and fathers.[42] Main et al.[32] have reported strong associations between adults' attachment history and the attachment styles of their own young children; however, some parents do manage to develop a better attachment style with their own children than they experienced as children. This and other evidence of multiple life course pathways evolving from similar infant attachment patterns[44] again suggests potential plasticity in attachment style over the life course based on differentials in environmental experience and in other relationships.

Secure attachment style has been empirically linked to greater social competence, more friends, and more social support in childhood[45,46] and adolescence.[47] Research is now linking differences in attachment style to differences in the formation and maintenance of romantic partner relationships.[42,48–50] Quality of attachment to mothers at a young age may also influence lifelong patterns of closeness between mothers and daughters[19] and daughters' caregiving motivation and consequences.[51,52]

Temperament (i.e. constitutional differences in reactivity and self-regulation[53]) is another biologically-based characteristic that influences inter-individual differences in relationships, including mother–daughter attachment. Although there is considerable controversy about the exact dimensions of temperament in infants and the mechanisms whereby temperamental dispositions become translated through culture and life experience into particular dimensions of adult personality,[54] there is some consensus that there are inter-individual temperamental differences due to genetic patterning at birth in sociability/inhibition (perhaps related to later extraversion) and negative emotionality (perhaps related to later neuroticism).[55–57] Both of these temperamental characteristics influence the development, quality, and maintenance of social relationships over the life course. Research on adult twins suggesting that genetic factors predict between 28% and 52% of the variance in perceived support and formal affiliative interaction[58] is also consistent with the proposition that aspects of relatively enduring temperament and personality play a role in the development and maintenance of social relationships.

Unanticipated family life transitions can also influence girls' social development. Children who lose a mother to death typically display more troubled emotional and behavioural expressions,[59–61] more struggles with social competence and self-perception,[62] and more anxiety about forming and maintaining other close relationships[63] than non-bereaved peers. Problems in each of these emotional and behaviour areas can influence future social relationships. Depression, whether due to parental loss or other factors, can elicit negative reactions from social network members and also result in decreased social support[64–66] and poorer marital quality.[67]

Living with a single mother during childhood can also alter mother–daughter relationships and women's social trajectories. It is increasingly common for children to be born to an unmarried mother[68] and/or to live at least part of their lives in a household with only their mother present due to parental divorce.[68,69] Divorce and living in a mother-headed household are associated with greater risk of poverty, lower school quality, living in a neighbourhood of poorer quality, more residential moves, a decline in mother involvement, a decline in supervision and mother–child talks, poorer psychological well-being, greater propensity to drop out of high school (lowering a woman's own SES), a greater propensity to engage in earlier sexual activity, and greater risk of experiencing a teenage birth (increasing a woman's own potential to become a young, single parent).[68–73] Although during the initial period after parental divorce boys appear to display more negative effects than girls, evidence suggests girls experience more delayed effects, for example, more distress if their mothers remarry and problems in establishing emotional commitments in early adulthood.[74–76] Adult women whose parents divorced in childhood also have been found to have poorer psychological well-being,[70,77] to be more likely to be depressed as adults,[67,78] and to experience poorer marital quality.[67,77]

However, not all divorces have the same impact on children, and research suggests a number of moderating effects.[70,72] For example, adults who experience only one divorce during childhood that does not lead to a decline in their relationship with both parents report similar psychological and social well-being to those who grew up in very happily intact families, and they report better psychological and social well-being than adults who report they grew up in unhappily intact families.[77]

Mothers and daughters tend to retain a close (if sometimes also conflictual) relationship over the life course. Chodorow[18] hypothesized that daughters do not need to disconnect from their mothers as much as sons during identity development, which leads to continued strong mother–daughter ties, as well as the ongoing socialization of a schema for identity that emphasizes nurturance and embeddedness in close relationships. Of the four possible family dyad ties, mother–daughter, mother–son, father–daughter, father–son, the mother–daughter tie evokes the highest levels of normative obligation, affectional support, and instrumental support across adulthood.[19]

Overall, mothers continue to provide a range of financial, emotional, and instrumental support to daughters across the adult years.[19,79,80] Beginning in early adulthood, there is also a considerable amount of reciprocity in the relationship, especially in emotional and instrumental support. It is only after mothers become relatively older, typically in their 60s or 70s, that daughters are more likely to provide more support to mothers than they continue to receive.[19] Thus, mothers often remain a critical social resource to women, through early adulthood and into middle age.

There are, however, demographic differences in patterns of support from mothers. Mothers who have more income provide more financial support to daughters. There is more help provided to daughters by mothers across early and middle adulthood when daughters also report there was greater family cohesion in childhood; when there is current affective closeness and contact; when the mother is married; and when the daughter is single, not employed, younger, and has a lower income.[19,80] Greater help provided to mothers from daughters is likewise predicted by greater early family cohesion, greater current affective closeness, less geographic distance, poorer mother health, and mother being single.[19,81]

Low income persons and African Americans in the US receive less money, emotional support, and childcare from parents (mothers and fathers) than higher income persons and non-Hispanic Whites,[79] yet African American women are more likely to reside with their parents than Whites.[82,83] Strong kin ties may be culturally emphasized in many race ethnic families, but tight resources may not always allow for the high levels of compensatory intergenerational exchanges policy-makers often count upon.[79,84,85]

An important part of a woman's adult life is typically spent now in relationships with parents who are living to older ages and experiencing increasing functional limitation and disability prior to death. Men and women from contemporary midlife birth cohorts are likely to spend more years with one or more parents aged 65 and older than they are to spend with children under age 18.[86] By middle adulthood, many women are beginning to experience some caregiving demands from mothers and/or fathers.[87–90] A little over one in ten US women aged 35–64 report having lived with or cared for a disabled parent during the previous year.[90]

The hierarchical model of caregiving[91] suggests that if spouse care is not available, care from a child (typically a daughter, if she is available) is sought out next in most western societies. However, the need for care among ageing mothers varies significantly by SES. Due to consistent associations between lower SES and poorer physical and mental health,[39–40,92–95] lower SES mothers are more likely to become more functionally impaired at younger ages than higher SES mothers, and therefore require more care. Lower SES and ethnic minority mothers are more likely to be single due to earlier partner mortality or divorce,[96] and therefore more likely to seek care from a daughter. Additionally, lower SES children tend to live closer to their mothers and are therefore more able to provide instrumental and emotional support.[19,81]

Providing care to disabled elderly parents (as well as others) has been linked to considerable strain, burden, psychological distress, and sometimes poorer health[87,89,97–101] although caregiving can also be associated with psychological benefits.[101,102] Most studies suggest that women providing parent care experience more burden and distress than men, although the evidence is not entirely consistent.[103,104] Part of the stress of elder care for midlife women often comes from attempting to combine this typically unanticipated care with other role commitments to employment, children, and/or a spouse.[87,89,101,105]

Daughters' temperament and mothers' SES, marital quality, marital history, and mental and physical health trajectories influence the quality of early mother–daughter attachment and quality of the mother–daughter relationship over time. Early mother–daughter attachment has an important impact on the trajectory of women's quality of social relations with others across the life course. At midlife, middle-class White women are more likely to have healthier, married, more affluent mothers who can continue to provide emotional, financial, and instrumental support to them rather than vice versa. More highly educated women are also more likely to live more distant from kin, including mothers, which makes it less likely for them to become involved in intense hands-on caregiving. Lower SES women and women of Colour at midlife are more likely to have lost mothers to death, to have mothers who are less able to provide them with financial and other resources due to their own relatively restricted means, or to have mothers who have health needs that require daughters to participate in day-to-day caregiving and support.

12.3 Women's relationships with fathers

Fathers, too, have an important influence on women's lives and life course social development through their multifaceted roles as care providers, companions, spouses, protectors, models, moral guides, teachers, and breadwinners in families.[106] Although there is controversy whether biology predisposes women to be more optimally equipped for nurturant parenting than men,[107] considerable research has suggested there is nothing about the biological make-up of fathers that prevents them from becoming a critical secondary (or even primary) attachment figure for infants.[108] Most infants do become attached to their fathers, and this attachment is not necessarily the same style (i.e. secure or insecure) as to their mothers.[108]

Fathers tend to spend proportionately less time with children than mothers across childhood, and their style of interaction tends to emphasize play whereas mothers' style emphasizes caregiving.[109] Fathers tend to interact less with daughters than sons at all ages, but particularly during adolescence. Since fathers give infants and young children different types of social cues, having an involved father appears to aid a child's early development of interpersonal differentiation, social competence, and social understanding.[108,110–112] Couple interaction between mother and father are also predictive of both maternal and paternal responsiveness to a child, and, in turn, to socioemotional outcomes for daughters as well as sons.[113] Therefore, fathers positively influence their daughter's social development both through sensitive response to them directly, but also through sensitive responding and support provided to their mothers and other members of the family.

Loss of a father to death during childhood has been associated with greater anxiety, more somatic symptoms, and more problems in peer relationships.[62] Parental divorce, together with the negative effects noted previously, also usually critically disrupts the father–daughter tie. After a divorce between parents, children typically reside with their mother (about 86% do so in the US), and contact with a father tends to decline dramatically.[72,74,114] Non-resident divorced fathers also typically remarry, at which time contact with non-resident daughters tends to decline even more.[72,74] The effects of divorce on daughter–father relationships continues into adulthood. Divorced and remarried fathers are less likely to indicate positive attitudes towards parental obligation to adult children and are less likely to have contact with and provide financial, instrumental, and emotional support to adult daughters than are continuously married fathers.[19,79,115,116]

Overall, the father–daughter bond and reciprocity is much more sensitive to environmental and life course changes than the mother–daughter bond. Marital unhappiness among parents tends to realign family bonds even if divorce does not ensue, resulting in daughters typically remaining closer to an unhappily married mother than to an unhappily married father. This also extends to grandparent relationships: marital unhappiness among parents also tends to reduce children's contact with paternal grandparents.[19]

Due to gender differences in mortality, and the fact that fathers tend to be somewhat older than mothers, fathers tend to die before mothers.[95] Using recent US population data, Marks, Bumpass, and Jun[117] report that young adults (aged 25–39) are more than three times more likely to have a sole surviving mother than a sole surviving father. By midlife ages 40–59, less than one in ten adults reports a father alive; more than one quarter report the loss of both parents. Additionally, lower SES fathers die at younger ages than higher SES fathers,[95] and in the US African American fathers also die younger than non-Hispanic White fathers.[95,118]

The quality of mother–father social interaction and the mother–father partnering trajectory (e.g. continuously married, married and later divorced or separated, never married, divorced and remarried to another) have a critical influence on the development of early daughter–father attachment, daughter–father contact, and the quality of daughter–father relationships over the life course. Fathers, in turn, shape the life course of women's other social relationships in multiple ways, through their nurturing and attachment in infancy, through their different styles of interaction and social cues aiding in women's development of social understanding (i.e. the competent differentiation of social cues and the learning of appropriate social response to social cues), through their interactions with women's mothers in modelling adult social interaction, through economic support leading to women's opportunities for educational and occupational attainment, and through ongoing financial, emotional, and instrumental support in adulthood. Women who have disrupted ties with fathers through absence due to desertion, divorce, or death in childhood lose an important social capital and economic resource, which can influence a trajectory of other experiences (e.g. early sexuality, early birth) that can result in impoverished relationship quality at midlife—with a partner, with children, with friends, and with other family. Lower SES fathers and ethnic minority fathers are more likely to be under social constraints that do not allow them to fulfil all the roles of fatherhood as adequately as higher SES fathers, and they are more likely to become disabled and die at younger ages than high SES fathers—leaving mothers to the care of daughters, and reducing the multifaceted support adult daughters might otherwise experience from fathers.

12.4 Women's relationships with siblings

Sibling relationships are typically the longest enduring social relationships of individuals' lives. Most children have at least one sibling, and among current cohorts of midlife and elderly persons most have at least one living sibling.[119] Sibling relationships are relatively unique in that they typically involve sharing a common genetic heritage, cultural milieu, and early life experiences with parents. Quality within sibling relationships (as measured by dimensions of rivalry, conflict, control, and friendliness) varies greatly across sibling dyads and across time.[110] Sibling relationships in childhood are often intense and ambivalent; a high level of conflict often concurrently occurs with a high level of friendliness.

Birth order, temperament, gender mix, age differences, parental interaction patterns with both siblings, all influence sibling relations.[110] Individual differences in parent–child, marital, and parent–sibling relationships also have important effects on sibling relationships,[110] highlighting how the quality of social relationships are interconnected in the family system.

Sibling relationships offer young children the experience of a relationship that often combines some aspects of complementarity (e.g. an older sibling teaching a younger sibling) as well as reciprocity (e.g. both siblings playing together as equals), and may therefore be instrumental in a child's development of social understanding.[110,120]

From preschool age, children begin to develop connections with friends, and sibling ties may begin to diminish in prominence through middle childhood and adolescence. This process tends to continue as young adults leave home and begin to make decisions about individual life paths, education, employment, and partners. Early adulthood is the period during which sibling ties may be the least actively pursued.[119]

In middle adulthood, siblings may become closer again, especially after launching children and life events like a divorce, death of a spouse, or in the event of parent health issues.[121] Siblings are often considered 'in reserve' as sources of support if need arises, particularly for never-married childless women.[122] Norms of obligation to siblings are less than for most inner circle family members (i.e. parents, children, and spouse),[19] yet siblings provide emotional support and services when needed, especially if they live close by. Siblings are more likely to maintain active long-distance relationships than are friends. Sibling relationships with sisters tend to be emotionally closer than with brothers.[122–123] Sister–sister dyads tend to be particularly intense in inter-identification, often leading to intimacy, volatility, stress, and ambivalence.[124] Making decisions about caregiving sometimes brings siblings into more contact;[87,125] however, negative sibling interaction can also create more stress for women who are primary caregivers.[87,126]

Different cultural and ethnic communities vary in norms for sibling relationships.[122] In the US, African Americans and Mexican Americans exhibit more instrumental and emotional help exchange than do non-Hispanic Whites.[127,128]

As social circles narrow with age, siblings may value each other even more as kin and confidantes due to their long-shared history.[122] In some cases, especially if a spouse or an adult child is not available, a sibling may become caregiver for another sibling.[129] Sibling caregiving is also likely to occur if a sibling has a lifelong disability and parents are no longer able to provide care.[130]

Having one or more siblings reduces the likelihood of receiving support from mothers and fathers during adulthood.[19] Only children, however, are more likely to need to respond to the needs of ageing parents.[131]

Temperament, gender mix, age difference, and birth order, as well as the quality of parent–child, marital, and parent–sibling relationships influence the quality of early sibling relationships. Sibling relationships often provide rich (and challenging) opportunities for social learning and social development at young ages, which, in turn, influence the quality of later social relationships. At midlife, siblings are often part of a secondary layer of social support women may rely upon for companionship, emotional support, and sometimes services. Sister–sister bonds tend to be closer than sister–brother bonds, but both types of sibling relationships can be important resources for women at midlife. Sibling tensions tend to smooth out as women age; however, prior family histories, and ongoing challenges in meeting the needs of ageing parents can still influence the quality of midlife sibling relationships.

12.5 **Women's partner relationships**

Beginning in adolescence, partner relationships become prominent social relationships in women's lives. Yet there is great variance in the timing, quantity, and quality of partner relationships experienced by women.

Young women's involvement in dating and sexual relationships in early adolescence is significantly influenced by a biological factor, pubertal timing. Early maturing girls are at more risk of early sexual relations, earlier partnering, earlier childbearing, delinquency, and diminished educational attainment than later maturing girls.[132–136] This is critical for the life course of women and the evolution of their social relationship quality over time, since earlier childbearing, younger age at marriage, and less education are associated with a greater risk of poorer marital quality, divorce, and single parenting.[132]

Although there has been a great upheaval in the stability of marriage, most women continue to develop cohabiting or marital partnerships during their adult years. Due to increases in divorce rates, lowering of remarriage rates, and increases in women's longevity, the proportion of women's adult lives spent married now, compared with fifty years ago, however, is becoming smaller.[137,138] This is even more dramatically the case for African Americans in the US in comparison to Whites.[139] Marriage now, compared to fifty years ago, is typically occurring at older ages for both women and men.[137,138] Ever more commonly, contemporary marriages occur after a period of cohabitation.[140,141]

Historically, being married has been associated with lower mortality and less distress than being unmarried,[142–146] yet being in a unhappy marriage also has been associated with more psychological and physical health problems than being single.[143,147] As marriage has become more delayed, cohabitation more common, divorce more common, and a period of single living has become more typical and acceptable for young adults, there has been some speculation and even some evidence that marriage may have become less important for adult happiness.[148,149] Overall, however, population research continues to suggest that marriage is associated with better mental and physical health for both women and men.[150–152]

The mechanisms related to better health outcomes may differ by gender, however: marriage may be associated with health for men due to its offering men more support for positive health behaviours and more emotional support, while marriage may be associated with better health for women in large part due to the financial advantages of being married for women.[150,152]

Women generally report less satisfaction with their marriages than husbands. Better quality of marital relationships (as perceived by wives) and stability of marriage over time has been associated with higher SES (i.e. more woman's education, more husband's and family income, greater financial assets), fewer environmental stressors (e.g. not having an unemployed husband), positive childhood factors (e.g. having had a happy childhood, not having experienced a parental divorce), life course factors (e.g. no premarital pregnancy, no cohabitation prior to marriage) as well as more positive personality and mental health factors (e.g. less neuroticism, more extraversion, more conscientiousness, more agreeableness, less depression, more self-esteem).[153]

Temperament/personality factors, pubertal timing, socioeconomic factors from childhood and adulthood, race-ethnicity, childhood factors, and life course event trajectories all influence the likelihood, timing, quality of and duration of partner relationships for women. Marriage is associated with better health in most epidemiological work, but contemporary cohorts of women spend proportionately fewer of their adult years married than cohorts born in the early decades of the twentieth century. There is considerable variance among women now in the timing of marriage, the stability of marriages, the sequencing of serial periods of cohabitation and marriage across the life course, and the quality of marital and cohabiting partnerships.

12.6 Women's relationships with children

Although great advances in birth control across the last few decades have increasingly made it possible to separate sex from parenthood, and to allow for more options and timing of parenthood, about 90% of currently midlife women are biological, adoptive, or step-parents.[154] Children become social ties of lifelong significance and potential gratification, yet the demands in this relationship are very heavy for women.[89,155,156] Overall, evidence suggests that being a parent is associated with greater psychological distress than being childfree,[157,158] and that parenting is associated with more strains for women than men,[159,160] because of the greater normative and behavioural responsibility for children women maintain.[19,109]

However, many factors moderate the degree to which motherhood is distressing. Single parenting has been found to be more distressing than parenting with another parent.[157,158,161–163] Step-parenting has also generally been associated with increased distress.[164,165] Worries about child care exacerbate the stress of working mothers.[155] Poverty and residence in poor quality neighbourhoods add to the challenges of parenting.[89,96,156,166,167] Greater father involvement and better marital quality also reduce the distress of parenting for women.[155] Having older children, especially 'launched' non-residential adult children, has been associated with greater life satisfaction, meaning, and psychological health.[117,157,162,168]

Adolescent childbearing can create a sequelae of challenges for women, including poorer psychological functioning, lower rates of school completion, lower levels of marital stability, less stable employment, higher rates of poverty, more likelihood of subsequent non-marital births, and somewhat greater rates of health problems for mothers as well as children in contrast to women who postpone childbearing.[132] Yet, consistent with a life course perspective emphasizing ongoing developmental plasticity and moderating environmental factors, longitudinal studies have demonstrated that successful trajectories can result for some women who bear children as teens if family and social program support, opportunities to continue in school, solid employment, a good marriage, or some combination of these factors are available.[169,170]

Young children at home tend to reduce the social networks of mothers (especially in terms of friends and associates), reducing their reliable social support, and creating more localized networks than is the case for similar women without children.[171] Women's social networks as well as well-being also continue to be influenced by the life course development of adult children. A significant proportion of contemporary adult children continue to coreside with parents for some period of time to get their adult lives established or 'boomerang back' to the parental home after some period on their own. About 30% of all US parent householders with children or step-children aged 19 and older report a coresident adult child.[172] Most parents are not dissatisfied with this arrangement (selection plays a part in this), however, greater dissatisfaction with coresidence is evident when the parent is of higher SES and when the adult child is more economically dependent, returns home after a divorce, or returns home with a child.[173] Mothering a child with a lifelong disability such as mental retardation also typically entails extended parent-child coresidence and creates unique challenges as well as rewards for midlife mothers.[174]

Most women become mothers at some point during the life course. Mothering can be both distressing and meaningful for women. The distress and rewards of mothering across young adulthood and into midlife is moderated by a number of life course factors—timing of and number of births, ages of children, family SES and resources available to meet the demands and challenges of parenting, neighbourhood quality, marital status and marital history of the woman, marital quality, mother's employment, father's participation and support, and children's needs and developmental trajectories. Mothers of young children typically have more limited social networks than women who are not mothers. There is considerable variance in the 'launching' of children to independence. Continued coresidence or a return to the parental home by contemporary young adult children for some period of time is not uncommon.

12.7 **Women's relationships with other kin**

In childhood, girls' relationships to kin outside the immediate family are dependent upon parents' contact and quality of relationships with their kin. Mothers tend to maintain more contact with their families of origin than fathers do, so most children have more contact with maternal extended kin than paternal extended kin.[19] Grandparents are most likely to be an important part of children's lives, and sometimes aunts, uncles, and cousins. Paternal kin ties may be diminished further if divorce occurs, and daughters continue to reside with their mothers. Overall, relationships with kin beyond the immediate family do not appear to be a significant part of the daily social contact of most children's lives in industrialized societies.[175]

In adulthood, women name more kin (beyond parents and children), more kin types, and a greater proportion of their overall social network as kin than men.[171,176,177] Women (as well as men) with less education and less income tend to have an even higher proportion of kin (in contrast to non-kin) in their social networks than their peers with more education and more income.[171,177] Contrary to popular stereotype, there is also some evidence that African Americans and Mexican Americans in the US have smaller, less supportive, and more culturally confined kin networks than comparable non-Hispanic Whites.[171] Urbanicity also influences kin networks; urbanites in Fischer's social network study[171] reported 40% fewer relatives and almost 50% more non-relatives in their networks than respondents from less urban areas.

Grandchildren typically become new important kin ties for women in midlife,[154] and often bring new rewarding relationships into women's lives.[178] The experience of grand-mothering can vary significantly, though, depending upon the marital status, proximity, and economic need of the adult child parent.[19,178] Additionally, grandmothers sometimes become extensive caregivers, even custodial caregivers for grandchildren when their own adult children are unable to handle their parenting responsibilities. Over one in ten American grandparents report raising a grandchild at some point for at least 6 months, and usually for three or more years.[179] Undertaking custodial grandparent caregiving is associated with a greater risk for poor health.[180]

Overall, women report higher levels of normative obligation to 'kinkeeping' and kin work than men,[19] and they continue to predominate in the provision of emotional and instrumental support, including personal caregiving, to other kin.[19,88,90,176] Although providing support to other kin (in contrast to primary kin) may be somewhat more voluntary and therefore less likely to lead to a decline in well-being,[101] providing support to a larger number of other kin (beyond parents and children) has also been associated with more psychological distress.[176]

Thus ties to other kin in childhood are largely dependent on parents' ties to kin and parents' marital histories. In midlife, SES, race-ethnicity, urbanicity, and adult child marital and fertility trajectories influence the number of other kin ties reported by women. Women tend to have more other kin in their social networks than men. Some of these relationships offer important solidarity and support. Some kin relationships demand a fair amount of care and help. Overall, providing support for other kin may not be overly problematic for women. But at times, extended kin relationships may become emotionally draining and labour-intensive (e.g. custodial grandparenting) and problematic for women's mental and physical health, as well as women's pursuit of more equitable and rewarding social relationships with friends.

12.8 Women's relationships with friends

Friendships constitute a critical part of women's social networks across the life course. As noted previously, temperament, attachment style, and social understanding influence the quality of early peer relations. Beginning in the preschool years, and increasingly into school ages and adolescence, both boys and girls have been found to prefer same-sex friendships.[175,181] Therefore, girls tend to emphasize friendships with other girls beginning at young ages. Many studies do not find gender differences in the extensiveness of friendship networks during childhood and adolescence; some studies find boys have more non-kin interaction due to boys' greater likelihood of participating in large groups, such as teams.[175,182,183] Girls, by contrast, show a preference for dyadic interaction and for private settings, emphasizing more self-disclosure, intimacy, nurturance, and exclusivity in their friendships.[182,184]

In childhood and adolescence girls tend to seek more emotional help from friends and give more emotional help to friends than boys do. Girls' emphasis on self-disclosure and dyadic relationships may bring the emotional benefits of confidante relationships, but this same style of interaction may also make them more vulnerable to their peers when relationships do not go well. For example, girls' greater concerns about the faithfulness of friends and rejection by friends may, in part, reflect greater vulnerability due to greater self-disclosure in their friendships.[182] Boys also seek out friends when stressed, but more typically to engage in distracting activity.[182]

In adulthood, many of the same gendered patterns of friendship continue. Quantitatively, overall, women tend to name fewer non-kin in their social networks than men,[23,171,177] but this varies depending on their life stage. For example, Fischer[171] found that younger women, especially young mothers, had smaller social networks and fewer 'just friends' than younger men had; however, at midlife, women tended to rebuild their social ties to friends, and older women had more friends than older men. Unemployed women tended to know more neighbours; however, residential mobility (often occurring due to poverty or divorce) was likely to fracture social networks in the neighbourhood.

Moore[177] found that while at a bivariate level, US women in 1985 reported fewer types of non-kin (friends, coworkers, and advisors, although not neighbours) in their social networks than men, structural factors related to work (employment status and occupational status), marital status, and SES (education) accounted for this association. Moore, like Fischer,[171] interpreted her findings to suggest that men's quantitative advantage in terms of non-kin ties is structurally determined more than it is a result of dispositional or socialized gender preference.

Overall, SES is the factor most significantly linked to broader, deeper, and richer friendship networks.[171,177] More education is associated with larger networks, more companionship, more intimate relations and wider geographic range of ties. Even adjusting for education and other factors, more income is associated with more non-kin ties, and more secure and companionable support. Poorer people report fewer friends as well as relatives for support.[171] Among the affluent in contrast to the poor, friendship networks are less constrained by children, spatial separation from associates, and community characteristics.[171]

Qualitatively, adult women continue to report more emphasis on intimate ties, more confiding relationships, and more self-disclosure in friendships than men.[184,185] Although, overall, women report more satisfaction with friendships than family relationships,[23] not all friendships are of equal quality and support. Among lower-SES women, in particular, stress contagion[186] (i.e. the experience of greater stress after having contact with another person experiencing stress) among neighbours, relatives, and friends is likely to occur,[166,187] thus making even shared 'support' in efforts like child care potentially burdensome.[188]

Temperament, attachment style, and social understanding influence friendships in early childhood. Girls and women tend to invest intensely in close, intimate friendships, and in adulthood women tend to rate more satisfaction with their friends than with their family relationships. However, due to their greater kin responsibilities (e.g. in parenting), and their often-disadvantaged economic and labour market status, women are sometimes less likely to report as wide a range of the types of friendships and associational ties associated with advantage in occupational success, recreation, exercise, and leisure as men do. Under circumstances of economic disadvantage and neighbourhood deprivation where stress contagion is a common risk, even friends may become as much a burden as an asset for women's well-being.

12.9 Summary and implications for future research and policy

This chapter has reviewed biological, psychological, and social factors across the life course that influence the quality and quantity of women's social relationships at midlife, which, in turn, would be expected to influence women's health. It has explored how biologically-based factors (e.g. attachment, temperament, and pubertal timing) in interaction with psychosocial factors (e.g. mental health, personality, family structure, life events, childhood SES, adult SES, life course timing of partnering and parenting, family social support, and neighbourhood quality) influence women's social development and the quality of social ties.

There are a number of factors that can tilt a woman in the direction of cumulative disadvantage in social relationships at midlife (e.g. inhibited or difficult childhood temperament, lower SES parents, childhood with a single parent, childhood in a step-family, an insecure attachment style, loss of a parent (or parents) to death, divorce of parents, early pubertal maturation, early sexual relations, teen birth, marriage at a very young age, depression, lower adult SES) but none of these risk factors for diminished social relationship quality is definitive in determining the course of a woman's social relationships and social network. The plasticity of ongoing life course development is evident as there is also evidence that moderating factors (e.g. socially competent mother, father, or partner; school resources; neighbourhood resources; family and friend social support; rewarding employment; social service programs; mental and physical health services; income support) can mitigate the direction of trajectories and life course effects. Future social policy might usefully target interventions that provide support to girls and women at multiple junctures of life course risk to social developmental problems: e.g. infancy (especially for 'difficult' babies and mothers in poverty to facilitate secure attachment and the development of social competence), childhood (especially for girls suffering parent absence and economic deprivation to facilitate their mental health, social competence, and academic success), adolescence (especially for early-maturing girls, girls suffering parent absence, and girls in high-risk economic and neighbourhood circumstances to facilitate their mental health, social competence in developing partner relationships, and planful life course choices in education, occupation, and parenthood), and adulthood (especially for low SES women, single women, mothers of young children, caregivers, and women in poor quality marriages to provide resources to facilitate the maintenance of their mental and physical health and planful decisions about taking care of self as well as others).

Future research needs to pay particular attention to relationship quality (e.g. strains as well as gains, equity, and reciprocity) in each social relationship in social network analysis. It also would be beneficial for scholars to consider cumulative patterns of social relationships (e.g. marital histories, child in household histories, caregiving histories) as well as one point in time assessments of social networks in order to better gauge how social relationships influence women's health.

This review of some of the variance in the quantity and quality of women's social relationships over the life course suggests that policy-makers should not assume that because women tend to emphasize more intimacy and support in relationships than men, therefore, women's social relationships are necessarily more protective of their health than men's and women's social ties can compensate for women's often-disadvantaged status in families, labour markets, and society. This is particularly true for women of colour who may be triply disadvantaged by gender, race/ethnicity, and class.

Women's social relationships at midlife reflect a complex evolution of ties with family, friends, and neighbours that are determined by a range of biological, psychological, and social factors emerging from infancy to middle adulthood. Continued attention to these multiple factors and the cumulative relationship histories of women is important for a better understanding of the ways in which social relationships influence women's health.

Acknowledgements

Work on this chapter was supported by grants from the National Institute on Aging (AG12731) and the National Institute on Mental Health (MH61083).

Commentary on 'Life course influences on women's social relationships at midlife'

Stephen Stansfeld and Rebecca Fuhrer

The life course has not been a dominant theme in empirical studies of social support and health but is dispersed in diverse literature such as child development. This chapter brings together a range of different perspectives on social support and proposes a coherent set of hypotheses on the origins of social support in midlife. The authors address a number of very important themes. They demonstrate that patterns of attachment established with mothers and fathers may form the template for future relationships into adulthood. Thus, the structure of early relationships may have long term consequences influencing, on the one hand, the development of personality, and, on the other, the development of the ability to initiate and maintain relationships.

The chapter emphasizes the importance of the interaction between biological, social, and psychological factors influencing the development of, and need for, social relations. The authors propose that there is differential socialization of women and men which they explain as being due to greater responsibility of women for maintaining and providing social support. This is often associated with having to help others who are undergoing stressful life events within the immediate social network, with the consequent cost of being involved, and having to deal with, other people's problems. The universality of this proposition requires confirmation from more empirical evidence. The behaviours they attribute to girls and women may be more a reflection of gender patterning and cultural values that are indeed culture-specific. The chapter provides detailed descriptions of the relationship between women and their mothers, as well as their relationships with fathers and siblings. Partnership, relationships with children, and grandparents are also described. These relationships vary in importance at differing times in the life course. For example, the balance of support reciprocity with parents begins to change in midlife with support flowing from daughters to parents rather than vice versa.

The literature on social support and mental health has shown that the impact of early parental loss may have lifelong effects. However, it is often not the loss itself but the subsequent disruption of caring relationships which is most damaging. In a study of London women, early inadequate parenting was related to negative interaction in adult close relationships.[189] Early inadequate parenting was also related to negative evaluation of the self as an adult, which in turn was also related to negative interaction in adult relationships. It is possible that these disruptions in early relationships may have very long-term consequences, however this is not always the case. One study of young women reared in institutional settings showed that in their twenties they tended to have poor social functioning and poor parenting skills compared to a community sample of women.[190] However, good social relations and better parenting skills were seen among those who developed a good relationship with a non-deviant male partner. There may be scope for both reparative as well as damaging relationships across the life course.

The time around childbirth is a crucial period where women need social support. Lack of support during pregnancy is related to an increased incidence of postnatal depression.[191] Antenatal care, both provided by health services and non-statutory care has important supportive influences preparative to childbirth. Antenatal support has also been related to higher birth weight.[192] Postnatal support groups and statutory support such as health visitors, in the UK, may also play a helpful role for mothers with young children. Nevertheless, structured support interventions in pregnancy for mothers who are at risk of depression has not always proved effective.[193]

Much of the research quoted in the chapter originates from North America and it would be interesting to have a broader emphasis on cultural differences in social support. Regrettably, there are relatively few studies of cultural differences in social support,[194,195] especially where social support may influence health. Such comparisons would provide evidence that may partly explain why there are cultural differences in health, particularly mental health.[196] The importance of social support in the workplace needs further exploration, especially during the adult lifespan, and may have effects on health and well-being. Low levels of social support at work from supervisors and colleagues has been shown to be predictive of poor physical and mental health in the Whitehall II study of British government employees.[197]

Defining the distinctive quality of social support in women as opposed to men may help in the understanding of how lack of support impairs well-being and health and may explain differences in rates of diseases between women and men. Social support seems to be more protective against coronary heart disease in men than in women. Lack of social support, coupled with the greater responsibilities for providing support, may also contribute to the higher rates of minor psychiatric disorder in women. This chapter lays the foundation for an examination of the protective influences of support, and the damaging effects of lack of support across the life course in both women and men.

References

1 Berkman LF. The relationship of social networks and social support to morbidity and mortality. In: Cohen S, Syme SL, eds, *Social support and health*. Orlando (Florida): Academic Press, 1985: 241–59.

2 Ryff, CD, Singer, BH, eds, *Emotion, social relationships, and health*. New York: Oxford University Press, 2001.

3 Cohen SC. Psychosocial models of the role of social support in the etiology of physical disease. *Health Psychol* 1988;**7**:269–97.

4 House JS, Landis KR, Umberson DL. Social relationships and health. *Science* 1988;**241**:540–45.

5 Uchino BN, Cacioppo JT, Kiecolt-Glaser JK. The relationship between social support and physiological processes: a review with emphasis on underlying mechanisms and implications for health. *Psychol Bull* 1996;**119**:488–531.

6 Berkman LF, Syme SL. Social networks, host resistance, and mortality: a nine-year follow-up study of Alameda County residents. *Am J Epidemiol* 1979;**109**:186–204.

7 House JS, Robbins C, Metzner HL. The association of social relationships and activities with mortality: prospective evidence from the Tecumseh community health study. *Am J of Epidemiol* 1982;**116**:123–40.

8 Schoenbach VJ, Kaplan BH, Fredman L, Kleinbaum DG. Social ties and mortality in Evans County, Georgia. *Am J Epidemiol* 1986;**123**:577–91.

9 Orth-Gomer K, Johnson JV. Social network interaction and mortality: a six year follow-up study of a random sample of the Swedish population. *J Chron Dis* 1987;**40**:949–57.

10 Cohen S, Herbert TB. Health psychology: psychological factors and physical disease from the perspective of human psychoneuroimmunology. *Ann Rev Psychol* 1996;**47**:113–42.

11 Seeman TE, Berkman LF, Blazer D, Rowe J. Social ties and support and neuroendocrine function: the MacArthur studies of successful aging. *Ann Behav Med* 1994;**16**:95–106.

12 Seeman T, McEwen B. Impact of social environment characteristics on neuroendocrine regulation. *Psychosom Med* 1996;**58**:459–71.

13 Rook KS. The negative side of social interaction: impact on psychological well-being. *J Pers Soc Psychol* 1984;**46**:1097–108.

14 Fiore J, Becker J, Coppel DB. Social network interactions: a buffer or a stress? *Am J Comm Psychol* 1983;**11**:423–39.

15 Pagel MD, Erdly WW, Becker J. Social networks: we get by with (and in spite of) a little help from our friends. *J Pers Soc Psychol* 1987;**53**:793–804.

16 Schuster TL, Kessler RC, Aseltine RH. Supportive interactions, negative interactions, and depressed mood. *Am J Comm Psychol* 1990;**18**:423–38.

17 Gilligan C. *In a different voice.* Cambridge (Massachusetts): Harvard University Press, 1982.

18 Chodorow N. *The reproduction of mothering: psychoanalysis and the sociology of gender.* Berkeley (California): University of California Press, 1978.

19 Rossi AS, Rossi PH. *Of human bonding: parent-child relations across the life course.* New York: Aldine de Gruyter, 1990.

20 Kessler RC, McLeod JD. Sex differences in vulnerability to undesirable life events. *Am Sociol Rev* 1984;**49**:620–31.

21 Kessler RC, McLeod JD, Wethington E. The costs of caring: a perspective on the relationship between sex and psychological distress. In: Sarason IG, Sarason BR, eds, *Social support: theory, research, and applications.* Dordrecht: Martinus Nijhoff Publishers, 1985.

22 Shumaker SA, Hill DR. Gender differences in social support and physical health. *Health Psychol* 1991;**10**:102–11.

23 Antonucci T. A life-span view of women's social relations. In: Turner BF, Troll LI, eds. *Women growing older: psychological perspectives.* Thousand Oaks (California): Sage, 1994:239–69.

24 Kahn RL, Antonucci TC. Convoys over the life course: attachment, roles, and social support. In: Baltes PB, Brim OG, eds, *Life-span development and behavior.* New York: Academic Press, 1990:253–86.

25 Bowlby J. *Attachment and loss. Volume I: Attachment.* New York: Basic Books, 1969.

26 Bowlby J. *Attachment and loss. Volume II: Separation: anxiety and anger.* New York: Basic Books, 1973.

27 Bowlby J. *Attachment and loss. Volume III: Loss.* New York: Basic Books, 1980.

28 Ainsworth MDS, Blehar MC, Waters E, Wall S. *Patterns of attachment: a psychological study of the strange situation.* Hillsdale (New Jersey): Erlbaum, 1978.

29 Van Ijzendoorn MH, Sagi A. Cross-cultural patterns of attachment: universal and contextual dimensions. In: Cassidy J, Shaver PR, eds, *Handbook of attachment: theory, research, and applications.* New York: Guilford, 1999:713–34.

30 Main M, Solomon J. Discovery of a disorganized/disoriented attachment pattern. In: Brazelton TB, Yogman MW, eds, *Affective development in infancy.* Norwood (New Jersey): Ablex, 1986:95–124.

31 Cicchetti D, Toth SL. Child maltreatment and attachment organization: implications of intervention. In: Goldberg S, Muir R, Kerr J, eds, *Attachment theory: social, developmental and clinical perspectives.* Hillsdale (New Jersey): Analytic Press, 1995:279–308.

32 Main M, Kaplan N, Cassidy J. Security in infancy, childhood, and adulthood: a move to the level of representation. In: Bretherton I, Waters E, eds, *Growing points of attachment theory and research. Monographs of the Society for Research in Child Development*, 1985;**50**(1–2, Serial No. 3209):66–104.

33 Sroufe LA, Schork E, Frosso M, Lawroski N, LaFreniere P. The role of affect in social competence. In: Izard C, Kagan J, Zajonc R, eds, *Emotions, cognitions and behavior*. New York: Cambridge University Press, 1984:289–319.

34 Main M, Cassidy J. Categories of response to reunion with the parent at age 6: predictable from infant attachment classifications and stable over a 1-month period. *Dev Psychol* 1988;**24**:415–26.

35 Waters E. The reliability and stability of individual differences in infant-mother attachment. *Child Dev* 1978;**49**:520–616.

36 Egeland B, Sroufe LA. Attachment and early maltreatment. *Child Dev* 1981;**52**:44–52.

37 Vaughn B, Egeland B, Sroufe LA, Waters E. Individual differences in infant-mother attachment at twelve and eighteen months: stability and change in families under stress. *Child Dev* 1979;**50**:971–75.

38 Spieker SJ, Booth CL. Maternal antecedents of attachment quality. In: Belsky J, Nezworski T, eds, *Clinical implications of attachment*. Hillsdale (New Jersey): Erlbaum, 1988:95–135.

39 Kessler RC, McGonagle KA, Zhao S, Nelson CB, Hughes M, Eshleman S, Wittchen HU, Kendler KS. Lifetime and 12-month prevalence of DSM-III-R psychiatric disorders in the United States. *Arch Gen Psychiat* 1994;**51**:8–19.

40 Mirowsky J, Ross CE. *The social causes of psychological distress*. New York: Aldine de Gruyter, 1989.

41 Feeney JA, Noller P. Attachment style as a predictor of adult romantic relationships. *J of Pers Soc Psychol* 1990;**58**:281–91.

42 Hazan C, Shaver P. Romantic love conceptualized as an attachment process. *J Pers Soc Psychol* 1987;**52**:511–24.

43 Simpson JA. Influence of attachment styles on romantic relationships. *J Pers Soc Psychol* 1990;**59**:971–80.

44 Skolnick A. Early attachment and personal relationships across the life course. In: Baltes PB, Featherman DL, Lerner RM, eds, *Life-span development and behavior*. Vol. 7. Hillsdale (New Jersey): Erlbaum, 1986:173–206.

45 Waters E, Wippman J, Sroufe LA. Attachment, positive affect, and competence in the peer group: two studies of construct validation. *Child Dev* 1979;**50**:821–9.

46 Sroufe LA. Infant-caregiver attachment and patterns of adaptation in preschool: the roots of maladaptation and competence. In: Perlmutter M, ed. *Minnesota symposium on child psychology*. Vol. 16. Hillsdale (New Jersey): Erlbaum, 1983:41–81.

47 Kobak RR, Sceery A. Attachment in late adolescence: working models, affect regulation, and representations of self and others. *Child Dev* 1988;**59**:135–46.

48 Shaver PR, Hazan C. Adult romantic attachment: theory and evidence. In: Jones WH, Perlman D, eds, *Advances in personal relationships*. Vol. 4. London: Jessica Kingsley, 1993:29–70.

49 Kobak RR, Hazan C. Attachment in marriage: effects of security and accuracy of working models. *J Pers Social Psychol* 1991;**60**:861–9.

50 Reis HT, Patrick BC. Attachment and intimacy: component processes. In: Tory Higgins E, Kruglanski AW, eds, *Social psychology: handbook of basic principles*. New York: Guilford Press, 1996:523–63.

51 Cicirelli V. Adult children's attachment and helping behavior to elderly parents: a path model. *J Mar Fam* 1983;**45**:815–24.

52 Cicirelli VG. Attachment and obligation as daughters' motives for caregiving behavior and subsequent effect on subjective burden. *Psychol Aging* 1993;**8**:144–55.

53 **Rothbart MK, Derryberry D**. Development of individual differences in temperament. In: Lamb ME, Brown AL, eds, *Advances in developmental psychology*. Vol. 1. Hillsdale (New Jersey):1981:37–86.

54 **Halverson CF Jr., Kohnstamm GA, Martin RP, eds**. *The developing structure of temperament and personality from infancy to adulthood*. Hillsdale (New Jersey): Erlbaum, 1994.

55 **Robins RW, John OP, Caspi A**. Major dimensions of personality in early adolescence: the Big Five and beyond. In: Haverson CF Jr., Kohnstamm GA, Martin RP, eds, *The developing structure of temperament and personality from infancy to adulthood*. Hillsdale (New Jersey): Erlbaum, 1994:267–91.

56 **Ahadi SA, Rothbart MK**. Temperament, development, and the Big Five. In: Haverson CF Jr, Kohnstamm GA, Martin RP, eds, *The developing structure of temperament and personality from infancy to adulthood*. Hillsdale (New Jersey): Erlbaum, 1994:189–207.

57 **Kagan J**. Temperamental contributions to social behavior. *Am Psychol* 1989;**44**:668–74.

58 **Kessler RC, Kendler KS, Heath A, Neale MC, Eaves LJ**. Social support, depressed mood, and adjustment to stress: a genetic epidemiologic investigation. *J Pers Soc Psychol* 1992;**62**:257–272.

59 **Bowlby J**. The nature of the child's tie to his mother. *Int J Psychoanal* 1958;**39**:350–373.

60 **Kranzler EM, Shaffer D, Wasserman G, Davies M**. Early childhood bereavement. *J Am Acad Child Adolesc Psychiat* 1999;**29**:513–20.

61 **Gray RE**. Adolescent response to the death of a parent. *J Youth and Adolesc* 1987;**16**:511–25.

62 **Worden JW**. *Children and grief*. New York: Guilford, 1996.

63 **Harris M**. *The loss that is forever*. New York: Plume, 1995.

64 **Coyne JC**. Toward an interactional theory of depression. *Psychiatry* 1976;**39**:28–40.

65 **Kowalik DL, Gotlib IH**. Depression and marital interaction: concordance between intent and perception of communication. *J Abnorm Psychol* 1987;**96**:127–34.

66 **Turner RJ**. Social support as a contingency in psychological well-being. *J Health Soc Behav* 1981;**22**:357–67.

67 **McLeod JD**. Childhood parental loss and adult depression. *J Health Social Behav* 1991;**32**:205–20.

68 **Seltzer JA**. Families formed outside of marriage. *J Mar Fam* 2000;**62**:1247–68.

69 **McLanahan S, Sandefur G**. *Growing up with a single parent: what hurts, what helps*. Cambridge (Massachusetts): Harvard University Press, 1994.

70 **Amato PR**. The consequences of divorce for adults and children. *J Mar Fam* 2000;**62**:1269–87.

71 **Cherlin AJ, Furstenberg FF Jr., Chase-Lansdale PL, Kiernan KE, Robins PK, Morrison DR, Teitler JO**. Longitudinal studies of effects of divorce on children in Great Britain and the United States. *Science* 1991;**252**:1386–9.

72 **Hetherington EM, Stanley-Hagan MM**. The effects of divorce on fathers and their children. In: Lamb ME, ed, *The role of the father in child development*. 3rd edition. New York: Wiley and Sons, 1997:191–226.

73 **Wadsworth MEJ, Maclean M, Kuh D, Rodgers B**. Children of divorced parents: a summary and review of findings from a national long-term follow-up study. *Fam Pract* 1990;**7**:104–9.

74 **Furstenberg FF Jr**. Divorce and the American family. *Ann Rev Sociol* 1990;**16**:379–403.

75 **Chase-Lansdale PL, Hetherington EM**. The impact of divorce on life-span development: short and long term effects. In: Baltes PB, Featherman DL, Lerner RM, eds, *Life-span development and behavior*. Volume 10. Hillsdale (New Jersey): Erlbaum, 1990:105–150.

76 **Wallerstein JS, Blakeslee S**. *Second chances: men, women, and children a decade after divorce*. New York: Ticknor and Fields, 1989.

77 **Amato PR, Booth A**. Consequences of parental divorce and marital unhappiness for adult well-being. *Soc Forces* 1991;**69**:895–914.

78 **Brown GW**. Early loss and depression. In: Parkes CM, Stevenson-Hinde J, eds, *The place of attachment in human behavior*. New York: Basic Books, 1982:232–68.

79 **Eggebeen DJ, Hogan DP.** Giving between generations in American families. *Hum Nature* 1990;**11**:211–32.

80 **Cooney TM, Uhlenberg P.** Support from parents over the life course: the adult child's perspective. *Soc Forces* 1992;**71**:63–84.

81 **Wadsworth MEJ.** Social and historical influences on parent–child relations in midlife. In: Ryff CR, Seltzer MM, eds, *The parental experience in midlife.* Chicago: University of Chicago Press, 1996.

82 **Beck RW, Beck SH.** The incidence of extended households among middle-aged black and white women. *J Fam Issues* 1989;**10**:147–68.

83 **Hogan DP, Hao LX, Parish WL.** Race, kin networks, and assistance to mother-headed families. *Soc Forces* 1990;**68**:797–812.

84 **Hofferth SL.** Kin networks, race and family structure. *J Mar Fam* 1984;**46**:791–806.

85 **Roschelle AR.** No more kin: exploring race, class, and gender in family networks. Thousand Oaks (California): Sage, 1997.

86 **Watkins SC, Mencken JA, Bongaarts J.** Demographic foundations of family change. *Am Sociolog Rev* 1987;**50**:689–98.

87 **Brody EM.** Women in the middle: their parent-care years. New York: Springer, 1990.

88 **Stone R, Cafferata GL, Sangl J.** Caregivers of the frail elderly: a national profile. *Gerontologist* 1987;**27**:616–26.

89 **Graham H.** *Women, health and the family.* Harvester Press: Brighton, Sussex, 1984.

90 **Marks NF.** Caregiving across the lifespan: national prevalence and predictors. *Fam Relations* 1996;**45**:27–36.

91 **Cantor MH.** Neighbors and friends: an overlooked resource in the informal support system. *Res Aging* 1979;**1**:434–63.

92 **Wilkinson RG, ed.** *Class and health: research and longitudinal data.* London: Tavistock. 1986.

93 **Adler NE, Boyce WT, Chesney MA, Folkman S, Syme SL.** Socioeconomic inequalities in health: no easy solution. *J Am Med Assoc* 1993;**269**:3140–5.

94 **Marmot MG, Kogevinas M, Elston MA.** Social/economic status and disease. *Ann Rev Public Health* 1987;**8**:111–35.

95 **Geronimus AT, Bound J, Waidmann TA, Colen CG, Steffick D.** Inequality in life expectancy, functional status, and active life expectancy across selected black and white populations in the United States. *Demography* 2001;**38**:227–51.

96 **Seccombe K.** Families in poverty in the 1990s: trends, causes, consequences and lessons learned. *J Mar Fam* 2000;**62**:1094–1113.

97 **Schulz R, Visintainer P, Williamson GM.** Psychiatric and physical morbidity effects of caregiving. *J Gerontol: Psychol Sciences* 1990;**45**:P181–91.

98 **Kiecolt-Glaser JK.** Stress, personal relationships, and immune function: health implications. *Brain, Behav Immunity* 1999;**13**:61–72.

99 **Schulz R, O'Brien AT, Bookwala J, Fleissner K.** Psychiatric and physical morbidity effects of Alzheimer's disease caregiving: prevalence, correlates, and causes. *Gerontologist* 1995;**35**:771–91.

100 **Schulz R, Newsom J, Mittelmark M, Burton L, Hirsch C, Jackson S.** Health effects of caregiving: the caregiver health effects study: an ancillary study of the cardiovascular health study. *Ann Behav Med* 1997;**19**:110–16.

101 **Marks NF.** Does it hurt to care? Caregiving, work-family conflict, and midlife well-being. *J Mar Fam* 1998;**60**:951–66.

102 **Kramer BJ.** Gain in the caregiving experience: where are we? what next? *Gerontologist* 1997;**37**:218–32.

103 **Montgomery RJV**. Gender differences in patterns of child-parent caregiving relationships. In: Dwyer JW, Coward RT, eds, *Gender, families, and elder care*. Newbury Park (California): Sage, 1992:65–83.

104 **Yee JL, Schulz R**. Gender differences in psychiatric morbidity among family caregivers: a review and analysis. *Gerontologist* 2000;**40**:147–64.

105 **Neal MB, Chapman NJ, Ingersoll-Dayton B, Emlen AC**. *Balancing work and caregiving for children, adults, and elders*. Newbury Park (California): Sage, 1993.

106 **Lamb ME**. Fathers and child development: an introductory overview and guide. In: Lamb ME, ed. *The role of the father in child development*. 3rd edition. New York: Wiley and Sons, 1997:1–18.

107 **Rossi A**. Gender and parenthood. *Am Sociol Rev* 1984;**49**:1–18.

108 **Lamb ME**. The development of father-infant relationships. In: Lamb ME, ed. *The role of the father in child development*. 3rd edition. New York: Wiley and Sons, 1997:104–20.

109 **Pleck JH**. Paternal involvement: levels, sources, and consequences. In: Lamb ME, *The role of the father in child development*. 3rd edition. New York: Wiley and Sons, 1997:66–103.

110 **Dunn J**. *Young children's close relationships: beyond attachment*. Newbury Park (California): Sage, 1993.

111 **Lewis C**. Fathers and preschoolers. In: Lamb ME, ed. *The role of the father in child development*. 3rd edition. New York: Wiley and Sons, 1997:121–42.

112 **MacDonald K, Parke R**. Bridging the gap: parent-child play interaction and peer interactive competence. *Child Dev* 1984;**55**:1265–77.

113 **Cummings EM, O'Reilly AW**. Fathers in family context: effects of marital quality on child adjustment. In: Lamb ME, ed, *The role of the father in child development*. 3rd edition. New York: Wiley and Sons, 1997:49–65.

114 **Seltzer JA**. Relationships between fathers and children who live apart. *J Mar Fam* 1991;**53**:79–101.

115 **Marks NF**. Midlife marital status differences in social support relationships with adult children and psychological well-being. *J Fam Issues* 1995;**16**:5–28.

116 **Cooney TM, Uhlenberg P**. The role of divorce in men's relations with their adult children after mid-life. *J Mar Fam* 1990;**52**:677–88.

117 **Marks NF, Bumpass LL, Jun H**. Family roles and well-being during the middle life course. In: Ryff C, Kessler R, Brim B, eds, *Midlife development in the United States*. Chicago: University of Chicago Press, *forthcoming*.

118 **Sorlie PD, Backlund E, Keller JB**. US mortality by economic, demographic, and social characteristics: the national longitudinal mortality study, *Am J Pub Health* 1995;**85**:949–56.

119 **Cicirelli VG**. Sibling influence throughout the lifespan. In: Lamb ME, Sutton-Smith B, eds, *Sibling relationships: their nature and significance across the lifespan*. Hillsdale (New Jersey): Erlbaum, 1982:267–84.

120 **Bryant BK**. Sibling relationships in middle childhood. In: Lamb ME, Sutton-Smith B, eds, *Sibling relationships: their nature and significance across the lifespan*. Hillsdale (New Jersey): Erlbaum, 1982.

121 **Connidis IA**. Life transitions and the adult sibling tie: a qualitative study. *J Mar Fam* 1992;**54**:972–82.

122 **Bedford VH**. Sibling relationships in middle and old age. In: Blieszner RB, Bedford VH, eds, *Aging and the family: theory and research*. Westport (Connecticut): Praeger, 1996.

123 **Gold D**. Sibling relations in old age: a typology. *Int J Aging Hum Dev* 1989;**28**:37–51.

124 **Downing C**. *Psyche's sisters: reimaging the meaning of sisterhood*. San Francisco (California): Harper and Row, 1988.

125 Matthews SH, Rosner TT. Shared filial responsibility: the family as the primary caregiver. *J Mar Fam* 1988;**50**:185–95.

126 Suitor JJ, Pillemer K. Support and interpersonal stress in the social networks of married daughters caring for parents with dementia. *J Gerontol: Soc Sciences* 1993;**48**:S1–8.

127 Myers DR, Dickerson BE. Intergenerational interdependence among older, low-income African American, Mexican American, and Anglo siblings. *Fam Perspective* 1990;**24**:217–43.

128 Taylor RJ, Chatters LM, Mays VM. Parents, children, siblings, in-laws, and non-kin as sources of emergency assistance to black Americans. *Fam Relations* 1988;**37**:298–304.

129 Cicirelli VG. Siblings as caregivers in middle and old age. In: Dwyer JW, Coward RT, eds, *Gender, families, and elder care*. Newbury Park (California): Sage, 1992:84–101.

130 Seltzer GB, Begun A, Seltzer MM, Krauss MW. Adults with mental retardation and their aging mothers: impact of siblings. *Fam Relations* 1991;**40**:310–7.

131 Spitze G, Logan JR. Sibling structure and intergenerational relations. *J Mar Fam* 1991:**53**:871–84.

132 Coley RL, Chase-Lansdale PL. Adolescent pregnancy and parenthood: recent evidence and future directions. *Am Psychol* 1998;**53**:152–66.

133 Magnusson D, Stattin H, Allen VL. Differential maturation among girls and its relations to social adjustment: a longitudinal perspective. In: Baltes PB, Featherman DL, Lerner RM, eds, *Life-span development and behavior*. Vol. 7. Hillsdale (New Jersey): Erlbaum, 1986:135–72.

134 Simmons RG, Blyth D. *Moving into adolescence: the impact of pubertal change and school context*. New York: Aldine de Gruyter, 1987.

135 Caspi A, Moffit TE. Individual differences are accentuated during periods of social change: the sample case of girls at puberty. *J Pers Soc Psychol* 1991;**58**:250–58.

136 Caspi A, Lynam D, Moffitt TE, Silva PA. Unraveling girls' delinquency: biological, dispositional, and contextual contributions to adolescent misbehavior. *Dev Psychol* 1991;**29**:19–30.

137 Schoen R, Urton WL, Woodrow K, Baj J. Marriage and divorce in 20th century American cohorts. *Demography* 1985;**22**:101–14.

138 Schoen R, Weinick RM. The slowing metabolism of marriage: figures from 1988 US marital status life tables. *Demography* 1993;**30**:737–46.

139 Castro-Martin T, Bumpass LL. Recent trends and differentials in marital disruption. *Demography* 1989;**26**:37–51.

140 Bumpass L, Sweet JA. National estimates of cohabitation: cohort levels and union stability. *Demography* 1989;**26**:615–25.

141 Bumpass L, Lu H-H. Trends in cohabitation and implications for children's family contexts in the US. *Pop Stud* 2000;**54**:29–41.

142 Booth A, Amato P. Divorce and psychological stress. *J Health Soc Behav* 1991;**32**:396–407.

143 Gove WR, Hughes M, Style CB. Does marriage have positive effects on the well-being of the individual? *J Health Soc Behav* 1983;**24**:122–31.

144 Pearlin LI, Johnson JS. Marital status, life-strains and depression. *Am Sociol Rev* 1977;**42**:704–15.

145 Gove WR. Sex, marital status and mortality. *Am J Sociol* 1973;**79**:45–67.

146 Litwak E, Messeri P. Social supports and mortality rates: a disease specific formulation. In: Steinmetz SK, ed. *Family and support systems across the life span*. New York: Plenum, 1988:257–81.

147 Renne K. Health and marital experience in an urban population. *J Mar Fam* 1971;**33**:338–48.

148 Glenn ND, Weaver CN. The changing relationship of marital status to reported happiness. *J Mar Fam* 1988;**50**:317–24.

149 Lee G, Seccombe K, Shehan C. Marital status and marital happiness: an analysis of trend data. *J Mar Fam* 1991;**53**:839–44.

150 Hahn BA. Marital status and women's health: the effect of economic marital acquisitions. *J Mar Fam* 1993;**55**:495–504.

151 Marks NF, Lambert JD. Marital status continuity and change among young and midlife adults: longitudinal effects on psychological well-being. *J Fam Issues* 1998;**19**:652–86.

152 Waite L. Trends in men's and women's well-being in marriage. In: Waite LJ, ed. *The ties that bind: perspectives on marriage and cohabitation*. Hawthorne (New York): Aldine de Gruyter, 2000:368–92.

153 Karney BR, Bradbury TN. The longitudinal course of marital quality and stability: a review of theory, method, and research. *Psychol Bull* 1995;**118**:3–34.

154 Marks NF. Social demographic diversity among American midlife parents. In: Ryff CD, Seltzer MM, eds, *When children grow up: development and diversity in midlife parenting*. Chicago: University of Chicago Press, 1996:29–75.

155 Arendell T. Conceiving and investigating motherhood: the decade's scholarship. *J Mar Fam* 2000;**62**:1192–1207.

156 Graham H. *Hardship and health in women's lives*. Hertfordshire: Harvester Wheatsheaf, 1993.

157 McLanahan SS, Adams J. Parenthood and psychological well-being. *Ann Rev Sociol* 1987;**13**:237–57.

158 McLanahan SS, Adams J. The effects of children on adults' psychological well-being: 1957–1976. *Soc Forces* 1989;**68**:124–46.

159 Simon RW. Parental role strains, salience of parental identity, and gender differences in psychological distress. *J Health Soc Behav* 1992;**33**:25–35.

160 Scott J, Alwin DF. Gender differences in parental strain: parental role or gender role. *J Fam Issues* 1989;**10**:482–503.

161 Aneshensel CS, Frerichs RR, Clark VA. Family roles and sex differences in depression. *J Health Soc Behav* 1981;**22**:379–93.

162 Umberson D, Gove WR. Parenthood and psychological well-being. *J Fam Issues* 1989;**10**:440–62.

163 Hope S, Power C, Rodgers B. Does financial hardship account for elevated psychological distress in lone mothers? *Soc Sci Med* 1999;**29**:381–89.

164 Coleman M, Ganong L, Fine M. Reinvestigating remarriage: another decade of progress. *J Mar Fam* 2000;**62**:1288–307.

165 White LK, Booth A. The quality and stability of remarriages: the role of stepchildren. *Am Sociolog Rev* 1985;**59**:689–98.

166 Belle D. The stress of caring: women as providers of social support. In: Goldberger L, Breznitz S, eds, *Handbook of stress: theoretical and clinical aspects*. New York: Free Press, 1982:296–505.

167 Burton LM, Jarrett RL. In the mix, yet on the margins: the place of families in urban neighborhoods and child development research. *J Mar Fam* 2000;**62**:1114–35.

168 White L, Edward JN. Emptying the nest and parental well-being: an analysis of national panel data. *Am Sociolog Rev* 1990;**55**:235–42.

169 Furstenberg FF Jr., Brooks-Gunn J, Morgan SP. *Adolescent mothers in later life*. New York: Cambridge University Press, 1987.

170 Horwitz SM, Klerman LV, Ko HS, Jekel JF. School-age mothers: predictors of long-term education and economic outcomes. *Pediatrics* 1991;**87**:862–67.

171 Fischer CS. *To dwell among friends*. Chicago: University of Chicago Press, 1982.

172 Aquilino WA. The likelihood of parent-adult child coresidence: effects of family structure and parental characteristics. *J Mar Fam* 1999;**52**:405–19.

173 Aquilino WA. Predicting parents' experiences with coresident adult children. *J Fam Issues* 1991;**12**:323–42.

174 **Seltzer MM, Krauss MW, Choi SC, Hong J**. Midlife and later-life parenting of adult children with mental retardation. In: Ryff CD, Seltzer MM, eds, *The parental experience in midlife*. Chicago: University of Chicago Press, 1996:459–89.

175 **Feiring C, Lewis M**. The child's social network: sex differences from three to six years. *Sex Roles* 1987;**17**:621–36.

176 **Gerstel N, Gallagher SK**. Kinkeeping and distress: gender, recipients of care, and work-family conflict. *J Mar Fam* 1993;**55**:598–607.

177 **Moore G**. Structural determinants of men's and women's personal networks. *Am Sociol Rev* 1990;**55**:726–35.

178 **Cherlin A, Furstenberg FF Jr**. *The new American grandparent*. New York: Basic Books, 1986.

179 **Fuller-Thomson E, Minkler M, Driver D**. A profile of grandparents raising grandchildren in the United States. *Gerontologist* 1997:**37**:406–11.

180 **Minkler M, Fuller-Thomson E**. The health of grandparents raising grandchildren: results of a national study. *Am J Pub Health* 1999;**89**:1384–89.

181 **Douvan E, Adelson J**. *The adolescent experience*. New York: Wiley, 1966.

182 **Belle D**. Gender differences in children's social networks and supports. In: Belle D, ed, *Children's social networks and social supports*. New York: Wiley, 1989:173–88.

183 **Berndt TJ, Perry TB**. Children's perceptions of friendship as supportive relationships. *Dev Psychol* 1986;**22**:640–48.

184 **Maccoby EE**. Gender and relationships: a developmental account. *Am Psychol* 1990;**45**:513–20.

185 **Blieszner R, Adams RG**. *Adult friendship*. Newbury Park (California): Sage, 1992.

186 **Wilkins W**. Social stress and illness in industrial society. In: Gunderson E, Rahe R, eds, *Life stress and illness*. Springfield (Illinois): Charles C. Thomas, 1974:242–54.

187 **Stack C**. *All our kin: Strategies for survival in a black community*. New York: Harper and Row, 1974.

188 **Goldsteen K, Ross CE**. The perceived burden of children. *J Fam Issues* 1989;**10**:504–26.

189 **Brown GW, Bifulco A, Veiel HOF, Andrews B**. Self-esteem and depression. II. Social correlates of self-esteem. *Soc Psychiat Psychiatric Epidemiol* 1991;**25**:225–34.

190 **Quinton D, Rutter M, Liddle** C. Institutional rearing, parenting difficulties and marital support. *Psychol Med* 1984;**14**:107–24.

191 **Paykel ES, Emms EM, Fletcher J, Rassaby ES**. Life events and social support in puerperal depression. *Br J Psychiat* 1980;**136**:339–46.

192 **Oakley A**. Social support in pregnancy: the 'soft' way to increase birthweight? *Soc Sci Med* 1985;**21**:1259–68.

193 **Brugha TS, Wheatley S, Taub NA, Culverwell A, Friedman T, Kirwan P, Jones DR, Shapiro DA**. Pragmatic randomized trial of antenatal intervention to prevent post-natal depression by reducing psychosocial risk factors. *Psychol Med* 2000;**30**:1273–81.

194 **Antonucci TC, Fuhrer R, Jackson JS**. Social support and reciprocity: a cross-ethnic and cross-national perspective. *J Soc Pers Relationships* 1990;**7**:519–30.

195 **Antonucci TC, Lansford JE, Schaberg L, Smith J, Baltes M, Akiyama H, Takahasi K, Fuhrer R, Dartigues JF**. Widowhood and illness: a comparison of social network characteristics in France, Germany, Japan and the United States. *Psychol Aging* 2001;**16(4)**:655–65.

196 **Halpern D**. Minorities and mental health. *Soc Sci Med* 1993;**36**:597–607.

197 **Stansfeld SA, Fuhrer R, Shipley MJ, Marmot MG**. Work characteristics predict psychiatric disorder: prospective results from the Whitehall II study. *Occupation Environment Med* 1999;**56**:302–7.

Chapter 13

A life course perspective on women's health behaviours

Mary Schooling and Diana Kuh

Adult behaviours such as smoking, alcohol consumption, diet, and exercise are sources of risk for many chronic diseases and the need to change unhealthy behaviours remains a key aspect of health promotion policies. Intervention studies have not been very successful despite, or perhaps because of, considerable population changes in these behaviours and their social distribution over the past hundred years. It follows that successful health promotion strategies need to address the social context of women's lives and understand what drives behavioural change in groups who are the quickest and the slowest to change their behaviours in response to health messages.

The difficulty of changing adult behaviours has led to a growing interest in the origins and development of individual behaviours and healthy lifestyles. An interdisciplinary life course perspective seeks to integrate into a broad developmental framework alternative approaches to the study of health behaviour which currently focus either on individual characteristics or on the social context. We review evidence for the long-term effects of the childhood social environment on adult behaviour and for role modelling and behavioural tracking, pathways through which behaviours are conventionally thought to be initiated and maintained into adult life. There is a need for more research to identify specific adverse and protective early experiences that affect maintenance of, and change in, adult health behaviours and to look for processes beyond role modelling and tracking. A better understanding of the development of autonomy and choice in childhood and adolescence will come from studying how cultural norms and images, stressful life experiences, parental practices and peer exposure interact with the development of individual attributes like competence, self-esteem and decision-making skills and the construction of self-identity.

13.1 **Introduction and background**

The early post war epidemiological studies of mainly white middle-aged men, drawing on aetiological clues from the inter-war studies, were successful in confirming the longstanding idea that the causes of many adult chronic diseases are to be found in the way people live and their daily activities.[1] Smoking, diets rich in saturated fats, heavy alcohol consumption, obesity and inactivity are now established risk factors for coronary heart disease, and most of these are also implicated in hypertension and stroke.[2] Smoking is the major risk factor for lung cancer and chronic obstructive lung disease, and fruit and vegetable consumption protects against some cancers and other chronic diseases.[3,4] Despite the lack of attention paid until recently to whether these behaviours have similar effects in women, adult lifestyle became the prevailing aetiological model for chronic disease in women as well as men after the Second World War. A World Health Organisation study estimated that in 1990 15% of all deaths and 12% of disability adjusted life years (DALYS) in established market economies were attributable to tobacco use. The comparable figures for alcohol use were 1% and 10%, and for physical activity were 12% and 5%.[5]

In most developed countries, the state began to take more responsibility for the health of its citizens, including their health education, with the rise of the public health movement in the nineteenth century. The initial focus was on legislation to provide clean water, sewage disposal, and drainage. From the 1880s, a broadly based educational movement gathered momentum; its aim was the education of mainly working class and poor women, seen as the 'agents of cleanliness', about domestic hygiene and preventive health practices, in particular infant and child care.[6–8] Thus for a long time public health has had an interest in the daily habits of women not so much for their own health but for the health of their families and the next generation. In contrast, the state was more reluctant to tell men what they should or should not do for their health and to be seen as interfering in individual 'liberties', restricting widely acceptable and glamorized social behaviours. While the dangers of smoking were outlined in reports published by the Royal College of Physicians in 1962[9] and the Surgeon General in 1964,[10] it was not until the middle of the 1970s (spurred on by spiralling health care costs) that health promotion strategies that focused on adult lifestyle gained a higher profile.[11–13]

Health education (rather than fiscal policies or regulatory measures) remains the main preventive strategy in most established market economies.[14,15] The no smoking health education message is clear. The message on alcohol is moderation, if at all, though the definition of moderation is evolving. Since 1990 in the USA, moderate drinking has been defined as 1 unit per day for women.[16] In the UK the recommended limit was 14 units a week[17] but is now 3 units a day.[18] In the UK dietary messages initially focused on reducing fat and saturated fat and increasing fibre,[17,19] but now there is more emphasis on eating five portions of fruit and vegetables a day,[14] as in the USA.[20] The recommended intake of fat is 35% of energy in the UK,[17] and 30% in the USA.[20] Internationally accepted guidelines in 1990 of vigorous activity for 20 minutes or more three times a week, while ideal for cardiac benefit, were later revised to 30 minutes or more of moderate activity at least five times a week.[21]

In the 1970s and 1980s large scale intervention studies were set up, designed to assess whether specific intervention programmes could persuade (mainly) middle-aged men to change their health-related behaviours. Research findings have generally shown rather disappointing results, both of risk factor change and subsequent reductions in mortality and morbidity.[22] The difficulty encountered in changing health damaging behaviours in adult life gave rise to three developments relevant to a life course perspective. The first was to stimulate research (Section 13.4) into the childhood and adolescence origins of these behaviours so that strategies to prevent the initiation of unhealthy lifestyles could be developed.[23] The second was a growing recognition that the sociocultural context that shapes the initiation and maintenance of health behaviours needs to be addressed by health promotion interventions.[24] The third was to draw attention to the long-term trends in health behaviours[25] (Section 13.3) and to ask what drove these changes.

13.2 Current perspectives on the study of health behaviours

The difficulties of changing adult health behaviours encouraged a new field of study called health psychology or behavioural health.[26,27] Health psychologists emphasize the role of individual characteristics (such as personal attitudes, feelings, knowledge, and beliefs) in shaping health behaviour. Most health behaviour models assume that 'behaviour and decisions are based upon elaborate, but subjective, cost-benefit analysis of the likely outcomes of differing courses of action',[28] i.e. some reflection of attitudes and feelings. Models employ different sets of motivating forces, such as attitudes, perceived susceptibility, benefits, barriers to action, cues to action, health motivation, health locus of control, behavioural control, self-efficacy, and norms. Recent reviews[29,30] have found several of these models to be moderately effective in predicting intentions and/or behaviour, though a common framework and standardized concepts are needed.[31] From a life course perspective, these models provide no sense of an individual's development and change, nor how that individual acquired the relevant personal qualities. The models often lack a social and temporal perspective.[32,33]

The importance of social context in shaping behaviour is emphasized by sociologists, anthropologists, and social epidemiologists. Graham's detailed analysis of smoking among young women with children living on low income provides a well-known example of the impact of social context on individual behaviour. For these women cigarettes were a 'cheap' luxury and an effective coping mechanism for economic stress.[34] Researchers from these disciplines have a longstanding interest in socioeconomic differences in adult lifestyle as measured by social class, educational level or income. They seek explanations for behavioural choices both in material circumstances (at the household and neighbourhood level[35,36]) and in psychosocial processes (such as the adverse effects of stress[37,38] and the protective effects of social support[39]). Until recently little attention was paid to whether childhood socioeconomic circumstances had long-term effects on adult health behaviours.

A life course approach seeks to integrate these alternative approaches into a broad developmental framework. It considers how environmental and personal factors in earlier life shape adult health behaviours (Section 13.4), and how these relationships may be modified by, or help to create, the social changes in behaviours and the socioeconomic differences observed at the population level (Section 13.3).

13.3 The social and temporal context in women's health behaviours

Economic and social development associated with growing industrialization, urbanization, and international trade triggered the 'epidemiological transition' with its associated changes in lifestyle (see Chapter 16). Cultural forces (traditions and fashions) influenced the timing and speed of these changes in lifestyle in different countries and social groups. Historically women's smoking started in the 1920s in the US and the UK,[40,41] somewhat later elsewhere in northern Europe and later still in southern Europe, for example in the mid 1960s in parts of Spain[42] and Italy.[43] Women's smoking peaked about 40 years later, so rates are declining in northern Europe and the US but not (yet) in southern Europe.[41,44] In a few countries such as Japan smoking among women has remained low at around 15% of the female population.[45] Men's smoking started earlier, reached higher levels and peaked earlier. The decline in smoking has also been less marked in women than in men so prevalence rates for men and women are converging.[41,46] Thus, smoking is changing from being predominantly a masculine activity to being a feminine activity, possibly because it is a more socially acceptable way for women to relieve stress than alcohol or food consumption.

Currently smoking is more prevalent among women of lower socioeconomic status in the US, the UK and northern Europe, but not necessarily in southern Europe.[41,47–49] The upward and downward trends in smoking prevalence are best explained by a diffusion process led by younger, more educated women of higher socioeconomic status who were the first to start smoking and have been the first to give up.[44,50,51] In countries where women adopted the smoking habit early, an initial positive social gradient in smoking (where women of higher socioeconomic status smoked more) has now become an inverse social gradient (where women of lower socioeconomic status smoke more).[52,53] In countries such as Spain, where women adopted smoking later, a positive social gradient still exists.[49]

Alcohol use declined to a low point in the 1930s but has risen steadily since the Second World War in the UK and US.[54,55] Generally, alcohol consumption is declining in southern Europe, but increasing in parts of northern Europe.[56] Women drink much less men[57–59] due to their smaller size and possibly the constraints of their roles. Nevertheless, since the Second World War it has become more socially acceptable for women to drink alcohol and to have greater access to alcohol, and women's alcohol consumption has gone up in several northern European countries.[58,60]

Alcohol use has been and is more common for women from higher socioeconomic status groups[49,58,61,62] although this can vary between countries and over time.[59,63] In Sweden, the positive relationship between moderate to high levels of alcohol use and social class in the 1970s was replaced by an inverse relationship in the 1990s.[63] As with smoking, a diffusion process may be driving these trends.[64] Cultural factors strongly influence women's use of alcohol. For example, ethnic minority women in the US and UK drink less alcohol than other women.[65,66]

In the UK, per capita fruit consumption increased throughout the twentieth century and per capita fat consumption increased until the 1970s since when it has started to fall.[54] The proportion of energy from fat has declined only modestly because of a similar fall in total energy intake. Long-term trends in fat intake in many other developed countries are broadly similar but vary in their timing.[67,68] Although fruit, vegetable, and cereal consumption has traditionally been higher and fat intake lower in southern compared with northern European countries, in the last 20–30 years there has been some convergence in dietary patterns across Europe.[46] Women's diets are constrained more than men's by family needs[69,70] and considerations of social acceptability, in terms of what they are seen to eat and in relation to body image. For these reasons women are seen and see themselves as eating healthier diets; women eat less than men and may be less likely to meet their recommended daily allowance for micronutrients,[71,72] but the proportion of fat in their diets is similar.[67,73]

Historically higher status socioeconomic groups ate a more varied diet with more fat, protein, fruit and vegetables.[74] Many studies show that women of higher socioeconomic status still eat healthier foods such as low fat products, wholemeal bread, low salt, or fruit and vegetables.[35,53,75–78] and have higher intakes of some essential micronutrients, such as calcium and vitamin C than other women.[79] In the UK the decline in fat consumption has been strongest in more affluent households[80] and more recent studies which allow for the social acceptability bias in dietary reporting find little evidence for a socioeconomic gradient in fat intakes.[81,82] Cultural influences and acculturation rates of ethnic minorities complicate the relationship between socioeconomic status and dietary patterns.

In contrast to the other health-related behaviours, little is known about trends in adult physical activity within and between countries. The increased prevalence of obesity (see Chapter 14) and the downward trend in energy intake reported in some but not all national dietary studies[80,83] suggest that physical activity has fallen.[84] This is partly due to the shift from manual to non manual occupations, the greater use of motor vehicles and labour saving devices at work and at home, and more time spent watching television. In recent years, participation in sports and leisure activities may have increased slightly.[85–87] Levels of inactivity are higher in southern Europe than northern Europe.[46] Girls are less physically active than boys and women participate less than men in leisure exercise.[85,88,89] Socially accepted norms for a feminine role have only recently included sport[90] and time pressures may reduce women's participation in sport. There is less public provision for women's sports, less prominence given to women's professional sport, and less acceptance of a well-muscled, athletic body as consistent with ideals of femininity.

Historically sports and pastimes have been more common among the upper social groups[91] and for privately educated girls.[92] Women from higher socioeconomic groups are more likely than those from lower socioeconomic groups to be physically active in their leisure time[35,53,93–96] but not during the working day. Although they are less likely to be inactive, they are no more likely to have high activity levels that meet current guidelines.[93] In the US, women from ethnic minorities are particularly inactive in leisure time, allowing for socioeconomic status,[89] but this is less marked if occupational activity is allowed for.[97]

One of the reasons why the initial intervention studies to change behaviour had little effect on risk factor change was because the trials were 'outrun by the pace of social change'.[25] Women from the upper socioeconomic groups generally have healthier behaviour than other women. This was not always so and appears to be due to their quicker response to health education messages. In terms of changing health behaviours at the population level it is necessary to understand what drives social change and the importance of health promotion and other types of interventions relative to factors such as economic forces and fashion trends. This is a broad research agenda, which has still to be thoroughly investigated, and there is little agreement or understanding of how fashions spread.[98,99] Diffusion is a retrospective interpretation; if it is correct, then the forces that drive diffusion need to be harnessed to make health education effective and equitable,[64] and to change the norms of socially acceptable behaviour, as has been done for smoking, through initiatives like smoke free worksites and public spaces.

We also need to understand the material, cultural, or psychosocial processes underlying individual and group differences in health behaviours. Are there factors at each life stage that are particularly important?

13.4 **A developmental life course framework for health behaviour**

A life course perspective studies the environmental and personal factors at each life stage that are associated with initiation, maintenance and change in health behaviours across the entire life course, and explores underlying mechanisms. It specifically tests the hypothesis that adult health behaviours and their associated adult risk and protective factors are linked to environmental influences in childhood and adolescence and to individual attributes established during those sensitive developmental stages. The key elements of a life course framework are illustrated in Fig. 13.1 and defined and discussed in the following sections.

A life course approach recognizes adolescence and young adulthood as a particularly important life stage for behavioural development. During this time, smoking and alcohol drinking are initiated, and decisions about physical activity and eating become increasingly the responsibility of the young person. Smoking, alcohol use, and physical activity peak in late adolescence or early adulthood and then decline, though not necessarily uniformly.[57,100–103] The healthiness (or otherwise) of these behavioural choices may be of less importance compared with other functions they serve. They may be markers of transition into the adult world; for gaining admission to peer groups or making oneself attractive to the opposite sex; as a sign of personal identity, independence, and autonomy; as a coping mechanism for adolescent anxiety, failure, or stress; or simply because certain activities are fun.

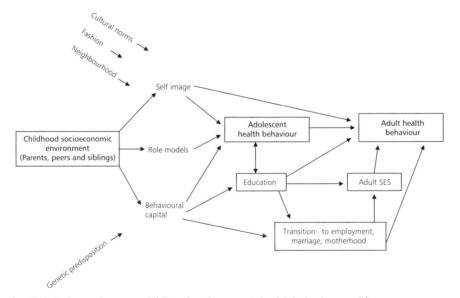

Fig. 13.1 Pathways between childhood and women's health behaviours: a life course framework.

13.4.1 **Socioeconomic environment in childhood and the initiation and maintenance of health behaviours**

In regard to the *initiation* of health behaviours, recent reviews in the predominately English-speaking world and northern Europe agree that teenage smoking is related to lower parental socioeconomic status.[104–107] However, the relationship is not always evident for girls[76,108,109] and, as expected, is not consistent for girls across historic time[25,110] or culture. Girls from minority ethnic groups in the US are generally less well off than white girls but are less likely to start smoking.[111] Children from lower socioeconomic families are more likely to eat unhealthy food, such as confectionery, soft drinks and crisps to have higher fat intakes and lower intakes of fruit, vegetables, and fibre.[107,112–114] Parental socioeconomic status is not consistently related to exercise or alcohol consumption,[107–109,115] although exercise in girls in some studies is associated with higher parental socioeconomic status.[109,112,116] Inconsistency may be due to the inaccuracy of self reported physical activity data or because socioeconomic differences vary depending on the type of activity, for example, supervised sports show much stronger differentials than unsupervised activity.[117]

Educational characteristics such as low aspirations, earlier school leaving, and poor educational performance are associated with teenage female smoking,[76,104,105,118] less healthy eating,[113,114] less exercise,[76] and more alcohol use.[119] The adoption of a healthy lifestyle in adolescence has been shown to precede educational attainment[120] suggesting it is not educational attainment in itself that is responsible for better health behaviour but common factors, which we describe as 'behavioural capital' (Section 13.4.4), that increase the chance of better outcomes in both these domains.

In regard to the *maintenance* of health behaviours, several studies have investigated whether childhood markers of socioeconomic status have a long lasting effect on adult behaviour independent of adult socioeconomic status. Findings for women are inconsistent for smoking, exercise, or drinking,[121–123] perhaps because of trends, cohort effects, and differences between countries. We re-analysed data from the British 1946 birth cohort[79,94,124] to look at the joint effects on health behaviours at age 36 of child and adult social class and education. Women from manual origins were more likely to smoke, remain a smoker, be inactive, and have an unhealthy diet (in terms of fibre and vitamin C but not in terms of fat intake) but were less likely to drink high amounts of alcohol than women from non manual origins. These effects remained after adjusting for current social class, which showed similar associations (Table 13.1). The effect of educational qualifications was stronger than the effect of child or adult social class on all these health behaviours except alcohol consumption. The additional inclusion of educational qualifications in the multivariate model reduced all the social class effects, but childhood social class remained associated (at the 5% level) with inactivity and quitting smoking, and adult social class remained associated with smoking, quitting smoking, vitamin C, and fibre intake (Table 13.1, fully adjusted models). The independent associations of adult health behaviours with educational characteristics and parental social class suggest that lifelong attachment to cultural norms, psychosocial processes and living conditions in childhood play a role in the maintenance of these health behaviours in addition to current adult circumstances. These are discussed further below.

13.4.2 Role models

According to social learning theory[125] adolescent health behaviours may be modelled on the behaviours of others or transmitted through their attitudes and values towards these behaviours. There are also competing developmental theories that postulate either parental influences or strong genetic and peer influences on behaviour.[126–128]

Research studies frequently investigate the relationship between specific parental health behaviours and adolescent behaviours; fewer have investigated the transmission of a healthy

Table 13.1 Health behaviours at age 36 years according to socioeconomic indicators in childhood and adult life. Odds ratio (95% confidence intervals (CI)) for manual vs non manual and low education (up to O-level) vs high education (A-levels and above). Women from the British 1946 birth cohort study

Socioeconomic indicator	Smoking (n=1442)						Quitting smoking (n=973)					
	Unadjusted OR (95% CI)	p-value	Adjusted[1] OR (95% CI)	p-value	Adjusted[2] OR (95% CI)	p-value	Unadjusted OR (95% CI)	p-value	Adjusted[1] OR (95% CI)	p-value	Adjusted[2] OR (95% CI)	p-value
Father's social class	1.66 (1.33–2.08)	<0.001	1.40 (1.10–1.78)	0.005	1.22 (0.95–1.57)	0.115	0.49 (0.38–0.63)	<0.001	0.56 (0.43–0.74)	<0.001	0.62 (0.47–0.83)	0.001
Adult social class	1.91 (1.53–2.38)	<0.001	1.72 (1.36–2.17)	<0.001	1.54 (1.23–1.91)	<0.001	0.53 (0.41–0.68)	<0.001	0.63 (0.48–0.83)	<0.001	0.69 (0.53–0.92)	0.011
Education	2.18 (1.66–2.85)	<0.001			1.67 (1.24–2.26)	<0.001	0.46 (0.34–0.63)	<0.001			0.65 (0.46–0.90)	0.010

Socioeconomic indicator	Inactivity (n=1442)					
	Unadjusted OR (95% CI)	p-value	Adjusted[1] OR (95% CI)	p-value	Adjusted[2] OR (95% CI)	p-value
Father's Social class	1.80 (1.45–2.23)	<0.001	1.61 (1.28–2.02)	<0.001	1.35 (1.06–1.71)	0.045
Adult social class	1.65 (1.37–2.10)	<0.001	1.43 (1.14–1.8)	0.002	1.24 (0.98–1.56)	0.071
Education	2.40 (1.87–3.09)	<0.001			1.93 (1.45–2.60)	<0.001

	% fat (>40%) (n=1070)						Fibre (lowest third) (n=1070)					
			Model[1]		Fully adjusted[2]				Model[1]		Fully adjusted[2]	
	OR (95% CI)	p	OR (95% CI)	p	OR (95% CI)	p	OR (95% CI)	p	OR (95% CI)	p	OR (95% CI)	p
Father's social class	0.85 (0.66-1.10)	0.223	0.91 (0.7-1.18)	0.463	0.96 (0.73-1.27)	0.796	1.42 (1.08-1.87)	0.011	1.17 (0.88-1.56)	0.287	1.61 (1.23-2.08)	<0.001
Adult social class	0.79 (0.61-1.01)	0.066	0.81 (0.62-1.05)	0.120	0.85 (0.65-1.12)	0.265	1.58 (1.20-2.06)	<0.001	1.33 (1.01-1.77)	0.043	1.74 (1.34-2.25)	<0.001
Education	0.75 (0.56-0.99)	0.042			0.81 (0.59-1.11)	0.118	2.08 (1.47-2.96)	<0.001			2.50 (1.82-3.42)	<0.001

	Vitamin C (<40 mg) (n=1070)						Alcohol (>14 units) (n=1070)					
			Model[1]		Fully adjusted[2]				Model[1]		Fully adjusted[2]	
	OR (95% CI)	p	OR (95% CI)	p	OR (95% CI)	p	OR (95% CI)	p	OR (95% CI)	p	OR (95% CI)	p
Father's social class	1.60 (1.23-2.07)	<0.001	1.43 (1.09-1.88)	0.010	1.28 (0.96-1.7)	0.091	0.52 (0.35-0.76)	<0.001	0.59 (0.39-0.87)	0.008	0.66 (0.43-1.00)	0.052
Adult social class	1.65 (1.28-2.14)	<0.001	1.50 (1.14-1.96)	0.003	1.36 (1.03-1.80)	0.030	0.55 (0.42-0.96)	0.003	0.66 (0.42-0.96)	0.033	0.71 (0.46-1.09)	0.117
Education	1.88 (1.39-2.53)	<0.001			1.49 (1.06-2.09)	0.020	0.51 (0.35-0.72)	<0.001			0.69 (0.44-1.05)	0.090

Father's social class when study member was aged 15 years. Head of household social class at age 36 years. Educational qualifications by age 26 years.

[1] Model including both social class measures.

[2] Fully adjusted model including both social class measures and education.

lifestyle.[129] Generally children show similarities with their parents, and are more likely to smoke,[115,130–132] drink,[115] have a healthy diet,[133] or exercise[116,134] if their parents do, though parental influence may be moderated by the relationship with the parent, particularly for drinking. Recently there has been investigation of whether these similarities are due to cultural transmission or shared genes. Most studies find some evidence of genetic effects (alongside environmental effects) for smoking,[48,135] drinking,[136,137] and physical activity.[138] Genetic influences on healthy food choices or nutrient intakes have yet to be investigated in detail.

During later childhood and adolescence there is a growing impact of peers on behavioural choices. Peer influence on smoking and drinking initiation has been confirmed in many studies[104,106,139,140] and shown for exercise[134] though it may be less marked on diet.[141] The influence of parents and peers are not independent. Peer factors may reduce parental influences on smoking and alcohol use,[142] and parental practices (Section 13.4.4) may modify or exacerbate the influence of peers by affecting their offspring's peer orientation[128] or risk of forming deviant affiliations.[143] Overall, it is not clear which transmission route—parents, genes, peers—is most important, how they interact and whether they have the same effects on male and female adolescents. For example, there are some suggestions from twin studies that genetic effects are weaker for girls,[144] and were weaker for women when there was less social acceptability of smoking.[48]

13.4.3 Tracking of health behaviours through childhood and adolescence and into adult life

Tracking is the stability of behaviour over time or the predictability of a measurement of a risk factor later in life for values of the same risk factor earlier in life.[145] Childhood and adolescence are seen as formative stages for shaping lifelong behaviour patterns,[23] as they are for biological development, and are appropriate times to provide health education.

Smoking is known to be addictive. It has been shown in longitudinal studies to track strongly in adolescence,[146] and up until the late twenties.[145] This is consistent with the observation that currently those who do not smoke regularly in their teens are unlikely to smoke in adult life[100] and that those who initiate smoking at younger ages, or smoke more heavily, are less likely to give up.[147–149] In contrast, longitudinal follow-up through adolescence and into young adult life shows that alcohol use,[145] diet,[150–152] and physical activity[96,145,153] do not track as strongly from adolescence into young adult life. Physical inactivity may track more strongly than physical activity.[154]

Given that adolescence and young adulthood is a time of experimentation and change when a number of life transitions occur, it may not be surprising that tracking is only moderate during this life stage. We might expect, as women settle into their adult social roles, to see more similarity between childhood and adult rankings of eating and exercise patterns. Skills instilled in childhood or adolescence may be put to use again. Several prospective studies have shown that those who participated in sports activities (particularly organized sports) when they were young were more likely to be doing so in their late twenties,[155] thirties,[94] and beyond.[156]

13.4.4 Adverse and protective childhood environments and the development of behavioural capital

We now move beyond the use of simple markers of childhood socioeconomic circumstances to consider the kinds of adverse and protective childhood experiences with short- and possibly long-term effects on behavioural choices and the underlying mechanisms through which they may operate. We suggest that these mechanisms include the development of what we have called 'behavioural capital' as well as the more conventionally accepted routes of role modelling and behavioural tracking already discussed (Fig. 13.1). By behavioural capital we mean the accumulation of positive individual attributes such as social competence, decision-making and problem-solving skills, coping strategies, personal efficacy, self-esteem, attitudes and values that help the individual remain resilient in times of adversity or take advantage of talents and opportunities. Many of these attributes are more easily acquired during child and adolescent development, and although they may be acquired later, it is often harder to do so.[157] In turn behavioural capital is likely to lead to healthy behavioural choices throughout life, either directly or indirectly by influencing many aspects of adult life that shape adult behaviour (such as education, social support, and employment opportunities).[158] As many aspects of behavioural capital affect educational aspirations and achievement as well as the choice of health behaviours the relationships observed between educational achievement and health behaviours may reflect their common origins.

Adverse experiences such as family or parental conflict, parental mental health and social problems, and child abuse are related to smoking and drinking in adolescence[118,159] and smoking in adult life, independent of education.[160,161] These outcomes may be the direct result of the stressful experience or associated lifetime psychosocial orientations such as hopelessness, depression, or cynical hostility.[162] Smoking, drinking, and comfort eating may be used by some as coping strategies whereas others may have more recourse to healthier coping mechanisms. They may also be mediated or moderated by parental practices.

The mediating role of parental practices has been examined using measures of the warmth of the parent–child relationship (attachment, support, connectedness, bonding, responsiveness) and of parental supervision (control, demandingness, monitoring, supervision), or combined into a typology of parenting styles. Authoritative parenting (responsive and demanding) has the best adolescent outcomes.[163,164] Parental support and control are associated with less smoking and drinking and more fruit and vegetable consumption in adolescence.[114,128,132,165–167] Positive parenting practices may develop emotional resilience in times of adversity.[168] Their effects on these health behaviours in adult life or on other health behaviours at any stage of life have not yet been thoroughly investigated. A life course perspective would also pay attention to material and social factors (including intergenerational factors) that promote or inhibit the development of good parenting skills.[169,170]

Many aspects of the child's behavioural capital, such as competence, self-esteem, coping skills, decision-making skills, and personal efficacy are associated with less smoking,[105,106,171] less drinking,[172–174] and more exercise in adolescence.[175] As yet little is known about diet.[176] The relative importance of these different aspects of behavioural capital is difficult to assess because of the wide range of measures used and because many studies lack a theoretical framework.[104] More theoretically based research is needed on how these attributes are acquired,[177] how they shape the development of choice in childhood, and their effects on adult health behaviour. The health psychology literature is replete with examples of associations between adult measures of these attributes and health behaviours.[28] Such attributes would be expected to show some stability throughout life, as do some personality traits.[178,179]

13.4.5 **Identity in adolescence**

The section on trends in health behaviours (Section 13.3) indicated that at a population level, there are differences in behaviour between men and women, and that social acceptability, which changes over time, may constrain women's behaviour. The role of social acceptability has been investigated in more detail[180] using the concepts of self-presentation and self-identity from sociology.[181,182] This approach recognizes that women are concerned about how they present themselves, beyond purely physical considerations. It postulates that behavioural choices are the result of an interaction between how women want to present themselves and the image represented by a particular activity. Anthropology and cross-cultural psychology[183,184] provide dimensions of cultural identity, beyond gender-identity, such as conformity, sociability, and religiosity. Initial findings, using a British cohort that have been followed since their birth in 1946[124] suggest that health behaviour in adult life is influenced by how closely these aspects of identity (measured in adolescence) match the social image of that health behaviour. For example, alcohol use has more masculine connotations and women who behaved in adolescence in a rough, competitive, or aggressive manner (seen as presenting a more masculine identity) have a heavier alcohol consumption in adulthood at age 36 than their peers, independent of education, current and parental socioeconomic status. Drinking and exercise are often social activities, and women who were popular or good at making friends in adolescence (seen as projecting a more sociable identity) were more likely (at age 36) to drink more alcohol and participate in leisure exercise, independent of education, current and parental socioeconomic status.

This study extends previous studies which have found a relationship between femininity and less drinking,[60,185] or between sociability and being more likely to take physical activity.[116,186] by demonstrating that an identity developed in adolescence can affect health behaviours 20 years later. From a preventive perspective, it highlights that rather than changing individuals, it is also important to change the social context. These findings provide a novel perspective that now needs to be replicated in other studies. We need to know, for example, how women construct their identities, and the role peers play in re-enforcing identities. Such an approach may also offer insight in how to change the image of a behaviour at the societal level.

13.4.6 **Adult transitions and health behaviours**

According to the argument presented so far, women entering adult life bring with them a set of health behaviours, constraints from their childhood environment, and their accumulated behavioural capital and identity. These will shape the adult social environment which, as we have seen (Section 13.3), has strong effects on adult health behaviours. They may also influence their ability and motivation to change in response to changing circumstances or changing messages.

Given current socioeconomic variations in health behaviour, the effect of entry into the workforce on health behaviours probably depends on the nature and type of employment and facilities available. Becoming unemployed does not seem to raise the risk of smoking[187] or consistently change drinking habits[188,189] although it has been associated with more drinking among specific groups, such as highly educated, single women during a recent recession in Finland.[190] Marriage is associated with drinking reductions[62,189,191] and may help a woman quit smoking if her husband is a non-smoker.[192] There is little evidence of marriage having much effect on nutrient intake or exercise.[75,89,193] Conversely, marital break-up is associated with increased alcohol consumption,[188] alcohol abuse,[194] and smoking.[195] In pregnancy, women are advised to give up smoking and drinking. Although pregnant women have lower smoking rates than other women,[22,196] many women (up to 75%[41]) go back to smoking after pregnancy. Women of higher socioeconomic status are generally more likely to give up in pregnancy than other women.[197,198] Childcare has been shown to have both positive and negative influences on health behaviours.[75,199,200] There may be pressure from children to adopt a healthy lifestyle, but the financial, time, and emotional demands of childcare may make it more difficult to do so, and may be moderated by living in a child-friendly neighbourhood. In middle-age, there may be more time for active leisure activities when children leave home unless it is taken up by caring for frail parents.[201] There is little evidence of a change in habits associated with the menopause[202] or of different factors relating to health behaviour before or after midlife. The onset of chronic illness, such as diabetes, will force some women to change their health habits, depending on the nature and severity of the illness.[203–205] Retirement or spouse's retirement is another opportunity for change but has been little studied. Its effect on health behaviour may be different for those living on a state pension compared with those with a good occupational pension.

From a life course perspective, these changes give women an opportunity to rewrite their script and reinvent themselves. However, it is not clear that many women do so, or to what extent their behavioural response to new opportunities or constraints is conditioned by previous experiences, behavioural capital, and identity. This is an area ripe for further research.

13.5 Conclusions

Promoting healthy lifestyles requires both a population strategy to shift cultural norms towards the healthier options and a targeted strategy for individuals most engaged in harmful health behaviour. A life course approach encourages a temporal and social perspective, highlighting the considerable population changes in diet, smoking, drinking, and exercise that have taken place in the twentieth century and studying their diffusion with respect to gender and socioeconomic group. This has been most striking for smoking but recent evidence indicates that changes in the socioeconomic distribution of alcohol consumption may be occurring. Health promotion strategies that address the social context of women's health behaviours and provide local and accessible facilities that help to promote healthy behaviour are likely to be more effective than simple health education messages.

The study of health behaviour is a relatively new research field that has attracted several different disciplines that focus on different explanations for behaviour. A life course approach encourages a developmental perspective in which to organize current theories. Role modelling and tracking of health behaviours have been the main explanations for the links between childhood and adult life, although with the exception of smoking, tracking into adult life is only moderate. This suggests that socially sensitive health promotion in childhood should be offered on a comprehensive basis, not targeted to certain groups.

Evidence to date suggests that the early socioeconomic environment has long-term effects on adult behaviours independent of the strong effects of the adult environment. We need longitudinal studies to move beyond simple socioeconomic indicators and study how stressful experiences, individual development and social context interact to influence the child's behaviour as well as their physical and mental health in ways that may be lifelong.

For example, adult psychosocial orientations are strongly related to health behaviour and may have their origins in childhood. How do protective factors, such as parental practices or intervention policies in childhood, and new opportunities in adult life moderate any long-term behavioural effects of early stress? In these ways we may begin to account for the socioeconomic differences observed in health behaviours. From a policy point of view, interventions to ameliorate the effects of stressful circumstances would need to be targeted towards vulnerable young girls and women and offer support for managing all life domains, not just those to do with health behaviours.

We also need to understand more fully how children learn to make choices as part of normal development and how environmental and personal factors affect this in ways that promote or prevent the development and maintenance of healthy lifestyles. Part of this process, and one that has important implications for health behaviours, is the construction of self-identity in adolescence. Understanding how young women construct their identities and the role of parents, peers, and the wider society in this process may also offer insight into how to change the image of certain behaviours at a societal level and thus have implications for population health.

Acknowledgements

Mary Schooling would like to thank Professor Michael Wadsworth and Dr Rebecca Hardy for their advice and support as tutors for her doctoral dissertation.

Commentary on 'A life course perspective on women's health behaviours'

Hilary Graham

The chapter provides a life course perspective on lifestyles, setting the cluster of health behaviours implicated in the aetiology of chronic disease in the context of the pathways which women follow across their lives. It is an important and timely chapter. To date, neither research on health behaviour nor research on life course epidemiology has given detailed consideration to how cigarette smoking, alcohol consumption, diet, and physical activity are shaped by experiences in early and later life. The ways in which gender makes a difference to life course pathways and to their associated lifestyles have received even less attention.

Schooling and Kuh address this gap in two ways. First, they provide a review of evidence on trends in women's health behaviour over time, between countries and across socioeconomic groups, focusing primarily on Europe and the US. They note how the epidemiological transition which accompanied the process of industrialization has been associated with changes in health behaviour which, like the uptake of smoking and the increase in alcohol consumption among women, challenged accepted gender norms. The socioeconomic profile of these behaviours has shifted over time and varies across ethnic groups. However, in post-industrial societies, socioeconomic advantage is typically associated with health promoting behaviours: women in higher socioeconomic groups smoke less, have healthier diets, and are more physically active in their leisure time than women in more disadvantaged circumstances.

Secondly, the authors outline a life course framework for understanding these contemporary patterns of health behaviour (Fig. 13.1). In this framework, adolescence and early adulthood are the formative life stage: the time for (not) taking up cigarette smoking and drinking alcohol and for taking over responsibility for diet and exercise from parents and teachers. Adolescent health behaviour in this key transition is seen as influenced by childhood socioeconomic circumstances and, in turn, as shaping health behaviour in adulthood. The framework is supported by new analyses of the British 1946 birth cohort study of the joint effects of childhood social class, education, and adult social class on health behaviours at age 36. While confirming the established associations between adult lifestyles and adult social class, these analyses also found independent associations between adult lifestyles and parental social class and, particularly, educational qualifications.

Schooling and Kuh's life course framework identifies the mechanisms that may underlie the associations between childhood social class, education, and adult lifestyles. These mechanisms include the modelling of adolescent health behaviour on parents and peers and the development of what the authors term 'behavioural capital'. This refers to psychological resources—like social competence, personal efficacy, and self-esteem—which support healthy behavioural choices, both directly and indirectly by influencing educational careers. The authors point to evidence that children with greater behavioural capital smoke less, drink less, and take more exercise in adolescence. Evidence is presented that parenting practices—with respect to parental support and supervision for example—are important for the development of behavioural capital.

As this brief overview suggests, the authors provide a generic framework for understanding the life course influences on women's health behaviours. It is a framework which emphasizes psychosocial mechanisms, identifying the psychological characteristics and capacities of the adolescent as central to the pathways which run between childhood origins and adult lifestyles. This psychological orientation is in accord with related fields of life course research, where cognitive and behavioural development in childhood is identified as having lifelong effects on socioeconomic position and health in adult life.[157] However, as the authors note, these psychological processes are framed by the broader structures of class, gender, and ethnic inequality—structures which are complex, dynamic, and hard to measure in the longitudinal studies which resource life course perspectives.

An important next stage for life course research on women's health behaviour may therefore be to locate analyses derived from longitudinal studies within research on the changing economic and cultural contexts of their lives. The disciplinary reach of life course perspectives could be extended to incorporate insights from qualitative studies, from ethnographies, and from cultural and class analyses on the formative transition from childhood to adulthood. Qualitative studies, for example, have recorded how young women negotiate (and resist) their class and sexual identities through their health behaviours.[206,207] Ethnographic studies of young women and young mothers have suggested that the development and maintenance of health-promoting behaviours—not smoking, eating well, keeping fit—is both a product and a display of privilege: it reflects a past and current class position which enables 'work on the self'.[208] Linked to this seam of research are analyses which suggest that, in post-industrial societies, class is defined less in terms of the means of production and more in terms of modes of consumption—including food, cigarettes, alcohol, and exercise.[209,210]

Schooling and Kuh have provided a state-of-the-art review of life course research on women's health behaviour. They have generated a framework for understanding the relationship between the childhood environment, adolescent health behaviour, and lifestyles in adult life which is grounded in evidence from cross-sectional and longitudinal studies. An important challenge is to connect the pathways they uncover with the broader social hierarchies which structure women's lives.

References

1 **Kuh D, Davey Smith G**. The life course and adult chronic disease: an historical perspective with particular reference to coronary heart disease. In Kuh D, Ben-Shlomo Y, eds. *A life course approach to chronic disease epidemiology: tracing the origins of ill-health from early to adult life*. Oxford: Oxford University Press, 1997, pp. 15–44.

2 **Cardiovascular Review Group Committe on the Medical Aspects of Food Policy**. *Nutritional Aspects of Cardiovascular Disease*. Department of Health Report on Health and Social Subjects 46. London: HMSO, 1994.

3 **Working Group on Diet and Cancer of the Committee on Medical Aspects of Food and Nutrition Policy**. *Nutritional Aspects of the Development of Cancer*. Department of Health Report on Health and Social Subjects 48. London: The Stationery Office, 1998.

4 **World Health Organization Study Group**. *Diet, nutrition, and the prevention of chronic diseases*. Technical Report Series No. 797. Geneva: World Health Organization, 1990.

5 **Murray CJL, Lopez AD**. *The global burden of disease: a comprehensive assessment of mortality and disability from diseases, injuries and risk factors in 1990 and projected to 2020*. WHO & World Bank. Cambridge, Mass.: Harvard University Press, 1996.

6 **Hoy S**. *Chasing dirt. The American pursuit of cleanliness*. New York: Oxford University Press, 1995.

7 **Hardy A**. *The Epidemic Streets*. Oxford: Clarendon Press, 1993.

8 **Dwork D**. *War is Good for Babies and Other Young Children. A History of the Infant and Child Welfare Movement in England 1898–1918*. London: 1987.

9 **Royal College of Physicians**. *Smoking and Health*. London: Pitman, 1962.

10 **United States Public Health Service**. *The Health Consequences of Smoking. A Public Health Service Review*. Washington: U.S. Department of Health, Education and Welfare, 1967.

11 **Department of Health and Social Security**. *Prevention and health, eating for health*. London: HMSO, 1978.

12 **Lalonde M**. *A new perspective in the health of Canadians*. Ottawa: Canadian Government Printing Office, 1974.

13 **United States Department of Health Education and Welfare**. *Forward Plan for Health*. Washington DC: US Government Printing Office, 1975.

14 **Department of Health**. *The NHS Plan: a plan for investment—a plan for reform*. London: The Stationery Office, 2000.

15 **US Department of Health and Human Services**. *Healthy People 2010*. Washington, DC: US Department of Health & Human Services, 2000.

16 **Dufour MC**. If you drink alcoholic beverages do so in moderation: what does this mean? *J Nutr* 2001;**131**:552S–61S.

17 **Department of Health**. *The health of the nation—a strategy for health in England*. London: HMSO, 1992.

18 **Department of Health**. Inter-Departmental Working Group. *Sensible drinking*. London: 1995.

19 **Committee on Medical Aspects of Food Policy**. *Diet and Cardiovascular Disease*. London: HMSO, 1984.

20 **Dietary Guidelines Advisory Committee**. *Report of the dietary guidelines advisory committee on the dietary guidelines for Americans*. Washington, DC: U.S. Department of Agriculture Human Nutrition Information Service, 2000.

21 **Killoran A**. *Moving on: international perspectives on promoting physical activity*. London: Health Education Authority, 1995.

22 **Ebrahim S, Smith GD**. Systematic review of randomised controlled trials of multiple risk factor interventions for preventing coronary heart disease. *Br Med J* 1997;**314**:1666–74.

23 **United States Department of Health and Human Services**. Health People. Surgeon-General's Report on Health *Promotion and Disease Prevention*. Washington DC: US Government Printing Office, 1979.

24 **Emmons KM**. Health Behaviors in a Social Context. In Berkman LF, Kawachi I, eds. *Social Epidemiology*. New York: Oxford University Press, 2000:242–66.

25 **Susser M**. The tribulations of trials- intervention in communities. *Am J Public Health* 1995;**85**:156–8.

26 **Matarazzo J**. *Behavioral health*. New York: Wiley, 1984.

27 **Gochman DS**. Health behavior: plural perspectives. In Gochman DS, ed. *Health behavior*, New York: Plenum, 1988:3–18.

28 **Connor M, Norman P**. *Predicting health behaviours*. Oxford: OUP, 1995.

29 **Sutton S**. Predicting and explaining intentions and behaviour: how well are we doing? *J Appl Soc Psychol* 1998;**28**:1317–38.

30 **Floyd DL, Prentice-Dunn S, Rogers RW**. A meta-analysis of research on protection motivation theory. *J Appl Soc Psychol* 2000;**30**:407–29.

31 **Stroebe W, Stroebe MS**. *Social psychology and health*. Buckingham: Open University Press, 1995.

32 **Bunton R, Murphy S, Bennett P**. Theories of behavioural change and their use in health promotion: some neglected areas. *Health Ed Res: Theory Pract* 1991;**6**:153–62.

33 **Levy J**. A conceptual meta-paradigm for the study of health behaviour and health promotion. *Health Ed Res: Theory Pract* 1991;**6**:195–202.

34 **Graham H**. *When life's a drag*. London: HMSO, 1994.

35 **Bartley M, Sacker A, Firth D, Fitzpatrick R**. Understanding social variation in cardiovascular risk factors in women and men: the advantage of theoretically based measures. *Soc Sci Med* 1999;**49**:831–45.

36 **Diez-Roux AV, Nieto FJ, Muntaner C, Tyroler HA, Comstock GW, Shahar E** *et al*. Neighborhood environments and coronary heart disease: a multilevel analysis. *Am J Epidemiol* 1997;**146**:48–63.

37 **House JS, Strecher V, Metzner HL, Robbins CA**. Occupational Stress and health among men and women in the Tecumseh Community Health Study. *J Health Soc Behav* 1986;**27**:62–77.

38 **Kivimaki M, Vahtera J, Pentti J, Ferrie JE**. Factors underlying the effect of organisational downsizing on health of employees: longitudinal cohort study. *Br Med J* 2000;**320**:971–5.

39 **Berkman LF, Glass T, Brissette I, Seeman TE**. From social integration to health: Durkheim in the new millennium. *Soc Sci Med* 2000;**51**:843–57.

40 Todd GF. *Statistics of Smoking*. London: Tobacco Manufacturers Standing Committee, 1959.

41 Husten RF, Malarcher AM. Cigarette Smoking: Trends, Determinants, and Health Effects. In Goldman MB, Hatch MC, eds. *Women and Health*, San Diego, Calif., London: Academic Press, 2000:563–77.

42 Borras JM, Fernandez E, Schiaffino A, Borrell C, La Vecchia C. Pattern of Smoking Initiation in Catalonia, Spain, From 1948–1992. *Am J Public Health* 2000;**90**:1459–62.

43 La Vecchia C, Decarli A, Pagano R. Patterns of smoking initiation in Italian males and females from 1955 to 1985. *Prev Med* 1995;**24**:293–6.

44 Graham H. Smoking prevalence among women in the European Community 1950–90. *Soc Sci Med* 1996;**43**:243–54.

45 Honjo K, Kawachi I. Effects of market liberalisation on smoking in Japan. *Tob Control* 2000;**9**:193–200.

46 Rayner M, Petersen S. *European cardiovascular disease statistics*. London: British Heart Foundation, 2000.

47 Jarvis MJ, Wardle J. Social patterning of individual health behaviours: the case of cigarette smoking. In Marmot M, Wilkinson RG, eds. *Social Determinants of Health*, Oxford: OUP, 1999:240–55.

48 Kendler KS, Thornton LM, Pedersen NL. Tobacco consumption in Swedish twins reared apart and reared together. *Arch Gen Psychiatry* 2000;**57**:886–92.

49 Borrell C, Dominguez-Berjon F, Pasarin MI, Ferrando J, Rohlfs I, Nebot M. Social inequalities in health related behaviours in Barcelona. *J Epidemiol Community Health* 2000;**54**:24–30.

50 Rogers EM. *Diffusion of Innovations*. London: Collier Macmillan, 1983.

51 Waldron I. Patterns and causes of gender differences in smoking. *Soc Sci Med* 1991;**32**:989–1005.

52 Pekkanen J, Uutela A, Valkonen T, Vartiainen E, Tuomilehto J, Puska P. Coronary risk factor levels: Differences between educational groups in 1972–87 in eastern Finland. *J Epidemiol Community Health* 1995;**49**:144–9.

53 Bennett S. Cardiovascular risk factors in Australia: trends in socioeconomic inequalities. *J Epidemiol Community Health* 1995;**49**:363–72.

54 Swerdlow A, dos Santos Silva I, Doll R. *Cancer incidence and mortality in England and Wales: trends and risk factors*. Oxford: Oxford University Press, 2001.

55 Russell M, Testa M, Wilsnack S. Alcohol use and abuse. In Goldman MB, Hatch MC, eds. *Women and health*, New York: Academic Press, 2000:589–98.

56 Simpura J. Trends in alcohol consumption and drinking patterns: lessons from worldwide development. In Holder HD, Edwards G, eds. *Alcohol and public policy: evidence and issues*, Oxford: OUP, 1995:9–37.

57 Johnson FW, Gruenewald PJ, Treno AJ, Taff GA. Drinking over the life course within gender and ethnic Groups: a hyperparametric analysis. *J Stud Alcohol* 1998;**59**:568–80.

58 Knibbe RA, Drop MJ, van Reek J, Saenger G. The development of alcohol consumption in the Netherlands: 1958–1981. *Br J Addict* 1985;**80**:411–9.

59 Bobak M, McKee M, Rose R, Marmot M. Alcohol consumption in a national sample of the Russian population. *Addiction* 1999;**94**:857–66.

60 Hammer T, Vaglum P. The increase in alcohol consumption among women: a phenomenon related to accessibility or stress? A general population study. *Br J Addict* 1989;**84**:767–75.

61 Edwards G, Chandler J, Hensman C. Drinking in a London Suburb. *Quart J Stud Alcohol* 1972;**S6**:69–93.

62 Caetano R, Clark CL. Trends in alcohol consumption patterns among whites, blacks and hispanics: 1984–1995. *J Stud Alcohol* 1998;**58**:659–68.

63 **Romelsjo A, Lundberg M**. The changes in the social class distribution of moderate and high alcohol consumption and of alcohol-related disabilities over time in Stockholm County and in Sweden. *Addiction* 1996;**91**:1307–23.

64 **Ferrence R**. Diffusion theory and drug use. *Addiction* 2001;**96**:165–73.

65 **Guendelman S, Abrams B**. Dietary, alcohol, and tobacco intake among Mexican-American women of childbearing age: results from HANES data. *Am J Health Prom* 1994;**8**:363–72.

66 **Williams R, Shams M**. Generational continuity and change in British Asian health and health behaviour. *J Epidemiol Community Health* 1998;**52**:558–63.

67 **Stephen AM, Wald NJ**. Trends in individual consumption of dietary fat in the United States, 1920–1984. *Am J Clin Nutr* 1990;**52**:457–69.

68 **Law M, Wald N**. Why heart disease mortality is low in France: the time lag explanation. *Br Med J* 1999;**318**:1471–80.

69 **Pill R, Parry O**. Making changes—women, food and families. *Health Ed J* 1989;**48**:51–4.

70 **Charles N, Kerr M**. *Women, Food and Families*. Manchester: Manchester University Press, 1988.

71 **Zive MM, Nicklas TA, Busch EC, Myers L, Berenson GS**. Marginal vitamin and mineral intakes of young adults: the Bogalusa Heart Study. *J Adolesc Health* 1996;**19**:39–47.

72 **Millen BE, Quatromoni PA, Franz MM, Epstein BE, Cupples LA, Copenhafer DL**. Population nutrient intake approaches to dietary recommendations: 1991 to 1995 Framingham Nutrition Studies. *J Am Diet Assoc* 1997;**97**:742–9.

73 **Stephen AM, Sieber GM**. Trends in individual fat consumption in the UK 1900–1985. *Br J Nutr* 1994; **71**:775–88.

74 **Boyd Orr J**. *Food Health and Income*. London: Macmillan, 1937.

75 **Roos E, Lahelma E, Virtanen M, Prattala R, Pietinen P**. Gender, socioeconomic status and family as determinants of food behaviour. *Soc Sci Med* 1998;**46**:1519–29.

76 **Karvonen S, Rimpela A**. Socio-regional Context as a determinant of adolescents' health behaviour in Finland. *Soc Sci Med* 1996;**43**:1467–74.

77 **Irala-Estevez JD, Groth M, Johansson L, Oltersdorf U, Prattala R, Martinez-Gonzales MA**. A systematic review of socioeconomic differences in food habits in Europe: consumption of fruit and vegetables. *Eur J Clin Nutr* 2000;**54**:706–14.

78 **Li R, Serdula M, Bland S, Mokdad A, Bowman B, Nelson D**. Trends in fruit and vegetable consumption among adults in 16 US states: Behavioral Risk Factor Surveillance System, 1990–1996. *Am J Public Health* 2000;**90**:777–81.

79 **Braddon FEM, Wadsworth MEJ, Davies JMC, Cripps HA**. Social and regional differences in food and alcohol consumption and their measurement in a national birth cohort. *J Epidemiol Community Health* 1988;**42**:341–9.

80 **Charlton J, Quaife K**. Trends in diet 1841–1994. In Charlton J, Murphy M, eds. *The health of adult Britain 1841–1994*. London: ONS, HMSO, 1997:93–113.

81 **Lindstrom M, Hanson BS, Brunner E, Wirfalt E, Elmstahl S, Mattisson I et al**. Socioeconomic differences in fat intake in a middle-aged population: report from the Malmo Diet and Cancer Study. *Int J Epidemiol* 2000;**29**:438–48.

82 **Stallone DD, Brunner EJ, Bingham SA, Marmot MG**. Dietary assessment in Whitehall II: the influence of reporting bias on apparent socioeconomic variation in nutrient intakes. *Eur J Clin Nutr* 1997;**51**:815–25.

83 **Harnack LJ, Jeffery RW, Boutelle KN**. Temporal trends in energy intake in the United States: an ecologic perspective. *Am J Clin Nutr* 2000;**71**:1478–284.

84 **Durnin JVGA**. Physical activity levels past and present. In Norgan N, ed. *Physical activity and health*. Cambridge: Cambridge University Press, 1992:20–7.

85 **Office of Population Censuses and Surveys.** *General Household Survey 1990*. London: HMSO, 1992.

86 **Office of Population Censuses and Surveys.** *General Household Survey 1983*. London: HMSO, 1985.

87 **Jacobs DRJ, Hahn LP, Folsom AR, Hannan PJ, Sprafka JM, Burke GL.** Time trends in leisure-time physical activity in the upper midwest 1957–1987:University of Minnesota studies. *Epidemiology* 1991;2:8–15.

88 **Armstrong N, Welsman J.** *Young people and physical activity*. Oxford: Oxford University Press, 1997.

89 **Crespo CJ, Smit E, Andersen RE, Carter-Pokras O, Ainsworth BE.** Race/ethnicity, social class and their relation to physical inactivity during leisure time: results from the Third National Health and Nutrition Examination Survey, 1988–1994. *Am J Prev Med* 2000;**18**:46–53.

90 **Gottlieb NH, Baker JA.** The relative influence of health beliefs, parental and peer behaviors and exercise program participation on smoking, alcohol use and physical activity. *Soc Sci Med* 1986;**22**:915–27.

91 **Malcomson RW.** Sports in Society: a historical perspective. *Br J Sports History* 1984;**1**:60–72.

92 **Atkinson P.** Strong minds and weak bodies: sports, gymnastics and the medicalization of women's education. *Br J Sports History* 1985;**2**:62–71.

93 **Erens B, Primatesta P.** *Health Survey for England: cardiovascular disease '98*. London: Her Majesty's Stationery Office, 1999.

94 **Kuh DJL, Cooper C.** Physical activity at 36 years: patterns and childhood predictors in a longitudinal study. *J Epidemiol Community Health* 1992;**46**:114–9.

95 **Crespo CJ, Ainsworth BE, Keteyian SJ, Heath GW, Smit E.** Prevalence of physical inactivity and its relation to social class in U.S. adults: results from the Third National Health and Nutrition Examination Survey, 1988–1994. *Med Sci Sports Exerc* 1999;**31**:1821–7.

96 **Anderssen N, Jacobs Jr DR, Sidney S, Bild DE, Sternfeld B, Slattery ML** *et al.* Change and secular trends in physical activity patterns in young adults: a seven-year longitudinal follow-up in the Coronary Artery Risk Development in Young Adults Study (CARDIA). *Am J Epidemiol* 1996;**143**:351–62.

97 **Brownson RC, Eyler AA, King AC, Brown DR, Shyu Y-L, Sallis JF.** Patterns and correlates of physical activity among US women 40 Years and older. *Am J Public Health* 2000;**90**:264–70.

98 **Lindbladh E, Lyttkens H, Hanson BS, Ostergren P-O.** The diffusion model and the socio-hierarchical process of change. *Health Prom Int* 1997;**12**:323–30.

99 **Wadsworth M.** Early life. In Marmot M, Wilkinson RG, eds. *Social determinants of health*. Oxford: OUP, 1999:44–63.

100 **US Department of Health and Human Services.** *Preventing tobacco use among young people*. A report of the Surgeon General, Public Health Service, Centers for Disease Control and Prevention, Office on Smoking and Health. Washington,DC: US Department of Health & Human Services, 1994.

101 **Fillmore KM.** Women's drinking across the adult life course as compared to men's. *Br J Addict* 1987;**82**:801–11.

102 **Sillitoe KK.** *Planning for Leisure*. London: HMSO, 1969.

103 **Stephens T.** Secular trends in adult physical activity: exercise boom or bust? *Res Q Exerc Sport* 1987;**58**:94–105.

104 **Tyas SL, Pederson LL.** Psychosocial factors related to adult smoking: a critical review of the literature. *Tob Control* 1998;7:409–20.

105 Derzon JH, Lipsey MW. Predicting tobacco use to age 18: a synthesis of longitudinal research. *Addiction* 1999;**94**:995–1006.

106 Conrad KM, Flay BR, Hill D. Why children start smoking cigarettes: predictors of onset. *Br J of Addiction* 1992;**87**:1711–24.

107 Batty D, Leon DA. *Socioeconomic position and coronary heart disease risk factors in children and young people—evidence from UK epidemiological studies.* British Heart Foundation, 2002.

108 Leino M, Porkka KVK, Raitakari OT, Laitinen S, Taimela S, Viikari JSA. Influence of Parental Occupation on Coronary Heart Disease Risk Factors in Children. The Cardiovascular Risk in Young Finns Study. *Int J Epidemiol* 1996;**25**:1189–95.

109 Tuinstra J, Groothoff GW, van den Heuvel WJA, Post D. Socioeconomic differences in health risk behaviour in adolescence: do they exist? *Soc Sci Med* 1998;**47**:67–74.

110 Bewdley BR, Day I, Ide L. *Smoking by children in Great Britain—A review of the literature.* London: Social Science Research Council—Medical Research Council, 1973.

111 Johnson RA, Hoffman JP. Adolescent cigarette smoking in U.S. racial/ethnic subgroups: findings from the National Education Longitudinal Study. *J Health Soc Behav* 2000;**41**:392–407.

112 Van Lenthe FJ, Boreham CA, Twisk JW, Strain JJ, Savage JM, Smith GD. Socioeconomic position and coronary heart disease risk factors in youth. Findings from the Young Hearts Project in Northern Ireland. *Eur J Public Health* 2001;**11**:43–50.

113 Sweeting H, Anderson A, West P. Socio-demographic correlates of dietary habits in mid to late adolescence. *Eur J Clin Nutr* 1994;**48**:736–48.

114 Neumark-Sztainer D, Story M, Resnick MD, Blum RW. Correlates of inadequate fruit and vegetable consumption among adolescents. *Prev Med* 1996;**25**:497–505.

115 Green G, MacIntyre S, West P, Ecob R. Like parent like child? Associations between drinking and smoking behaviour of parents and their children. *Br J Addict* 1991;**86**:745–58.

116 Vilhjalmsson R, Thorlindsson T. Factors relating to physical activity: a study of adolescents. *Soc Sci Med* 1998;**47**:665–75.

117 Offord DR, Lipman EL, Duku EK. *Sports, the arts and community programs: rates and correlates of participation.* Ottawa: report from the National Longitudinal Survey of Children and Youth, ~W-98–18E. Ottawa: Human Resources Development Canada, 1998.

118 Isohanni M, Moilanen I, Rantakallio P. Determinants of teenage smoking with special reference to non-standard family background. *Br J Addict* 1991;**86**:391–8.

119 Lifrak PD, McKay JR, Rostain A, Alterman AI, O'Brien CP. Relationship of perceived competencies, perceived social support, and gender to substance use in young adolescents. *J Am Acad Child Adolesc Psychiatry* 1997;**36**:933–40.

120 Koivusilta L, Rimpela A, Rimpela M. Health related lifestyle in adolescence predicts adult educational level: a longitudinal study from Finland. *J Epidemiol Community Health* 1998;**52**:794–801.

121 Brunner E, Shipley MJ, Blane D, Davey Smith G, Marmot MG. When does cardiovascular risk start? Past and present socioeconomic circumstances and risk factors in adulthood. *J Epidemiol Community Health* 1999;**53**:757–64.

122 van de Mheen H, Stronks K, Looman CWN, Mackenbach JP. Does childhood socioeconomic status influence adult health through behavioural factors? *Int J Epidemiol* 1998;**27**:431–7.

123 Leino M, Raitakari OT, Porkka KV, Taimela S, Viikari JS. Associations of education with cardiovascular risk factors in young adults: the Cardiovascular Risk in Young Finns Study. *Int J Epidemiol* 1999;**28**:667–75.

124 Wadsworth MEJ, Kuh DJL. Childhood influences on adult health: a review of recent work in the British 1946 national birth cohort study, the MRC National Survey of Health and Development. *Paediatr Perinat Epidemiol* 1997;**11**:2–20.

125 Bandura A. *Social Learning Theory*. Englewood Cliffs, New Jersey: Prentice Hall, 1977.

126 Harris RE, Zang EA, Anderson JI, Wynder EL. Race and sex Differences in lung cancer risk associated with cigarette smoking. *Int J Epidemiol* 1993;**22**:592–9.

127 Vandell DL. Parents, peer groups, and other socializing influences. *Dev Psychol* 2000;**36**:699–710.

128 Bogenschneider K, Wu MY, Raffaelli M, Tsay JC. Parent influences on adolescent peer orientation and substance use: the interface of parenting practices and values. *Child Dev* 1998;**69**:1672–88.

129 Wickrama KAS, Conger RD, Wallace LE, Elder GHJr. The intergenerational transmission of health risk behaviours: adolescent lifestyles and gender moderating effects. *J Health Soc Behav* 1999;**40**:258–72.

130 Murray M, Kiryluk S, Swan AV. Relation between parents' and children's smoking behaviour and attitudes. *J Epidemiol Community Health* 1985;**39**:269–74.

131 Osler M, Clausen J, Ibsen KK, Jensen G. Maternal smoking during childhood and increased risk of smoking in young adulthood. *Int J Epidemiol* 1995;**24**:710–4.

132 Chassin L, Presson CC, Todd M, Rose JS, Sherman SJ. Maternal socialization: the intergenerational transmission of parenting and smoking. *Dev Psychol* 1998;**34**:1189–201.

133 Rossow I, Rise J. Concordance of parental and adolescent health behaviors. *Soc Sci Med* 1994;**38**:1299–305.

134 Anderssen N, Wold B. Parental and peer influences on leisure-time physical activity in young adolescents. *Res Q Exerc Sport* 1992;**63**:341–8.

135 Swan GE. Implications of genetic epidemiology for the prevention of tobacco use. *Nicotine Tob Res* 1999;**1**(Suppl1):S49–56.

136 Koopmans JR, Boomsma DI. Familial resemblances in alcohol use: genetic or cultural transmission? *J Stud Alcohol* 1996;**57**:19–28.

137 Viken RJ, Kaprio J, Koskenvuo M, Rose RJ. Longitudinal analyses of the determinants of drinking and of drinking to intoxication in adolescent twins. *Behav Genet* 1999;**29**:455–61.

138 Beunen G, Thomis M. Genetic determinants of sports participation and daily physical activity. *Int J Obes Relat Metab Disord* 1999;**23**(Suppl 3):S55–63.

139 West P, Sweeting H, Ecob R. Family and friends' influences on the uptake of regular smoking from mid-adolescence to early adulthood. *Addiction* 1999;**94**:1397–411.

140 Wilks J, Callan VJ, Austin DA. Parent, peer and personal determinants of adolescent drinking. *Br J of Addiction* 1989;**84**:619–30.

141 Feunekes GI, de Graaf C, Meyboom S, van Staveren WA. Food choice and fat intake of adolescents and adults: associations of intakes within social networks. *Prev Med* 1998;**27**:645–56.

142 Glendinning A, Hendry L, Shucksmith J. Lifestyle, health and social class in adolescence. *Soc Sci Med* 1995;**41**:235–48.

143 Fergusson DM, Horwood LJ. Prospective childhood predictors of deviant peer affiliations in adolescence. *J Child Psychol Psychiatry* 1999;**40**:581–92.

144 Han C, McGue MK, Iacono WG. Lifetime tobacco, alcohol and other substance use in adolescent Minnesota twins: univariate and multivariate behavioral genetic analyses. *Addiction* 1999;**94**:981–93.

145 Twisk JWR, Kemper HCG, van Mechelen W, Post GB. Tracking of risk factors for coronary heart disease over a 14-year period: a comparison between lifestyle and biologic risk factors with data from the Amsterdam Growth and Health Study. *Am J Epidemiol* 1997; **145**:888–98.

146 Kelder SH, Perry CL, Klepp K-I, Lytle LL. Longitudinal tracking of adolescent smoking, physical activity, and food choice behaviors. *Am J Public Health* 1994;**84**:1121–6.

147 Wald N, Kiryluk S, Barby S, Doll R, Pike M, Peto R. U.K. *Smoking Statistics*. Oxford: Oxford University Press, 1988.

148 Breslau N, Peterson EL. Smoking cessation in young adults: age at initiation of cigarette smoking and other suspected influences. *Am J Public Health* 1996;**86**:214–20.

149 Coambs RB, Li S, Kozlowski LT. Age interacts with heaviness of smoking in predicting success in cessation of smoking. *Am J Epidemiol* 1992;**86**:214–20.

150 Dunn JE, Liu K, Greenland P, Hilner JE, Jacobs Jr DR. Seven-year tracking of dietary factors in young adults: The CARDIA Study. *Am J Prev Med* 2000;**18**:38–45.

151 Post GB, de Vente W, Kemper HCG, Twisk JWR. Longitudinal trends in and tracking of energy and nutrient intake over 20 years in a Dutch cohort of men and women between 13 and 33 years of age: the Amsterdam Growth and Health longitudinal study. *Br J Nutr* 2001;**85**:375–85.

152 Cusatis DC, Chinchilli VM, Johnson-Rollings N, Kieselhorst K, Stallings VA, Lloyd T. Longitudinal nutrient intake patterns of U.S. adolescent women: The Penn State Young Women's Health Study. *J Adolesc Health* 2000;**26**:194–204.

153 Telama R, Yang X, Laakso L, Viikari J. Physical activity in childhood and adolescence as predictor of physical activity in young adulthood. *Am J Prev Med* 1997;**13**:317–23.

154 Raitakari OT, Porkka KV, Taimela S, Telama R, Rasanen L, Viikari JS. Effects of persistent physical activity and inactivity on coronary risk factors in children and young adults. The Cardiovascular Risk in Young Finns Study. *Am J Epidemiol* 1994;**140**:195–205.

155 Glenmark B, Healberg G, Jansson E. Prediction of physical activity level in adulthood by physical characteristics, physical performance and physical activity in adolescence: an 11-year follow-up study. *Eur J Appl Physiol* 1994;**69**:530–8.

156 Scott D, Willits FK. Adolescent and adult leisure patterns: a 37-year follow-up study. *Leisure Sci* 1989;**11**:323–35.

157 Hertzman C, Wiens M. Child development and long-term outcomes: a population health perspective and summary of successful interventions. *Soc Sci Med* 1996;**43**:1083–95.

158 Kuh D, Power C, Blane D, Bartley M. Social pathways between childhood and adult health. In Kuh D, Ben-Shlomo Y, eds. *A life course approach to chronic disease epidemiology: tracing the origins of ill-health from early to adult life*, Oxford: Oxford University Press, 1997:169–200.

159 Goddard D. *Why Children Start Smoking*. London: HMSO, 1990.

160 Wolfinger NH. The effects of parental divorce on adult tobacco and alcohol consumption. *J Health Soc Behav* 1998;**39**:254–69.

161 Anda RF, Croft JB, Felitti VJ, Nordenberg D, Giles WH, Wlliamson DF *et al*. Adverse childhood experiences and smoking during adolescence and adulthood. *J Am Med Assoc* 1999;**282**:1652–8.

162 Lynch JW, Kaplan GA, Salonen JT. Why do people behave poorly? Variation in adult health behaviours and psychosocial characteristics by stages of the socioeconomic lifecourse. *Soc Sci Med* 1997;**44**:809–19.

163 Baumrind D. Rearing competent children. In Damon W, ed. *Child development today and tomorrow*. San Francisco: Jossey-Bass, 1989:349–78.

164 Darling N, Steinberg I. Parenting styles as context: an integrative model. *Psychol Bull* 1993;**113**:487–96.

165 Stice E, Barrera M. A Longitudinal Examination of the reciprocal relations between perceived parenting and adolescents' substance use and externalizing behaviours. *Dev Psychol* 1995;**31**:322–34.

166 Weiss LH, Schwarz JC. The relationship between parenting types and older adolescents' personality, academic achievement, adjustment, and substance use. *Child Dev* 1996;**67**:2101–14.

167 **Foxcroft DR, Lowe G**. Adolescent drinking behaviour and family socialization factors: a meta-analysis. *J Adolesc* 1991;**14**:255–73.

168 **Tiet QQ, Bird HR, Davies M, Hoven C, Cohen P, Jensen PS** *et al*. Adverse life events and resilience. *J Am Acad Child Adolesc Psychiatry* 1998;**37**:1191–200.

169 **Dunn J, Davies LC, O'Connor TG, Sturgess W**. Parents' and partners' life course and family experiences: links with parent-child relationships in different family settings. *J Child Psychol Psychiatry* 2000;**41**:955–68.

170 **De Garmo DS, Forgatch MS, Nartubez CR**. Parenting of divorced mothers as a link between social status and boys' academic outcomes: unpacking the effects of socioeconomic status. *Child Dev* 1999;**70**:1231–45.

171 **Epstein JA, Griffin KW, Botvin GJ**. Competence skills help deter smoking among inner city adolescents. *Tob Control* 2000;**9**:33–9.

172 **Epstein JA, Griffin KW, Botvin GJ**. Role of general and specific competence skills in protecting inner-city adolescents from alcohol use. *J Stud Alcohol* 2000;**61**:379–86.

173 **Loveland-Cherry CJ, Leech S, Laetz VB, Dielman TE**. Correlates of alcohol use and misuse in fourth-grade children: psychosocial, peer, parental, and family factors. *Health Educ Q* 1996;**23**:497–511.

174 **Jackson C, Henriksen L, Dickinson D, Levine DW**. The early use of alcohol and tobacco: its relation to children's competence and parents' behavior. *Am J Public Health* 1997;**87**:359–64.

175 **Dwyer JJ, Allison KR, Makin S**. Internal structure of a measure of self-efficacy in physical activity among high school students. *Soc Sci Med* 1998;**46**:1175–82.

176 **Baranowski T, Cullen KW, Baranowski J**. Psychosocial correlates of dietary intake: advancing dietary intervention. *Annu Rev Nutr* 1999;**19**:17–40.

177 **Keating DP, Miller FK**. Individual pathways in competence and coping: from regulatory systems to habits of mind. In Keating DP, Hertzman C, eds. *Developmental health and the wealth of nations. Social, biological and educational dynamics*. New York: The Guilford Press, 2001:220–33.

178 **Finn SE**. Stability of personality self-ratings over 30 years: evidence for an age/cohort interaction. *J Pers Soc Psychol* 1910;**50**:813–8.

179 **Gest SD**. Behavioural Inhibition: Stability and associations with adaptation from childhood to early adulthood. *J Pers Soc Psychol* 1997;**72**:467–75.

180 **Schooling, M**. *Health behaviour in a social and temporal context*. Unpublished PhD thesis, Royal Free and University College London. 2001.

181 **Goffman E**. *The presentation of self in everyday life*. London: Penguin, 1990.

182 **Giddens A**. *Modernity and self-identity, self and society in the late modern age*. Cambridge: Polity Press, 1991.

183 **Douglas M**. *Thought styles*. London: Sage, 1996.

184 **Hofstede G**. *Culture's consequences. International differences in work-related values*. London: Sage, 1980.

185 **Huselid RF, Cooper ML**. Gender roles as mediators of sex differences in adolescent alcohol use. *J Health Soc Behav* 1992;**33**:348–62.

186 **Ryckman RM, Hamel J**. Female adolescents' motives related to involvement in organised team sports. *Int J Sport Psychol* 1992;**23**:147–60.

187 **Osler M**. Unemployment and change in smoking behaviour among Danish adults. *Tob Control* 1995;**4**:53–6.

188 **Temple MT, Fillimore KM, Hartka E, Johnstone B, Leino EV, Motoyoshi M**. A meta-analysis of change in marital and employment status as predictors of alcohol consumption on a typical occasion. *Br J Addict* 1991;**86**:1269–81.

189 **Hajema K-J, Knibbe RA**. Changes in social roles as predictors of changes in drinking behaviour. *Addiction* 1998;**93**:1717–27.

190 **Luto R, Poilkolainen K, Uutela A**. Unemployment, sociodemographic background and consumption of alcohol before and during the economic recession of the 1990s in Finland. *Int J Epidemiol* 1998;**27**:623–9.

191 **Leonard KE, das Eiden R**. Husband's and wife's drinking: unilateral or bilateral influences among newlyweds in a general population sample. *J Stud Alcohol* 1999;**13**(**Suppl**):130–8.

192 **Osler M, Prescott E**. Psychosocial, behavioural and health determinants of successful smoking cessation: a longitudinal study of Danish adults. *Tob Control* 1998;**7**:262–7.

193 **Kemmer D, Anderson AS, Marshall DW**. The 'Marriage Menu': life, food and diet in transition. In Murcott A, ed. *The Nation's Diet*. London: Longman, 1998:197–208.

194 **Richards M, Hardy R, Wadsworth M**. The effects of divorce and separation on mental health in a national UK birth cohort. *Psychol Med* 1997;**27**:1121–8.

195 **Umberson D**. Gender, marital status and the social control of health behavior. *Soc Sci Med* 1992;**34**:907–17.

196 **Owen L, McNeill A, Callum C**. Trends in smoking during pregnancy in England, 1992–7: quota sampling surveys. *Br Med J* 1998;**317**:728.

197 **Cnattingius S, Lindmark G, Meirik O**. Who continues to smoke while pregnant? *J Epidemiol Community Health* 1992;**46**:218–21.

198 **Mas R, Escriba V, Colomer C**. Who quits smoking during pregnancy? *Scan J Soc Med* 1996;**24**:102–6.

199 **Jarvis MJ**. The association between having children, family size and smoking cessation in adults. *Addiction* 1996;**91**:427–34.

200 **Sternfeld B, Ainsworth BE, Quesenberry CP**. Physical activity patterns in a diverse population of women. *Prev Med* 1999;**28**:313–23.

201 **Wilcox S, Castro C, King AC, Housemann R, Brownson RC**. Determinants of leisure time physical activity in rural compared with urban older and ethnically diverse women in the United States. *J Epidemiol Community Health* 2000;**54**:667–72.

202 **Do KA, Green JR, Dudley EC, Burger HG, Dennerstein L**. Longitudinal study of risk factors for coronary heart disease across the menopausal transition. *Am J Epidemiol* 2000;**151**:584–93.

203 **Freund KM, D'Agostino RB, Belanger AJ, Kannel WB, Stokes 3rd J**. Predictors of smoking cessation: the Framingham Study. *Am J Epidemiol* 1992;**135**:957–64.

204 **Hebert JR, Ebbeling CB, Olendzki BC, Hurley TG, Ma Y, Saal N** *et al*. Change in women's diet and body mass following intensive intervention for early-stage breast cancer. *J Am Diet Assoc* 2001;**101**:421–31.

205 **Neil HA, Roe L, Godlee RJ, Moore JW, Clark GM, Brown J** *et al*. Randomised trial of lipid lowering dietary advice in general practice: the effects on serum lipids, lipoproteins, and antioxidants. *Br Med J* 1995;**310**:569–73.

206 **Lesko, N**. The curriculum of the body. In Roman, LG, Christian-Smith. L, eds. *Becoming Feminine: the Politics of Popular Culture*, London: Falmer Press, 1988.

207 **Pavis S, Cunningham-Burley S**. Male youth street culture: understanding the context of health-related behaviours. *Health Ed Res: Theory Pract* 1999;**14**:583–96.

208 **Skeggs, B**. *Formations of Class and Gender*. London: Sage, 1997.

209 **Bourdieu, P**. *Distinction*. London: Routledge, 1984.

210 **Bauman, Z**. *Work, Consumerism and the New Poor*. Buckingham: Open University Press, 1998.

Chapter 14

Overweight and obesity from a life course perspective

Chris Power and Tessa Parsons

Obesity is an increasing problem in the UK and other developed countries, in adults and in children. Women who are obese experience adverse health consequences throughout life, though it is in relation to adult chronic disease that the effects of obesity are best documented. Undesirable socioeconomic consequences, such as lower educational attainment and income, have also been observed for obese women. Research on the causes of obesity implicates factors at different life stages, but increasingly emphasizes early life, in particular social factors, parental adiposity, intrauterine growth, timing of maturation, diet, physical activity and behavioural and psychosocial factors. Diet and physical activity are suspected as the primary underlying factors and, although direct evidence is weak, there are indications that activity attenuates weight gain. The most consistent findings are for parental fatness and tracking of fatness from childhood to adulthood: women born to fatter parents and who themselves were fat in childhood, have increased risks of obesity in adult life. There are, in addition, several adult life factors, such as smoking habit, pregnancy, and menopause, which may influence obesity risk among women, but for many of these factors effects appear to be modest. Early life may therefore offer the greatest potential for policies aimed at reducing the prevalence of obesity and its associated social and health burden.

14.1 Introduction

The World Health Organisation (WHO) recently pronounced that obesity should be regarded as today's principal neglected public health problem, with adverse effects on multiple health outcomes, including mortality due to non-insulin dependent diabetes, coronary heart disease, and certain cancers.[1] Dramatic increases in the prevalence of obesity have occurred worldwide, both in women and in men, particularly in developed countries. The rapid increase in prevalence and distribution of obesity is associated with urban western culture; environment and lifestyles therefore provide a focus of research. Although many of the trends in obesity are similar for women and men, some differing patterns on the associated health consequences and causes of obesity are apparent. In this overview of obesity among women, we consider the causes of obesity from a life course perspective. Our emphasis is on factors that affect a woman's vulnerability to obesity, particularly those from childhood since it is suspected that obesity risk starts early in life. Although only a brief outline is provided on the consequences of obesity, here too several life stages are involved. Our review is not exhaustive, neglecting for example, some of the macro cultural and economic influences, such as the trends in urbanization and globalization, that shape the environment and lifestyles of women in developed countries. Though genetic factors may be important, they are also omitted as unlikely to account for the dramatic rise in prevalence of obesity, although genetic factors may interact with the lifestyle and environmental factors described here. The management and treatment of obesity are beyond the scope of this chapter, and research on body image was discussed in Chapter 9.

14.1.1 Definitions

Obesity is defined as an excess of body fat, which may be estimated using various alternative methods, the current gold standard being a multi-compartment model involving several detailed measurements of body composition.[2] Large epidemiological studies that may extend over long time periods require easily obtained measures such as weight relative to height, skinfold thicknesses, or body circumferences. Body mass index (BMI), defined as weight/height[2], a simple proxy measure of body fat and the most convenient measure to obtain, has become a standard for obesity assessment in adults.[1] The current definition for obesity in adults as proposed by WHO[1] (Table 14.1), is derived from comparisons of BMI with health outcomes, and the observation that mortality, and the risk of co-morbidities (e.g. hypertension, hyperlipidaemia) increase with BMI over 25 kg/m[2] and particularly with BMI over 30 kg/m[2].[1] Although the cut-offs apply to both sexes, women are known to have more body fat, on average, than men at identical levels of BMI.[3]

For life course studies, the measurement of obesity is most difficult in childhood, when the amount of body fat changes over different stages of growth and maturation. Despite its shortcoming, BMI has become more widely accepted for use in children,[1,4] although the cut-off for obesity has been arbitrary, with little standardization across studies. The approach taken to establish cut-offs in adults is less easily applied to children, although a recent study has plotted an international distribution of BMI, from early childhood to late

Table 14.1 WHO classification of BMI[(1)]

	BMI, (kg/m²)
Underweight	<18.5
Normal range	18.5–24.9
Preobese (or overweight)	25.0–29.9
Obese class 1	30.0–34.9
Obese class 2	35.0–39.9
Obese class 3	≥40.0

adolescence, and identified centiles that pass through the adult BMI cut-offs of 25 kg/m^2 and 30 kg/m^2 at age 18.[5]

Although these new standards for childhood overweight and obesity are likely to be useful in future life course studies, so far, a number of cut-offs have been used, both in children and adults, and studies quoted throughout this chapter use varying definitions of obesity.

Cut-offs for BMI, or any measure of body fat, present some problems. Changes in body fat occur not only in childhood, but also in adult life; during the first 18 years of the Framingham study about 75% of women experienced fluctuation in weight of 7 kg or more.[6] Whatever cut-off point is used, people will continually be crossing it to be above or below the threshold. Additional limitations of a weight/height based measure include the fact that a large range of percentage body fat may occur for a given BMI, that a high BMI may result from a high muscle mass, and that BMI does not indicate fat distribution. Excess abdominal fat, in contrast to excess fat around the hips and thighs, is an independent risk factor for diabetes, coronary heart disease, and premature death.[1] None the less, in adults, BMI predicts (cross-sectionally) external validity criteria, such as diastolic blood pressure and serum glucose, as well as other measures of body fat, including densitometry and skinfold thicknesses.[7]

14.1.2 Prevalence and time trends

The WHO MONICA (MONItoring of trends and determinants of CArdiovascular disease) study shows that in many countries women are more likely than men to be obese, whereas men are more likely to be overweight.[1] In most populations participating in the study, 50–75% of women aged 35–64 years were overweight or obese during the period 1983–1986. Secular trends suggest the problem may be even worse today. The prevalence of obesity in adults and children is rapidly increasing, not only in developed, but also in developing countries, where higher rates are associated with urban, more affluent populations. In general, industrialized countries have higher rates of obesity than developing countries, with countries undergoing transition falling in between, suggesting that obesity is associated with modern lifestyles and affluence. Good quality, nationally representative secular trend data for adults are available for North America, Brazil, parts of Europe, Australia, Japan, Samoa, and China. All data sets show alarmingly fast increases in rates of obesity. As examples, US data spanning 35 years (1960–1994) show an increase among women from 15% to 25%,[8] and the increase has continued until the end of the 1990s.[9,10] In Britain, 8% of women were obese in 1980;[11] in England only, 16.4% were obese in 1993 and 20.9% in 1999.[12] A Danish study suggests that BMI increases are highest for younger women,[13] and data from the MONICA study suggest that social inequalities in obesity in women are widening.[14] Women may not only be getting fatter, but changing in shape, towards a more centralized fat pattern, as indicated by secular increases in waist-hip ratio in Sweden and Finland.[15,16]

It is only more recently that obesity has become a recognized problem in children, with increasing trends seen in many countries. In England, the proportion of obese girls (4–11 years) has increased from 1.5% in 1974 to 2.6% in 1994.[17] Among 7–13 year-old Canadian girls, the prevalence of obesity doubled from 5% to 12% between 1981 and 1996.[18] In Japan, since 1970 the prevalence of obese girls has also doubled, to reach approximately 5% of 6–8 year-olds and 8% of 10–14 year-olds.[19] Even among preschool girls, the prevalence of overweight and obesity is increasing.[20]

14.2 **Social and health burden related to obesity**

The social and disease burden associated with obesity extends across the life span (Table 14.2; see also Chapters 2–7 and 9), starting with negative attitudes shown towards fatter body shapes in preschool girls.[21] Fatter girls show subsequently poorer self-esteem and cognitive outcomes during adolescence, and lower social and economic consequences in adulthood.[22,23] There is also an unfavourable biological profile associated with obesity in childhood,[24,25] which, later in life, predicts disease burden especially in relation to cardiovascular disease. Obesity that is acquired in adolescence and young adulthood has also been directly related to increased adult cardiovascular[26] and mortality[27] risks.

With increasing age, the disease burden associated with obesity becomes extensive (Table 14.2).[1,28,29] During the reproductive life stage, extremes of body weight are associated with reproductive irregularities, including increased risk of infertility and menstrual problems.[30,31] Obese women also have elevated risks of diabetes, gallbladder disease, hypertension, coronary heart disease, cancer (breast cancer, endometrial cancer, cervical cancer), respiratory problems, and arthritis.[1,28,29] Relative risks for some diseases are much higher for obese women than men, for example, 12.7 versus 5.2 for diabetes, 4.2 versus 2.6 for hypertension, and 3.2 versus 1.5 for myocardial infarction.[32] The risk of death from all causes, cardiovascular disease, cancer or other diseases, increases throughout the range of

Table 14.2 Social and disease burden associated with obesity among women

Lifestage	Biological/disease burden[1]		Social, economic / psychological burden
Childhood /adolescence	polycystic ovaries menstrual irregularities increased anaesthetic risk		social stigma, prejudice poor school performance[23] self-esteem fewer years of school[22]

Adulthood -early	breast, endometrial, cervical and colon cancers
	reproductive hormone abnormalities
	impaired fertility
	obstetric complications/fetal defects
	  (caesarean operation, large babies,
	  neural tube defects)
	low back pain
			less likely to marry[22]
			lower income[22]

-later	**non-insulin dependent diabetes dyslipidaemia breathlessness coronary heart disease osteoarthritis (knees)** varicose veins deep vein thrombosis haemorrhoids	**insulin resistance gallbladder disease sleep apnoea hypertension gout**	

[1] Adapted from Jung[121] and WHO[1]

Conditions in bold text are those identified by the WHO for which the risk is considerably increased with obesity (relative risk ≥2)[1]

moderate to severe overweight.[29] Overweight is regarded as a fundamental avoidable cause of female cancers, with an estimated 6% of all incident cancers in the European Union potentially preventable if there were no women with a BMI greater than 25 kg/m[2].[33] Some studies report waist-hip ratio or waist circumference to be stronger predictors of mortality,[34] coronary heart disease,[35] and diabetes than BMI[36] although possibly less predictive of cancer incidence.[34]

14.3 **Changes in fatness (BMI) over the lifespan**

During the first year of life, BMI increases rapidly, but then decreases, reaching a minimum at approximately 5 or 6 years. This point of minimum BMI has been called the adiposity rebound,[37] since BMI then starts to increase again (Fig. 14.1). Age trends in BMI are due in part to changes in proportion of body fat, but also to changing weight-for-height relationships, and therefore may not replicate exactly with other measures; some studies show a rebound effect with skinfold thicknesses,[38] whereas others do not.[39]

During adulthood, BMI increases most rapidly in early adulthood, as illustrated in the Health Survey for England (Fig. 14.2), and this is followed by a steady increase to the mid-fifties (55–64 years). Thereafter, the increase in BMI is more gradual and then declines in the oldest age groups. However, the change of BMI with age does not reveal the tendency for lean body mass to be lost with increasing age: older persons have a relatively greater percentage body fat than younger age groups of comparable BMI.[3] Also, among women, the distribution of body fat changes with increasing age. Before menopause women tend to accumulate fat peripherally rather than centrally, with a result that they accumulate more body fat before reaching the amount of abdominal fat that is generally found in

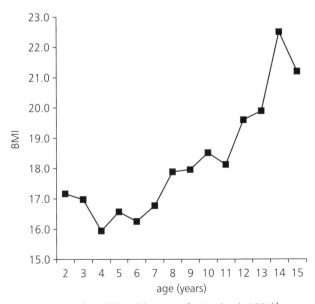

Fig. 14.1 BMI and age in English girls (Health Survey for England, 1991)[1].

[1]Data available from HSE website http://www.doh.gov.uk/stats/trends1.htm.

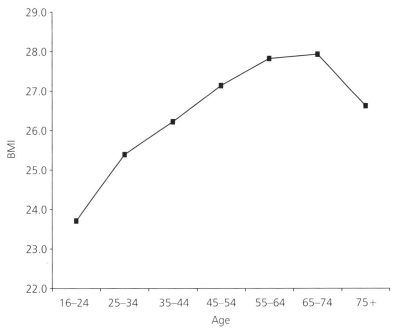

Fig. 14.2 BMI and age in English women (Health Survey for England, 1999)[1].

[1]Data available from HSE website http://www.doh.gov.uk/stats/trends1.htm.

men.[40] Then, around the time of the menopause there is accelerated visceral fat deposition.[41]

14.4 Causes of obesity: explanations across the life course

The lifespan patterns described above, provide some clues for the timing of possible causes of obesity. Childhood has been studied extensively, as it is suspected that there may be critical periods of development when environmental influences on obesity are most marked. Three stages have been identified as potentially important; the prenatal period, the adiposity rebound (second rise in adiposity occurring at about 6 years), and puberty.[42] With many studies now focusing on childhood factors, evidence is likely to be forthcoming on whether critical periods exist. But there are other reasons why childhood attracts interest. First, lifestyles established during childhood may track, albeit modestly, through to adult life (see Chapter 13),[43] and second as we describe below, adult obesity is related to earlier patterns of growth, most obviously to childhood fatness.

14.4.1 Childhood and adolescence

In a recent review of childhood factors and adult obesity we assessed the role of several potential influences, including parental fatness, patterns of growth and maturation, social factors, childhood diet, physical (in)activity and behavioural/psychosocial factors.[44] Table 14.3 summarizes the main findings from studies included in the review, and from more recent longitudinal studies, reporting data for females.

Table 14.3 Childhood predictors of obesity: evidence from longitudinal studies of at least 1 year duration

Predictor	Number of studies (to adulthood)[1]	Extra studies (to adulthood)[2]	Summary of main findings
Genetic–inheritance of phenotype	2(46;122) (2)(46,122)		Consistent evidence that offspring fatness increases with parental fatness. Evidence from few longitudinal studies supported by numerous family, twin and adoption studies. Relationship may be stronger between mother and offspring, stronger in younger children, and parental obesity may increase tracking of offspring obesity. Proportion of inherited fatness due to genetic and environmental components is unclear.
Intra-uterine growth	9(47;50;82;100;123–126) (3)(47;100)	3(48;127;128) (3)(48;127;128)	Consistent evidence from some large, some smaller studies for positive relationship between birthweight and subsequent fatness. Some J-shape relationships reported in adulthood.
Maturation	16(37;56;62;127;129–141) (14)(37;56;62;127;129–139)	3(57;58;142) (3)(57;58;142)	Consistent evidence from some large, some smaller studies for earlier or faster maturation being associated with increased subsequent fatness. Relationship holds true for variety of maturation markers; age of menarche, pubertal stage, skeletal age, adiposity rebound.
Social factors	8(100;126;143–148) (5)(100;143–146)		Consistent evidence from mostly large studies for a higher risk of fatness associated with a lower social group.
Dietary factors (i) infant feeding	3(149–151) (1)(150)	4(69–72)	Some large, some small studies arguing both for a protective effect of breast feeding and for no effect.
(ii) post-weaning energy intake	2(75;76) (1)(76)	1(77)	Few studies suggesting lower or higher energy intake may be associated with greater . subsequent fatness.
% energy from fat	1(76) (1)(76)	1(77)	One small, one large study suggesting no relationship between % energy intake from fat and subsequent fatness.
% energy from carbohydrate	1(76) (1)(76)		One small study suggesting a positive relationship between % energy intake from carbohydrate and subsequent fatness.
% energy from protein	1(76) (1)(76)		One small study suggesting no relationship between % energy intake from protein and subsequent fatness.

Physical activity (i) pre-walking	1[152]		Few studies/poor evidence suggesting no relationship between infant activity and childhood fatness.
(ii) post walking	6[76;83;152–155] (2)[76,83]	1[77]	Mostly small studies showing either no association between activity and fatness, or lower activity level predicting greater fatness. One study reports no effect of TV viewing, one study reports unfavourable effect on obesity.
Behavioural and psychological factors	3[85–87] (1)[86]		Few diverse studies, suggesting possible relationships between achievement motivation, physical appearance, social acceptance, behavioural conduct and fatness (and no effect of various other factors)

[1] Adapted from Parsons et al.[44] to include only studies presenting data separately for females. Studies searched for up to March–May 1998.

[2] Additional studies identified since review completed and discussed in this chapter.

14.4.1.1 Parental fatness

Parental fatness is known to increase the risk of obesity among their offspring, although the magnitude of the genetic, as compared with the environmental contribution is still debated. Children may inherit a susceptibility to fatness through genes shared with their parents, but they also inherit lifestyle factors, such as dietary, physical activity and/or socioeconomic patterns that may promote obesity. Inherited genes and lifestyle factors potentially operate across the life course, though we might expect their impact to be greatest in childhood and then diminish. One study demonstrates this trend with parental fatness having a greater impact on offspring fatness before six years, and becoming less important with increasing age of offspring.[45] Parental obesity also appears to influence the child's tracking of obesity through to adult life, which is much stronger if both parents are obese.[46]

14.4.1.2 Patterns of early growth and child-adult tracking of fatness

Intrauterine and childhood growth and maturation differ for boys and girls, for example female fetuses grow more slowly than male fetuses, and girls enter puberty earlier. In turn, certain patterns of early growth are suspected to influence the development of obesity. Birthweight is often used to indicate fetal growth, with several studies showing a consistent positive relationship with later BMI (Table 14.3). A J-shaped or U-shaped relationship is also seen, with a higher prevalence of obesity at the lowest and highest birthweights,[47–49] but less in childhood than in adulthood, suggesting a more complex association between fetal growth and obesity. Maternal fatness appears to influence the relationship[50] and may be the main underlying explanation for the association between birthweight and BMI.[49]

In monozygotic twins, birthweight differences are unrelated to adult differences in relative weight, suggesting that, after allowing for genetic factors, the fetal environment is not a significant contributor to adult fatness.[51] Studies of prenatal exposure to famine seem to refute this argument. The Dutch Famine Study showed adverse effects on body weight, BMI, and waist circumference at age 50 in women exposed to famine in early gestation, whereas famine in the last trimester and postnatally was associated with a reduced obesity risk.[52] Studies of maternal smoking in pregnancy also suggest that the fetal environment is important, with girls born to smokers experiencing rapid weight gain and increased fatness in childhood.[53]

Postnatally, childhood fatness is an important factor, due to tracking of fatness through to adulthood. Fatter girls have a high risk of going on to become fat women, although risk estimates depend on the measures used and study duration.[54,55] To illustrate, 12% of all women in the 1958 British birth cohort were obese adults (33 years) but among those with a BMI above the 95th centile at age 7 or age 16 the prevalence was greater (44% and 56% respectively).[56]

Earlier and faster maturation is also associated with obesity risk in women. Some argue that an earlier adiposity rebound increases the risk of later fatness, possibly independently of BMI at the age of rebound (which is greater in those with an early rebound) or parental obesity (more prevalent in those with an early rebound).[57] But age of rebound may add little to the prediction of adult obesity, if BMI at age seven years, i.e. following rebound, and height in childhood are known.[58] Links with other measures of maturation, particularly during puberty have long been noted: those more advanced in biological maturation tend to be taller, heavier and fatter than average and later maturing individuals of the same chronological age.[59,60] The greater subsequent fatness of early maturing girls is a remarkably consistent finding (Table 14.3), which seems to apply to measures of central adiposity as well as BMI.[61] Fatness earlier in childhood is also related to maturation, at least after three to four years of age,[44] foreshadowing the pattern seen in adulthood.[56] Activity levels, energy intake and protein intake are higher in late, than early maturing girls,[62] but how such relationships evolve across the life course is uncertain.

14.4.1.3 Social factors

Research on childhood growth has pointed to the possibility that early life may be an important life stage in the development of obesity risk, and there is now some support for this from work in developed countries on social factors at different life stages. Longitudinal studies consistently show that a lower socioeconomic position in childhood increases the risk of fatness in adulthood; seven of eight studies in Table 14.3 found this negative relationship, one study found no relationship.[44] Thus socioeconomic position in childhood seems to influence the development of obesity in adulthood, which cannot be explained by the reverse relationship whereby obesity affects the achievement of adult social position (Section 14.2). Being born into a particular social class cannot itself 'cause' obesity, but characteristics of socioeconomic groups related to material circumstances and behaviour or knowledge, which ultimately influence energy balance, might.

Further clues are provided by studies that distinguish between effects of alternative socioeconomic indicators at different life stages. Socioeconomic position early in life and education are related to adult BMI,[63] arguing for early childhood being an important life stage in determining obesity risk as well as adulthood. Specific social factors, such as family structure and functioning, age of mother at the birth of her child, residential area, and scholarly abilities in childhood are only rarely examined and the results are inconsistent.[44] However, one study suggested that parental neglect during childhood was a key factor, increasing the risk of obesity in early adulthood (21 years) by seven-fold in comparison with children assessed as having the support of their parents.[64]

Obesity rates in children and adults vary within countries by geographical location and ethnic group, although how much this variation is due to social and biological factors is uncertain. In the US pre-pubescent Black girls are not fatter than White girls, but longitudinal data suggest that between 9 and 19 years, Black girls become progressively fatter than White girls.[65] Obesity prevalence among Black women is greater than among White, which does not seem to be explained by differences in socioeconomic status.[66]

14.4.1.4 Diet

Energy intake and the specific dietary constituents are an important consideration in studies on obesity. Different stages of childhood have been investigated, but the main distinction is between feeding method in infancy and the post weaning diet.

Arguments about infant feeding have centred around whether the infant's ability to regulate its intake, and/or the mother's encouragement to feed, differs between breast and formula feeding. Formula (bottle) feeding is frequently cited as a contributor to obesity, since in earlier studies, formula-fed infants were larger than breastfed infants.[67] Relationships with obesity may have changed over time, with changes in the composition of infant formulas, and parental attitudes to feeding.[67] Modern formulas resemble breast milk more closely and infants fed old-style formulas consumed significantly more energy than those fed modern formulas or breast milk.[67] Length of breastfeeding and age of introduction of solid foods might also influence the infant's regulation of energy intake, since the introduction of solid foods may lead to excess energy intake by increasing the energy density of the diet.[68] The evidence for an effect of infant feeding method on later risk of obesity is inconclusive (Table 14.3). In boys and girls combined, two recent large studies argue for a protective effect of breastfeeding on obesity,[69,70] but others argue this is due to confounding with other factors, such as social class, or maternal fatness.[71–73]

There is more general acceptance that the post weaning diet is involved in obesity development, but even here the evidence is sparse and controversial. Higher energy intake may plausibly increase energy storage and body fat, but paradoxically energy intakes in adolescents, in the US, have decreased[74] while the prevalence of obesity has doubled.[1] Very few studies have investigated the effect of energy intake or macronutrient composition of the diet in childhood on subsequent fatness in women. Studies included in our review[44] suggest that increasing absolute energy intake is associated with *decreasing* fatness, (Table 14.3)[75,76] but not after adjustment for physical activity.[76] In contrast, a large and more recent study reports that the one-year change in BMI in adolescent girls was greater in those who consumed more calories (BMI increased by 0.006 kg/m^2 for each extra 100 kcals/day consumed) after adjusting for activity.[77] Overall, evidence is weak for an effect of any aspect of childhood diet on fatness in adult women,[44] which may seem surprising given the belief that there is tracking in food preferences and eating habits, in addition to any postulated physiological effects.

14.4.1.5 Physical (in)activity

Sedentary lifestyles require less energy expenditure than active ones and are thus implicated in the development of obesity. As obesity rates have increased, activity levels in developed countries have declined, as indicated by crude markers of (in)activity which show increased transport use and time spent watching television. Walking and cycling by children aged 14 years and under have declined by 20% and 26% respectively in the UK between 1985 and 1992[78] and by 40% in the US between 1977 and 1995.[79] In contrast, car travel by children in the UK increased concurrently by 40%.[78] Figures for television viewing in 1999 show girls in the UK watch 18 hours of television per week,[80] slightly more in the US. Activity and energy expenditure are not synonymous, and direct evidence of decreasing energy expenditure is lacking. Physical activity tracks to a moderate effect through the life course, although estimates may be stronger with more objective measures (e.g. heart rate monitoring rather than self report).[81] Yet activity patterns change; younger children are highly active, and much of their activity is play, which is sporadic and spontaneous in nature, whereas older children are less active, and their activity tends to be structured. Marked decreases in activity levels occur during adolescence, starting earlier in girls than in boys[82] and girls are less active than boys throughout the teenage years.[43,82]

Two studies identified for our review[44] included the adolescent period and both found activity to protect against increased fatness measured by skinfold thicknesses,[83,84] although Twisk *et al.*[84] also found an unfavourable effect on waist-hip ratio. A larger study of approximately 6000 girls (9–14 years) reports both a protective effect of activity, and an adverse effect of inactivity (watching television and playing computer/video games) on change in BMI over one year.[77] For each extra hour per day of television watched, BMI increased by 0.037 kg/m^2, and for each extra hour per day of physical activity (outside of school gym class) BMI decreased by 0.028 kg/m^2.[77] Several small studies of younger children are roughly divided between finding either no effect or a protective effect of activity, although findings sometimes depended on outcome or method of analysis (Table 14.3). Differences in methods and measures of physical activity may lead to inconsistencies between studies, particularly as it is unclear whether some types or aspects of physical activity (intensity, duration) are more relevant to obesity than others. Overall, however, the evidence suggests a protective effect of activity and adverse effect of inactivity on fatness.

14.4.1.6 Behavioural and psychological factors

Research on behavioural or psychological factors and obesity is largely cross-sectional, hence the direction of causality cannot be determined. The few longitudinal studies identified[44] describe a range of factors, some in infancy, and others in childhood. In studies looking at boys and girls combined, infant feeding style, feeding problems (undefined) and temperament were inconsistently related to subsequent fatness.[44] Gender differences perhaps become more critical in adolescence. For example, there is no relationship between self-esteem in three to six year old girls and later fatness,[85] but some evidence that girls with poorer achievement motivation (the need and will to achieve) at 13–16 years,[86] or poorer physical appearance and social acceptance self esteem at 12–15 years,[87] experience greater increases in central body fat[86] or BMI[87] over a three-year period.

14.4.2 **Adulthood**

Contemporary factors in adulthood are also likely to affect the development of obesity, as well as influences originating earlier in the life course. The fact that only a small proportion of fat adults are fat in childhood, suggests that influences in adulthood are important.[54,55] Some suspected factors are almost exclusive to adulthood, including marriage, pregnancy, hormone replacement therapy (HRT) and menopause, whilst others, such as smoking, weight cycling and dieting, are most common in adulthood. Another group of factors, including parental adiposity, diet, physical activity, social class, and education, probably continue to impact on adiposity throughout life.

14.4.2.1 Diet

Ecological data (per capita availability of energy and nutrients) suggest that energy intake has actually increased over the past few decades,[88] although reported adult energy intakes show a decrease. Also paradoxically, dietary surveys show lower energy intakes to be associated with higher BMIs in western countries. Firstly, these findings may be confounded by other factors, particularly energy expenditure. Secondly, under-reporting, both of total energy, and of fat and/or carbohydrate rich foods, is known to be a problem in the obese and may be becoming a more serious problem in the general population.[89] This may be a result of public health messages increasing awareness of a healthy diet. Energy intake may not be the most important aspect of diet that contributes to obesity; metabolic studies suggest that energy dense diets, which tend to be high in fat, play a role, since fat is preferentially stored in the body.

Energy, fat, protein, and carbohydrate intakes have all been positively related to weight gain in women, though generally associations are weak and inconsistent.[90] Given that diet and adiposity are difficult to measure and relationships may be weak, the influence of diet on fatness may only become apparent when comparing distinct groups, or when diet is acting in combination with other factors. Numerous studies (though not all), in child and adulthood, observe lower relative body weights in female vegetarians,[91] vegans, macrobiotics[92] and Seventh Day Adventists[93] compared with omnivores. Higher intakes of fibre[91,92] or carbohydrate,[94] or lower intakes of fat or energy,[92] might partly explain the differences in body fatness, but other factors associated with alternative diets, such as higher levels of physical activity, lower levels of smoking and alcohol consumption and generally increased health consciousness, may also contribute.

14.4.2.2 Behavioural factors

Various inter-related food consumption patterns are related to weight gain in women, including dieting, weight cycling, binge eating disorder, dietary restraint, and smoking for weight control. In Europe and North America, considerably more women (and girls) than men are concerned about their weight, and dieting or attempting to lose weight[82,95] (see Chapter 9). Many who lose weight then regain it, and this repeated loss and regain of weight has been termed 'weight cycling' or 'yo-yo dieting'. A relationship between weight cycling and increased morbidity and mortality has caused concern, but weight cycling is inconsistently defined, and intentional weight loss is frequently not distinguished from unintentional loss. Thus, the US National Task Force on the Prevention and Treatment of Obesity concluded that the evidence was insufficient to override the benefits of moderate weight loss.[96]

Some women suffer from binge eating disorder, which is more common among the obese than the general population, and characterized by regular binge eating, but distinct from bulimia nervosa since starvation or compensatory behaviours are absent. In obese women, binge eating disorder is associated with earlier onset obesity, a history of weight cycling, greater levels of psychopathology, dieting, and other eating behaviours,[97] including lower or higher dietary restraint (an individual's conscious effort to restrict food intake) and greater disinhibition (impulsive eating).[97,98]

Current smokers tend to show a lower prevalence of overweight and mean BMI than other groups (never smokers, quitters),[99] though not all studies show this relationship.[100] However, smoking cessation appears to increase average weight gain; sustained quitters gained 3.8 kg more than continuous smokers between 1971 and 1984 in the US.[101] Correspondingly, the relative risk of large weight gain ($>$13 kg) is increased among quitters compared with women continuing to smoke, by 5.8 (95% confidence interval (CI), 3.7, 9.1).[101] Women smokers generally have greater weight concerns in relation to quitting than men, and adolescent girls (not boys) attempting to lose weight are more likely to start smoking.[102]

14.4.2.3 Physical (in)activity

The decline in activity levels observed in adolescence continues into early adulthood, although in mid-adulthood levels become more stable.[103] Adult levels of physical activity in industrialized countries are low, and starting in adolescence, women are less physically active than men.[104] On the basis of dramatic increases over recent decades in time spent watching television and car ownership, it is argued that physical activity is a primary factor underlying the current high rates of obesity.[105] Few studies relate individual levels of activity and obesity prospectively in women, and although findings are somewhat varied, on balance it appears that activity attenuates weight gain.[90]

Energy expenditure is a complex exposure comprising exercise and non-exercise activity. A recent experimental study of overfeeding in adults suggests that non-exercise activity, i.e. activities of daily living, fidgeting, spontaneous muscle contraction and maintaining posture when not recumbent may be an important factor in resisting weight gain.[106] A 10-fold difference in fat storage was largely accounted for by non-exercise activity; those who increased their non-exercise activity most, gained less fat. Exercise activity itself is difficult to measure, as mentioned above, and non-exercise activity poses additional problems.

14.4.2.4 Reproduction: biological and social factors

Reproduction and child-rearing factors may also influence the development of obesity in women. Marriage is one potential social factor: overweight women are less likely to marry than other women,[22] though evidence is less consistent for a reverse effect of marriage on obesity.[107] Some studies do, however, show relationships with parity. For example, among 36-year-old British women who had had three or more pregnancies, 10.5% were obese, compared with 6.1% of those with fewer pregnancies.[100] A general population sample in Stockholm found a net mean weight gain associated with a pregnancy of 0.5 kg, but with a wide range: 30% lost weight, 13% gained 5–10 kg and 1.5% gained more than 10 kg.[108] Many women (40–50% in one Swedish study) report that pregnancies had triggered the development of their obesity.[108] Cumulative weight gain *during* successive pregnancies is suspected as an important factor, although women of high parity (four or more) also gain weight *between* pregnancies.[109]

After the childbearing period, weight may increase with onset of menopause, although this may reflect age-related weight gain. In a study of healthy non-obese women, for example, BMI was higher on average among the postmenopausal than the premenopause group (23.5 versus 22.1 kg/m^2) with postmenopausal women having a 20% greater fat mass.[41] Also at the time of the menopause, body fat is redistributed from the hips and thighs to the abdomen,[41] and some women commence hormone replacement therapy (HRT) to alleviate menopausal symptoms. Effects of HRT on fatness may be small: a review of 22 randomized control trials found that mean weight gain in users of HRT did not differ from that in non-users, but data were insufficient to evaluate effects on BMI, waist-hip ratio, fat mass, or skinfold thickness.[110] An observational study following long-term (15 year) users of HRT, found that hormone users tended to be leaner when commencing HRT, but effects on weight gain and central adiposity, if any, were small.[111]

14.5 Cumulating and interacting factors across the life course

Obesity, therefore, has both multiple causes and multiple health-related consequences among women, which are apparent onwards from early life throughout the lifespan. Effects of potential causal factors may cumulate over time. It is possible, for example, that small differences in dietary intake may be substantial over a long period, representing a cumulative 'dose'. Both parental, and own childhood obesity status are established risks for adult obesity, and whilst conventionally interpreted as representing genetic susceptibility, they may also indicate cumulative effects of diet or (in)activity patterns. (Furthermore, we would argue that small effects may have considerable importance at the population level).

In addition to cumulative effects of a particular factor over time, it is possible that with multiple causes the life course sequence and combination(s) of factors are important. A further issue is *how* factors combine, that is whether effects cumulate or interact. One example, suggesting that diet and physical activity interact, is evident from the observation that weight gain is dependent on dietary fat only among sedentary women, and that together, a low fat diet and higher physical activity have a greater protective effect on weight gain than separately.[112] Higher levels of physical activity have also been shown to attenuate many of the health risks associated with obesity.[113] Another example of interacting factors is suggested by the Dutch Hunger Winter Study, showing adverse effects on body weight, BMI, and waist circumference at age 50 in women exposed to famine prenatally, but who grew up at a time of increasing affluence and abundant diet.[52] With few exceptions,[100] studies of obesity risk among women rarely assess cumulative effects spanning from childhood to adulthood. Yet, several relevant biological and social factors do cluster across the life course and thence, may exert cumulative effects. Of the factors discussed here, this applies to lifestyles, parental obesity, social origins, and education level. To illustrate, social trajectories starting with poorer socioeconomic origins are, relative to others, more likely to be followed by lower educational achievement, less favourable dietary and activity patterns, and higher parity. Life course patterns of risk are therefore potentially important in future research on obesity.

14.6 Policy implications

As the prevalence of obesity continues to rise, so costs and the burden of ill-health associated with obesity escalate. The cost implications for health services and economies across the world are both direct (e.g. diagnosis and treatment costs) and indirect (e.g. loss of earnings and productivity due to absenteeism, disability pensions, and premature death). Chronic non-fatal disease contributes more to total cost than mortality, and overweight more than obesity, simply because more people are involved. The most important non-fatal diseases in cost terms in the UK and Canada are hypertension, coronary heart disease, and type 2 diabetes.[32,114] In the UK, direct costs of obesity (not including overweight) for 1998 were estimated at £480 million, equivalent to 1.5% of National Health Service expenditure, and the total cost at £2.6 billion, or 0.3% of Gross Domestic Product.[32] In Canada, a conservative estimate for the direct costs of obesity in 1997 was $1.8 billion, 2.4% of health care expenditure.[114] Data from other European countries and North America estimate that 1–5% of total health care costs are attributable to obesity.

   Two approaches to tackle the problem of obesity are available; treatment and prevention. Treatment is clearly beneficial because weight loss is likely to avert the social and health burden related to obesity, with benefits seen for example, in blood pressure and serum lipids.[115,116] In general, lifestyle treatment for weight loss (dietary, physical activity, or behavioural) can be successful in the short term (up to one year), with a combined approach being more effective.[116,117] However, post-intervention follow-up suggests that weight is often regained, and longer-term benefits are uncertain.[117] Evidence for treatment effectiveness in children is very limited,[4,117] although the earlier obesity is treated the greater the potential for social and health benefit.

   Given the problems associated with treatment, prevention is an attractive option and the earlier in life prevention is achieved the better, with some data suggesting that children are more responsive to prevention than adults.[118] The tracking of fatness across the life course, and also to some extent of lifestyle patterns, adds to the argument that childhood is an important period for obesity prevention. Prevention strategies are further informed by prevalence and trend data. In Finland for example, rates are levelling off in women in high and medium education groups, but continue to rise steeply in the low education group,[119] demonstrating successful weight control in some sections of the population. The sharp decrease in physical activity among teenage girls and young women suggest this to be a potential period for prevention. Studies showing some success are generally multifactorial in approach[115,120] and such approaches should enable healthy eating and physical activity patterns to be adopted and maintained throughout life.

14.7 Conclusions

Obesity has costs to individuals and to society. Women who are obese encounter a double jeopardy, involving their social and economic lives, as well as their physical functioning and life expectancy. This social and health burden is not confined to short periods, but is a long-term problem. Life course perspectives have been invaluable in establishing when health-damaging effects of obesity commence: studies in childhood show adverse effects on multiple cardiovascular risks, including blood pressure and lipid levels, with relationships resembling those seen later in adulthood. Some important questions are relatively neglected, particularly on whether fatness in childhood has long-term health consequences. In adulthood, obese women encounter adverse risks of disease which are greater, in some instances, than risks for men. Whilst disease consequences emerge primarily in adult life, the causes of obesity are seen as acting onwards from early life. Life course studies suggest that many of the early influences on obesity are common to women and to men. Generally accepted ideals of faster and greater childhood growth may have adverse consequences for obesity, and whilst the triggers for this pattern of growth are not fully understood, several potential factors are under investigation, including maternal nutrition in pregnancy and other prenatal influences, weaning in infancy, post-weaning diet, and activity. Studies showing an effect of socioeconomic circumstances in childhood, also argue for the importance of early life, although several issues remain outstanding on critical periods of growth and the development of obesity. Parental obesity and own status in childhood influence obesity risk in adulthood, but for women and for men the role of diet and physical activity has proved difficult to establish from observational studies. In adulthood, reproduction may be an added influence on obesity risk in women, although research is lacking on how such adult influences combine with those from earlier in life. This provides a challenge for future life course research on women.

Acknowledgement

This chapter draws on the research funded by the Department of Health and other material. The views expressed are the authors' own.

Commentary on 'Overweight and obesity from a life course perspective'

William H. Dietz

Power and Parsons provide a good review of the factors in childhood, adolescence, and adulthood that affect the risk of overweight and obesity in women. Overweight, defined as a body mass index (BMI) above the 95th percentile for children of the same age and gender now affects 10–15% of children and adolescents in the United States.[155] Between 1980 and 1994, the prevalence of overweight in the paediatric age group almost doubled.[156] Sixty per cent of all overweight 5–10 year old children have at least one cardiovascular disease (CVD) risk factor, such as elevated blood pressure or hyperlipidaemia, and 25% of children have two or more CVD risk factors.[24] Childhood onset obesity appears to exert a disproportional effect on adult severity. Although obesity that begins in childhood accounts for one third of adult obesity, 70–80% of adults who were more than 100 pounds overweight were overweight as children.[157] Women appear to be particularly vulnerable. In the United States, more women than men are overweight or obese, and 3% of Caucasian, 4% of Mexican American, and 7% of African American women have a BMI above 40 kg/m^2.[8] Although the changes in the prevalence and consequent effects of obesity on chronic diseases are more pronounced in the United States, the trends in prevalence seen in the United States have occurred throughout the world. Every country that has examined changes in the prevalence of obesity has found increases. As Power and Parsons illustrate, obesity confers a wide variety of adverse health effects on women. The rapid increase in obesity is likely to increase the frequency and severity of these complications further.

The development of effective interventions must begin not only with the identification of periods at risk for the development of obesity considered by Power and Parsons, but also the causal factors that operate at these periods. The prenatal period, adolescence, and pregnancy appear to constitute periods of risk for the development of obesity in females. The increase in weight with age suggests additional factors that characterize the ageing process may contribute to weight gain. The effect of pregnancy on the development of obesity in both the fetus and the mother poses a particularly interesting and potentially productive opportunity. For example, does pregnancy pose a greater risk for the mother-child dyad than it does for the fetus or mother separately? Do comparable risks suggest familial characteristics that affect susceptibility or comparable physiological mechanisms? Excessive weight gain during pregnancy might be expected to increase the risk of subsequent obesity for both mother and fetus, but studies to date have only examined the mother or the fetus. For both fetus and mother, is weight gain during pregnancy more important than postpartum weight gain for the infant, or postpartum weight retention for the mother? Are the weight changes subsequent to birth synchronous in mother and infant? If excessive maternal weight gain during pregnancy presages later obesity for both the mother and the fetus, control of weight gain during pregnancy becomes a much higher priority than interventions directed at postpartum weight retention. Most of these questions cannot be answered with the studies performed to date, and emphasize the need for prospective studies that allow simultaneous examinations of maternal and child data.

Demonstration of the existence of periods of risk for obesity represents only the first step in the development of preventive interventions. The next essential step is identification of the factors that affect energy balance at those periods. Even less information exists to help us decide whether we should focus on energy intake or energy expenditure at these periods, and more specifically the factors that promote increased energy intake or reduced energy expenditure. The techniques by which we assess energy intake and expenditure require reconfiguration. For example, the historical focus of dietary analyses has been on nutrient intake rather than patterns of dietary intake. From the population standpoint, analyses of patterns of food intake that demonstrate the association of fast food, fizzy drinks, meal frequency, or variety, are likely to be more helpful in linking food intake to the development of obesity, and in the design of interventions. Gender may modify the influence of many of these relationships. For example, mothers who are restrained eaters may exert more control over their daughters' food intake than over their sons'.[158] Meal-skipping among girls as well as other behaviours adopted to control weight may paradoxically predispose to weight gain.[159]

Obesity exerts a major influence on health. Because women appear disproportionally affected by obesity, identification of the periods of risk for the development of obesity and the factors that mediate these periods must become a high priority if effective strategies to prevent and treat obesity are to be developed.

References

1 **World Health Organisation**. *Obesity: preventing and managing the global epidemic*. Report of a WHO consultation, Geneva, 3–5 June 1997. WHO/NUT/98.1. 1998. Geneva, WHO.

2 **Withers RT, Laforgia J, Heymsfield SB**. Critical appraisal of the estimation of body composition via two-, three-, and four-compartment models. *Am J Hum Biol* 1999;**11**:175–85.

3 **Gallagher D, Visser M, Sepulveda D, Pierson RN, Harris T, Heymsfield SB**. How useful is body mass index for comparison of body fatness across age, sex, and ethnic groups? *Am J Epidemiol* 1996;**143**:228–39.

4 **Barlow SE, Dietz WH**. *Obesity evaluation and treatment: Expert Committee recommendations*. Pediatrics 1998;**102**(3):E29-http://www.pediatrics.org/cgi/content/full/102/3/e29.

5 **Cole TJ, Bellizzi MC, Flegal KM, Dietz WH**. Establishing a standard definition for child overweight and obesity worldwide: international survey. *Br Med J* 2000;**320**:1–6.

6 **Garrow JS**. Significance of within person weight variation. *Obesity: The Report of the British Nutrition Foundation Task Force*. Oxford: Blackwell Science, 1999, pp. 132–8.

7 **Spiegelman D, Israel RG, Bouchard C, Willett WC**. Absolute fat mass, percent body fat, and body-fat distribution: which is the real determinant of blood pressure and serum glucose? *Am J Clin Nutr* 1992;**55**:1033–44.

8 **Flegal KM, Carroll MD, Kuczmarski RJ, Johnson CL**. Overweight and obesity in the United States: prevalence and trends, 1960–1994. *Int J Obes* 1998;**22**:39–47.

9 **Mokdad AH, Serdula MK, Dietz WH, Bowman BA, Marks JS, Koplan JP**. The spread of the obesity epidemic in the United States, 1991–1998. *J Am Med Assoc* 1999;**282**:1519–22.

10 **Mokdad AH, Serdula MK, Dietz WH, Bowman BA, Marks JS, Koplan JP**. The continuing epidemic of obesity in the United States [letter]. *J Am Med Assoc* 2000;1650–1.

11 **Knight I**. *The heights and weights of adults in Great Britain*. 1984. London, HMSO.

12 **Erens B, Primatesta P, Prior G, eds**. *Health Survey for England: The Health of Minority Ethnic Groups 99*. 2001. London, The Stationery Office. Website *http://www.doh.gov.uk/public/hse99.htm*

13 **Heitmann BL**. Ten-year trends in overweight and obesity among Danish men and women aged 30–60 years. *Int J Obes* 2000;**24**:1347–52.

14 **Molarius A, Seidell JC, Sans S, Tuomilehto J, Kuulasmaa K**. Educational level, relative body weight, and changes in their association over 10 years: an international perspective from the WHO MONICA Project. *Am J Public Health* 2000;**90**:1260–8.

15 **Lahti-Koski M, Pietinen P, Mannisto S, Vartiainen E**. Trends in waist-to-hip ratio and its determinants in adults in Finland from 1987 to 1997. *Am J Clin Nutr* 2000;**72**:1436–44.

16 **Lissner L, Bjorkelund C, Heitmann BL, Lapidus L, Bjorntorp P, Bengtsson C**. Secular increases in waist-hip ratio among Swedish women. *Int J Obes* 1998;**22**:1116–20.

17 Chinn S, Rona RJ. Prevalence and trends in overweight and obesity in three cross sectional studies of British Children, 1974–94. *Br Med J* 2001;**322**:24–6.

18 Tremblay MS, Willms JD. Secular trends in the body mass index of Canadian children. *Can Med Assoc J* 2000;**163**:1429–33.

19 Murata M. Secular trends in growth and changes in eating patterns of Japanese children. *Am J Clin Nutr* 2000;**72(Suppl 5)**:1379S-83S.

20 Bundred P, Kitchiner D, Buchan I. Prevalence of overweight and obese children between 1989 and 1998: population based series of cross sectional studies. *Br Med J* 2001;**322**:326–8.

21 Turnbull JD, Heaslip S, McLeod HA. Pre-school children's attitudes to fat and normal male and female stimulus figures. *Int J Obes* 2000;**24**:1705–6.

22 Gortmaker SL, Must A, Perrin JM, Sobol AM, Dietz WH. Social and economic consequences of overweight in adolescence and young adulthood. *N Engl J Med* 1993;**329**:1008–12.

23 Sargent JD, Blanchflower DG. Obesity and stature in adolescence and earnings in young adulthood. Analysis of a British birth cohort. *Arch Pediatr Adolesc Med* 1994;**148**:681–7.

24 Freedman DS, Dietz WH, Srinivasan SR, Berenson GS. The relation of overweight to cardiovascular risk factors among children and adolescents: the Bogalusa Heart Study. *Pediatrics* 1999;**103**:1175–82.

25 Morrison JA, Sprecher DL, Barton BA, Waclawiw MA, Daniels SR. Overweight, fat patterning, and cardiovascular disease risk factors in black and white girls: The National Heart, Lung, and Blood Institute Growth and Health Study. *J Pediatr* 1999;**135**:458–64.

26 Lauer RM, Lee J, Clarke WR. Factors affecting the relationship between childhood and adult cholesterol levels: the Muscatine Study. *Pediatrics* 1988;**82**:309–18.

27 Nieto FJ, Szklo M, Comstock GW. Childhood weight and growth rate as predictors of adult mortality. *Am J Epidemiol* 1992;**136**:201–13.

28 Must A, Jacques PF, Dallal GE, Bajema CJ, Dietz WH. Long-term morbidity and mortality of overweight adolescents. A follow-up of the Harvard Growth Study of 1922 to 1935. *N Engl J Med* 1992;**327**:1350–5.

29 Calle EE, Thun MJ, Petrelli JM, Rodriguez C, Heath-CW J. Body-mass index and mortality in a prospective cohort of U.S. adults. *N Engl J Med* 1999;**341**:1097–105.

30 Rich-Edwards JW, Goldman MB, Willett WC, Hunter DJ, Stampfer MJ, Colditz GA *et al*. Adolescent body mass index and infertility caused by ovulatory disorder. *Am J Obstet Gynecol* 1994;**171**:171–7.

31 Lake JK, Power C, Cole TJ. Women's reproductive health: the role of body mass index in early and adult life. *Int J Obes* 1997;**21**:432–8.

32 National Audit Office. *Tackling Obesity in England*. HC 220. 15–2–2001. London, The Stationery Office.

33 Bergstrom A, Pisani P, Tenet V, Wolk A, Adami HO. Overweight as an avoidable cause of cancer in Europe. *Int J Cancer* 2001;**92**:927.

34 Folsom AR, Kushi LH, Anderson KE, Mink PJ, Olson JE, Hong CP *et al*. Associations of general and abdominal obesity with multiple health outcomes in older women: the Iowa Women's Health Study. *Arch Intern Med* 2000;**160**:2117–28.

35 Folsom AR, Stevens J, Schreiner PJ, McGovern PG. Body mass index, waist/hip ratio, and coronary heart disease incidence in African Americans and whites. Atherosclerosis Risk in Communities Study Investigators. *Am J Epidemiol* 1998;**148**:1187–94.

36 Wei M, Gaskill SP, Haffner SM, Stern MP. Waist circumference as the best predictor of noninsulin dependent diabetes mellitus (NIDDM) compared to body mass index, waist/hip ratio and other anthropometric measurements in Mexican Americans: a 7-year prospective study. *Obes Res* 1997;**5**:16–23.

37 Rolland-Cachera MF, Deheeger M, Bellisle F, Sempe M, Guilloud-Bataille M, Patois E. Adiposity rebound in children: a simple indicator for predicting obesity. *Am J Clin Nutr* 1984;**39**:129–35.

38 Tanner JM, Whitehouse RH. Revised standards for triceps and subscapular skinfolds in British children. *Arch Dis Child* 1975;**50**:142–5.

39 Garn SM, Clark DC. Trends in fatness and the origins of obesity Ad Hoc Committee to Review the Ten-State Nutrition Survey. *Pediatrics* 1976;**57**:443–56.

40 Lemieux S, Prud'homme D, Bouchard C, Tremblay A, Despres JP. Sex differences in the relation of visceral adipose tissue accumulation to total body fatness. *Am J Clin Nutr* 1993;**58**:463–7.

41 Ley CJ, Lees B, Stevenson JC. Sex- and menopause-associated changes in body-fat distribution. *Am J Clin Nutr* 1992;**55**:950–4.

42 Dietz WH. Critical periods in childhood for the development of obesity. *Am J Clin Nutr* 1994;**59**:955–9.

43 Kemper HC, Post GB, Twisk JW, Van Mechelen W. Lifestyle and obesity in adolescence and young adulthood: results from the Amsterdam Growth And Health Longitudinal Study (AGAHLS). *Int J Obes* 1999;**23**(Suppl 3):S34–S40.

44 Parsons TJ, Power C, Logan S, Summerbell CD. Childhood predictors of adult obesity: a systematic review. *Int J Obes* 1999;**23**(Suppl 8):S1-S107.

45 Whitaker RC, Wright JA, Pepe MS, Seidel KD, Dietz WH. Predicting obesity in young adulthood from childhood and parental obesity. *N Engl J Med* 1997;**337**:869–73.

46 Lake JK, Power C, Cole TJ. Child to adult body mass index in the 1958 British birth cohort: Associations with parental obesity. *Arch Dis Child* 1997;**77**:376–81.

47 Curhan GC, Chertow GM, Willett WC, Spiegelman D, Colditz GA, Manson JE *et al*. Birthweight and adult hypertension and obesity in women. *Circulation* 1996;**94**:1310–5.

48 Fall CH, Osmond C, Barker DJ, Clark PM, Hales CN, Stirling Y *et al*. Fetal and infant growth and cardiovascular risk factors in women. *Br Med J* 1995;**310**:428–32.

49 Parsons TJ, Power C, Manor O. Fetal and early life growth and body mass index from birth to early adulthood in the 1958 British cohort: a longitudinal study. *Br Med J* 2001;**323**:1331–5.

50 Maffeis C, Micciolo R, Must A, Zaffanello M, Pinelli L. Parental and perinatal factors associated with childhood obesity in north-east Italy. *Int J Obes* 1994;**18**:301–5.

51 Allison DB, Paultre F, Heymsfield SB, Pi Sunyer FX. Is the intra-uterine period really a critical period for the development of adiposity? *Int J Obes* 1995;**19**:397–402.

52 Ravelli AC, van Der M, Osmond C, Barker DJ, Bleker OP. Obesity at the age of 50 y in men and women exposed to famine prenatally. *Am J Clin Nutr* 1999;**70**:811–6.

53 Vik T, Jacobsen G, Vatten L, Bakketeig LS. Pre- and post-natal growth in children of women who smoked in pregnancy. *Early Hum Dev* 1996;**45**:245–55.

54 Power C, Lake JK, Cole TJ. Measurement and long-term health risks of child and adolescent fatness. *Int J Obes* 1997;**21**:507–26.

55 Serdula MK, Ivery D, Coates RJ, Freedman DS, Williamson DF, Byers T. Do obese children become obese adults? A review of the literature. *Prev Med* 1993;**22**:167–77.

56 Power C, Lake JK, Cole TJ. Body mass index and height from childhood to adulthood in the 1958 British born cohort. *Am J Clin Nutr* 1997;**66**:1094–101.

57 Whitaker RC, Pepe MS, Wright JA, Seidel KD, Dietz WH. Early adiposity rebound and the risk of adult obesity. *Pediatrics* 1998;**101**:E5.

58 Freedman D, Kettel KL, Serdula M, Srinivasan S, Berenson G. BMI rebound, childhood height and obesity among adults: the Bogalusa Heart Study. *Int J Obes* 2001;**25**:543–9.

59 Bayley N. Size and body build of adolescents in relation to rate of skeletal maturity. *Child Dev* 1943;**14**:47–90.

60 Bayley N. Skeletal maturing in adolescence as basis for determining percentage of completed growth. *Child Dev* 1943;**14**:1–46.

61 Van Lenthe FJ, Kemper HC, Van Mechelen W, Post GB, Twisk JW, Welten DC *et al*. Biological maturation and the distribution of subcutaneous fat from adolescence into adulthood: the Amsterdam Growth and Health Study. *Int J Obes* 1996;**20**:121–9.

62 Post GB, Kemper HC. Nutrient intake and biological maturation during adolescence. The Amsterdam growth and health longitudinal study. *Eur J Clin Nutr* 1993;**47**:400–8.

63 Hardy R, Wadsworth M, Kuh D. The influence of childhood weight and socioeconomic status on change in adult body mass index in a British national birth cohort. *Int J Obes* 2000;**24**:725–34.

64 Lissau I, Sorensen TI. Parental neglect during childhood and increased risk of obesity in young adulthood. *Lancet* 1994;**343**:324–7.

65 Kimm SY, Barton BA, Obarzanek E, McMahon RP, Sabry ZI, Waclawiw MA *et al*. Racial divergence in adiposity during adolescence: the NHLBI growth and health study. *Pediatrics* 2001;**107**:E34.

66 Kumanyika S. Obesity in black women. *Epidemiol Rev* 1987;**9**:31–50.

67 Whitehead RG, Paul AA. Growth charts and the asessment of infant feeding practices in the western world and in developing countries. *Early Hum Dev* 1984;**9**:187–207.

68 *Present-day practice in infant feeding*. Report of a working party of the panel on child nutrition. 1974. London, The Stationery office. Report on Health and Social Subjects 9.

69 von Kries R, Koletzko B, Sauerwald T, von Mutius E, Barnert D, Grunert V *et al*. Breastfeeding and obesity: cross sectional study. *Br Med J* 1999;319:147–50.

70 Gillman MW, Rifas-Shiman SL, Camargo CA, Jr., Berkey CS, Frazier AL, Rockett HR *et al*. Risk of overweight among adolescents who were breastfed as infants. *J Am Med Assoc* 2001;**285**:2461–7.

71 Hediger ML, Overpeck MD, Kuczmarski RJ, Ruan WJ. Association between infant breastfeeding and overweight in young children. *J Am Med Assoc* 2001;**285**:2453–60.

72 Wadsworth M, Marshall S, Hardy R, Paul A. Breastfeeding and obesity. Relation may be accounted for by social factors [letter]. *Br Med J* 1999;**319**:1576.

73 Parsons TJ, Power C, Manor O. Infant feeding and body mass index through the lifecourse in the 1958 British cohort, forthcoming.

74 Cavadini C, Siega-Riz AM, Popkin BM. US adolescent food intake trends from 1965 to 1996. *Arch Dis Child* 2000;**83**:18–24.

75 Griffiths M, Payne PR, Stunkard AJ, Rivers JP, Cox M. Metabolic rate and physical development in children at risk of obesity. *Lancet* 1990;**336**:76–8.

76 Van Lenthe FJ, Van Mechelen W, Kemper HC, Post GB. Behavioral variables and development of a central pattern of body fat from adolescence into adulthood in normal-weight whites: the Amsterdam Growth and Health Study. *Am J Clin Nutr* 1998;**67**:846–52.

77 Berkey CS, Rockett HR, Field AE, Gillman MW, Frazier AL, Camargo CA *et al*. Activity, dietary intake, and weight changes in a longitudinal study of preadolescent and adolescent boys and girls. *Pediatrics* 2000;**105**:E56.

78 DiGuiseppi C, Roberts I, Li L. Influence of changing travel patterns on child death rates from injury: trend analysis [published erratum appears in *Br Med J* 1997;**314**:1385]. *Br Med J* 1997;**314**:710–3.

79 Department of Transportation, Federal Highway Administration, Research and Technical Support Center. *Nationwide personal transportation survey*. 1997. Lantham, MD, Federal Highway Administration.

80 Matheson J, Summerfield C, eds. *Social Trends 31*. 2001. London, The Stationery Office.

81 Riddoch C. *Physical activity outcomes 1. Young and Active*? Draft policy framework for young people and health enhancing physical activity. Health Education Authority, 1997.

82 Prescott-Clarke P, Primatesta P, eds. *Health Survey for England: The Health of Young People '95—97*. 1998. London, The Stationery Office. Website *http://www.doh.gov.uk/public/hs9597.htm*

83 Raitakari OT, Porkka KV, Taimela S, Telama R, Rasanen L, Viikari JS. Effects of persistent physical activity and inactivity on coronary risk factors in children and young adults. The Cardiovascular Risk in Young Finns Study. *Am J Epidemiol* 1994;**140**:195–205.

84 Twisk JW, Van Mechelen W, Kemper HC, Post GB. The relation between 'long-term exposure' to lifestyle during youth and young adulthood and risk factors for cardiovascular disease at adult age. *J Adolesc Health* 1997;**20**:309–19.

85 Klesges RC, Haddock CK, Stein RJ, Klesges LM, Eck LH, Hanson CL. Relationship between psychosocial functioning and body fat in preschool children: a longitudinal investigation. *J Consult Clin Psychol* 1992;**60**:793–6.

86 Van Lenthe FJ, Snel J, Twisk JWR, Van Mechelen W, Kemper HCG. Coping, personality and the development of a central pattern of body fat from youth into young adulthood: The Amsterdam Growth and Health Study. *Int J Obes* 1998;**22**:861–8.

87 French SA, Perry CL, Leon GR, Fulkerson JA. Self-esteem and change in body mass index over 3 years in a cohort of adolescents. *Obes Res* 1996;**4**:27–33.

88 Harnack LJ, Jeffery RW, Boutelle KN. Temporal trends in energy intake in the United States: an ecologic perspective. *Am J Clin Nutr* 2000;**71**:1478–84.

89 Heitmann BL, Lissner L, Osler M. Do we eat less fat, or just report so? *Int J Obes* 2000;**24**:435–42.

90 Williamson DF. Dietary intake and physical activity as 'predictors' of weight gain in observational, prospective studies of adults. *Nutr Rev* 1996;**54**:S101–S109.

91 Appleby PN, Thorogood M, Mann JI, Key TJ. Low body mass index in non-meat eaters: the possible roles of animal fat, dietary fibre and alcohol. *Int J Obes* 1998;**22**:454–60.

92 Dagnelie PC, van Dusseldorp M, van Staveren WA, Hautvast JGAJ. Effects of macrobiotic diets on linear growth in infants and children until 10 years of age. *Eur J Clin Nutr* 1994;**48**(Suppl 1): S103–S112.

93 Sabate J, Lindsted KD, Harris RD, Johnston PK. Anthropometric parameters of schoolchildren with different life- styles. *Am J Dis Child* 1990;**144**:1159–63.

94 Janelle KC, Barr SI. Nutrient intakes and eating behavior scores of vegetarian and nonvegetarian women. *J Am Diet Assoc* 1995;**95**:180–6.

95 Serdula MK, Mokdad AH, Williamson DF, Galuska DA, Mendlein JM, Heath GW. Prevalence of attempting weight loss and strategies for controlling weight. *J Am Med Assoc* 1999;**282**:1353–8.

96 National Task Force on the Prevention and Treatment of Obesity. Weight cycling. *J Am Med Assoc* 1994;**272**:1196–202.

97 Yanovski SZ. Binge eating disorder: current knowledge and future directions. *Obes Res* 1993;**1**:306–24.

98 Pinto BM, Borrelli B, King TK, Bock BC, Clark MM, Roberts M *et al*. Weight control smoking among sedentary women. *Addict Behav* 1999;**24**:75–86.

99 Flegal KM, Troiano RP, Pamuk ER, Kuczmarski RJ, Campbell SM. The influence of smoking cessation on the prevalence of overweight in the United States. *N Engl J Med* 1995;**333**:1165–70.

100 Braddon FE, Rodgers B, Wadsworth ME, Davies JM. Onset of obesity in a 36 year birth cohort study. *Br Med J* 1986;**293**:299–303.

101 Williamson DF, Madans J, Anda RF, Kleinman JC, Giovino GA, Byers T. Smoking cessation and severity of weight gain in a national cohort. *N Engl J Med* 1991;**324**:739–45.

102 French SA, Perry CL, Leon GR, Fulkerson JA. Weight concerns, dieting behavior, and smoking initiation among adolescents: a prospective study. *Am J Public Health* 1994;**84**:1818–20.

103 Caspersen CJ, Pereira MA, Curran KM. Changes in physical activity patterns in the United States, by sex and cross-sectional age. *Med Sci Sports Exerc* 2000;**32**:1601–9.

104 Gordon-Larsen P, McMurray RG, Popkin BM. Determinants of adolescent physical activity and inactivity patterns. *Pediatrics* 2000;**105**:E83.

105 Prentice AM, Jebb SA. Obesity in Britain: gluttony or sloth? *Br Med J* 1995;**311**:437–9.

106 Levine JA, Eberhardt NL, Jensen MD. Role of nonexercise activity thermogenesis in resistance to fat gain in humans. *Science* 1999;**283**:212–4.

107 Sobal J, Rauschenbach BS, Frongillo-EA J. Marital status, fatness and obesity. *Soc Sci Med* 1992;**35**:915–23.

108 Rossner S. Weight gain in pregnancy. *Hum Reprod* 1997;**12**(Suppl 1):110–5.

109 Harris HE, Ellison GT, Holliday M. Is there an independent association between parity and maternal weight gain? *Ann Hum Biol* 1997;**24**:507–19.

110 Norman RJ, Flight IHK, Rees MCP. *Oestrogen and progestogen hormone replacement therapy for peri-menopausal and post-menopausal women: weight and body fat distribution* (Cochrane Review). In: The Cochrane Library, Issue 1. Oxford: Update Software, 2001.

111 Kritz-Silverstein D, Barrett-Connor E. Long-term postmenopausal hormone use, obesity, and fat distribution in older women. *J Am Med Assoc* 1996;**275**:46–9.

112 Lissner L, Heitmann BL, Bengtsson C. Low-fat diets may prevent weight gain in sedentary women: prospective observations from the population study of women in Gothenburg, Sweden. *Obes Res* 1997;**5**:43–8.

113 Blair SN, Brodney S. Effects of physical inactivity and obesity on morbidity and mortality: current evidence and research issues. *Med Sci Sports Exerc* 1999;**31**(11 Suppl):S646–S662.

114 Birmingham CL, Muller JL, Palepu A, Spinelli JJ, Anis AH. The cost of obesity in Canada. *Can Med Assoc J* 1999;**160**:483–8.

115 Douketis JD, Feightner JW, Attia J, Feldman WF. Periodic health examination, 1999 update: 1. Detection, prevention and treatment of obesity. *Can Med Assoc J* 1999;**160**:513–25.

116 Expert Panel on the Identification and Treatment of Overweight in Adults. *Clinical guidelines on the identification, evaluation, and treatment of overweight and obesity in adults: The Evidence Report*. 98–4083. 1998. USA, National Heart, Lung and Blood Institute. Website *http://www.nhlbi.nih.gov/guidelines/obesity/e_txtbk/index.htm*

117 Glenny AM, O'Meara S, Melville A, Sheldon TA, Wilson C. The treatment and prevention of obesity: a systematic review of the literature. *Int J Obes* 1997;**21**:715–37.

118 Epstein LH, Valoski AM, Kalarchian MA, McCurley J. Do children lose and maintain weight easier than adults: a comparison of child and parent weight changes from six months to ten years. *Obes Res* 1995;**3**:411–7.

119 Pietinen P, Vartiainen E, Mannisto S. Trends in body mass index and obesity among adults in Finland from 1972 to 1992. *Int J Obes* 1996;**20**:114–20.

120 Campbell K, Waters E, O'Meara S, Summerbell CD. *Interventions for preventing obesity in children* (Cochrane Review). In: The Cochrane Library, Issue 2. Oxford: Update Software, 2001.

121 Jung RT. Obesity as a disease. *Br Med Bull* 1997;**53**:307–21.

122 Kaplowitz HJ, Wild KA, Mueller WH, Decker M, Tanner JM. Serial and parent-child changes in components of body fat distribution and fatness in children from the London Longitudinal Growth Study, ages two to eighteen years. *Hum Biol* 1988;**60**:739–58.

123 Barker M, Robinson S, Osmond C, Barker DJ. Birthweight and body fat distribution in adolescent girls. *Arch Dis Child* 1997;**77**:381–3.

124 Fomon SJ, Rogers RR, Ziegler EE, Nelson SE, Thomas LN. Indices of fatness and serum cholesterol at age eight years in relation to feeding and growth during early infancy. *Pediatr Res* 1984;**18**:1233–8.

125 Guillaume M, Lapidus L, Beckers F, Lambert A, Bjorntorp P. Familial trends of obesity through three generations: the Belgian-Luxembourg child study. *Int J Obes* 1995;**19**(Suppl 3):S5–9.

126 Seidman DS, Laor A, Gale R, Stevenson DK, Danon YL. A longitudinal study of birthweight and being overweight in late adolescence. *Am J Dis Child* 1991;**145**:782–5.

127 Miller FJ, Billewicz WZ, Thomson AM. Growth from birth to adult life of 442 Newcastle upon Tyne children. *Br J Prev Soc Med* 1972;**26**:224–30.

128 Valdez R, Athens MA, Thompson GH, Bradshaw BS, Stern MP. Birthweight and adult health outcomes in a biethnic population in the USA. *Diabetologia* 1994;**37**:624–31.

129 Burke GL, Savage PJ, Manolio TA, Sprafka JM, Wagenknecht LE, Sidney S *et al.* Correlates of obesity in young black and white women: the CARDIA Study. *Am J Public Health* 1992;**82**:1621–5.

130 Garn SM, LaVelle M, Rosenberg KR, Hawthorne VM. Maturational timing as a factor in female fatness and obesity. *Am J Clin Nutr* 1986;**43**:879–83.

131 Guo SS, Chumlea WC, Roche AF, Siervogel RM. Age- and maturity-related changes in body composition during adolescence into adulthood: the Fels Longitudinal Study. *Int J Obes* 1997;**21**:1167–75.

132 Freeman JV, Power C, Rodgers B. Weight-for-height indices of adiposity: relationships with height in childhood and early adult life. *Int J Epidemiol* 1995;**24**:970–6.

133 Stark O, Peckham CS, Moynihan C. Weight and age at menarche. *Arch Dis Child* 1989;**64**:383–7.

134 Prokopec M, Bellisle F. Adiposity in Czech children followed from 1 month of age to adulthood: analysis of individual BMI patterns. *Ann Hum Biol* 1993;**20**:517–25.

135 Rolland-Cachera MF, Deheeger M, Guilloud-Bataille M, Avons P, Patois E, Sempe M. Tracking the development of adiposity from one month of age to adulthood. *Ann Hum Biol* 1987;**14**:219–29.

136 St.George IM, Williams S, Silva PA. Body size and the menarche: the Dunedin Study. *J Adolesc Health* 1994;**15**:573–6.

137 Sherman B, Wallace R, Bean J, Schlabaugh L. Relationship of body weight to menarcheal and menopausal age: implications for breast cancer risk. *J Clin Endocrinol Metab* 1981;**52**:488–93.

138 Van Lenthe FJ, Kemper CG, Van Mechelen W. Rapid maturation in adolescence results in greater obesity in adulthood: the Amsterdam Growth and Health Study. *Am J Clin Nutr* 1996;**64**:18–24.

139 Wellens R, Malina RM, Roche AF, Chumlea WC, Guo S, Siervogel RM. Body size and fatness in young dults in relation to age at menarche. *Am J Hum Biol* 1992;**4**:783–7.

140 Knishkowy BN, Palti H, Adler B, Gofin R. A follow-up study of adiposity and growth of Jerusalem schoolchildren from age 6 to 14 years. *J Adolesc Health Care* 1989;**10**:192–9.

141 Hediger ML, Scholl TO, Schall JI, Cronk CE. One-year changes in weight and fatness in girls during late adolescence. *Pediatrics* 1995;**96**:253–8.

142 Guo SS, Huang C, Maynard LM, Demerath E, Towne B, Chumlea WC *et al.* Body mass index during childhood, adolescence and young adulthood in relation to adult overweight and adiposity: the Fels Longitudinal Study. *Int J Obes* 2000;**24**:1628–35.

143 Arnesen E, Forsdahl A. The Tromso heart study: coronary risk factors and their association with living conditions during childhood. *J Epidemiol Community Health* 1985;**39**:210–4.

144 Garn SM, Hopkins PJ, Ryan AS. Differential fatness gain of low income boys and girls. *Am J Clin Nutr* 1981;**34**:1465–8.

145 **Goldblatt PB, Moore ME, Stunkard AJ**. Social factors in obesity. *J Am Med Assoc* 1965;**192**:97–101.

146 **Power C, Matthews S**. Origins of health inequalities in a national population sample. *Lancet* 1997;**350**:1584–9.

147 **Lindgren G**. Height, weight and menarche in Swedish urban school children in relation to socioeconomic and regional factors. *Ann Hum Biol* 1976;**3**:501–28.

148 **Spiegelaere Md, Dramaix M, Hennart P**. The influence of socioeconomic status on the incidence and evolution of obesity during early adolescence. *Int J Obes* 1998;**22**:268–74.

149 **Birkbeck JA, Buckfield PM, Silva PA**. Lack of long-term effect of the method of infant feeding on growth. *Hum Nutr Clin Nutr* 1985;**39C**:39–44.

150 **Marmot MG, Page CM, Atkins E, Douglas JW**. Effect of breast-feeding on plasma cholesterol and weight in young adults. *J Epidemiol Community Health* 1980;**34**:164–7.

151 **Vobecky JS, Vobecky J, Shapcott D, Demers PP**. Nutrient intake patterns and nutritional status with regard to relative weight in early infancy. *Am J Clin Nutr* 1983;**38**:730–8.

152 **Ku LC, Shapiro LR, Crawford PB, Huenemann RL**. Body composition and physical activity in 8-year-old children. *Am J Clin Nutr* 1981;**34**:2770–5.

153 **Moore LL, Nguyen US, Rothman KJ, Cupples LA, Ellison RC**. Preschool physical activity level and change in body fatness in young children. The Framingham Children's Study. *Am J Epidemiol* 1995;**142**:982–8.

154 **Robinson TN, Hammer LD, Killen JD, Kraemer HC, Wilson DM, Hayward C *et al.***. Does television viewing increase obesity and reduce physical activity? Cross-sectional and longitudinal analyses among adolescent girls. *Pediatrics* 1993;**91**:273–80.

155 **Shapiro LR, Crawford PB, Clark MJ, Pearson DL, Raz J, Huenemann RL**. Obesity prognosis: a longitudinal study of children from the age of 6 months to 9 years. *Am J Public Health* 1984;**74**:968–72.

156 **Troiano RP, Flegal KM, Kuczmarski RJ, Campbell SM, Johnson CL**. Overweight prevalence and trends for children and adolescents. *Arch Pediatr Adolesc Med* 1995;**149**:1085–91.

157 **Rimm IJ, Rimm AA**. Association between juvenile onset obesity and severe adult obesity in 73,532 women. *Am J Public Health* 1976;**66**:479–81.

158 **Johnson SL, Birch LL**. Parents' and children's adiposity and eating style. *Pediatrics* 1994;**94**:653–61

159 **Stice E, Cameron RP, Killen JD, Hayward C, Taylor CB**. Naturalistic weight-reduction efforts prospectively predict growth in relative weight and onset of obesity among female adolescents. *J Consult Clin Psychol* 1999;**67**:967–74.

Chapter 15

Sexually transmitted infections and health through the life course

Ronald H. Gray, Maria J. Wawer, and
David Serwadda

Sexually transmitted infections (STIs) are common, particularly in developing countries, and are acquired at younger ages in women than men. STIs have acute and long-term consequences for adult health, particularly in women, and via infections during pregnancy, directly affect infant health at birth and during the life course.

15.1 Introduction

Infectious diseases can affect health throughout the life course and are important public health problems, particularly in sub-Saharan Africa, where such diseases are prevalent and generally go undiagnosed and untreated. Transmission of infections *in utero*, at time of delivery or via breast milk can affect survival of newborns, and have consequences for later disease and disability in adult life. During adolescence and sexual debut, women are at particular risk of STIs and human immunodeficiency virus (HIV) which affect subsequent reproduction (e.g. causing pelvic inflammatory disease, infertility, and ectopic pregnancy), and the health and survival of women during their reproductive lives. There is increasing evidence that infectious diseases acquired at younger ages are linked to chronic disease in adulthood. Examples include human papilloma virus (HPV) the cause of cervical cancer,[1,2] hepatitis B which causes cirrhosis and cancer of the liver,[3,4] helicobacteria which leads to gastric ulceration and gastric cancer,[5,6] Kaposi's sarcoma human herpes virus type 8 (KSHV or HHV-8) which causes Kaposi's sarcoma,[7–9] and *Chlamydia pneumoniae* which has been linked to coronary atherosclerosis and myocardial infarction.[10] Similarly renal infections such as pyelonephritis in childhood or adolescence is a major cause of renal failure and hypertension in adulthood.[11] Tuberculosis (TB) often acquired in childhood, may be reactivated at older ages, causing active TB and premature death.[11–13] These problems have been exacerbated in sub-Saharan Africa by the HIV epidemic which, in addition to HIV risk *per se*, has facilitated secondary epidemics of other diseases such as HPV and cervical cancer,[1] herpes simplex type 2 (HSV-2)[14,15] and pulmonary TB.[16,17] Thus, there is a life course continuum of risk from infections of childhood and adolescence leading to morbidity and mortality at later ages.

Women are particularly vulnerable to these long-term sequelae, partly because they are more likely to acquire sexually transmitted infections, and possibly because the burden of repeated pregnancy and lactation may undermine nutritional status. In addition, social discrimination against women may impair their ability to obtain medical care and support to cope with illness.

A full review of the complex effects of infections at different life stages on the full range of adult health outcomes is beyond the scope of the chapter. We will focus on the role of STIs and HIV, because these are serious public health concerns for which there is a paucity of representative data or official statistics. We will illustrate our review using selected examples drawn from our ongoing population-based cohort studies in rural Rakai District, south-western Uganda. We also highlight some the social and behavioural risk factors for disease, as well as the social and health consequences of disease (see also Chapter 17).

There are no studies that have directly assessed the effects of STIs on health of women and their children throughout the life course, and there are difficulties with empirical investigations. Most importantly, such studies would require reliable diagnosis of infection in large and representative populations of infants or women of reproductive age, with long-term follow-up to determine sequelae. However, non-invasive and feasible diagnostic tests using sensitive and specific immunological or molecular amplification methods for most of these infections have only been developed during the past 10–15 years. Thus, accurate diagnosis early in life and prospective follow-up to assess the long-term consequences of these diseases has not yet been possible. Based on incomplete information, one can only infer the long-term consequences of STIs. A schematic framework is given in Fig. 15.1.

15.2 **The Rakai Cohort Study**

The Rakai Project was established in 1989 and conducted descriptive epidemiological studies of HIV until 1992. Between 1994 and 1998 the Rakai Project conducted a large

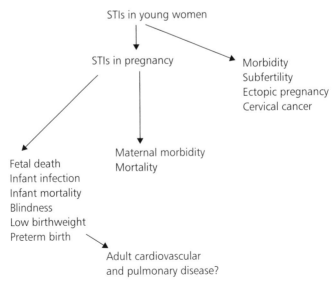

Fig. 15.1 Consequences of sexually transmitted diseases in young women: a schematic framework.

community-randomized trial of sexually transmitted disease (STD) control for HIV Prevention, and since 1999 the project has conducted community molecular epidemiological studies.[18,19] The project undertakes annual surveillance in a population of over 12 000 adults aged 15–19 resident in 56 communities located on secondary roads in this rural area. Participants are followed up over time (annual follow-up rates 77%), and in this open cohort, newly age eligible and immigrants are enrolled at each survey round. This maintains complete, longitudinal observation of the resident population. All data collection is conducted in the home. This has allowed close monitoring of demographic, behavioural, and health characteristics of the population. In addition, diseases monitoring has employed innovative, minimally invasive methods and advanced laboratory testing, to measure the frequency of infections in a representative general population. For example, we pioneered the use of self-collected vaginal swabs, obtained by women in the home, to diagnose trichomonas, bacterial vaginosis (BV), chlamydia, gonorrhoea, and HPV infections in a representative female population. This series of studies provides a unique opportunity to assess the health consequences of STIs.

The Rakai setting is typical of rural populations in east and southern Africa, and is generalizable to 80% of the sub-Saharan African population that live in rural settings. Although the epidemiology of STIs has not been well studied in representative rural African populations, we draw parallels between the observations in Rakai and other investigations in comparable populations elsewhere. These rural communities differ markedly from urban settings in which commercial sex plays a more important role in transmission, and where urban labour migration, predominantly of single individuals, may place them at particularly high risk of STIs and HIV.[20]

15.2.1 Sexually transmitted infections in rural Rakai

STIs are important to consider from a life course perspective because these infections are often acquired at younger ages, particularly in women, and can cause long-term morbidity in the woman, as well as posing a risk to the newborn. The STIs of most concern are viral infections (HIV, HSV-2, HPV), bacterial infections (chlamydia, gonorrhoea, BV, chancroid), and protozoal infections (trichomonas).

In the Rakai population, the median age of menarche is around 15 years. The median age of first intercourse for women is approximately 15.5 years, and often involves sexual relationships with older men.[21] This age disparity in sexual partners is also observed in urban populations.[20] Unfortunately, sexual debut in many instances is coercive, and 30% of women report that their first sexual encounter was rape. Overall, 24.2% of women report sexual coercion in the year prior to interview, and the risk is markedly increased among women under age 25 (adjusted odds ratio (OR) = 1.56, 95% confidence interval (CI), 1.19–2.05), and among women who report their first sexual experience under the age of 15 years (OR = 1.54, 95% CI, 1.20–1.96).[22] This early onset of female sexual activity with older males places younger women at particularly high risk of STIs. Other factors predictive of sexual coercion include the male partner's frequent use of alcohol (OR = 2.82, 95% CI, 2.15–3.70), the man having non-marital partners (OR = 1.52, 95% CI, 1.09–2.12), and the woman's perception that the male partner is likely to be at risk of having HIV (OR = 2.89, 95% CI, 2.09–3.99).[22]

The prevalence of HIV in Rakai is 19% in women and 14% in men. This suggests a mature, generalized HIV epidemic and prevalence is lower than in urban areas of

East-Central Africa, but higher than the prevalence rates observed in West Africa.[20] Figure 15.2 shows the age-specific prevalence of viral STIs, HIV, HSV-2, and HPV. Female prevalence of HIV and HSV-2 increase rapidly during adolescence and young adulthood, whereas the male prevalence of these infections is delayed to older ages and is generally lower than the rates in women. The consequences for women and their children are substantial. HIV infection will prove fatal to the mother within a decade, because of the absence of antiretroviral therapy in this rural setting.[23] HIV also impairs fertility, both by reducing the likelihood of conception and increasing the likelihood of spontaneous abortion or stillbirth. In Rakai, pregnancy rates among HIV-positive women are reduced by 55% (OR = 0.45, 95% CI, 0.35–0.57), and spontaneous abortion rates are increased by 50% (OR = 1.50, 95% CI, 1.01–2.27).[24] The impairment of fertility is most marked in symptomatic HIV-positive women (OR = 0.23, 95% CI, 0.11–0.48), and recent findings suggest that HIV-infected women with blood viral loads above 50 000 viral copies/ml have markedly reduced fertility.[25] Subfertility among HIV-positive women can lead to marital dissolution, because the inability to bear children is a common cause of divorce and separation in this society; the annual rates of marital dissolution are 7.3% in HIV-positive women compared with 3% in HIV-negative women.[26] Separated and divorced women are more likely to enter into new relationships and to have multiple sexual partners, which further facilitates transmission of HIV. In addition, separated, widowed, and divorced women are often economically disadvantaged female heads of household, and command fewer resources than are available to male household heads. In Rakai, women who head households have almost twice the age-adjusted mortality compared with male heads of households (relative risk (RR) = 1.98), whereas among non-household heads, male and female mortality are comparable (RR = 0.91).[27]

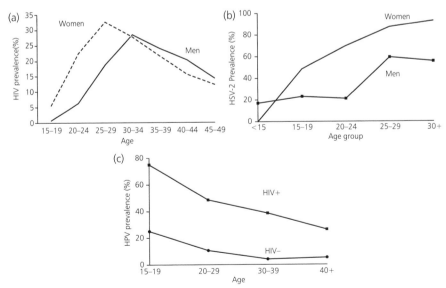

Fig. 15.2 Age-specific prevalence of (a) HIV (b) HSV-2 and (c) HPV (by HIV status). Rakai cohort, southwestern Uganda.[29]

Herpes type 2 (HSV-2) infections result in recurrent ulceration, which in itself is a risk factor for HIV acquisition.[28] In addition, women co-infected with HIV and HSV-2 experience more frequent, severe and persistent herpetic ulceration, which increases the genital tract shedding of both viruses.[14,15] Such higher genital viral shedding is likely to increase the transmission to male partners. These two infections interact, such that HSV-2 increases the risk of HIV infection, and HIV increases shedding and thus transmission of HSV-2 to sexual partners. A similar pattern is observed with HPV infections which are common in younger women, especially if they have co-infection with HIV.[29] In addition, shedding of HPV in the genital tract is increased among HIV-infected women, thus facilitating spread of HPV in the population (Fig. 15.3). Most women clear HPV infections by acquired immunity, but persistent HPV infection causes cervical cancer, and persistence is exacerbated by HIV.[1] In addition, the immunodeficiency caused by advanced HIV infection, promotes the more rapid progression of cervical cancers. There are approximately 500 000 new cases of cervical cancer annually, most in the developing countries where screening and treatment facilities are least adequate.[1] Cervical cancer is the main cause of female cancer deaths in the world, and Uganda has one of the highest cervical cancer rates in the world.[30]

Syphilis is an endemic STI in this population, and high rates of serological syphilis were documented during the colonial period. Because serum positivity (rapid plasma reagin (RPR) and Treponema pallidum hemagglutination assay (TPHA)/fluorescent treponemal antibody absorption test (FTA)) persists for many years, and is even lifelong with untreated syphilis, the overall syphilis seroprevalence rates rise progressively with age in this population, and are comparable in men and women (Fig. 15.4). This does not necessarily reflect active syphilis, particularly primary, secondary, and early latent infections, which constitute the greatest risk of transmission, particularly from mother to child. The diagnosis of active syphilis is based on a RPR titre of more than 1 : 8 and, as shown in Fig. 15.4, the age-specific prevalence of active syphilis increases up to age 39 in both sexes, although male rates tend to exceed female rates. However, at older ages, active syphilis continues to increase among males, but not among females. This probably reflects the higher frequency of extramarital relationships in older men, and suggests, as with HIV, that older men may be a source of infection for younger women.

Figure 15.5 shows the age-specific prevalence of the cervical bacterial STIs, (gonorrhoea and chlamydia). Chlamydia prevalence is highest in adolescence and declines with age as

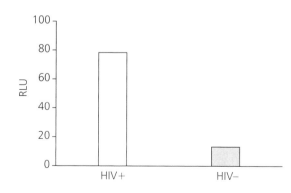

Fig. 15.3 HPV shedding (median relative light units (RLU)) in HIV+ and HIV− women less than 30 years old. Rakai cohort, southwestern Uganda.

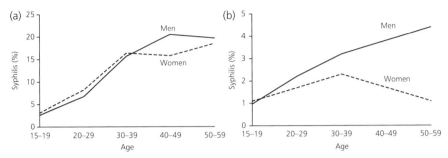

Fig. 15.4 Age-specific prevalence of (a) syphilis and (b) active syphilis (RPR > 1:8). Rakai cohort, southwestern Uganda.

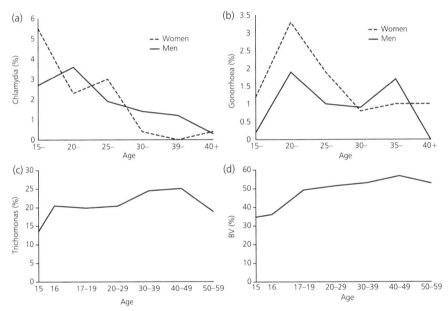

Fig. 15.5 Age-specific prevalence of (a) chlamydia, (b) gonorrhea, (c) trichomonas (females only) and (d) bacterial vaginosis (females only). Rakai cohort, southwestern Uganda.

women acquire immunity, but persistent asymptomatic infections are an important cause of tubal infertility.[32] Gonorrhoea prevalence peaks in young adulthood, where female infections exceed male infections, probably because male-to-female transmission of gonorrhoea is more efficient than transmission from females to males.[33] During pregnancy, both chlamydia and gonorrhoea are associated with poor pregnancy outcomes, and gonorrhoea in particular is a cause of blindness due to neonatal ophthalmia.[34]

The vaginal infections of bacterial vaginosis (BV) and trichomonas were only measured in women, using self-collected vaginal swabs, so male rates are not available. BV is a disturbance of the vaginal microbiology in which the normally beneficial lactobacilli are replaced by anaerobic organisms.[36] The causes of BV are unknown and are currently under investigation. BV is a sexually associated condition, and increases among women at time of sexual debut, or after recent changes in partners, but direct sexual transmission has not been demonstrated. One hypothesis is that the depletion of lactobacilli may be attributable to a viral bacteriophage, and the virus itself may be sexually transmitted, although this has not yet been demonstrated in humans. Personal hygiene, particularly douching, is associated with increased risk in US women, but no specific hygienic practices have been implicated in Rakai.[37] The normal vagina is acidic as a consequence of the hydrogen peroxide produced by lactobacilli, and this acidic environment is protective against infections from a wide variety of other organisms. However, with BV, the anaerobic overgrowth leads to an alkaline vaginal milieu and the anaerobes have been implicated as a cause of tubal infection, leading to infertility. As shown in Fig. 15.5, BV is extremely common in Rakai, affecting 50% of women. BV prevalence increases after sexual debut, and remains high throughout the reproductive ages. BV is also common in other rural and urban sub-Saharan African populations.[38,39]

Trichomonas rates increase among the young and remain high, diminishing somewhat in older women (Fig. 15.5). Trichomonas is highly infectious and there is little acquired immunity, so the persistent high rates probably reflect lack of treatment and re-infection.[40]

The complex transmission of HIV and STIs is illustrated in Fig. 15.6. Among women, the prevalence of both infections increases markedly if they have multiple sexual partners, particularly if these partners come from outside of the community of residence. Approximately 4% of women report having multiple extramarital relationships per year, most of which are concurrent relationships and often are an economic necessity.[41] In essence, these women constitute a 'core group' of transmitters, but they are not identifiable as conventional commercial sex workers or bar girls who commonly form core groups in urban settings. These are predominantly economically disadvantaged single women, who depend on multiple relationships with men for support. Rates of these infections do not increase markedly among men with multiple sexual partners. In this population, 25% of men report multiple partners each year, and most contacts are casual relationships. Because such casual sex is relatively frequent and more 'normative' behaviour among males, it is less predictive of disease risk. These men probably have relationships predominantly with the minority of women reporting multiple partnerships.

In summary, STIs are common in this population, and rates are higher than hitherto estimated in studies such as the WHO Global Burden of Disease. Earlier studies which used less

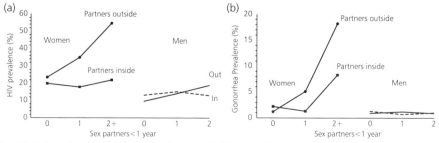

Fig. 15.6 Prevalence of (a) HIV prevalence and (b) gonorrhea by sex partners and location. Rakai cohort, southwestern Uganda.

sensitive diagnostic methods, often in selected clinic populations, seriously underestimate the frequency of these infections.

15.3 Consequences of maternal sexually transmitted infections for the newborn

STIs during pregnancy present a serious hazard to the fetus and newborn.[42] The rates of maternal infection during pregnancy and infections of newborn are shown in Table 15.1. These data are derived from the control arm of a randomized trial to evaluate the impact of STD control during pregnancy in the Rakai cohort.[35] The prevalence of HIV among pregnant woman was 12.8%, which is lower than the prevalence in all women of reproductive-age (19%), because HIV infection suppresses fertility.[24] In Rakai, the rate of HIV transmission from mother-to-child either *in utero* or at delivery is 20%, and rates of breast milk transmission are approximately 12%, which is comparable to transmission rates observed in urban populations of sub-Saharan Africa.[43] Thus, on average 32% of babies born to HIV-infected mothers are themselves infected. The mortality among HIV-positive

Table 15.1 Maternal HIV and STI infections during pregnancy, and infant ocular infections in the control arm of the STD Control for Maternal and Child Health Study[35]

Maternal and Infant STDs	Infections/ Number tested	Prevalence (%)
Prevalence of Maternal Infections		
HIV	176/1374	12.8
Syphilis	46/1376	3.3
Trichomonas	248/1569	15.9
Bacterial Vaginosis	764/1576	48.5
Gonorrhoea	24/1394	1.7
Chlamydia	38/1394	2.7
Gonorrhoea and/or Chlamydia	60/1394	4.3
Upper genital tract infection	63/1808	3.5
Prevalence of Infant Ocular Infections		
Gonorrhoea	17/1008	1.7
Chlamydia	11/1008	1.1
Gonorrhoea or Chlamydia	28/1008	2.8

infants is very high; 310 per 1000 during the first year of life and 515 per 1000 by the end of the second year.[44] The high transmission and mortality rates reflect the absence of treatment in the population, although programmes have now been established to prevent mother-to-child transmission, using home-based maternal self-medication with nevirapine. (Most deliveries occur in the home, and mothers must take the medication at onset of labour, and provide a infant syrup within 72 hours of birth, so self-medication is the only feasible mode of service delivery). Maternal HIV infection also increases the risk of low birthweight and preterm birth twofold or more in infants born to HIV-positive mothers.[35,45] This is in part a consequence of *in utero* HIV infection of the fetus, and possibly an effect of poor maternal nutrition, consequent upon immunodeficiency and opportunistic infections. In addition, HIV-infected mothers are more likely to have placental malaria, which itself increases the risk of low birthweight.[46]

There are also social factors affecting infant survival. Children born to HIV-positive mothers in polygamous marriages had twice the mortality of children born to HIV-infected mothers in monogamous marriages, but no effects of polygamy on child survival is observed in HIV-negative women.[47] This suggests possible paternal stigmatization and disadvantage of HIV-infected wives and their offspring in polygamous relationships.

HIV incidence among pregnant women is high (3.3 per 100 person years), and maternal mortality in HIV-positive mothers is 1686 per 100 000 births, which is five times higher than maternal mortality in HIV-negative mothers.[35] Orphaned children of mothers who die are also at markedly increased risk of death.

The prevalence of syphilis in pregnancy was 10% at the enrollment baseline survey, but declined to 3% after provision of testing and treatment.[35] Syphilis among pregnant women was 3.3% in the Rakai control arm population, because for ethical reasons, all pregnant women were screened and treated with penicillin for syphilis during pregnancy. Approximately 50–70% of infants born to mothers with active syphilis will either die *in utero* or during infancy, be born at low birthweights or prematurely, or develop congenital syphilis. The effects on birthweight and preterm birth probably reflect infection of the fetus and newborn. This treatable disease is still a significant cause of morbidity in children, in settings where screening is inadequate.

The prevalence of maternal gonorrhoea during pregnancy was 1.7%, and 45% of infants born to infected mothers develop gonorrhoeal ophthalmia, which is a common cause of blindness in the new born. Chlamydia infection was 2.7%, and 45% of babies born to infected mothers were found to have ocular infections. Gonorrhoea and chlamydia are both associated with low birthweight and preterm birth, because ascending genital tract infections cause inflammation of the placental membranes (chorioamnionitis), which weakens the connective tissues resulting in premature and often preterm rupture of membranes.[49]

In Rakai, BV was very common during pregnancy (48.5%) and similar findings have been reported from other African studies.[38,39] BV has been implicated as a common cause of preterm and low birthweight births via chorioamnionitis and premature rupture of membranes.[50] Several, but not all, clinical trials have shown that treatment of BV during pregnancy can reduce the rates of these adverse pregnancy outcomes.[35] Trichomonas was markedly reduced by treatment in the intervention arm, but the link between trichomonas and low birthweight/preterm delivery is less clearly established.[51] Postpartum upper genital tract infection is difficult to diagnose under these circumstances, and was lower in the intervention arm, although this was not statistically significant.

The randomized trial of STD control in Rakai treated all bacterial STDs among pregnant women in the intervention arm. The control arm women received syndromic management for symptomatic STIs, and screening and treatment for syphilis. Thus, with the exception of syphilis (which was comparable in the intervention and control arms), the trial allowed an estimate of the impact of treatable STIs on pregnancy outcome. The treatment reduced the risk of low birthweight (RR = 0.68, 95% CI, 0.53–0.86), preterm birth (RR = 0.77, 95% CI, 0.56–1.05), neonatal death (RR = 0.83, 95% CI, 0.71–0.97), and infant ophthalmia due to gonorrhoea or chlamydia (RR = 0.33, CI 0.20–0.70).[35] This provides an indication of the importance of maternal STIs for the health and survival of infants.

15.4 Long-term consequences of sexually transmitted diseases through the life course

Infections such as gonorrhoea, chlamydia, and the anaerobes of BV that are known to invade the upper genital tract causing pelvic inflammatory disease and tubal scarring, are also known risk factors for infertility and ectopic pregnancy. Other infections, such as HIV and untreated syphilis have consequences for long-term health. In the absence of treatment, the median adult survival time for HIV is approximately 10 years following infection, and the disease is almost universally fatal.[52] Studies of untreated syphilis in the pre-antibiotic era suggests that one third of cases progressed to tertiary syphilis, developing disseminated disease affecting the central nervous system, cardiovascular system, skin, eyes, bones, and internal organs.[48] Although HPV is common in younger women (approximately 16%), persistent infections are found in approximately 5% among women aged 30–35. Such persistent infections are likely to progress to pre-malignant cervical lesions in 15–25% of women over two to four years, and such lesions are likely to progress to cancer in 20–30% of women. Cervical cancer has a relatively early age of onset (late thirties and early forties). Five-year survival rates in the US are over 70%, but in developing countries survival is much lower, because women present with advanced disease and treatment options are limited.[1]

The long-term consequences of infant infections are known to some degree. Among HIV-infected infants, the median survival time in the absence of treatment is approximately two years. Among children born to mothers with active syphilis, approximately 20% are likely to die during infancy, and 20% will have active syphilis resulting in serious morbidity, handicap, and death, if untreated.[48]

As noted earlier, many STIs (e.g. gonorrhoea, chlamydia, BV, syphilis, and HIV) result in low birthweight and preterm birth, both of which are associated with higher risks of infant mortality. Infections during pregnancy have also been implicated as serious risk factors for cerebral palsy and impairment of brain development resulting in mental handicap.[54] In addition, there is a growing body of epidemiological evidence suggesting that infants born with low birthweight or prematurely, have higher rates of cardiovascular disease (hypertension, diabetes, and myocardial infarction,[11,55] and see Chapters 5 and 6), and are at greater risk of chronic obstructive lung disease in adulthood. However, there is controversy in the interpretation of these associations, partly because of concerns over uncontrolled confounding due to genetic influences and other factors such as the importance of prenatal or postnatal growth.[56] In addition, there have been no studies of the association between low birthweight and subsequent cardiovascular disease in African populations, so the long-term consequences cannot be determined for these populations. The causes of low birthweight observed in African populations may differ from those observed in industrialized countries, or the survival of infants may be poorer, so the consequences for adult cardiovascular disease may not be applicable in this context.

Quantifying the effects of STIs on health during the life course will be an important subject for future research. Nevertheless, given the frequency of these infections, even a modest increase in the relative risk of long-term sequelae could be of profound public health importance.

Commentary on 'Sexually transmitted infections and health through the life course'

Andrew J. Hall

This paper elegantly describes the high rates of infection with a plethora of infectious agents in Ugandan women. Even more horrifying is the violence that frequently leads to their acquisition. Gray, Wawer, and Serwadda point out two of the important consequences of these infections. First the high rates of perinatal transmission of some of these infections—notably HIV and syphilis—which leads to serious morbidity and mortality in the children. Second the long-term consequences of many of these infections, especially the persistent viruses HIV, HBV, and HPV on the health of the women. The impact of STI on the subsequent fertility of the women is also well-known and deserves mention. In many African societies this infertility is stigmatized and can lead to social isolation.

From a life course perspective STIs are an interesting example because the vast bulk of exposure occurs over a relatively limited period of life. Nevertheless age at infection may turn out to be a critical factor in determining outcome. For hepatitis B virus the evidence is very strong that the risk of persistence, with the associated chronic liver disease including primary liver cancer, is very high early in life. By the age of six years it is down to the relatively low levels of adult life, at around 6% of infections leading to carriage. In fact in Uganda, as throughout Africa, the long-term sequelae of hepatitis B virus are not associated with sexual transmission at all but with childhood transmission by close contact. There is now a suggestion that early age at infection with a pathogenic papillomavirus may be a particularly high risk for cervical cancer. This makes the findings in these studies from Rakai particularly worrying.

A second point that may be rewarded by longitudinal study is the effect of the sequence of infection by different agents. We know that many infections may modify response to subsequent infections both by the same agent and by others. HIV because of its profound effects on the immune system is the classical example of this. However infections such as measles and respiratory syncytial virus also modify immune responses over a period of weeks and possibly longer. Reproductive tract infections may also have direct physical effects making the woman more susceptible to subsequent infection. This interplay of infections has been studied to some extent in the transmission of HIV but it would be interesting to relate it to the natural history of infection and in particular to long-term effects. Viral load is an increasingly useful intermediary variable for this purpose.

The maturation and competence of the immune system both locally and systemically is another important factor when considering the impact of infections. The timing and sequence of infections may again be important here. This effect may be particularly important early in life when the immune system is still plastic. The effect of early life infection as a protective factor against atopy is a clear example of this. This programming of the immune system may determine the response to acute infection as well as the ability to deal with persistent infection. An interesting aspect of this in Africa is the pattern of mixing of children at a young age that differs markedly from western Europe where most studies of atopy have been conducted. Studies of the age at acquisition of infection in African villages in relation to family size and mixing patterns would be of interest. These would lay the ground for studies of their effect when infection is acquired in adolescence and adulthood. In much of Africa every child has acquired persistent infections with Epstein Barr virus, Herpes simplex, and cytomegalovirus by the age of three years. Since much of the circulating T cell pool, even in Europeans, is devoted to these agents the impact of this on subsequent infections deserves study.

The immune system's functional capacity is also dependent on nutrition. Mucosal surfaces require micronutrients such as vitamin A to maintain optimal protective integrity. A number of dietary elements are key to the optimal function of phagocytes and lymphocytes. The role of dietary deficiency in childhood, adolescence and at the time of a sexually acquired infection may be critical to the outcome. Supplementation trials are now addressing some of these issues in the context of HIV.

However the starkest message from this article is the violence of sexual debut for many women in this society and the repetitive nature of that sexual violence. This is clearly the issue that is most deserving of a life course approach, in terms of the childhood background that leads to an acceptance of this by society and a continuation of it by men. Understanding the intergenerational effects in relation to psychology and societal values that lead to the persistence of the phenomenon may clarify ways of interrupting it. This may be the best way forward in addressing the burden of STIs in these women.

References

1 **Schiffman MH, Brinton LA, Devesa SS, Fraumeni JF**. Cervical Cancer. In: Schottenfeld D, Fraumeni JF, eds. *Cancer epidemiology and prevention*. Second ed. New York; Oxford: Oxford University Press,1996, pp. 1090–116.

2 **Herrero R, Hildesheim A, Bratti C, Sherman ME, Hutchinson M, Morales J** *et al*. Population-based study of human papillomavirus infection and cervical neoplasia in rural Costa Rica. *J Natl Cancer Inst* 2000;**92**:464–74.

3 **Francis DP**. Hepatitis B virus and its related diseases. In: Walsh JA, Warren KS, eds. *Strategies for primary health care*. Chicago: University of Chicago Press,1986, pp. 289–97.

4 **Kane M, Clements J, Hu D**. Hepatitis B. In: Jamison DT, Mosley WH, eds. *Disease control priorities in developing countries*. New York: Oxford University Press for the World Bank, 1993.

5 **Nomura A, Stemmermann GN, Chyou PH, Kato I, Perez-Perez GI, Blaser MJ**. Helicobacter pylori infection and gastric carcinoma among Japanese Americans in Hawaii. *N Engl J Med* 1991;**325**:1132–6.

6 Parsonnet J, Friedman GD, Vandersteen DP, Chang Y, Vogelman JH, Orentreich N *et al*. Helicobacter pylori infection and the risk of gastric carcinoma. *N Engl J Med* 1991;**325**:1127–31.

7 Lyall EG, Patton GS, Sheldon J, Stainsby C, Mullen J, O'Shea S *et al*. Evidence for horizontal and not vertical transmission of human herpesvirus 8 in children born to human immunodeficiency virus-infected mothers. *Pediatr Infect Dis J* 1999;**18**:795–9.

8 Antman K, Chang Y. Kaposi's sarcoma. *N Engl J Med* 2000;**342**:1027–38.

9 Beral V, Newton R, Sitas F. Human herpesvirus 8 and cancer. *J Natl Cancer Inst* 1999;**91**:1440–1.

10 Gaydos CA, Quinn TC. The role of Chlamydia pneumoniae in cardiovascular disease. *Adv Intern Med* 2000;**45**:139–73.

11 Mosley WH, Gray RH. Childhood precursors of adult morbidity and mortality in developing countries: implications for health programs. In: Gribble JN, Preston SH, eds. *The epidemiologic transition: policy and planning implications for developing countries*. Washington, DC: National Academy Press, 1993:69–100.

12 Murray CJL, Styblo K, Rouillon A. Tuberculosis. In: Jamison DT, Mosley WH, eds. *Disease control priorities in developing countries*. New York: Oxford University Press for the World Bank, 1993.

13 Frost WH. The age selection of mortality from tuberculosis in successive decades. *Am J Hygiene* 1939;**30**:91–6.

14 Schacker T, Zeh J, Hu HL, Hill E, Corey L. Frequency of symptomatic and asymptomatic herpes simplex virus type 2 reactivations among human immunodeficiency virus-infected men. *J Infect Dis* 1998;**178**:1616–22.

15 Schacker T, Ryncarz AJ, Goddard J, Diem K, Shaughnessy M, Corey L. Frequent recovery of HIV-1 from genital herpes simplex virus lesions in HIV-1-infected men. *J Am Med Assoc* 1998;**280**:61–6.

16 Dye C, Scheele S, Dolin P, Pathania V, Raviglione MC. Consensus statement. Global burden of tuberculosis: estimated incidence, prevalence, and mortality by country. WHO Global Surveillance and Monitoring Project. *J Am Med Assoc* 1999;**282**:677–86.

17 von Reyn CF. The significance of bacteremic tuberculosis among persons with HIV infection in developing countries. *AIDS* 1999;**13**:2193–5.

18 Wawer MJ, Gray RH, Sewankambo NK, Serwadda D, Paxton L, Berkley S *et al*. A randomized, community trial of intensive sexually transmitted disease control for AIDS prevention, Rakai, Uganda. *AIDS* 1998;**12**:1211–25.

19 Wawer MJ, Sewankambo NK, Serwadda D, Quinn TC, Paxton LA, Kiwanuka N *et al*. Control of sexually transmitted diseases for AIDS prevention in Uganda: a randomised community trial. Rakai Project Study Group. *Lancet* 1999;**353**:525–35.

20 Buve A, Carael M, Hayes RJ, Auvert B, Ferry B, Robinson NJ *et al*. The multicentre study on factors determining the differential spread of HIV in four African cities: summary and conclusions. *AIDS* 2001;**15 (Suppl 4)**:S127–S131.

21 Kelly RJ, Gray RH, Sewankambo NK, Serwadda D, Wabwire-Mangen F, Lutalo T *et al*. Age differences in Sexual Partners and Risk of HIV-1 Infection in Rural Uganda. J *AIDS Retrovirol* 2001;Submitted.

22 Koenig MA, Lutalo T, Zhao F, Kiwanuka N, Wabwire-Mangen F, Kigozi G *et al*. Prevalence of and risk factors for coercive sex in Rakai, Uganda. *Bull World Health Org* 2001, Submitted.

23 Sewankambo NK, Gray RH, Ahmad S, Serwadda D, Wabwire-Mangen F, Nalugoda F *et al*. Mortality associated with HIV infection in rural Rakai District, Uganda. *AIDS* 2000;**14**:2391–400.

24 Gray RH, Wawer MJ, Serwadda D, Sewankambo N, Li C, Wabwire-Mangen F *et al*. Population-based study of fertility in women with HIV-1 infection in Uganda. *Lancet* 1998;**351**:98–103.

25 Nguyen RHN, Gange SJ, Quinn TC, Serwadda D, Wabwire-Mangen F, Wawer MJ, Gray RH. Association between HIV-RNA Viral Load and Subfertility: Rakai, Uganda (Abstract).

39th Annual Meeting of the Infectious Diseases Society of America, October 25–28, 2001, San Francisco, CA. ABSTRACT 201916

26 Porter LE, Hao L, Bishai D, Gray RH, Serwadda D, Lutalo T, *et al.* IV Status and Union Dissolution in Uganda (Abstract). Annual Meeting of the Population Association of America, May 9–11, 2002, Atlanta, GA.

27 Nalugoda F, Gray RH, Serwadda D, Sewankambo NK, Wabwire-Mangen F, Kiwanuka N *et al.* HIV infection among heads and non-heads of rural households in Rakai, Uganda. *J AIDS Retrovirol* 2002; Submitted.

28 Gray RH, Wawer MJ, Sewankambo NK, Serwadda D, Li C, Moulton LH *et al.* Relative risks and population attributable fraction of incident HIV associated with symptoms of sexually transmitted diseases and treatable symptomatic sexually transmitted diseases in Rakai District, Uganda. Rakai Project Team. *AIDS* 1999;**13**:2113–23.

29 Serwadda D, Wawer MJ, Shah KV, Sewankambo NK, Daniel R, Li C *et al.* Use of a hybrid capture assay of self-collected vaginal swabs in rural Uganda for detection of human papillomavirus. *J Infect Dis* 1999;**180**:1316–9.

30 Wabinga HR, Parkin DM, Wabwire-Mangen F, Mugerwa JW. Cancer in Kampala, Uganda, in 1989–91: changes in incidence in the era of AIDS. *Int J Cancer* 1993;**54**:26–36.

31 Schulz KF, Cates W, Jr., O'Mara PR. Pregnancy loss, infant death, and suffering: legacy of syphilis and gonorrhoea in Africa. *Genitourin Med* 1987;**63**:320–5.

32 Stamm WE. Chlamydia trachomatis infections of the adult. In: Holmes KK, Sparling PF, Mardh P, Lemon SM, Stamm WE, Piot P *et al.*, eds. *Sexually transmitted diseases.* Third ed. New York, NY: McGraw-Hill, 1999, pp. 407–22.

33 Hook III EW, Hansfield HH. Gonococcal infections in the adult. In: Holmes KK, Sparling PF, Mardh P, Lemon SM, Stamm WE, Piot P *et al.*, eds. *Sexually transmitted diseases.* Third ed. New York, NY: McGraw-Hill, 1999, pp. 451–66.

34 Gutman LT. Gonococcal disease in infants and children. In: Holmes KK, Sparling PF, Mardh P, Lemon SM, Stamm WE, Piot P *et al.*, eds. *Sexually transmitted diseases.* Third ed. New York, NY: McGraw-Hill, 1999, pp. 1145–53.

35 Gray RH, Wabwire-Mangen F, Kigozi G, Sewankambo NK, Serwadda D, Moulton LH *et al.* Randomized Trial of presumptive STD Therapy During Pregnancy in Rakai, Uganda. *Am J Obstet Gynecol* 2001;**185**:1209–17.

36 Hillier S, Holmes KK. Bacterial vaginosis. In: Holmes KK, Sparling PF, Mardh P, Lemon SM, Stamm WE, Piot P *et al.*, eds. *Sexually transmitted diseases.* Third ed. New York, NY: McGraw-Hill, 1999, pp. 563–86.

37 Mead PB. Epidemiology of bacterial vaginosis. *Am J Obstet Gynecol.* 1993;**169**:446–9.

38 Taha TE, Hoover DR, Dallabetta GA, Kumwenda NI, Mtimavalye LA, Yang LP *et al.* Bacterial vaginosis and disturbances of vaginal flora: association with increased acquisition of HIV. *AIDS* 1998;**12**:1699–706.

39 Cohen CR, Duerr A, Pruithithada N, Rugpao S, Hillier S, Garcia P *et al.* Bacterial vaginosis and HIV seroprevalence among female commercial sex workers in Chiang Mai, Thailand. *AIDS* 1995;**9**:1093–7.

40 Krieger JN, Alderete JF. Trichomonas vaginalis and Trichomoniasis. In: Holmes KK, Sparling PF, Mardh P, Lemon SM, Stamm WE, Piot P *et al.*, eds. *Sexually transmitted diseases.* third ed. New York, NY: McGraw-Hill, 1999, pp. 587–604.

41 Kelly RJ, Gray RH, Sewankambo NK, Serwadda D, Wabwire-Mangen F, Valente TW *et al.* The risk of prevalent and incident HIV with concurrent and non-concurrent sexual partnerships. *Sex Transm Dis* 2001; Submitted.

42 Hitchcock PJ, MacKay HT, Wasserheit JN, Binder R. *Sexually Transmitted Disease and Adverse Outcomes of Pregnancy.* Washington, DC: American Society of Microbiology Press, 2001.

43 Nduati R, John G, Mbori-Ngacha D, Richardson B, Overbaugh J, Mwatha A *et al.* Effect of breastfeeding and formula feeding on transmission of HIV-1: a randomized clinical trial. *J Am Med Assoc* 2000;**283**:1167–74.

44 Brahmbhatt H, Wabwire-Mangen F, Kigozi G, Wawer MJ, Rakai Project Team, Gray RH. Association of maternal HIV and child survival in Rakai, Uganda (Abstract). Global Strategies Conference, Sept. 2001, Kampala, Uganda.

45 Taha TE, Dallabetta GA, Canner JK, Chiphangwi JD, Liomba G, Hoover DR *et al.* The effect of human immunodeficiency virus infection on birthweight, and infant and child mortality in urban Malawi. *Int J Epidemiol* 1995;**24**:1022–9.

46 Wabwire-Mangen F, Gray RH, Wawer MJ, Sewankambo N, Serwadda D. HIV-1 infection and malaria parasitaemia. Lancet 2001;**357**:233.

47 Brahmbhatt H, Bishai D, Wabwire-Mangen F, Kigozi G, Wawer MJ, Gray RH. Polygyny, Maternal HIV status and child survival: Rakai, Uganda. *Soc Sci Med* 2001, Submitted.

48 Sanchez PJ. Syphilis and Pregnancy. In: Hitchcock PJ, MacKay HT, Wasserheit JN, Binder R, eds. *Sexually transmitted disease and adverse outcomes of pregnancy*. Washington, DC: American Society of Microbiology Press; 1999, pp. 125–50.

49 Morse SA, Beck-Sague CM. Gonorrhoea. In: Hitchcock PJ, MacKay HT, Wasserheit JN, Binder R, eds. *Sexually transmitted disease and adverse outcomes of pregnancy*. Washington, DC: American Society of Microbiology Press, 1999, pp. 151–74.

50 Eschenbach DA. Bacterial Vaginosis. In: Hitchcock PJ, MacKay HT, Wasserheit JN, Binder R, eds. *Sexually transmitted disease and adverse outcomes of pregnancy*. Washington, DC: American Society for Microbiology, 1999, pp. 103–24.

51 Klebanoff MA, Carey JC, Hauth JC, Hillier SL, Nugent RP, Thom EA *et al.* Failure of metronidazole to prevent preterm delivery among pregnant women with asymptomatic Trichomonas vaginalis infection. *N Engl J Med* 2001;**345**:487–93.

52 Morgan D, Malamba SS, Maude GH, Okongo MJ, Wagner HU, Mulder DW *et al.* An HIV-1 natural history cohort and survival times in rural Uganda. *AIDS* 1997;**11**:633–40.

53 Wu YW, Colford JM, Jr. Chorioamnionitis as a risk factor for cerebral palsy: A meta-analysis. *J Am Med Assoc* 2000;**284**:1417–24.

54 Barker JP, Godfrey KM, Fall C, Osmond C, Winter PD, Shaheen SO. Relation of birth weight and childhood respiratory infection to adult lung function and death from chronic obstructive airways disease. *Br Med J* 1991;**303**:671–5.

55 Poulter NR. Birthweights, maternal cardiovascular events, and the Barker hypothesis. *Lancet* 2001;**357**:1990–1.

56 Susser M, Levin B. Ordeals for the Fetal programming hypothesis; the hypothesis largely survives one ordeal but not another. *Br Med J* 1999;**318**:885–6.

Part IV

Explaining health and disease patterns

Chapter 16

Disease trends in women living in established market economies: evidence of cohort effects during the epidemiological transition

Diana Kuh, Isabel dos Santos Silva, and
Elizabeth Barrett-Connor

At a population level life course explanations for disease trends need to be sought in the differential life experiences of successive birth cohorts. In this chapter we chose to investigate birth cohort effects in all-cause mortality, breast cancer, and cardiovascular disease trends that may reflect long-term influences of early life experience. A positive relationship between all-cause child and adult mortality has been observed in a number of birth cohorts of established market economies. For example, birth cohort effects in all-cause mortality observed in England and Wales for cohorts born from 1766 to 1906 reflected successive cohort declines in mortality from diseases such as tuberculosis, stomach cancer, and rheumatic heart disease that were related to similar declines in childhood infections. These 'early life infection' diseases are still common in developing countries. Cohort effects that may be due to early growth are also evident in the increase in breast cancer mortality and the decline in stroke mortality. Trends in these diseases are more compatible with trends in postnatal growth indicators such as adult height and age at menarche than with prenatal growth indicators such as birthweight for which there is little evidence of a secular trend. These explanations enrich the traditional epidemiological transition theory which has focused on general environmental improvements, lifestyle modifications, and developments in medical care. Further research using cohort incidence or disability data is to be preferred in high life expectancy countries.

16.1 Extending a life course perspective to population health

Much of the initial emphasis of life course epidemiology has been on understanding individual variation in chronic disease risk (see Part II of this book). Recently, more attention has been given to the potential of a life course approach to aid in understanding variations in the health and disease of populations over time, across countries, and between social groups.[1–4] This is important as factors that explain the variation in risk between individuals may not explain the level of disease in a population or its change over time.[5] This chapter examines trends in all-cause mortality and in coronary heart disease (CHD), stroke, breast and lung cancer. These diseases show very different patterns over time and place but all had a significant impact on women's health in the twentieth century. The first three are the classic 'life course diseases' affected by factors operating at every stage of life and which may have interactive effects on individual disease risk (see Chapters 3 and 5).[2,6] Trends in lung cancer are also considered given the importance of this disease for cohorts of women born in the twentieth century.

A life course approach starts from the premise that various factors throughout life, independently, cumulatively, and interactively, affect health outcomes in later life. Thus, at the population level, explanations for disease trends need to be sought in the differential life experiences of successive birth cohorts or generations. Disentangling the effects of various risk factors at different life stages on mortality and disease trends poses considerable challenges and can be attempted by different approaches. Environmental factors in early life may have more effect on short- and long-term health than they would in later life, partly through their influence on growth. We have therefore chosen to focus on childhood risk factors such as living conditions and growth indicators such as birthweight, height and age at menarche, and investigate their influence on all-cause mortality and on disease-specific trends later in life. We studied populations of women living in established market economies where data on disease trends were deemed relatively reliable. Data on long-term trends in birthweight, age at menarche, and adult stature were derived from a number of sources as they have not been routinely monitored over a long period of time in these countries.

One way to investigate childhood influences on women's disease trends is to look for birth cohort effects which can occur if the disease impact of an environmental change (such as an improvement (or a deterioration) in living standards) depends on age at exposure. Although this may reflect an early life effect, birth cohort effects can occur for other reasons, for example, if new treatments are more effective at some ages than others. Cohort differences in adult disease can also occur if there are cohort variations in later risk factors such as childbearing characteristics or in the adoption of habits such as smoking. The interpretation of observed cohort effects as an early life effect will depend on whether cohort trends in adult mortality and disease rates are consistent with cohort trends in the childhood risk factors of interest or perhaps more consistent with cohort trends in these later risk factors. The change in some risk factors may be described as a period effect, for example the epidemic of obesity in the 1990s which affected all age groups[7] but it may play out in a cohort fashion on disease trends if duration of exposure to obesity affects disease risk.

16.1.1 Investigating temporal trends and cohorts effects

Interpretation of variation in disease-specific mortality trends has various difficulties.[8] The observed changes may be real, due to changes in disease incidence or case fatality, or artefactual, due to changes in clinical diagnosis or the quality of the data (for example in terms of coverage or accuracy). Quality of the data permitting, age-specific death rates (usually from official statistics) allow international comparison of disease trends. Changes in death rates may provide clues to aetiology particularly where case-fatality ratio is high. This ratio is not only affected by the natural history of the disease, but also by the effectiveness of treatment that may change over time and vary between countries. The increasing effectiveness of medical interventions for some chronic diseases[9,10] and rapid declines in adult mortality in recent years have further limited the use of mortality data to understand disease trends.

A cohort effect in disease trends is evident when age-specific rates rise and fall in parallel when plotted against year of birth. In contrast, period effects are evident when there is a parallel shift in rates for each age group during a particular calendar period. Age-cohort and age-period models provide summary measures for describing the data and identifying possible cohort or period effects. More complex age-period-cohort models can be fitted to help distinguish these effects but require assumptions in order to estimate the parameters of the model because of the linear dependency among the three factors.[11,12] Period and cohort effects are easiest to distinguish when disease trends have accelerated, decelerated, or changed direction. Where they are steady and linear they cannot be reliably assigned as a period or cohort effect.[8] This is a serious limitation that cannot be overcome.

16.1.2 The epidemiological transition: a common framework for studying time trends

Over the last two hundred years, economic and social development, including the pace of urbanization and industrialization in what are now called the established market economies, triggered the epidemiological transition. The epidemiological transition theory,[13] recently reformulated by Omran as a five stage/five model theory,[14] encompasses changes in disease and health patterns, fertility and population ageing, lifestyles, health care patterns, and the environment. By the second half of the nineteenth century, countries of northern and western Europe had moved through the first two transition stages of the western transition model (age of pestilence and famine and age of receding pandemics) and were entering the third stage (the age of degenerative, stress, and man-made diseases). They were followed somewhat later by southern Europe, Germany, the US, and Australia, and even later by Japan and the USSR (the transition in these last two countries is described as a semi-western/ accelerated model). The common feature of the epidemiological transition in its first three stages was a shift from a high mortality, low life expectancy regime where infectious diseases, occurring mainly in children and young adults, were the main causes of death, to a high life expectancy regime, where chronic diseases of adulthood and old age became the most frequent causes of death. This transition was essentially complete by the end of the Second World War for all western countries. The fourth stage (age of declining cardiovascular mortality, population ageing, lifestyle modification, emerging and resurgent diseases) began around 1970 for western countries and Japan. It has yet to occur in some of the countries of eastern Europe and the former USSR where there has been a continuing rise in cardiovascular mortality associated with social and economic change. Omran discusses briefly the expected fifth stage of the epidemiological transition (around the mid twenty-first century), questioning whether longevity gains will be matched by improvements in the quality of life or the compression of morbidity, or socioeconomic disparities within or between countries will be reduced.[14]

The transition from infectious to degenerative diseases benefited the health of women more than the health of men. In the pre-modern era females generally had a lower or equal life expectancy compared with males but by the nineteenth century the sex differential had shifted in favour of females in the developed countries.[14,15] Mortality rates for women of reproductive age in England and Wales remained higher than for their male peers until the middle of the nineteenth century.[16] They were persistently worse for adolescent girls until the end of the nineteenth century in these countries[16] and even later in other European countries such as Italy.[17] The relative improvement in female mortality was not due, at least at first, to the decline in maternal mortality which did not start its sustained decline in western countries until the late 1930s.[18] Rather women benefited more from the decline in respiratory tuberculosis (an important contributor to the overall decline in infectious disease, particularly at ages 15–44 years), and suffered less from the emerging degenerative diseases. For example, between 1900 and 1960 the age standardized excess mortality of US men over US women rose from 8% to 55% for respiratory diseases, 4 to 150% for respiratory tuberculosis, and 8% to 71% for cardiovascular diseases.[13] Cancers, for which there had been a female excess of 79% in 1900, turned into a male excess of 25% by 1960. From the mid 1970s (coinciding with the fourth stage of transition) the female advantage in life expectancy has lessened[19] in most industrialized countries, mainly because improvements in male death rates between the ages of 25 and 59 years have been more rapid for men than women. This may be because men modified their lifestyles earlier than women (see Chapter 13) or benefited more from new medical treatments.

Although the relative impact of cardiovascular diseases and cancers increased as infectious diseases declined, it is important to differentiate the chronic diseases such as ischaemic heart disease, lung cancer, and breast cancer for which death rates increased from diseases such as stomach cancer and stroke where death rates decreased during the third stage of the epidemiological transition. In association with the shift to a high life expectancy regime dominated by chronic disease and excess male mortality, the populations of established market economies experienced secular trends in body size, and significant changes in childbearing patterns, diet, smoking, and activity levels (see Chapters 1, 13, and 14). These are all common features of the epidemiological transition; however, the timing, speed, and duration of the transition has differed across countries[20,21] and by socioeconomic group, ethnicity, and other population subgroups.[14,22] A life course perspective enriches the epidemiological transition theory by investigating possible links between a cohort's experience at younger ages and its disease and mortality risk at older ages. It suggests explanations for the transition in addition to the general environmental improvements, lifestyle modifications, and developments in medical care described by Omran.[14]

16.2 The role of childhood living conditions in the decline in mortality during the epidemiological transition

16.2.1 Nineteenth century birth cohorts

We know from vital registrations from Nordic countries and from detailed analyses by historical demographers of parish registers in France and England that the secular decline in mortality for these countries had begun by the second half of the eighteenth century.[21,23] Heterogeneity rather than homogeneity was a feature of the mortality decline among European countries,[24] and there were periods of stagnation particularly in countries like England and Scotland which experienced rapid urbanization. The causes of the mortality decline have been the topic of longstanding interdisciplinary research and debate.

McKeown[25,26] argued that the most important reason for the decline was the improved resistance to infections caused by better nutrition which particularly reduced mortality from tuberculosis. Others have argued that the provision of clean water, sewerage, and drainage by public health authorities,[27] and changes in personal behaviour and hygiene[28] made much larger contributions to the mortality decline.

One of the features common to the mortality decline in all countries was that it occurred earlier and was greatest in the youngest age groups with the notable exception of infant mortality.[13,29,30] This is illustrated in Fig. 16.1 with data on official death rates for females from England and Wales from 1841. Whether the decline in infant and child mortality would weaken or strengthen the subsequent health of the surviving adult population was a matter of great debate in the early twentieth century[31] and remains so today.[32] In the early twentieth century, public health reformers argued that lower mortality in early life would improve population health whereas the eugenicists claimed it would lead to the physical degeneration of the population. Early cohort analysis of official mortality statistics between 1845–1921 in England and Wales provided some of the first evidence to support the positive public health view by showing one of the earliest cohort effects.[31,33–35] Age-specific death rates plotted by year of birth rather than year of death declined in parallel indicating that the mortality risk of each successive generation was lower at all subsequent ages (Fig. 16.2a).[33]

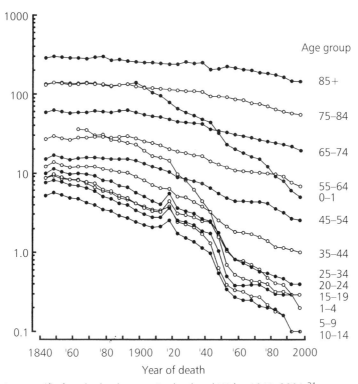

Fig. 16.1 Age-specific female death rates. England and Wales 1841–2001.[31]

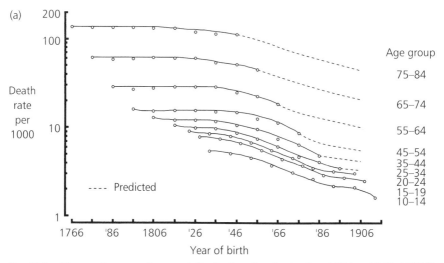

Fig. 16.2a Changes in generation mortality for females. England and Wales, 1841–1925.[31]

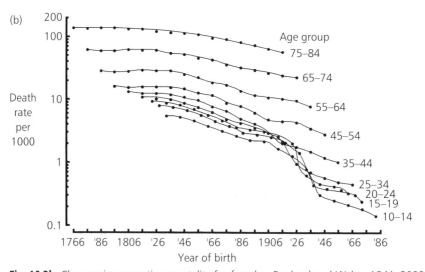

Fig. 16.2b Changes in generation mortality for females. England and Wales, 1841–2000.[31]

In 1934 this cohort effect was also shown by Kermack and his colleagues[34] who concluded that 'the expectation of life was determined by the conditions which existed during a child's earlier years'. They responded to the concerns of eugenicists such as Karl Pearson[36,37] when they noted:

> in a favourable environment the standard of health for survival through the younger age-periods would be lower than a less favourable one. Thus one would expect that a larger number of weaker individuals would go on to the higher age-groups. Nevertheless there is no indication in the statistics that the death rates in the higher age-groups are adversely affected by the presence therein of those weaker individuals. Possibly the persistence of a favourable environment may

counterbalance this effect and facilitate the survival of those weaker individuals so that their presence is not statistically noticeable.[34]

Was this cohort effect seen in other countries? According to Caselli,[38,39] Italian articles on these cohort effects in Sweden had been published several years earlier than the Kermack paper. Kermack and his colleagues also detected a cohort effect using Scottish and Swedish mortality data, although the relative mortalities in Sweden did not show the same simple regularities as those for England, Wales, and Scotland, and their interpretation of the mortality data was later disputed.[40] Preston and Van de Walle[41] have shown that the improvement in female mortality from the mid-nineteenth century in three urban centres of France also proceeded in a cohort specific fashion.

These cohort effects appear to reflect the importance of conditions throughout childhood rather than only the first few years of life *per se*, which is the focus of recent debate.[35] Infant mortality did not conform to the cohort effect observed in the nineteenth century because it did not resume its fall in France until 1895[21] and in Britain until the early years of the twentieth century (Fig. 16.1) well after the fall in child mortality. Kermack and his colleagues[34] argued that the fall in infant mortality was dependent upon the generational improvement in the health of women of childbearing age.

In Britain the decline in deaths from tuberculosis would have made a significant contribution to the cohort effect for all-cause mortality observed for cohorts born before 1920. For example, in women aged 15–44 years, 'respiratory' tuberculosis was the main cause of death in the second half of the nineteenth century and between 1848–72 and 1901–10 deaths from this disease declined by two thirds.[42] Adults dying from tuberculosis often acquired their initial infection early in life. The existence of cohort effects in tuberculosis has long been recognized.[43–45] Age-specific death rates from this disease show falls for successive cohorts born from at least the beginning of the nineteenth century in England and Wales.[46] Tuberculosis is strongly related to poor living conditions and its decline would have followed improvements in nutrition, housing conditions and standards of hygiene for most of the century; however these conditions stagnated or worsened in the second quarter of the nineteenth century.[47] Mercer[46] suggested that the cohort effect was due also to a secondary benefit from smallpox vaccination that became widespread in Britain in the first half of that century. According to Preston and Van de Walle,[41] the cohort improvement in French female mortality from the middle of the nineteenth century cannot be attributed to tuberculosis which did not play such a large role in the mortality decline. Rather they argued that improved sanitation and nutritional standards decreased the risk of diarrhoeal disease in childhood and hence the risk of other infectious diseases; this led to improved growth and development, protective against later mortality from many causes. Detailed investigation of early life and contemporary conditions on adult Swedish mortality at ages 55–80 years between 1760 and 1895 suggests that infections in infancy had an important impact.[48] Stomach cancer and rheumatic heart disease are other examples of diseases where childhood infection is associated with adult mortality. Rheumatic heart disease is a long-term consequence of acute rheumatic fever which usually occurs in children.[49] The decline in stomach cancer mortality showed marked cohort effects,[2,50–52] probably due to a lower exposure in successive cohorts to *Helicobacter pylori*, an infection usually acquired in childhood and related to crowded living conditions.[53,54] The declines in these diseases made substantial contributions to the overall mortality decline for cohorts born in the nineteenth as well as the start of the twentieth centuries.

16.2.2 **Twentieth century birth cohorts**

The cohort effect of declining all-cause mortality did not continue for the generations born in England and Wales in the twentieth century (Fig. 16.2b).[31,35] The mortality rates for women in midlife who had been born at the beginning of the twentieth century levelled off (possibly because of the increase in CHD mortality, Section 16.6) and did not parallel the reductions seen at earlier ages. Rates for cohorts who were young adults (15–34 years) at the time of the 1918 influenza epidemic worsened relative to those aged 35–44 years, and later cohorts had a faster decline at ages 15–34 than at ages 10–14. From the 1940s epidemiological and public health interest in early life effects on adult mortality waned and attention turned to risk factors associated with adult life that were thought to be responsible for the epidemics of heart disease and cancer.[55]

Demographers continued to ask whether cohorts exposed during childhood to high death rates subsequently experienced a mortality advantage or disadvantage.[38,39,56,57] For example, in an analysis of death rates in Italian cohorts born between 1882 and 1953, Caselli[38,39] showed that higher mortality up to age 15 was associated with higher mortality at adult ages up to 45 years and lower mortality at later ages. Findings were stronger for men but were also apparent for women. However, Preston and colleagues[56] found that area based measures of living conditions associated with child survival were also associated with survival to an advanced age (85 years and above) in a cohort of African Americans born between 1885–1900. Thus this study suggests a positive relationship between child and adult mortality even at older ages.

Other research has highlighted twentieth century birth cohorts with particularly adverse or favourable adult mortality experiences. For example, women and men born in Italy during the First World War subsequently had higher adult mortality than expected,[38,39] suggesting long-term adverse effects of poor early living conditions. Excess adult mortality was also seen in men but not women who were young adolescents in Italy, Germany, or France in the First World War or in Italy, Germany, or Japan in the Second World War.[39,58,59] Various reasons have been suggested, including the active participation of these young men in the wars in at least some of these countries,[17] or the greater vulnerability of men than women to malnutrition during adolescence which may have led to weaknesses of the blood vessel structures and a subsequent increase in deaths from haemorrhage.[59] In contrast, research using British mortality data shows no long-term adverse mortality effects for men who were adolescents during the Second World War. Indeed, the annual rate of improvement in mortality was higher for men and women born between 1925 and 1945 than the rates for those born earlier or later.[60] In comparison with the preceding generations they had better childhood health and benefited more from the introduction of antibiotic treatment for infectious disease from the 1930s. Most would have been too young to participate actively in the war but benefited from arrangements put in place to safeguard living standards and the improved educational and occupational opportunities after the conflict ended.

Epidemiologists see only a limited use in studying cohort effects in all-cause mortality and its association with early social and economic indicators. Their interest in early life effects was revived in the 1980s when ecological analyses linked infant mortality (and various components of infant mortality) in cohorts born in the inter-war period with adult mortality from cardiovascular and respiratory disease 60 or 70 years later.[61,62] One of the questions that remained from such ecological analyses was whether these associations reflected some factor acting in the prenatal or postnatal period, or continuity of living conditions across the life course.[63] A recent ecological analysis of 27 countries[64] found a

Table 16.1 Relation of adult mortality (age 65–74 years in 1991–1993) with infant mortality at time of birth and at time of death for 27 countries* (Women)

	Infant mortality 1921–3		Infant mortality 1991–3	
	Coefficient	P-value	Coefficient	P-value
Pearson correlation coefficients				
All causes	0.51	0.007	0.63	<0.001
Respiratory tuberculosis	0.73	<0.001	0.33	0.09
Stomach cancer	0.82	<0.001	0.44	0.02
Lung cancer	−0.48	0.01	−0.23	0.24
Coronary heart disease	0.16	0.42	0.28	0.16
Stroke	0.63	<0.001	0.64	<0.001
Breast cancer	−0.60	<0.001	−0.33	0.08
Partial correlation coefficients[†]				
All causes	0.28	0.17	0.50	0.009
Respiratory tuberculosis	0.69	<0.001	−0.07	0.72
Stomach cancer	0.77	<0.001	0.04	0.87
Lung cancer	−0.43	0.03	0.02	0.92
Coronary heart disease	0.03	0.90	0.23	0.27
Stroke	0.45	0.02	0.48	0.01
Breast cancer	−0.53	0.01	−0.06	0.77

* Australia, Austria, Belgium, Bulgaria, Canada, Chile, Czechoslovakia, Denmark, Finland, France, Greece, Hungary, Ireland, Italy, Japan, Netherlands, New Zealand, Norway, Poland, Portugal, Romania, Russian Federation, Spain, Sweden, Switzerland, United Kingdom, United States.

† Correlations of adult mortality with infant mortality in one period adjusted for infant mortality in the other period.

Adapted from Leon, D.A., Davey Smith, G. (2000) Infant mortality, stomach cancer, stroke and coronary heart disease: ecological analysis. *British Medical Journal*, 320, 1705–1706.

strong correlation between infant mortality rates in the 1920s (used as a measure of living conditions when this population was young) and mortality from a number of adult diseases at ages 65–74 years in 1991–93 (Table 16.1). In the case of respiratory tuberculosis and stomach cancer the positive correlations were hardly attenuated after adjusting for recent infant mortality rates. This suggests an important role for early life factors in the aetiology of these diseases, or it may be an artefact caused by the greater variability in past rather than more recent infant mortality rates. The negative correlation between infant mortality and breast cancer mortality also remained and evidence for cohort effects for this disease are discussed in Section 16.4.

16.3 **Lung cancer trends and cohort effects**

Lung cancer rates have been rising in all countries but the timing of the rise varied. The rise occurred earlier in the US and northern European countries and later in southern Europe. This is because of the earlier uptake of smoking in women in the former countries (see Chapter 13). There are clear cohort-related variations in lung cancer rates which correspond to estimates of lifetime cigarette consumption in different cohorts, illustrated for women in England and Wales in Fig. 16.3.[8] In the ecological analysis using 27 countries (described above)[64] there was a negative relationship between infant mortality in the 1920s and lung cancer mortality in women in the 1990s. As the authors pointed out this was probably because in most countries social reforms for mothers and children were associated

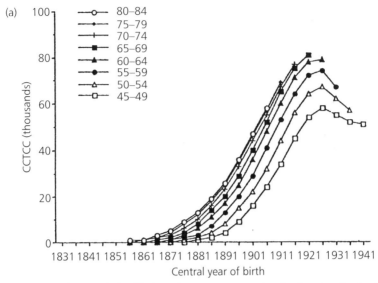

Fig. 16.3a Age-specific cumulative lifetime cigarette consumption for females, England and Wales, by year of birth 1831–1941.[8]

Notes: Prepared by Lung and Asthma Information Agency, St George's Hospital Medical School, London, from estimates of cumulative lifetime cigarette consumption by Lee *et al*.[128] CCTC: cumulative constant tar cigarette consumption.

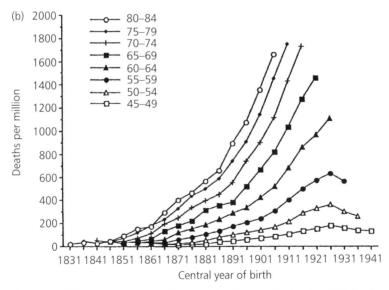

Fig. 16.3b Age-specific lung cancer mortality rates for females, England and Wales, by year of birth 1831–1941.[8]

Notes: Prepared by Lung and Asthma Information Agency, St George's Hospital Medical School, London, from mortality data published by the Office of Population Censuses and Surveys, London.

with improved educational, economic, and political opportunities for women, which were, in turn, associated with an increased uptake in smoking.

16.4 Breast cancer trends and cohort effects

Breast cancer was the most common cause of death in 1990 for women aged 45–59 years living in established market economies; it was also the seventh most important cause of disability adjusted life years in this age group.[65] Long-term changes in breast cancer incidence and mortality (shown for England and Wales in Fig. 16.4) have been much less dramatic than the change rates for other common cancers, such as stomach cancer or lung cancer[50] or the

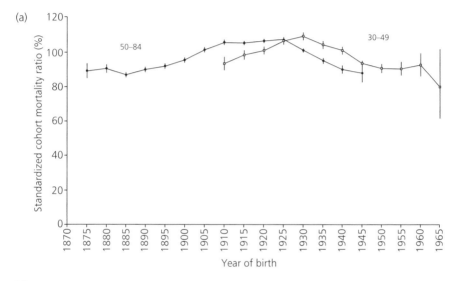

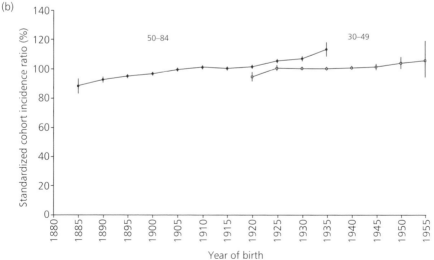

Fig. 16.4 Point estimates and 95% confidence intervals. Cancer of breast, female (pre-ICD classifications 'Breast'; ICD2 43; ICD3 47; ICD4&5 50; ICD6&7 170; ICD8&9 174): (a) birth cohort mortality 1960–92, by age; (b) birth cohort incidence 1971–87, by age.[50]

rates for cardiovascular diseases (Section 16.6). Trends in breast cancer mortality rates have been examined across countries[66-68] and within countries.[50,69-71] Rates increased between 1950 and 1990 but there was considerable variation in these trends as well as in the rates themselves, particularly at the beginning of this period. Even in 1990 there was a twofold difference in rates among European countries. In countries with historically high rates (such as the US, UK, The Netherlands, Australia, and Canada) rates have levelled off, decreased, or remained fairly constant. In countries with historically low rates (such as Spain, Greece, and Japan) or intermediate rates (such as France and Italy) there has been a stronger upward trend.

Age-specific mortality rates by birth cohort show that the upward trend in mortality began for cohorts born around 1900 for England and Wales, the United States, Canada, and Japan.[50,72,73] Hermon and Beral[66] published cohort-specific mortality ratios (from an age-cohort model) of breast cancer mortality for women aged 30–79 years born between 1875

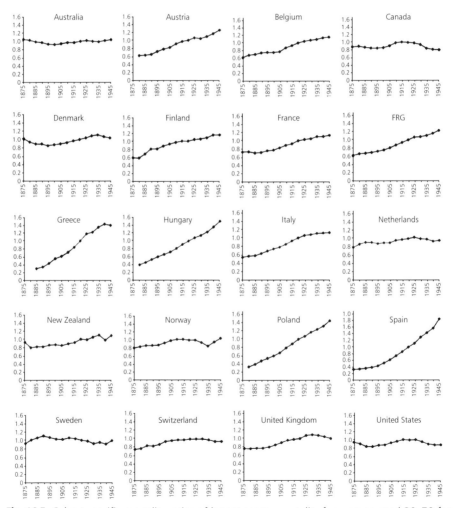

Fig. 16.5 Cohort-specific mortality ratios of breast cancer mortality for women aged 30–79 for cohorts with a central year of birth from 1875 to 1945 (1920=1.00) in 20 countries in Europe, North America, Australia and New Zealand.[66]

and 1945 in 20 countries and these are reproduced in Fig. 16.5. For many countries there was either a slight downturn or a slowdown in the rate of increase in the cohort mortality ratios for cohorts born around 1920–25. Tarone and colleagues[74] using age-period-cohort models also showed a reduction in mortality risk for cohorts born around this time in the US (for both White and Black women) and Canada.

Historically, the long-term mortality trends are thought to reflect secular trends in breast cancer incidence but interpretation must be cautious as there is a wide variation in the ratio of mortality to incidence and trends in incidence have mirrored trends in mortality in some countries but not others.[68] For example, long-term trends in mortality and incidence data by birth cohorts in England and Wales (Fig. 16.4) have not run parallel.[50] Whereas mortality rates increased to a peak for the cohort born in 1925–29 (or 1930–34 for those under 50) and then declined, breast cancer incidence has shown a generally increasing trend. Age-period-cohort models also show increases in breast cancer incidence for successive cohorts born between 1860 and 1950 in Denmark,[75] and between 1880 and 1950 in Sweden.[76]

For cohorts born since the 1950s, age-period-cohort models show a marked decrease in breast cancer mortality for 30–39 year-old US White women[74] which appears to reflect a decline in incidence in invasive breast cancer.[77] In contrast, breast cancer incidence and mortality rose slightly for women age 30–49 years born in England and Wales in the early post war years (Fig. 16.4).

Treatment and screening make the interpretation of breast cancer trends and comparisons across countries particularly difficult. For instance, the decline in breast cancer mortality in England and Wales, which began in the 1970s at premenopausal ages and in the 1990s at older ages, has been attributed to improvements in survival consequent to improvements in treatment.[10] In more recent years, the decline in mortality in the older age groups may also reflect screening activities as the national breast screening programme was introduced in 1988.[78] Similar organized screening programmes have been introduced in many western countries over the last 20 years, which may have contributed to initial rises in the incidence of this tumour in the targeted age groups followed by subsequent declines in mortality. Even in countries where organized national programmes have never been set up there has been a shift towards early detection and treatment. In the US, breast physical examinations by physicians increased during the 1970s whereas mammographic screening increased substantially in the 1980s.[79] These diagnostic changes together with the introduction of new treatments seem to have accounted for some of the recent breast cancer trends in the US.[74,77]

16.4.1 Do breast cancer trends parallel trends in fertility?

A number of studies have considered whether breast cancer trends parallel trends in fertility. Within cohorts, nulliparity and an older age at first birth increase the risk of breast cancer whereas a younger age at first birth and, to a lesser extent, parity are protective (see Chapter 3). For cohorts born from the turn of the century to the late 1920s in England and Wales the increase in breast cancer incidence and mortality parallels the decreasing fertility at young ages but is in opposition to decreasing nulliparity over most of that period. Most but not all of the countries that experienced a fall in breast cancer mortality for cohorts born after 1920 had parallel falls in nulliparity and mean age at first birth,[66] and a number of researchers have confidently linked the moderation of the risk of breast cancer mortality in cohorts born from 1925 to 1940 in North America to their low rates of childlessness[69,80] or their higher fertility rates at ages 20–24.[81] Childbearing patterns in these and earlier cohorts are less consistent with trends in breast cancer incidence.[50,82,83] Women born in the post war period have had lower fertility levels which are consistent with the small rise in incidence and mortality rates in young women in England and Wales (Fig. 16.5) but not with the decline in these rates seen in the US.[69] In Japan the increase in breast cancer mortality since the 1960s is compatible with a declining fertility rate and an increasing age at first birth but is counter to the trend of increased nulliparity.[71] In summary, trends in breast cancer do not relate very well to changes in cohort fertility.

16.5 Do breast cancer trends parallel secular changes in growth?

In Chapter 3 it was suggested that hormonal or nutritional factors associated with prenatal and postnatal growth could increase the risk of breast cancer in adult life. Could secular changes in growth lie behind the increase in breast cancer incidence rates in western countries? The answer is complicated partly because there has been little synchrony in the secular patterns of various growth indicators such as birthweight, height, and age at menarche suggesting their underlying causal mechanisms differ.[84]

16.5.1 Secular changes in birthweight

Information on trends in birthweight from the nineteenth century is available from hospital records in various European, North American, and Australian cities.[85–87] They suggest that although mean birthweight fluctuated by around 500 g in response to fluctuating economic conditions, there has been little evidence of a positive secular trend. Maternal birthweight is an important influence on offspring's birthweight[88] and would constrain rapid change over time.[89] For post war cohorts in England and Wales, the percentage of births of low birthweight has remained fairly stable but there have been changes in the birthweight distribution (Fig. 16.6). Up to 1970 the proportion of live births weighing 2.5–3.4 kg was rising while the proportion weighing 3.5 kg or more was falling. Since the 1980s these trends have reversed with the percentage of live births weighing between 2.5–3.4 kg falling by just under 5% and the percentage of births weighing at least 3.5 kg rising correspondingly. Comparative data on birthweight distributions for different countries also suggest recent increases in birthweight in the US (for Blacks as well as Whites) and in Sweden.[89] Japanese birthweight rose by 300 g between 1945 and 1964[90] and has been attributed to the increase in protein in the Japanese diet, but since 1970 the median birthweight has fallen consistently.[89]

The lack of a secular trend in birthweight is not consistent with the long-term increase in breast cancer incidence for cohorts born before the Second World War. In England and Wales the slight decline in the mean birthweight up to 1970 does not parallel the apparently increasing breast cancer incidence in the immediate post war cohorts.[50] In contrast, the increase in Japanese birthweight between 1945 and the 1960s is compatible with recent increase in breast cancer mortality since the 1960s. As yet we do not know the breast cancer rates of cohorts born since 1970. The slight increase in the birthweight since 1970 in the US, the UK, and Sweden would predict a small increase in disease risk, whereas the decrease in Japanese birthweight since 1970 would predict a small decrease in risk.

16.5.2 Secular changes in age at menarche

Age at menarche has declined by about two months per decade since the last century according to a comprehensive review of historical records.[91] The greatest decline occurred

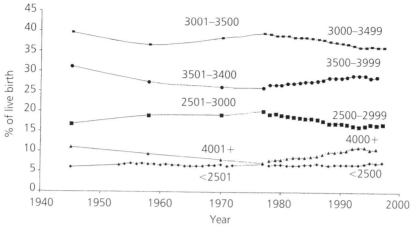

Fig. 16.6 Birthweight of live births, England and Wales, 1945–97.[50]

in the Scandanavian countries (at 3.2 months per decade) and the smallest (at 1.1 months per decade) in France. In England and Wales age at menarche was 14.7 years at the beginning of the twentieth century and fell to around 12.8 years by the 1950s, but has been stable since.[50] Evidence from a number of countries suggests the decline in age at menarche slowed or even reversed in developed countries.[84,91,92] Whereas evidence from the US suggests that the age of developing pubertal characteristics, such as breast development, has declined in Black and White girls,[93] perhaps due to increased childhood obesity (see Chapter 14), there is as yet, no evidence of a further decline in age at menarche. Causal factors for age at menarche may operate near the time of birth (see Chapters 2 and 3), but the mechanisms involved are still unclear.[84]

The long-term decline in the age at menarche until the Second World War indicates a change in postnatal growth tempo compatible with the observed increase in breast cancer mortality and incidence in pre war cohorts. It would not, however, have contributed to any moderation of risk seen in those born from around the middle of the 1920s. Whether the recent slowdown in the decline in age at menarche in most developed countries has moderated the risk of breast cancer in later birth cohorts remains to be seen. The continued decline in age at menarche in Japan (from 15.1 years in 1950 to 12.5 years in 1980) may account for some of their rapid increase in breast cancer mortality, an increase that has not yet levelled off.[71]

16.5.3 Secular changes in adult height

There is a dearth of data on the secular changes in women's heights but historical data, mainly on male conscripts, show a positive secular trend in adult stature in Europe, North America, and Australia since the nineteenth century,[47,94] amounting to about 1 cm per decade.[95] Whilst some countries, notably France, Netherlands, and Sweden, showed a steady improvement, others such as the UK, the US, Australia, and Italy experienced a decline in stature in the middle or second half of the nineteenth century during rapid industrialization or urbanization.[94,96] Were these trends similar for women? Recently analysed data from

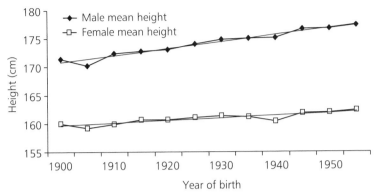

Fig. 16.7 Mean adult height of parents and study members of the 1946 and 1958 British birth cohorts, by year of birth, England and Wales 1900–1960.[98]

the records of English female prisoners suggest that heights of men and women fell in unison from the 1830s to the 1850s.[97] Height data of Australian born female and male army recruits[98] and of parents and study members of the 1946 and 1958 British birth cohorts[99] suggest the subsequent secular increase was weaker for women compared with men. For example, this last data set, illustrated in Fig. 16.7, shows the mean height for women born between 1892 and 1958 (at 0.4 cm per decade) was only a third of that for men (1.1 cm a decade).[99] The recent review by Cole[84] concludes that the secular trend in adult height has its origins in the first two years of life, most probably through increased leg length. He suggests that growth during this time is likely to depend on an interaction between growth factors (set by genetics and the intrauterine environment) and the quality of the diet and exposure to infection in the postnatal period.

This modest secular trend in height for women since the end of the nineteenth century is compatible with the observed small increase in breast cancer incidence and mortality. The continuation of the secular trend in height in post war cohorts would suggest a continued increase in the risk of breast cancer which has been seen for the immediate post war cohorts in England and Wales and Scandanavia but not in the US.

16.6 Cardiovascular disease trends and cohort effects

Figure 16.8 shows trends in age standardized rates for coronary heart disease for women aged 45–64 years between 1950–87 in 16 established market economies.[100] These correspond to cohorts born between 1886 and 1942. CHD mortality in the early post war period was particularly high in Ireland, the US, Canada, Scotland, Australia, New Zealand, and Finland. It was intermediate in Sweden, Italy, England and Wales, Denmark, and Japan, and low in the Netherlands, Norway, Spain, and France. Trends in some countries show a fall, rise, and subsequent fall (notably in Scotland and England and Wales, Finland, Australia, New Zealand, Denmark, Norway), whereas in others there has been a continuous decline (notably in US, Sweden, Italy, and Japan). Generally declines accelerated in the 1970s and continued through the 1990s.[101] Mortality rates were higher in men than in women in all these countries but the male : female ratio for 45–64 year-olds rose from between 1.5–3.5 in 1950–54 to around 3.5–5.5 in 1984–87. Sex differentials are particularly high in Finland,

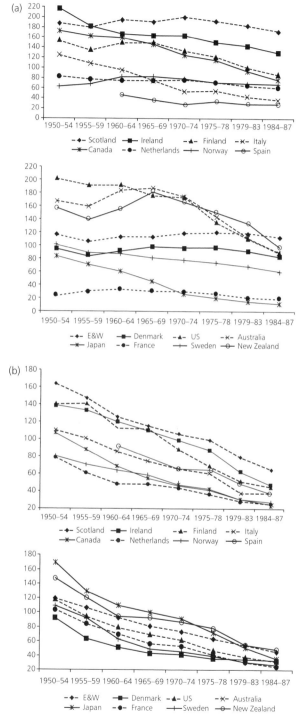

Fig. 16.8 (a) CHD mortality rates and (b) cerebrovascular mortality rates per 100 000 for females aged 45–64 years (age adjusted) in 16 established market economies for seven time periods, 1950–85.[99]

France, Norway, Italy, Spain, and Sweden (all above 4.5 in 1984–87) and low in Japan, Australia, Ireland, Scotland, and the US (all below 3.5).

Data from England and Wales going back to 1921 indicate that CHD mortality rose sharply from 1921–40 and then fell slightly before rising again to a more modest peak in the mid-1970s.[6] In the US, there was a similar increase in the inter-war period.[102] While increasing mortality in the earlier period almost certainly reflected increasing incidence, it is harder to distinguish whether the post war decline was caused by decreasing incidence or case fatality. Evidence from the US and Europe suggests that declines in mortality have been greater than declines in incidence due to improvements in treatment and secondary prevention.[103–105]

Examination of the age-specific death rates in British men and women show that the rise in CHD mortality occurred around the same time at all ages suggesting a period effect.[6] Studies have generally concluded that increases in dietary intake of saturated fat and smoking and their possible interactive effects were responsible for the initial adverse trends in CHD mortality from the 1920s.[6,106] However, birth cohort effects are evident in the decline in CHD mortality in England and Wales. The decline began earlier for younger compared with older women (in the 1970s for women aged 35–44 but only in the 1980s for women aged 65–74) and death rates have been lower for each successive generation born during or after the Second World War.[6] Modelling the death rates on age, period of death, and period of birth confirmed that although age and period of death explained more of the variation in CHD mortality than age and cohort, there was evidence of a small cohort effect.[6] This birth cohort effect in CHD mortality decline is not observed across all countries or in both sexes. For example in Norway there were birth cohort effects for men but none for women.[107]

Time trends in cerebrovascular mortality contrast with trends in CHD mortality despite common adult risk factors like hypertension, obesity, smoking, inactivity, and diabetes.[2] It fell in all the sixteen countries illustrated in Fig. 16.8.[100] Historically, Japan had a very high rate that declined rapidly after the Second World War. Stroke mortality rates in most established market economies have continued to decline into the 1990s albeit at a slower rate in North America. In Norway and Denmark rates have reversed.[108] Population registers of recent stroke incidence show little significant decline.[109,110] Most of the decline has been in ischaemic stroke (which is more common in older populations) rather than in haemorrhagic stroke.[111] Cerebrovascular mortality rates are more similar between men and women than rates for CHD mortality although there has been some widening over time because the decline in cerebrovascular mortality has generally been more rapid in women. More long-term data from England and Wales and the US show that the decline in stroke mortality began at least from the start of the twentieth century (see Chapter 5),[6,112] and probably earlier. In England and Wales stroke was responsible for more deaths until the late 1920s and again in the 1950s whereas CHD was responsible for more deaths in the 1930s and since the 1960s.[8] Debate about the reasons for the secular declines in stroke mortality have focused on the role of treatment of hypertension [110,113,114] but this would not explain the long-term decline in stroke in the US and the UK at least since the beginning of the twentieth century. The contribution of environmental improvements that accompanied economic and social development, such as the reduction in salt intake as refrigeration became more widespread, has also been discussed.[108,115]

There is evidence of birth cohort effects as well as a strong period effect in the decline in stroke mortality. For example, mortality data, between 1940 and 1991 from the US[116] and between 1951 and 1995 from Spain,[117] show a reduction in stroke mortality in successive generations across all age groups. In Spain this effect was more marked among women than men. Wolfe and Burney[118] used age-period-cohort modelling for mortality data between 1931 and 1985 for England and Wales and identified significant cohort as well as period and age effects. For cohorts born between 1870 and 1910 there was a deceleration in mortality risk followed by an acceleration of risk in cohorts born since 1910, so far until age 65 years, once period effects had been taken into account. This recent acceleration of risk is unlikely to have been due to early life factors. The authors attributed it to the increased survival of those with diabetes and CHD, increased heavy alcohol consumption in later born cohorts, and the fact that cohorts with higher proportions of immigrants (and with a higher incidence of cerebrovascular disease) had reached the age of increased risk.

Other types of ecological analysis also link a cohort's stroke mortality in adult life to conditions that prevailed when the cohort was young. For example, the ecological analysis of 27 countries discussed earlier[64] found that stroke mortality at ages 65–74 years in 1991–3 showed strong correlations with infant mortality rates in the 1920s as well as with current infant mortality (Table 16.1). This suggests that conditions in early life as well as in adult life are important in the aetiology of stroke. In contrast correlations between infant mortality and ischaemic heart disease in this same data set were weak.

16.7 Do cardiovascular disease trends parallel trends in growth?

Indicators of impaired growth are associated with a higher risk of CHD and stroke mortality in individuals (see Chapter 5) but can they explain the trends in these diseases? Certainly the increase in CHD mortality and the dominance of period effects observed in industrialized countries in the twentieth century are not compatible with the secular increase in indicators of postnatal growth. It is conceivable that the secular increases in growth tempo and final height made a small contribution to the subsequent decline in CHD mortality since the 1970s, given the small cohort effect observed in England and Wales for generations born from the 1930s. The apparent lack of any consistent trend in birthweight makes it an unlikely candidate to explain this small cohort effect.

The decline in stroke trends is broadly consistent with improvements in child survival and growth 50–70 years previously. More specifically, the British cohorts of 1870–1910 with a decelerating risk of stroke mortality showed generational increases in growth tempo and final height, and striking decreases in child mortality. This suggests a role for some as yet unidentified early life factor associated with improved nutrition or less infection in early life.[115] The delayed fall in infant mortality and the lack of any strong secular trends in birthweight in most industrialized countries would point to childhood rather than fetal factors.

16.8 Conclusions

There is evidence of a cohort effect in the decline of all-cause mortality in certain established market economies during the third stage of the epidemiological transition. This reflected cohort declines in mortality from diseases such as tuberculosis, stomach cancer, and rheumatic heart disease that are known to be related to childhood infections. Improvements in childhood living conditions in successive cohorts would have reduced the risk of these infections and their consequences for later health. Although these 'early life infection' diseases are uncommon in established market economies they are still significant causes of death in many developing countries (see Chapters 1 and 15). Cohort effects were also evident in the decline in mortality from stroke and the increase in mortality from breast cancer. Temporal trends in these diseases were compatible with secular trends in postnatal growth indicators but did not relate so well to changes in birthweight (or cohort fertility in the case of breast cancer). These findings, although preliminary and inconclusive, suggest that further research, using more sophisticated modelling techniques, into the role of early life factors on these disease trends would be worthwhile. In contrast the increase or stagnation in CHD mortality in the middle of the twentieth century was mainly a period effect and was not compatible with prenatal or postnatal growth trends. Age-period-cohort models of mortality and incidence data from other developed and developing countries, where available, would advance this field of research. Incidence data, where available, are to be preferred to mortality data, especially in high life expectancy countries where advances in medical care have led to improved survival from chronic diseases.

Examination of the role of life course influences during the fourth and fifth stage of the epidemiological transition needs to give more emphasis to cohort changes in morbidity, disability, and quality of life after diagnosis. The relationship between trends in mortality and morbidity at each stage of the epidemiological transition is a matter of debate[119] and there are few sources of reliable data.[120] Whether the cohorts now entering midlife and later life are healthier than previous cohorts is an important research area with enormous policy implications,[121–124] and one that will benefit from a life course approach.[125,126] We return to this theme in the last chapter.

Acknowledgements

We would like to thank Professor George Davey Smith very much for his helpful comments on an earlier draft of this chapter.

Commentary on 'Disease trends in women living in established market economies: evidence of cohort effects during the epidemiological transition'

David A. Leon

Modern epidemiology is preoccupied with differences in disease risk between individuals, while as a discipline it is defined as being concerned with the study of causes and distribution of disease in populations. Formally speaking there is no contradiction. Epidemiology studies individuals only in aggregate, as for example as members of exposed and unexposed populations. However, the term 'population' used in this way denotes a reified concept that bears little necessary relationship to geographically or socio-demographically defined populations such as countries, regions, or social classes. Analyses that compare disease rates between countries or over time are usually classified as descriptive or at best hypothesis-generating, as in the case of ecological studies. While the study of disease aetiology often requires a focus on more analytical and individual-level designs, such as cohort and case-control studies, the task of understanding and explaining time trends, international and socio-demographic differences as ends in themselves are relatively neglected. This is despite the fact that epidemiology is regarded as the science underlying public health, which in turn is primarily concerned with patterns and trends of disease in such real populations.

The emergence of a life course perspective on adult disease provides a stimulus to take a fresh look at the problems of developing and applying aetiological insights from epidemiology (and other disciplines) to explain real population trends and differences. One of the most promising diseases to look at in this respect is female breast cancer. Compared to many other causes of morbidity and mortality in middle and high income countries there exists abundant evidence that risk is related to a wide range of factors across the entire life course. These include (in reverse chronological order) postmenopausal obesity, number of children, age at first birth, age at menarche, and possibly rate of growth in early childhood and even *in utero*. Despite the depth of insight at the level of individual risk factors, taken individually they do not seem to provide explanations for secular trends in middle and high income countries. This chapter found little correlation between secular trends in breast cancer and trends in risk factors such as fertility patterns, age at menarche, and growth.

What do these disappointing findings concerning breast cancer tell us? It is instructive to compare breast with lung cancer. Lung cancer trends in a population are largely driven by its historical smoking profile. Historical data on smoking is relatively plentiful in countries such as the UK, and can be related to later lung cancer rates. As shown in this chapter, birth cohort patterns for smoking are very similar to those for lung cancer. This powerfully illustrates that birth cohort effects *per se* do not necessarily indicate the operation of biological exposures around the time of birth or even in childhood. In the case of lung cancer, they simply reflect how smoking habits in adult life have been socially patterned according to generation. In the case of breast cancer, however, there is no single variable equivalent to smoking that we can measure even though there may in principle be a common underlying exposure trend (such as endogenous hormone profiles) which may provide an important part of the explanation. Instead, our life course risk factors may operate by each making an independent contribution to this underlying cumulative exposure.

The fact that reproductive history or age at menarche may be exposure proxies is not a problem in itself in explaining trends. The more serious problem is that the social and economic changes driving the epidemiological (and other) transitions are tending to affect many, if not all, of these risk factors simultaneously—and not necessarily in the same direction with respect to their relationship to disease risk. The approach required to deal with this sort of situation would be to model the effects of the whole raft of risk factors simultaneously rather than looking at each one in turn. This of course presupposes adequate time series data is available for the pertinent exposures. This multivariate approach has not generally been adopted by epidemiologists. It has been economic historians and demographers, such as Preston,[127] who have used modelling approaches of this sort to explain population disease patterns and trends, although the explanatory variables they have employed have been social and economic rather than more proximal biological markers that would be of interest to epidemiologists.

Whatever the difficulties that may exist, both practical and methodological, in trying to develop more sophisticated aetiologically informed analyses of population differences and trends in diseases it is an important area to pursue if epidemiology is to realize its full potential as the underlying science of public health. The pronounced differences in disease patterns and mortality among women (and men) between western and eastern (former communist) Europe is a particular challenge. For example, in the late 1980s mortality rates of female breast cancer were generally lower and showed less variation in Eastern European countries than among those in Western Europe. There has been little attempt to examine the reasons for these differences.

Finally, the eastern European experience, particularly that of Russia and other parts of the former Soviet Union, provides a powerful illustration of the fact that major changes in disease rates and mortality can occur in populations as an almost immediate response to abrupt and massive societal disruption. The sharp changes in mortality from circulatory disease mortality, for example, among Russian women (and men) appear to follow-on from events such as the collapse of the Soviet Union. There is nothing in the life course perspective which prevents it incorporating such acute effects. Some of the more intriguing questions may relate to the influence of early life on adult health; however, the life course approach legitimately spans the contribution of influences on health acting at all ages irrespective of whether their effect is acute or delayed.

References

1 **Leon DA**. Common Threads: underlying components of inequalities in mortality between and within countries. In Leon D, Walt G, eds. *Poverty, inequality and health: an international perspective*. Oxford: Oxford University Press, 2000:58–87.

2 **Davey Smith G, Gunnell D, Ben-Shlomo Y**. Life-course approaches to socioeconomic differentials in cause specific adult mortality. In Leon D, Walt G, eds. *Poverty, inequality and health: an international perspective*. Oxford: Oxford University Press, 2000:88–124.

3 **Keating D, Hertzman C**. Developmental health and the wealth of nations: social, biological and educational dynamics. New York: The Guilford Press, 1999.

4 **Rutter M, Smith DJ**. Psychosocial Disorders in Young People: Time Trends and Their Causes. Chichester: John Wiley and Sons Ltd, 1995.

5 **Rose G**. Sick individuals and sick populations. *Int J Epidemiol* 1985;**14**:32–8.

6 **Charlton J, Murphy M, Khaw K-T, Ebrahim S, Davey Smith G**. Cardiovascular diseases. In Charlton J, Murphy M, eds. *The health of adult Britain 1841–1994*. London: ONS, HMSO, 1997:60–81.

7 **Flegal KM**. Obesity. In Goldman M, Hatch M, eds. *Women and Health*. Academic Press, 2000:830–8.

8 **Strachan DP, Perry IJ**. Time trends. In Kuh D, Ben-Shlomo Y, eds. *A life course approach to chronic disease epidemiology*. Oxford: Oxford University Press, 1997:101–20.

9 **Tunstall-Pedoe H, Vanuzzo D, Hobbs M, Mahonen M, Cepaitis Z, Kuulasmaa K** *et al*. Estimation of contribution of changes in coronary care to improving survival, event rates, and coronary heart disease mortality across the WHO MONICA Project populations. *Lancet* 2000;**355**:688–700.

10 **Peto R, Boreham J, Clarke M, Davies C, Beral V**. UK and USA breast cancer deaths down 25% in year 2000 at ages 20–69 years. *Lancet* 2000;**355**:1822.

11 **Holford TR**. Understanding the effects of age, period, and cohort on incidence and mortality rates. *Ann Rev Pubic Health* 1991;**12**:425–57.

12 **Robertson C, Gandini S, Boyle P**. Age-period-cohort models: a comparative study of available methodologies. *J Clin Epidemiol* 1999;**52**:569–83.

13 **Omran AR**. A century of epidemiologic transition in the United States. *Preventative Medicine* 1977;**6**:3–51.

14 **Omran AR**. The epidemiologic transition revisited thirty years later. *World Health Stat Q* 1998;**53**:99–119.

15 **Russell JC**. Late ancient and medieval population. *Trans Am Philosophical Society*. 1958;June, Part 3.

16 **Woods R, Shelton N**. *An atlas of Victorian mortality*. Liverpool: Liverpool University Press, 1997.

17 **Pinelli A, Mancini P**. Gender mortality differences from birth to puberty 1887–1940. In Corsini CA, Viazzo PP, eds. *The decline of infant and child mortality. The European experience 1750–1940*. The Hague: Martinus Nijhoff Publishers Kluwer Law International, 1997:73–93.

18 **Loudon I**. The transformation of maternal mortality. *Br Med J* 1992;**305**:1557–60.

19 **Trovato F. Lalu NM**. Narrowing sex differentials in life expectancy in the industrialised world: early 1970s to early 1990s. *Soc Biol* 1996;**43**:20–37.

20 **Caselli G**. Health transition and cause-specific mortality. In Schofield R, Reher D, Bideau A, eds. *The decline of mortality in Europe*. Oxford: Clarendon Press, 1991:68–96.

21 **Vallin J**. Mortality in Europe from 1720 to 1914: long-term trends and changes in patterns by age and sex. In Schofield R, Reher D, Bideau A, eds. *The decline of mortality in Europe*. Oxford: Clarendon Press, 1991:38–67.

22 **Gaylin DS, Kates J**. Refocusing the lens: epidemiologic transition theory, mortality differentials, and the AIDS pandemic. *Soc Sci Med* 1997;**44**:609–21.

23 **Wrigley EA, Schofield RS**. *The population history of England 1541–1871*. Cambridge, Mass.: Harvard University Press, 1981.

24 **Schofield R, Reher D, Bideau A**. *The decline of mortality in Europe*. Clarendon Press: Oxford, 1991.

25 **McKeown T**. *The modern rise of population*. London: Arnold, 1976.

26 **McKeown T**. The role of medicine: dream, mirage or nemesis? Oxford: Basil Blackwell, 1979.

27 **Szreter S**. The importance of social intervention in Britain's mortality decline c.1850–1914: a reinterpretation of the role of public health. *Soc Hist Med* 1988;**1**:1–37.

28 **Hardy A**. *The Epidemic Streets*. Oxford: Clarendon Press, 1993.

29 **Omran AR**. The epidemiologic transition: a theory of the epidemiology of population change. *Milbank Q* 1971;**49**:509–38.

30 **Caselli G**. *Long-term trends in European mortality*. Studies on medical and population subjects No. 56. London: HMSO, 1991.

31 **Kuh D. Davey Smith G**. When is mortality risk determined? Historical insights into a current debate. *Soc Hist Med* 1993;**6**:101–23.

32 **Preston SH, Hill ME, Drevenstedt GL**. Childhood conditions that predict survival to advanced ages among African-Americans. *Soc Sci Med* 1998;**47**:1231–46.

33 **Derrick VPA**. Observations on (1) errors on age on the population statistics of England and Wales and (2) the changes in mortality indicated by the national records. *J Inst Actuaries* 1927;**58**:117–59.

34 **Kermack WO, McKendrick AG, McKinlay PL**. Death rates in Great Britain and Sweden: Some general regularities and their significance. *Lancet* 1934;**226**:698–703.

35 **Davey Smith G, Kuh D**. William Ogilvy Kermack and the childhood origins of adult health and disease. *Int J Epidemiol* 2001;**30**:696–703.

36 **Pearson K**. The intensity of natural selection in man. *Proc R Soc Lond* 1912;**85**:469–76.

37 **Pearson K**. *Darwinism, Medical Progress and Eugenics*. The Cavendish Lecture. London: Eugenics Laboratory Lecture Series IX, 1912.

38 **Caselli G, Capocaccia R**. Age, period, cohort and early mortality: an analysis of adult mortality in Italy. *Pop Stud* 1989;**43**:133–53.

39 **Caselli G**. The influence of cohort effects on differentials and trends in mortality. In Vallin J, Dsouza S, Palloni A, eds. *Measurement and analysis of mortality-new approaches*. Clarendon Press: Oxford, 1990:229–49.

40 **Hobcraft J, Gilks W**. Age, period and cohort analysis in mortality studies. In Vallin J, Pollard JH, Heligman L, eds. *Methodologies for the collection and analysis of mortality data*. Liege: IUSSP, Ordina Editions, 1984:245–62.

41 **Preston S, van de Walle E**. Urban French mortality in the nineteenth century. *Popul Stud* 1978;**32**:275–98.

42 **Charlton J, Murphy M**. Trends in all-cause *mortality*: 1841–94- an overview. In Charlton J, Murphy M, eds. *The health of adult Britain* 1841–1994. London: ONS, HMSO, 1997:31–55.

43 **Brownlee J**. Certain considerations regarding the epidemiology of phthisis pulmonalis. *Public Health* 1916;**29**:139–45.

44 **Frost WH**. The age selection of mortality from tuberculosis in successive decades. *Am J Hyg* 1939;**30**:91–6.

45 **Springett VH**. An interpretation of statistical trends in tuberculosis. *Lancet* 1952;**15**:521–5.

46 **Mercer A**. *Disease mortality and population in transition*. Leicester: Leicester University Press, 1990.

47 **Floud R, Wachter K, Gregory A**. *Height, health and history*. Cambridge studies in population; economy and society in past time. Nutritional status in the United Kingdom 1750–1980. Cambridge: Cambridge University Press, 1990.

48 **Bengtsson T, Lindstrom M**. Childhood misery and disease in later life: the effects of mortality in old age of hazards experienced in early life, southern Sweden, 1760–1894. *Popul Stud* 2000;**54**:263–77.

49 **Elo IT, Preston SH**. Effects of early-life conditions on adult mortality: a review. *Popul Index* 1992;**58**:186–212.

50 **Swerdlow A, dos Santos Silva I, Doll R**. *Cancer incidence and mortality in England and Wales: trends and risk factors*. Oxford: Oxford University Press, 2001.

51 **La Vecchia C, Negri E, Levi F, Decarli A, Boyle P**. Cancer mortality in Europe: effects of age, cohort of birth and period of death. *Eur J Cancer* 1998;**34**:118–41.

52 **Aragones N, Pollan MM, Lopez-Abente G, Ruiz M, Vergara A, Moreno C *et al***. Time trend and age-period-cohort effects on gastric cancer incidence in Zaragoza and Navarre, Spain. *J Epidemiol Community Health* 1997;**51**:412–7.

53 **Banatvala N, Mayo K, Megraud F, Jennings R, Deeks JJ, Feldman RA**. The cohort effect and Helicobacter pylori. *J Infect Dis* 1993;**168**:219–21.

54 **Whitaker CJ, Dubiel AJ, Galpin OP**. Social and geographical risk factors in Helicobacter pylori infection. *Epidemiol Infect* 1993;**111**:63–70.

55 **Kuh D, Davey Smith G**. The life course and adult chronic disease: an historical perspective with particular reference to coronary heart disease. In Kuh D, Ben-Shlomo Y, eds. *A life course approach to chronic disease epidemiology*. Oxford: Oxford University Press, 1997:15–44.

56 **Preston SH, Haines MR**. *Fatal years. Child mortality in late nineteenth century America*. Princeton, New Jersey: Princeton University Press, 1991.

57 **Harris B**. 'The child is the father of the man.' The relationship between child health and adult mortality in the nineteenth and twentieth centuries. *Int J Epidemiol* 2001;**30**:688–96.

58 **Okubo M**. Increase in mortality of middle-aged males in Japan. *NUPRI Research Paper Series 3* 1981;1–21.

59 Horiuchi S. The long-term impact of war on mortality: old age mortality of first world war survivors in the Federal Republic of Germany. *Pop Bull* 1983;**5**:80–92.

60 **Office of Population Censuses and Surveys.** *National population projections. 1992-based.* Series PP2 No.19. London: HMSO, 1995.

61 **Barker DJP.** *Fetal and infant origins of adult disease.* London: British Medical Publishing Group, 1992.

62 **Forsdahl A.** Living conditions in childhood and adolescence and important risk factor for arteriosclerotic heart disease? *Br J Prev Soc Med* 1977; **31**:91–5.

63 **Ben-Shlomo Y, Davey Smith G.** Deprivation in infancy or adult life: which is more important for mortality risk? *Lancet* 1991;**337**:530–4.

64 **Leon DA, Davey Smith G.** Infant mortality, stomach cancer, stroke, and coronary heart disease: ecological analysis. *Br Med J* 2000;**320**:1705–6.

65 **Murray CJL, Lopez AD.** *The global burden of disease: a comprehensive assessment of mortality and disability from diseases, injuries and risk factors in 1990 and projected to 2020.* WHO and World Bank. Cambridge, Mass.: Harvard University Press, 1996.

66 **Hermon C, Beral V.** Breast cancer mortality rates are levelling off or begining to decline in many western countries: an analysis of time trends, age-cohort and age-period models of breast cancer mortality in 20 countries. *Br J Cancer* 1996;**73**:955–60.

67 **La Vecchia C, Negri E, Levi F, Decarli A.** Age, cohort-of-birth, and period-of-death trends in breast cancer mortality in Europe. *J Natl Cancer Inst* 1997;**89**:732–3.

68 **Coleman MP, Esteve J, Damiecki P, Arslan A, Renard H.** *Trends in cancer incidence and mortality.* Geneva: World Health Organisation, 1993.

69 **Tarone RE, Chu KC, Gaudette LA.** Birth cohort and calendar period trends in breast cancer mortality in the United States and Canada. *J Natl Cancer Inst* 1997;**89**:251–6.

70 **Smith CL, Kricker A, Armstrong BK.** Breast cancer mortality trends in Australia: 1921 to 1994. *Med J Aust* 1998;**168**:11–4.

71 **Gersten O, Wilmoth JR.** The cancer transition in Japan since 1951. Demographic Research [online], (forthcoming). Available http://www.demographic-research.org.

72 **MacMahon B.** Breast cancer at menopausal ages: an explanation of observed incidence changes. *Cancer* 1957;**10**:1037–44.

73 **Stevens RG, Moolgavkar SH, Lee JAH.** Temporal trends in breast cancer. *Am J Epidemiol* 1982;**115**:759–77.

74 **Tarone RE, Chu KC.** Evaluation of birth cohort patterns in population disease rates. *Am J Epidemiol* 1996;**143**:85–91.

75 **Ewertz M, Carstensen B.** Trends in breast cancer incidence and mortality in Denmark, 1943–1982. *Int J Cancer* 1988;**41**:46–51.

76 **Persson I, Bergström R, Sparén P, Thörn M, Adami H-O.** Trends in breast cancer incidence in Sweden 1958–1988 by time period and birth cohort. *Br J Cancer* 1993;**68**:1247–53.

77 **Chu KC, Tarone RE, Kessler LG, Ries LAG, Hankey BF, Miller BA** *et al.* Recent trends in US breast cancer incidence, survival and mortality rates. *J Natl Cancer Inst* 1996;**88**:1571–8.

78 **Moss SM, Michel M, Patnick J, Johns L, Blank R, Chamberlain J.** Results from the NHS breast screening programme. *J Med Screening* 1995;**2**:186–90.

79 **Ursin G, Bernstein L, Pike MC.** Breast cancer. In Doll R, Fraumeni JF Jr, Muir CS, eds. *Trends in cancer incidence and mortality. Cancer Surveys.* Volume 19/20. New York: Cold Spring Harbour Laboratory Press, 1994:241–64.

80 **Blot WJ, Devesa SS, Fraumeni Jr JF.** Declining breast cancer mortality among young American women. *J Natl Cancer Inst* 1987;**78**:451.

81 Wigle DT. Breast cancer and fertility trends in Canada. *Am J Epidemiol* 1977;**105**:428–38.

82 MacMahon B. Cohort fertility and increasing breast cancer incidence. *Cancer* 1958;**11**:250–4.

83 Hahn RA, Moolgavkar SH. Nulliparity, decade of first birth, and breast cancer in Connecticut cohorts, 1855–1945: an ecological study. *Am J Public Health* 1989;**79**:1503–7.

84 Cole TJ. Secular trends in growth. *Proc Nutr Soc* 2000;**59**:317–24.

85 Rosenberg M. Birth weights in three Norwegian cities, 1960–84. Secular trends and influencing factors. *Ann Hum Biol* 1988;**15**:275–88.

86 McCalman J. *Sex and suffering: women's health and a women's hospital.* Melbourne: Melbourne University Press, 1998.

87 Ward PW. *Birth weight and economic growth.* Chicago: The University of Chicago Press, 1993.

88 Emanuel I. Intergenerational studies of human birth weight from the 1958 birth cohort. I. Evidence for a multigenerational effect. *Br J Obstet Gynaecol* 1992;**99**:67–74.

89 Alberman E. Are our babies becoming bigger? *J R Soc Med* 1991;**84**:257–60.

90 Gruenwald P, Funakawa H, Mitani S, Nishimura T, Takeuchi S. Influence of environmental factors on foetal growth in man. *Lancet* 1967;May 13th:1026–8.

91 Wyshak J. Evidence of a secular trend in age at menarche. *N Engl J Med* 1982;**306**:1033–5.

92 Whincup PH, Gilg JA, Odoki K, Taylor SJC, Cook D. Age at menarche in contemporary British teenagers: survey of girls born between 1982 and 1986. *Br Med J* 2001;**322**:1095–6.

93 Herman-Giddens M, Slora EJ, Wasserman RC, Bourdony CJ, Bhapkar MV, Koch GG *et al*. Secondary sex characteristics and menses in young girls seen in office practice: a study from the pediatric Research in Office Settings Network. *Pediatr* 1997;**99**:507–12.

94 Steckl RH, Floud R. *Health and welfare during industrialization.* Chicago: University of Chicago Press, 1997.

95 Tanner JM. *Growth at Adolescence.* Oxford: Blackwell, 1962.

96 Hermanussen M, Burmeister J, Burkhardt V. Stature and staure distribution in recent West German and historic samples of Italian and Dutch conscripts. *Am J Hum Biol* 1995;**7**:507–15.

97 Johnson P, Nicholas S. Health and welfare of women in the United Kingdom 1785–1920. In Steckl RH, Floud R, eds. *Health and welfare during industrialization.* Chicago: University of Chicago Press, 1997:201–50.

98 Whitwell G, De Souza C, Nicholas S. Height, health and economic growth in Australia, 1860–1940. In Steckl RH, Floud R, eds. *Health and welfare during industrialization.* Chicago: Chicago University Press, 1997:379–422.

99 Kuh D, Power C, Rodgers B. Secular trends in social class and sex differences in height. *Int J Epidemiol* 1991;**20**:1001–9.

100 Thom TJ, Epstein FH, Feldman JJ, Leaverton PE, Wolz M. *Total mortality and mortality from heart disease, cancer, and stroke from 1950 to 1987 in 27 countries: highlights of trends and their interrelationships among causes of death.* National Institutes of Health, National Heart, Lung and Blood Institute, NIH Publication No.92–3088, 1992.

101 Beaglehole R. International trends in coronary heart disease mortality and incidence rates. *J Cardiovasc Risk* 1999;**6**:63–8.

102 Woolsey TD, Moriyama IM. Statistical studies of heart diseases. II. Important factors in heart disease mortality trends. *Pub Health Rep* 1948;**63**:1247–73.

103 Sytkowski A, D'Agostino RB, Belanger A, Kannel WB. Sex and time trends in cardiovascular disease incidence and mortality: the Framingham Heart Study, 1950–1989. *Am J Epidemiol* 1996;**143**:338–50.

104 McGovern PG, Pankow JS, Shahar E, Doliszny KM, Folsom AR, Blackburn H *et al*. Recent trends in acute coronary heat disease. Mortality, morbidity, medical care, and risk factors. *N Engl J Med* 1996;**334**:884–90.

105 Tunstall-Pedoe H, Kuulasmaa K, Mahonen M, Tolonen H, Ruokokoski E, Amouyel P. Contribution of trends in survival and coronary-event rates to changes in coronary heart disease mortality: 10-year results from 37 WHO MONICA Project populations. *The Lancet* 1999;**353**:1547–57.

106 Jackson R, Beaglehole R. Trends in dietary fat and cigarette smoking and the decline in coronary heart disease in New Zealand. *Int J Epidemiol* 1987;**16**:377–82.

107 Sverre JM. Secular trends in coronary heart disease mortality in Norway 1966–86. *Am J Epidemiol* 1993;**137**:301–10.

108 Sarti C, Rastenyte D, Cepaitis Z, Tuomilehto J. International trends in mortality from stroke, 1968 to 1994. *Stroke* 2000;**31**:1588–601.

109 Bonita R. Stroke trends in Australia and New Zealand: mortality, morbidity and risk factors. *AEP* 1993;**3**:529–33.

110 Bonita R, Beaglehole R. Cerebrovascular Disease. *Lancet* 1993;**341**:1510–1.

111 Ebrahim S, Harwood R. Stroke. *Epidemiology, evidence, and clinical practice*. Oxford: Oxford University Press, 1999.

112 Higgins M, Thom T. Trends in Stroke Risk Factors in the United States. *AEP* 1993;**3**:550–4.

113 Ostfeld AM, Wilk E. Epidemiology of stroke, 1980–1990: a progress report. *Epidemiol Rev* 1990;**12**:253–6.

114 Klag MJ, Whelton PK, Seidler AJ. Decline in US stroke mortality. Demographic trends and antihypertensive treatment. *Stroke* 1989;**20**:14–21.

115 Gale CR, Martyn CN. The conundrum of time trends in stroke. *J R Soc Med* 1997;**90**:138–43.

116 Feinleib M, Ingster L, Rosenberg H, Maurer J, Singh G, Kochanek K. Time trends, cohort effects and geographic patterns in stroke mortality—United States. *AEP* 1993;**3**:458–65.

117 Olalla T, Medrano J, Sierra J, Almazan J. Time trends, cohort effect and spatial distribution of cerebrovascular disease. *Eur J Epidemiol* 1999;**15**:331–9.

118 Wolfe CA, Burney PGJ. Is stroke mortality on the decline in England? *Am J Epidemiol* 1992;**136**:558–65.

119 Riley JC. Mortality and morbidity: trends and determinants. *World Health Stat Q* 1998;**53**:177–90.

120 Elman C, Myers G. Age- and sex-differentials in morbidity at the start of an epidemiological transition: returns from the 1880 US Census. *Soc Sci Med* 1997;**45**:943–56.

121 Freedman VA, Martin LG. Contribution of chronic conditions to aggregate changes in old-age functioning. *Am J Public Health* 2000;**90**:1759–60.

122 Freedman VA, Martin LG. Understanding trends in functional limitations among older Americans. *Am J Public Health* 1998;**88**:1457–62.

123 Mathers CD, Robine JM. International trends in health expectancies: a review. *Aust J Aging* 1998;**17(Suppl)**:51–5.

124 Robine J-M, Mormiche P, Sermet C. Examination of the causes and mechanisms of the increase in disability-free life expectancy. *J Aging Health* 1998;**10**:171–91.

125 Manton KG, Stallard E, Corder L. Changes in the age dependence of mortality and disability: cohort and other determinants. *Demography* 1997;**34**:135–57.

126 Manton KG, Stallard E, Corder LS. The Dynamics of dimensions of age-related disability 1982 to 1994 in the U.S. elderly Population. *J Gerontol: Biol Sci* 1998;**53A**:B59–B70.

127 Preston SH. *Mortality patterns in national populations: with special reference to recorded causes of death*. New York, Academic Press, 1976.

128 Lee PN, Fry JS, Fory BA. Trends in lung cancer, chronic obstructive lung disease, and emphysema death rates for England and Wales 1941–85 and their relation to trends in cigarette smoking. *Thorax* 1990;**45**:657–65.

Chapter 17

The life course of Black women in South Africa in the 1990s: generation, age, and period in the decade of HIV and political liberation

Zena Stein, Quarraisha Abdool Karim, and Mervyn Susser

This chapter opens with discussion of cohort analysis and the life course. This perspective is applied to Black women in South Africa during the latter half of the twentieth century. We reconstruct and compare the life course of those born in the 1950s with those born in the 1970s. These theoretical cohorts of births, separated by two decades, will have experienced, each at very different ages, two eventful and concurrent circumstances of the 1990s: on the one hand, the socio-political transition from apartheid to democracy, and on the other, the advent of the human immunodeficiency virus (HIV) epidemic. That the effects of political change on the two cohorts differ is a reasonable if untested hypothesis. That the effects of the HIV epidemic differ among them is demonstrable.

The chapter is a preliminary sortie that lays out markers. Its aim is to see the contemporaneous process of political liberation and the evolution

---

A technical report[13,13a] prepared for publication and dissemination in August 2001, entitled '*The impact of HIV/AIDS on adult mortality in South Africa*' was not available to the public at the time of writing. Written by acknowledged professionals in the South Africa Medical Research Council and the University of Cape Town, its suppression by the Government was widely and vocally criticized by church groups, the large (1.8 million) members of the Council of South African Trade Unions, and Treatment Action Group, and the Media. Fortunately, a leaked version was excerpted by the press; moreover, a series of actuaries' projections was already available, covering similar ground. From these sources, we inferred that South Africa was clearly undergoing devastating results of the epidemic in terms of mortality; and, failing major changing in behaviour and/or the access of appropriate treatment for those infected, AIDS was transforming the demographic picture of the country. Figs 17.2, 17.3, and 17.5 give an illustrative selection of the data for the year 2000 for women. The figures convey better than words, the way in which the active population are being hit.

of the HIV epidemic through a multidimensional prism: are these events entirely coincidental and independent or can we discern interactions between them? More particularly, we consider if and how the socio-political forces have related to the development of the epidemic. Following the introduction, therefore, our first theme is the liberation, and our second the HIV epidemic.

17.1 Introduction: cohorts and life course

A life course perspective on epidemiology offers one distinct advantage over typical individual risk factor epidemiology. This advantage is to add to risk factors the dimension of time passing, as events in the individual life course impinge on development and health states. Much life course epidemiology, whether of individuals or groups, scarcely attends to the changing course of the historical environment in which personal development and its outcomes are nested. To measure such changes is usually a formidable task for which new technical means are still to be found. In South Africa at the time of writing, the context of extraordinary political change cannot be ignored. At the same time, the sustained worldwide HIV epidemic is wreaking the greatest devastation on the health of societies in modern times.

Cohort studies of populations defined by their social structure are simplified when the onset, progress and recession of supposedly causal happenings are sharply demarcated both in time and place. Such situations are exemplified by studies of the atomic bomb in Japan[1] and the after-effects of the Second World War famine in the Netherlands.[2] These instances are exceptional. Most environmental changes considered as putative causes of cohort differences in health status are gradual, as with socioeconomic environment,[3] and with health behaviour such as smoking or diet. Imprecision reduces the specificity of such inquiry. Thus one question we ask, namely, the interaction of age at exposure to a given environment with later outcome, is difficult if not impossible to answer.

Our first theme examines the effects of political liberation on the life course at particular age-periods. Liberation marks the transition from centuries-old colonial segregation consolidated by Apartheid to democratic government. During the decade of the 1990s, political apartheid finally ended in South Africa.[4] A government elected by the whole adult population took over for the first time in 1994. A society rigidly segregated by law and force now conferred the same legal rights and prospects on all racial groups. Black and White, women and men, young and old, rich and poor, rural and urban, faced a changed world. We ask if such a remarkable transition might leave distinctive and lasting effects on the health of survivors.

A brief history of the role of women in the liberation struggle provides the setting. We proceed on the assumption that the changes experienced by women of the two cohorts in the 1990s differed in impact depending on a woman's age.

Our second theme is the HIV epidemic that took hold in South Africa during the 1990s. We consider its explosive advent in terms of cohort morbidity and mortality rates in that period. In these respects, the cohort experience can be clearly differentiated by age. By contrast with social change, in so far as infectious diseases are putative causes of health effects in later life, they can be generally well-defined in both onset and duration.

The frequency and distribution of infectious disease clearly relates to the historical environment—physical, biological, and social—as it impinges at given periods on cohorts or generations at the societal level, and at given ages on the life course at individual level. In the study of cohort effects, most infectious diseases are well-enough characterized to be given individual attention (as indeed do all other specific events that impinge on cohorts). Over recent decades, the once everyday diseases of infancy have declined in frequency and severity or have virtually disappeared, and fatalities have been largely prevented by new knowledge, education, vaccines, chemotherapy, and antibiotics. By contrast, tuberculosis far from disappearing, in some places in recent years is resurgent in both children and adults in the wake of the emergent HIV epidemic.

In latter years, the interest of epidemiologists has emphasized changes over the life course in the later expression of early infections. For instance, individuals who escape certain early childhood infections often seem to suffer more severely if they contract the same infection at older ages, as with poliomyelitis and varicella. Supposedly they have lost some immunological advantages of childhood. In contrast, among those who were infected early in life, quite different forms of the same infection may become manifest after a lapse of years: measles can be followed by subacute panencephalitis, varicella by herpes zoster, and primary tuberculosis by its different adult forms.

In peptic ulcer disease, the marked cohort changes in frequency over the course of the twentieth century can now be seen, with the discovery of the role of *helicobacter pylori*, to bear a resemblance to the changes in poliomyelitis. Before the advent of effective sanitation, it is very probable that infection early in childhood by both polio virus and *helicobacter* was almost universally prevalent and conferred substantial immunity. As the sanitary environment improved and prevalence declined, non-immune individuals were left vulnerable to attack by the more severe form of paralytic poliomyelitis with poliovirus and by peptic ulcer with *helicobacter pylori*. (It seems possible, however, that lower rates of infection with *helicobacter pylori* may have led to lower frequencies of gastric ulcer.)

Tuberculosis was the infectious disease first and most often analysed in terms of cohorts. Wade Hampton Frost's analysis of 1939[5] (published posthumously) suggested that exposure to mycobacterium tuberculosis in childhood was in adulthood a predictor of the risk of breakdown and hence of mortality. Conversely, infected adults are a main source of infection of children. Exposure in childhood sharply declined in better developed societies as conditions improved in housing, nutrition, and later in treatment of the infected adult.

Depression of immunocompetence by HIV also raises the risk of subsequent infections. In those infected, the risk of re-activation of tuberculosis at any subsequent age is greatly enhanced (some 10-fold). Hence, today, where adult HIV is rampant, as it is in South Africa, tuberculosis is resurgent.[6,7] Thus, for tuberculosis in South Africa in 2001, two separable issues need consideration, namely, the current and delayed effects of infection in childhood, and the causal factors of new or re-activated disease in adults.

These examples of the manifestations of infections at various ages draw for explanation both on immunological and ecological processes. By contrast sexually transmitted diseases, like HIV, draw for explanation, as we discuss later, on sexual maturation and social interaction as well,[8,9] phenomena explicitly within the domain of epidemiology.

17.2 Women living under apartheid: the historical context

Apartheid dominated the political landscape prior to liberation. Disenfranchisement of non-Whites was virtually complete. Moreover, they were strictly segregated in place of residence and in education, limited in entry to occupations and in freedom of movement, discriminated against in law, and governed by an authoritarian state within a state. Disparities in wealth and resources were gross. Blacks suffered all the malign accompaniments of poverty. At all ages, divergences between races in death and survival were great and consistent.[10] In 1970 age-adjusted relative mortality risks for Blacks (compared with Whites) were as follows: infective and parasitic diseases 15; tuberculosis 27; homicides 20; nutritional (mainly infants and children) 62; infant and child mortality 10. Figure 17.1 shows how overall age-specific mortality faithfully mirrors the political and socioeconomic position of each race group.

Demographic data for Blacks were neither detailed nor accurate.[11,12] Life expectancy for Blacks continued to be much shorter than for Whites.[13,14] In the 1980s, infant mortality for urban Blacks as well as Whites declined steeply but not for rural Blacks. By the 1990s, infant mortality rates over the prior 10 years were 18.8 per 1000 for Whites, 38.7 for urban Blacks, and 53.5 for rural Blacks.[15] Socioeconomic status, disease and death remained highly congruent with race.

17.2.1 Human rights and women's resistance movements under apartheid

As in every social and political sphere in South Africa before liberation, human and political rights were sharply differentiated by race.[16] Sometimes, however, women's interests founded on gender clashed with those founded on race. For example, during the first decades of the twentieth century, and in parallel with suffragettes in Europe and the US, educated White women campaigned for the vote and won it in 1929. Women of Colour were denied the vote. Only a small radical minority of White women had opposed that restriction.

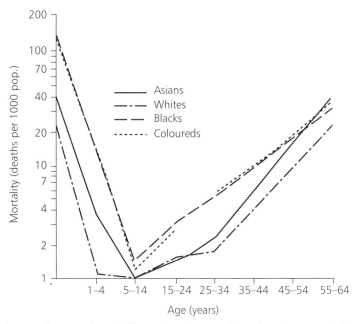

Fig. 17.1 Age-specific mortality of different 'race' groups for registration areas in South Africa in 1970. Adapted from reference.[10]

In one province, the Cape, the new law created an anomaly. In 1910 four provinces had been joined, in a parliamentary system on the British model, into the Union of South Africa. In the three northern provinces, White men alone were given an unqualified vote. Liberal leaders of the Cape Province, however, had been able to retain its formally colour-blind vote for all men, which was subject only to educational and property qualifications. The unqualified enfranchisement of all White women, including those in the Cape Province, thus placed White men at a disadvantage related to the women of the province and to all other Whites. In 1930 a further law removed this anomaly and gave all White men an unqualified vote. Thus, the principle of equal votes for White women was won at the cost of legalizing inequality between the races in the Cape.

In 1913, Indian women faced and met an issue of their marital rights. In accord with a new law, the Supreme Court ruled as null marriages solemnized by other than Christian rites. Protest by Indian women and men incensed by the voiding of their Hindu or Islamic unions led to the revocation of the law in the following year. This first taste of power for Indian women brought the newly formed Natal Indian Congress to recognize their political potential. In 1913 also, rural Black and Coloured women in the province of the Orange Free State protested an order that limited their movement. One consequence was the Bantu Women's League of the African National Congress formed in 1913/14, the first non-tribal and national organization of Black women.

Decades passed, however, before the multiracial Federation of South African Women (FSAW) was formed in 1953, after the 1948 election brought the Afrikaner nationalists to power. This was a vehicle for mainly urban left and liberal women opposed to the ideology of apartheid and its systematic imposition. The organizers represented the Congress Alliance of the African National Congress, the National Indian Congress, and the (White) Congress of Democrats. Those enrolled were mainly urban women. A Women's Charter set out their demands for political equality with men and added others—such as health services, schools, and housing—special to their roles in nurturing families and rearing children.[17,18]

In 1956 the organization led an historic demonstration to oppose the imposition of pass laws to Black women. Joined by unexpected numbers from rural areas, 2000 women defied the police and assembled outside the Prime Minster's offices in Pretoria. This excitement was soon snuffed out by the suppression of movements in open resistance to the government. Women were arrested, imprisoned, placed under house arrest, or exiled.

No women's protest as spectacular could occur again for another 30 years. None the less, the FSAW left an awareness of the relevance of political struggle to their own lives among Black women, such as those of the then young 1950s birth cohort. In later years, several politically active women of that cohort, like their elders, were either legally 'banned' from all political contact with others, or confined to remote rural areas, or forced into exile. (Mamphela Ramphela and others (see below) were later to assume prominent leadership roles in the new democracy). At the time of the teenage battles against the regime in the late 1970s, however, the birth cohorts of that decade were too young to have been politically engaged.

17.3 **The lives of Black women: the changed world since 1994**

In 1994, the constitution of the new democratic state conferred equal rights on all women for the first time. All could vote and stand for election. Several became leaders of elected bodies. Many of these were advocates in health matters, children's welfare, education, and women's particular needs. This was not to the exclusion of roles in other areas of government. Black women of our older birth cohort of the 1950s became a visible political force in the liberation government. Nkososane Dlamini-Zuma, who had completed her medical studies in exile in the UK, was Minister of Health in the first Mandela cabinet, and Minister of Foreign Affairs in the next Mbeki cabinet. Her successor as Minister of Health was Manto Tshabala-Msimang, who also graduated in exile as a primary care doctor in Soviet Russia. Others assumed influential positions in Parliament, the Executive and the provincial governments.

In this section, we first outline political and social change of the 1990s general to the Black population. We then turn to the cohorts of the 1950s and the 1970s. The outline of change in their general and reproductive health as well as in society at large should convey an idea of the significance of the period for their lives.

17.3.1 Political change

After 1994, the new right to vote in all elections was exercised by a very large majority. Many spoke of enhanced self-esteem, a sense of empowerment and of an entirely new sense of connection with government. By the end of the 1990s, much of importance had happened. Very large numbers continue to vote. Unsurprisingly, initial anticipations of equal social and political change have been disappointed. Constitutional safeguards and procedures to hold elected bodies and public officials to account are in place. At the same time, the very fact that ineffectuality, corruption, and cronyism are brought to light by the press and the courts gives rise to frustration.[20]

17.3.2 Social and economic change

Six years is all too brief a time for a nation to transform both its society and its economy. Standards of living have improved less than hoped. Unemployment, slums, and poverty remain widespread and little diminished.[21] Safe water has been supplied to large areas of the countryside for many, but more is still to be done. Much new housing has been built, but far from enough to meet the need. Pensions of the elderly, newly entitled, support many of their families, although some do not understand their claim to them.

Cyclic migrant labour, a fundamental and pernicious feature of the pre-liberation economy, has persisted with little change.[22,23] This century-old system was instituted by a compliant government to meet the demand of the powerful (and so-called primary) mining industry.[24] Hundreds of thousands of Black men are recruited for underground labour both from the large rural areas largely given over to subsistence farming and from other countries in the sub-Saharan region. In the past, many returned home annually after 9-month stints during which they lived in single-sex barracks. Nowadays, many rural men who find work in industry in towns nearby maintain the migratory pattern. They still shuttle between rural home and mine or factory while women and children remain at home.

Although the intervals between home visits tend to be shorter, the destabilizing of families seems hardly less than before. In these patriarchal societies, certain roles and decisions were reserved for the male head of the family. In his absence, women either failed to act or transcended tradition to do so. Although the hold of custom and tradition are eroded, in some degree the ill-consequences for families seem to persist.

Nowadays although a woman, free of the pass laws, may travel without let to towns or to her husband's work site, she often lacks the resources to do so. Some women deserted by their husbands settle in hope of work in urban areas, often to live in poverty in shacks without lights, roads, and piped water. If they find work, their children are likely to grow up unwatched in these slums.[25] These rural women, although more versed in modern city ways than before, are no less exposed to the hazards of poverty, to children unprotected, and to violence.

Many women, both rural and urban, complain of inability to control their children, and attribute it to the absence of husbands, the instability of the family structure, and the lesser weight of custom and tradition. Some of the bonds that ruled the lives of married women are undone; they live less well-protected from poverty and violence.

17.3.3 Education

Under apartheid, 'Bantu Education' legally restricted the content and level of the subject matter permitted for Black children.[26,27] This policy left an indelible mark on the complete schooling of 30 annual cohorts of scholars, and the partial schooling of about 20 others. The Act was quickly repealed by the new government, to the marked benefit of education for Blacks. Primary schooling is available everywhere, albeit often of poor quality, especially in rural areas and urban slums, for lack of both trained teachers and resources. If parents prefer, public transport conveys children to schools outside their home area. Some superior public schools are allowed to charge tuition; money, not race, limits this choice for some. People well understand the importance of education for future success. Many public high schools accessible to Black children, however, do not achieve high standards.

Higher education is open to all and indeed the best universities, all state-supported as before, encourage and compete for Blacks. Given the history of Bantu Education, and the handicaps Blacks still endure in its aftermath, the proportions admitted are remarkably high. In particular, young Black women are entering the 'learned' professions of medicine, law, and teaching in sharply increased proportion.

These improvements benefit Black women of the 1950s birth cohorts indirectly through their children. Well aware of the importance of education, these women grasped opportunities for their children they themselves never had.[15] The 1970s cohorts, many born to the 1950s cohort, thus benefited directly and substantially. Many such women convey a palpable sense of aspiration despite their inferior start under Bantu Education. Besides full-time university programmes, in the new era many extracurricular and part-time programmes, including distance learning, help to meet their aspirations. They have expanded opportunity and opened possibilities for careers. (The University of South Africa is said to be the largest distance-learning institution in the world, and other universities also provide programmes for further education. Women now in their twenties and thirties, for instance, nurses and clerks, frequently spend evenings and week-ends studying.)

17.3.4 Health

To say that the health care system still leaves much to be desired is not to understate the gains that have been achieved. In many rural areas reserved to Blacks, primary care was virtually non-existent. Now, for example, primary health care posts staffed by nurses are found in nearly all rural districts, the number of supervised deliveries is greater, and morbidity and mortality improved until reversed by the HIV epidemic. Health care for children under five years old also improved with the integration of all services in district health clinics. These gains are important to the parents in both cohorts as well as the grandparents in the older cohort.

Public and private health systems exist in parallel. The private system was largely rendered exclusive of Blacks by force of custom and cash. Now, it excludes them by virtue of cash alone. The minority who can pay includes almost all Whites and, now, a substantial number of Blacks insured through regular employment. The quality of much private care is thought to be reasonable.

Public care is better distributed than before but of doubtful quality outside tertiary-care hospitals. A recent survey of primary public care points to gross deficiencies both in trained staff and resources in general.[28] Nurses in the public services consider themselves underpaid and underappreciated; their attitude to patients, reported in several studies to be non-caring and authoritarian, perhaps reflects disaffection.[29–31]

Urban crime was a problem of the old regime, much of it at that time successfully confined to the urban African townships by an oppressive police force. Since the change in regime, however, crime has burst those bounds. Unpoliced robbery, murder, violence and, not least, rape pervade the society, and most of all the Black slums.[32,33]

Women of both the older and younger birth cohorts are of the ages that suffer the brunt of this social plague. Whether they are unpartnered, or have regular partners, or merely casual ones in the manner fostered by the migratory labour system, the severity and frequency of violence against women seems to amount to a new epidemic.[32,34] Male unemployment rates of 40% or more, predatory gangs, and the abuse of alcohol, as well as the inaction of the police, each surely plays its part.

We noted the rise of women's political activism during the resistance era. Their efforts concentrated on political oppression. The specific needs of women for legal protection, health rights, and their own general and reproductive health were secondary. Access to induced abortion was the single exception. Sporadically, women had raised this issue, and in an Act of 1975 the Government's modest response permitted abortion under specific circumstances only.[35–38]

After liberation in 1994, abortion reform figured prominently among women's demands. The resulting Choice of Termination of Pregnancy Act of 1996, as liberal as any law anywhere, in principle promised all women access to unconditional first trimester termination. In practice, it still awaits full implementation. The new Act, of greater import in the 1990s for the fertile younger women of the 1970s cohort, so far seems to have benefited rather few in the public sector.

Family planning, long intertwined with racist politics, is likewise a matter of concern chiefly for the younger cohort. Under the apartheid government, clinics designed for that single purpose were charged with the service. Under the new government, generic primary care facilities offer family planning as one among many services. These cover also prenatal and children's care, and therapeutic care for adults including sexually transmitted infection.[39] Family planning now operates with more resources and better trained health workers. Less beneficial is the continued exclusive use of injected hormones. Family planning services in South Africa as elsewhere promote the use of physical barriers only to prevent conception; their potential use to control sexually transmitted diseases including HIV is neglected.

Despite this limitation, since 1994 the rise in condom use by the women of the younger cohort has been marked if far from sufficient.[15] In a 1998 survey, 20% of teenage women reported using condoms at last sexual intercourse. Only about 4% of women over 40 years of age did so. In general, however, adolescent girls have not been well-served; many report that the older staff of primary care clinics even repulse them when in need of services connected with sexual activity. Thus risks are raised from sexually transmitted infections including HIV and unwanted pregnancy for the younger 1970s cohort.[40–43] For them, the new era has brought less radical change than might have been hoped for.

For women of all ages, the acquisition of rights in making their own decisions and empowerment generally seem, in practice, to have been slow to take effect. Activist women's groups are making more of such issues as rape and violence.[42] They do not forbear to criticize the representatives they have themselves elected. In sum, important post-liberation political developments for the women of both birth cohorts have been their aspirations and the realization of new political rights, together with unpecedented leadership roles for many. So too are new openings to education in schools and universities for themselves and their children.

Yet more is needed if women born in the 1970s are to improve the quality of their lives, and if those born in the 1950s (many the mothers of the younger cohort) are to overcome their historic handicaps. Perhaps most of all, the appalling apparition of the HIV epidemic must be faced and dealt with.

17.4 **HIV infection in South Africa in the 1990s**

Among the younger and older birth cohorts of Black women, the HIV epidemic is the period exposure of the 1990s we have chosen to contrast with that of concurrent liberation. In sub-Saharan Africa, sexual transmission is the predominant mode of epidemic spread and sexual behaviour is the key determinant of infection.[44]

Age is a predictor of sexual debut and also of the early rise and later fall of sexual activity. It affects the frequency of coition, the number of partners, the likelihood of protected or unprotected sex and, ultimately, the rates of viral transmission. A woman's age thus becomes a critical biological and social factor in defining the distribution and the limits of the risk of infection. Prevalence of infection, as expected, begins to rise in the teens and declines steeply from about 40 years of age.

At a given age in a cohort, prevalence of any persisting chronic disease is a rate that expresses the cumulation of incident cases among the survivors of the antecedent life course. Although prevalence can thus be only an imprecise indicator of incidence, in diseases such as HIV/AIDS it can be informative. (Indeed, a computed incidence can be derived from prevalence). Thus the available rates conform with our expectation that in the 1990s the force of the epidemic among older women born in the 1950s (or before) is less than in those born in the 1970s (or later). Further, birth cohort (and hence age) interacts with given periods (here the 1990s) to differentiate the epidemic pattern of successive generations. This interaction has implications for the trajectory of the epidemic.

17.4.1 **Incidence and prevalence**

The fastest growing HIV epidemic in the world now assails the southern African region, and in the region South Africa has by far the largest population.[45] HIV infection in South Africa was first reported in the early 1980s.[46] The HIV virus in this first relatively modest outbreak among men having sex with men was the Clade B variant and congruent with the US and European epidemics. (A related outbreak among patients treated by unscreened blood and blood products was promptly controlled by screening and quickly eliminated.)

The beginnings of the explosive epidemic of our concern, in the Black population, was first reported in 1985, among the population of men living in the mining compounds on the goldmines of the Witwatersrand.[47] Prevalence was about 1% overall among some 300 000 migrant Black goldminers on the Rand, but about 3% among the Malawians, an early signal of the epidemic incursion from the north (in the apartheid era, the northern borders were otherwise largely closed to migrants).

It is no accident that the epidemic reached the mines early in its course. As described above, in South Africa, miners typically shuttle every few months between place of work and rural home and back to the mine. Such conditions were and are still fertile ground for the rampant spread of sexually transmitted diseases.[48–50] In a classic paper of 1949 on the social pathology of syphilis, Sidney Kark first spelled out the mode of transmission of epidemic sexual disease and provided the dismaying data to demonstrate it.[48] Still today the route of migratory labour from city to tribal reserve creates the trellis for transmission of HIV.

From 1990, more or less in accord with expectation from mathematical projections, the epidemic grew fast. The main HIV variant in heterosexual transmission in South Africa is Clade C. In 1990 prevalence, established in antenatal clinics sampled across the country, was a little less than one per cent.[51] At the millennium, prevalence at the epicentre in Natal/KwaZulu antenatal clinics (some two years ahead of the rest of the country) had reached 40% without sign of stabilizing (Table 17.1 and Fig.17.2).[52,53] Its continuing course is foreshadowed in neighbouring countries (Botswana, Swaziland, Namibia, Zimbabwe). There, in some communities, the epidemic already affects more than half of those of reproductive age groups. Many women and men are wasting away, many have already died of AIDS; many children are orphaned, and many too have died.

In South Africa the infection, although found in all races, is spreading about 10 times more rapidly among Blacks than in other race groups. Women and especially young women have the highest incidence and prevalence rates. Countrywide anonymous seroprevalence testing, carried out annually among women attending public antenatal clinics, shows an

Table 17.1 Prevalence and computed annual incidence of HIV infection among antenatal clinic attenders, aged 15–49 in Hlabisa District, rural KwaZulu/Natal: 1992–1999 (Adapted from references[54,55])

Year	N	Prevalence (%) (95% CI)	Incidence per cent
1992	884	4.2 (2.0–5.7)	—
1993	709	7.9 (6.0–10.1)	2.3
1995	314	14.0 (10.4–18.4)	7.2
1997	4731	27.2 (25.9–28.5)	8.2
1998	3166	29.9 (28.4–3.16)	9.9
1999	3014	34.0 (32.3–35.7)	15.0

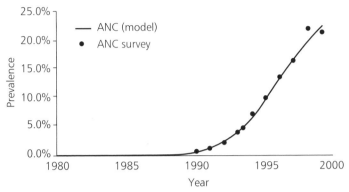

Fig. 17.2 HIV in South Africa: annual country-wide prevalence modelled from point prevalence anonymous surveys of attendees at representative antenatal clinics (ANC). Adapted from reference.[13]

Table 17.2 HIV point prevalence in women in rural South Africa (Hlabisa District) in five-year birth cohorts 1960–1979 (anonymous tests in antenatal clinics, 1992–1998) (Adapted from reference[54])

5 year Birth Cohorts	Year Prevalence (%) 1992–1998			
	1992	**1995**	**1997**	**1998**
1970–1974	6.9	21.1	34.7	39.3
1975–1979	2.7	18.8	27.8	36.4
1960–1964	1.4	15.0	23.4	23.4
1965–1969	0.0	3.4	12.9	23.0

extraordinarily accelerated rise in HIV-positive tests, from 4.2% in 1992 to 34% in 1998.[54] For young women the hazard is stark. The birth cohort of the 1970s remains the most affected (Table 17.2 and Fig. 17.3), although with the cumulation of incidence, prevalence by age necessarily shifts upward as those surviving grow older. Both statistical estimates and special ('detuned') laboratory tests confirm the recency of infection among many young women and the persistently high incidence among them.[55] The older women of the cohort born 20 years earlier, although not immune have, as anticipated, a lesser burden of infection.

The data from the national samples of representative public clinics capture poor Black women sexually active and reproducing, but some deficiencies should be noted.[56] The data do not reflect either the local variation across the country or the state of better-off pregnant women in private care. Infertility also reduces representation of older women and the very young. Among younger women too, reduced fertility induced by HIV infection removes them from the count in antenatal clinics. Similarly, those infertile because of other chronic sexually infections are unrepresented.

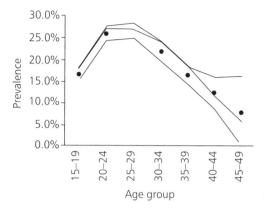

Fig. 17.3 Age-specific HIV prevalence (modelled with 95% confidence interval) in South Africa: antenatal attendees in 1999. Adapted from reference.[13]

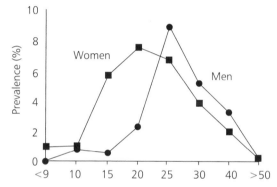

Fig. 17.4 Age and gender differences in HIV prevalence: rural KwaZulu-Natal in 1992. Adapted from reference.[8]

Representative local surveys give an independent picture of the prevalence but have their own shortcomings. In the rural district of Hlabisa, anonymous HIV tests were repeated at short intervals in routine surveys monitoring malaria.[57] In 1992, prevalence rates for young women already diverged sharply upward from those for men (Fig. 17.4). Women born in the 1970s and later predominated. Among women born in the 1950s and earlier, prevalence was relatively low. Thus, aside from the higher HIV ratio to be anticipated at the epicentre of the epidemic, these local distributions conform with those of the national antenatal clinic samples.

17.4.2 AIDS-related morbidity and mortality by birth cohort

It follows that when the manifestations of HIV infection appear, these too will have their main impact on the 1970s cohort rather than on that of the 1950s. The detection of HIV in an infant born to a seemingly healthy woman is often the first evidence of HIV infection in a woman. Other manifestations of HIV can be subtle and tend to be long deferred. Only as disease progresses and CD4 counts decline do symptoms emerge in the form of continuous bouts of diarrhoea, respiratory infections, a variety of skin lesions, infections of the ears and eyes, herpetic infections, weight loss, and other expressions of immunodeficiency. After the primary infection, these conditions tend to develop sooner in women than in men. Women

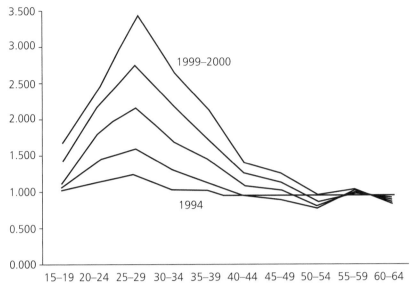

Fig. 17.5 Mortality in South Africa women by age (relative to 1983–85) rising for successive years from 1994 through 1996, 1997/98, 1998/9, 1999/2000, with a constant peak at ages 25–29. Adapted from reference.[13]

also experience relative or absolute infertility, as well as infections and malignancies of the cervix uteri. Tuberculosis, in South Africa the most common of presenting opportunistic infections related to HIV disease, is distributed as expected from the HIV pattern in the cohorts being compared.[6,7] In tuberculosis patients co-infected with HIV, fatality rates exceed those with HIV only.

Thus mortality is joined with the disproportionate burden of HIV infection and morbidity carried by the younger women of the 1970s cohort. Relative mortality rates for women for the period 1994 to 1999 (Fig. 17.5) have risen compared with 1985 and dramatically so for women aged 25–29 (the older segment of the 1970s cohort). The rise is far less for women aged 40 to 49, and absent for women of 50 and more. Women in their 60s, indeed, have lower death rates than those in their 20s.[13]

17.4.3 Cohorts and community impact

HIV prevalence in young women, as in the 1970s cohort, has importance for the whole community. The transmission of HIV from mother to child portends only tragedy. They not only themselves suffer the brunt of HIV mortality; they also leave orphaned infants and children to be cared for by others. Even if by good fortune the father is available to the family and a breadwinner, he too has a high likelihood of HIV infection and death.

Tragedy can be mitigated. Appropriate medication for the mother can control the ravages of the virus and avert transmission to the child. To do so across the nation requires the support or at least the acquiescence of government as well as local programmes that offer voluntary counselling and testing in antenatal clinics and discussion and advice for families.

Widespread stigma attaches to HIV infection. Some of the equally widespread violence against women seen to occur among the marginalized and poor of Black society has been attributed to stigma. For this reason and others, difficult decisions must be made about infant feeding practices. Formula and bottle feeding prevents transmission from mother to child. At the same time, it carries distinct risk for the untutored and those in the rural areas as yet without safe water supplies. In rural areas, where breastfeeding is still almost universal, moreover, not to do so can be stigmatizing because it rouses suspicions of HIV infection in the mother. Succour may come from a recent study that suggests that breastfeeding may be no less effective in preventing viral transmission than is formula feeding as long as it is strictly exclusive of any other intake at all by the infant.[58]

The older women of the birth cohorts of the 1950s and earlier, as noted, are less affected by sickness and death from HIV. They are the mothers of those who die and the grandmothers of their orphans. It is they who are left to care for the sick and dying and to sustain their families. Yet most will be without earnings, and nearly all entirely untaught in the tasks of nursing this disabling and painful chronic disease. Clearly, if or when the government makes appropriate treatment available, trained caretakers will be essential.

We leave till later the question of what has been done and what could have been done, given the socio-political changes.

17.5 Conclusion

The transition to liberal democracy is still very new, and judgements of gains and losses await confirmation in the long run. What we have described covers the elements of the transition over the past decade for two birth cohorts of women. We do the same for the HIV epidemic.

Our theme has been the comparative effects of the political, social, and epidemic changes on the life course experience of those born in the 1950s and the 1970s. Black women born in the 1950s were reared in the time of struggle and knew the apartheid regime as the enemy. Many who rebelled against injustice were restricted by banning orders, imprisoned, or forced into exile. They brought that experience to liberation. Virtually all rejoiced in that triumph, and many activists and returned exiles were rewarded with positions of authority. Ebullient as all were, the mass of ill-educated women in the large informal settlements of the city and in an unchanged countryside denuded of male migrant workers often found their families as poor, unstable, and lacking in resources as they had been before. Unemployment remained widespread or even increased. Access to health services and to schooling was distinctly improved. Still, overshadowing everything both wonderful and painful, the spectre of AIDS threatened the lives and livelihood of their families if not themselves.

Women born in the 1970s were less absorbed by and less aware of past struggles against apartheid than were the older cohort. The transition to a democracy and a Black majority government leaves almost untouched the patent differences between rich and poor. Such material inequalities largely but no longer entirely correspond to Black–White differences. These induce among many in the younger cohorts a sense of injustice unrelieved by a clear idea of who the enemy might be.

The new opportunities for education and self-improvement are eagerly taken up. Yet, schools with poor facilities and ill-educated teachers cannot change overnight. The upsurge in violence is resented and feared by all ages and classes, Black and White. The younger generation suffers the overriding impact of morbidity and mortality from AIDS. Overall, a national infection rate among these younger Black women in some areas has risen to about one third. In the sentinel areas of KwaZulu, it approaches one-half. Life expectation of Black women in the 1970s birth cohort has been reduced to a degree apparent even to individual consciousness.

Throughout recorded history, the *cri-de-coeur* of older generations about the shifting values and behaviour of the younger is a constant. But it is perhaps most acute in our rapidly changing, globally involved modern societies. What is unusual for Black women in South Africa today is the coincidence of a potentially liberating political context that is to the benefit of all with a stigmatizing, sexually transmitted epidemic devastating to the society at large, but which selectively maims and kills the young.

What might be the effects of the differing contemporaneous experiences of the older and younger cohorts on health later in the life course? Vulnerability to tuberculosis is an important likelihood. As noted above, Frost's 1939 paper suggested that youthful exposure to tubercle bacilli predicted a lifelong raised risk of the adult disease. Given the extra risks attendant on poor nutrition and overcrowded homes, an expectation of high prevalence at later ages would have attended the older cohort reared in the 1950s and 1960s. During the 1980s, improved living conditions and treatment for tuberculosis did somewhat ameliorate that expectation. In the 1990s however, HIV/AIDS emerged, and rates rose dramatically across the country. Epidemiological comparisons among older and younger cohorts of Black women of tuberculosis morbidity and mortality, using both clinical and molecular methods, might clarify this question.

Disorders presumed to be stress-related might also be found to differ by cohort if the diagnostic difficulties can be overcome. Mental disorders too, both mild and severe, might differ likewise. As compared with infectious diseases, or even with diet and the physical environment, speculation on these questions is hindered by a relative deficiency of firm knowledge about deferred effects of particular social or psychological experiences.

Pre-liberation political repression was directed at politically engaged persons. In the 1990s, repression was replaced by epidemic violence and rape as well as HIV. At different ages, the two cohorts discussed above have both experienced euphoria. Each, for different reasons, has also experienced despair. One might ask whether among the earlier and later cohorts the fears such experiences engender as well as the scars they leave differ in frequency and severity.

Finally we face, if briefly, a last question posed at the outset: what if any relationships, negative or positive, did the transition to liberation have on the trajectory of the epidemic for women of different ages? The epidemic was already present, if at low prevalence, in 1990. An important meeting, organised jointly by two anti-Apartheid groups (the Committee on Health in Southern Africa in the US, and the National Medical and Dental Association in South Africa) was held at Maputo in that year.[59] Representatives of the exiles and the then leaders of progressive health movements resident in South Africa met together. Prevalence data based on sample surveys and projections of the likely trajectory were discussed. South Africans in the country at that time felt strongly that nothing useful could be accomplished under the existing apartheid regime. Yet on that occasion Chris Hani, chief of the African National Congress armed forces in exile and assured of a prominent position in the new government then said:

> Those of us in exile are in the unfortunate situation of being in the areas where the prevalence is high. We cannot afford to allow the AIDS epidemic to ruin the realization of our dreams. Existing statistics indicate that we are still at the beginning of the AIDS epidemic in our country. Unattended, however, this will result in untold damage and suffering by the end of the century.

Commentators have asked 'what went wrong?' and our data show that is a fair question.[60,61] Tragically, Chris Hani was assassinated shortly before liberation was achieved. What could have been done and was not? We see four possibilities. First, the new government might have been much more forceful, in the manner of Thailand, in limiting the spread of the virus from critical high prevalence loci. Thailand contained the epidemic by stringent control of young men in military training and managers of public brothels. (Admittedly, these particular institutions do not exist in South Africa, nor could they be so easily achieved under the new democratic constitution). Second, after the model of Uganda, the president and government might have given strong moral leadership. To good effect, President Museveni has constantly and frequently repeated his call for citizens to respect and follow safe sexual practices. He urged those working in health, social, and educational institutions to initiate and oversee the critical steps of education, facilitation, and prevention. Third, government might have developed economic and social policies to induce a shift away from a migrant labour to a more settled labour force. Fourth, the government might have seriously addressed the possibilities of treatments, not for humanitarian reasons alone but for prevention: mother-to-child transmission certainly and sexual transmission quite probably, given reduction in viral load, can be prevented. In practice, no policy to contain the epidemic was ever approached with the needed foresight, urgency, and persistence.

On one count credit must be given to the government. The successful initiative to reduce the unaffordable prices of medications set by international pharmaceutical companies was courageous. Unaccountably, that success was followed by a policy that has denied the needed therapeutic and preventive medications to the public health services. The historic change achieved by the liberation forces were not harnessed to confront the epidemic, and the prophetic words of Chris Hani went unheeded.

Commentary on 'The life course of Black women in South Africa in the 1990s: generation, age, and period in the decade of HIV and political liberation'

Yoav Ben-Shlomo and George Davey Smith

The chapter by Zena Stein and her colleagues beautifully highlights the complexities and challenges that face an epidemiologist when trying to unravel life course and ecosocial determinants of health as well as psychosocial and material influences. They have chosen, unsurprisingly given the course of their own lives, to examine the experiences of two birth cohorts of Black women (1950s and 1970s). The older cohort who grew up during the apartheid regime faced political and racial oppression but knew 'the enemy'. Their struggles have led to victory and some resolution with the end of political apartheid. The younger cohort, who also experienced apartheid in childhood, is now empowered and enfranchised but continues to face the entrenched issues of poverty and sexism. Overlying this background is the emergence of the HIV epidemic during the mid 1980s period. The emergence of HIV as an exposure is both a period and a cohort effect given the strong association between age, birth cohort, and transmission of HIV through sexual behaviour.

The study of natural experiments in epidemiology is not new and one of the best such studies was the authors' earlier work on the survivors of the Dutch Hunger Winter.[2] Few studies, however, have used dramatic changes in the political structure of a society as their exposure, a potentially interesting and underexploited variable. One exception is the study by Sandiford and colleagues of the effect of the Sandanista regime on infant and child mortality in Nicaragua.[62] An obvious limitation of such an approach is that unless one chooses an acute outcome, it is unlikely that any benefits or harm of a new political system will be seen in the short-term. The increased uptake of higher education amongst South African Black women may soon show an observable benefit for child health,[63] a relatively short-term outcome. In the longer term, there may be even more marked benefits. For example, an analysis of mortality data from Japan between the late nineteenth and twentieth century observed a marked cohort effect for declining adult mortality beginning in the 1920s, twenty years after the mass uptake of education for Japanese girls (Professor Toshihiko Hasegawa—personal communication). Such potential benefits may be overridden in South Africa by the huge impact of the HIV epidemic. More recently, data on all-cause and cardiac mortality from the former USSR highlighted a marked period effect (1987–1994) with increased mortality associated with a period of state liberalization towards alcohol licensing and reduced cost.[64] Such major structural events provide fertile 'hypothesis testing' ground for advocates of an ecosocial model of disease aetiology[65] and may help overcome the methodological problems with statistically disentangling age, period, and cohort effects.[66] It is still too early to study the impact of the democratic liberation of Black women using such conventional approaches.

The authors also highlight the possible failing of the ANC government in its response to the HIV epidemic. The debate remains about the benefits of prepregnancy HIV screening, avoidance of breastfeeding in rural areas with poor access to clean water, and the use of pro-phylactic anti-retrovirals.[67] More importantly, but harder to change, are the important social and cultural issues around sexual abuse and rape of young women (see Chapter 15 and accompanying commentary) as well as the economic structure of a society that accepts the need for male migrant workers.

It is unclear to us whether one will ever be able to test if there were health benefits from fighting against an overt oppressive regime in the past, as compared to the frustrations of poor young Black rural women faced with state inertia in tackling the problems of poverty, poor housing, and lack of clean water. A cohort study of Welsh men observed that 'sup-pressed anger' was a better predictor of increased heart disease than overt anger,[68] from which one might conclude, depending on your political perspective, that political activism may yet have hidden benefits.

References

1 Neel JV, Schull WJ. *Effects of Exposure to the Atomic Bomb on Pregnancy Termination in Hiroshima and Nagasaki.* Washington, D.C.: National Research Council, 1956.

2 Stein Z, Susser M, Saenger G, Marolla F. *Famine and human Development: the Dutch Hunger Winter of 1944–1945.* New York: Oxford University Press, 1975.

3 McKeown T. *The modern rise of population.* London, England: Edward Arnold, 1976.

4 Sampson A. *Mandela: The Authorised Biography.* London: Harper Collins, 1999.

5 Frost WH. The age selection of mortality from tuberculosis in successive decades. *Am J Hygiene* 1939;**30**:91–6.

6 Wilkinson D, Davies GR. The increasing burden of tuberculosis in rural South Africa—impact of the HIV epidemic. *S Afr Med J* 1997;**87**:447–50.

7 Wilkinson D. TB research in South Africa. *S Afr Med J* 1999;**89**:155–9.

8 Abdool Karim Q, Frohlich J. Women try to protect themselves from HIV/AIDS in KwaZulu-Natal, South Africa. In: Turshen M, ed. *Women's Health in Africa.* Lawrenceville, NJ: Africa World Press, 2000:69–82.

9 Wilkinson D, Wilkinson N. HIV infection among patients with sexually transmitted diseases in rural South Africa. *Int J STD AIDS* 1998;**9**:736–9.

10 Susser M, Cherry V. Health and healthcare under apartheid. *J Public Health Pol* 1982;**3**:55–75.

11 Botha J, Bradshaw D. African vital statistics—a black hole? *S Afr Med J* 1985;**87**:977–81.

12 Katzenellenbogen J, Yach D, Dorrington RE. Mortality in a rural South African mission, 1837–1909: an historical cohort study using church records. *Int J Epidemiol* 1993;**22**:965–75.

13 Dorrington R, Dourne D, Bradshaw D, Laubscher R, Timaeus IM. *The impact of HIV/AIDS on adult mortality in South Africa.* Technical Report, Burden of Disease Research Unit, South African Medical Research Council, September 2001, Cape Town, South Africa.

13a An AIDS model of the Third Kind. *Actuarial Society of South Africa Transactions.* 1998;**13**:99–153.

14 Anderson N, Marks S. Apartheid and health in the 1980's. *Soc Sc Med* 1988;**27**:667–81.

15 South African Medical Research Council, Dept. of Health. *South Africa Demographic and Health Survey*, 1998, Preliminary Report.

16 Walker C, ed. *Women and gender in Southern Africa to 1945.* Cape Town: David Philip, 1990.

17 Bernstein H. *For their triumphs and for their tears: conditions and resistance of women in Apartheid South Africa.* London: International Defence and Aid Fund, 1975

18 Joseph H. Side by side: the autobiography of Helen Joseph. London: Zed Books, 1986.

19 Ramphele M. *A life.* Cape Town: David Philip, 1995.

20 Ramphele M. Citizenship challenges for South Africa's young democracy. In: *Why South Africa matters.* Cambridge, MA: Daedalus, Winter 2001. Issued as Volume 130, No. 1 of the Proceedings of the American Academy of Arts and Sciences, p. 1–17

21 Nattrass N, Seekings J. 'Two nations'? Race and economic inequality in South Africa today. In: *Why South Africa matters.* Cambridge, MA: Daedalus, Winter 2001. Issued as Volume 130, No. 1 of the Proceedings of the American Academy of Arts and Sciences, 45–70.

22 Wilson F. Minerals and migrants: how the mining industry has shaped South Africa. In: *Why South Africa matters.* Cambridge, MA: Daedalus, Winter 2001. Issued as Volume 130, No. 1 of the Proceedings of the American Academy of Arts and Sciences, 99–121.

23 Wilson F, Ramphele M. *Uprooting poverty: the South African challenge.* Cape Town: David Philip, 1989.

24 Walker C. Gender and development of the migrant labour system. 1850–1930: an overview. Cape Town: David Phillip Publishers, 1990:168–96.

25 **Susser I, Stein Z**. Culture, sexuality and women's agency in the prevention of HIV/AIDS in Southern Africa. *Am J Public Health* 2000;**90**:1042–48.

26 **Kallaway P**. *Apartheid and education: the education of Black South Africans*. Johannesburg: Raven Press, 1984.

27 **Asmal K, James W**. Education and democracy in South Africa today. In: *Why South Africa matters*. Cambridge, MA: Daedalus, Winter 2001. Issued as Volume 130, No. 1 of the Proceedings of the American Academy of Arts and Sciences, 185–204.

28 **McKoy D**. *Health Systems Trust Survey*: paper read to University of Witwatersrand History Department Conference: Issues on AIDS, 2001.

29 **Jewkes R, Abrahams N, Mvo Z**. Why do nurses abuse patients? Reflections from South African obstetric services. *Soc Sci Med* 1998;**47**:1781–95.

30 **Marks S**. *Divided Sisterhood*. New York: St. Martin's Press, 1994:173–174.

31 **Lubanga N**. Nursing in South Africa: Black women workers organization. In: Turshen M, ed. *Women and health in Africa*. Trenton, NJ: Africa World Press, 1991:51.

32 **Smith C**. *Proud of Me*. Penguin Books (South Africa), 2001.

33 **South African Institute of Race Relations**. *South African Survey, 1999–2000*. Johannesburg: South African Institute of Race Relations, 2000:79.

34 **Jewkes R**. Violence against women: an emerging health problem. *Int Clin Psychopharmacol* 2000;**Suppl 3**:S37–45.

35 **Walker E**. Abortion: *Some insights into power and partriarchy*. Occasional Paper No. 3. Johannesburg: Department of Sociology, University of Witwatersrand, 1994.

36 **Maforah F, Wood K, Jewkes R**. Backstreet abortion: women's experience. *Curations* 1997;**20**:79–82.

37 **Kaufman CE**. *Reproductive control in South Africa*. Policy Research Division Working Papers, Population Council, 1997.

38 **Krugman B**. *Balancing means and ends: population policy in South Africa*. University of Witwatersrand.

39 **Tint KS, Fonn S, Khuzwayo N, Robertson S**. Jeopardisation of preventive services of primary health care: a consequences of providing integrated services. *Women's Health Project Newsletter* 2000;**36**:15.

40 **Jewkes R, Vundule C, Maforah F, Jordaan E**. Relationship dynamics and teenage pregnancy in South Africa. *Soc Sc Med* 2001;**52**:733–44.

41 **Abdool Karim Q, Preston-Whyte E, Abdool Karim SS**. Teenagers seeking condoms at family planning services. Part I: A user's perspective. *S Afr Med J* 1992;**82**:356–9.

42 **Wood K, Maforah F, Jewkes R**. 'He forced me to love him': Putting violence on adolescent sexual health agenda. *Soc Sc Med* 1998;**47**:233–42.

43 **Vundule C, Naforah F, Jewkes R, Jordaan E**. Risk factors for teenage pregnancy among sexually active black adolescents in Cape Town. A case control study. *S Afr Med J* 2001;**91**:73–80.

44 **Piot P**. A gendered epidemic: women and the risks and burdens of HIV. *J Am Med Wom Assoc* 2001;**56**:90–1.

45 **Whiteside A, Wilkins N, Mason B, Wood G**. *The impact of HIV/AIDS on planning issues in KwaZulu/Natal*. Economic Research Unit, University of Natal, Durban, 1990.

46 **Sher R**. Acquired immune deficiency syndrome (AIDS) in the RSA. *S Afr Med J* 1986;**70**:23–36.

47 Proceedings, Third International AIDS Conference, Washington, DC.

48 **Kark SL**. The social pathology of syphilis in Africans. *S Afr Med J* 1949;**23**:77–84.

49 **Decosas J, Adrien A**. Migration and HIV. *AIDS* 1997;**11**(**Suppl A**):577–84.

50 Lurie M, Harrison A, Wilkinson D, Abdool Karim SS. Circular migration and sexual networking in rural KwaZulu/Natal: implications for the spread of HIV and other sexually transmitted diseases. *Health Transition Rev* 1997;7(**Suppl 3**):15–24.

51 Schall R. On the maximum size of the AIDS epidemic among the heterosexual black population in South Africa. *S Afr Med J* 1990;**78**:507–10.

52 Abdool Karim SS, Abdool Karim Q. Changes in HIV seroprevalence in a rural black community in KwaZulu. *S Afr Med J* 1992;**82**:484–5.

53 Coleman RL, Wilkinson D. Increasing HIV prevalence in a rural district of South Africa. *J AIDS Retrovirol* 1997;**16**:50–3.

54 Dept. of Health, RSA. Eleventh national HIV survey of women attending antenatal clinics of the public health services. Pretoria, 2001.

55 Williams B, Gouws E, Wilkinson D, Abdool Karim SS. Estimating HIV incidence rates from age prevalence data in epidemic situation. *Stat Med* 2001;**20**:2003–16.

56 Crookes Rl, Heyns AP. HIV seroprevalence—data derived from blood transfusion services. *S Afr Med J* 1992;**82**:484–5.

57 Abdool Karim Q, Abdool Karim SS, Singh B, Short R, Ngxongo S. HIV infection in rural South Africa. *AIDS* 1992;**6**:1535–9.

58 Coutsidis A, Pillay K Spooner E, *et al*. Influence of feeding patterns on early mother-to-child transmission of HIV-1 in Durban, South Africa. *Lancet* 1999;**354**:471–6.

59 Stein Z, Zwi A. *Action on AIDS in Southern Africa. Proceedings of Maputo Conference on health in transition in Southern Africa.* 1–16 April, 1990. CHISA and HIV Center for Clinical and Behavioral Studies, Columbia University.

60 Schneider H, Stein J. Implementing AIDS policy in post-apartheid South Africa. *Soc Sci Med* 2001;**52**:723–71.

61 Marais H. *To The Edge*. University of Pretoria, 2000.

62 Sandiford P, Morales P, Gorter A, Coyle E, Davey Smith G. Why do childhood mortality rates fall? An analysis of the Nicaraguan experience. *Am J Public Health* 1991;**81**:30–7.

63 Victora CG, Huttly SR, Barros FC *et al*. Maternal education in relation to early and late child health outcomes: findings from a Brazilian cohort study. *Soc Sci Med* 1992;**34**:899–905.

64 Leon DA. Chenet L. Shkolnikov VM. Zakharov S. Shapiro J. Rakhmanova G. Vassin S. McKee M. Huge variation in Russian mortality rates 1984–94: artefact, alcohol, or what? *Lancet*. 1997; **350**:383–8.

65 Susser M, Susser E. Choosing a Future for Epidemiology: II. From Black Box to Chinese Boxes and Eco-Epidemiology. *Am J Public Health* 1996;**86**:674–7

66 Holford TR. Analysing the temporal effects of age, period and cohort. *Stat Methods Med Res* 1992;**1**:317–37

67 Ades AE, Ratcliffe J, Gibb DM *et al*. Economic issues in the prevention of vertical transmission of HIV. *Pharmacoeconomics* 2000;**18**:9–22.

68 Gallacher JE. Yarnell JW. Sweetnam PM. Elwood PC. Stansfeld SA. Anger and incident heart disease in the Caerphilly study. *Psychosomatic Med* 1999;**61**:446–53.

Part V

Conclusions

Chapter 18

A life course approach to women's health: linking the past, present, and future

Diana Kuh and Rebecca Hardy

Evidence reviewed in this book suggests that adverse physical and psychosocial environments in early life affect biological and psychological developmental processes with long-term consequences for a number of diseases, disorders, and damaging health behaviours common in older women. In studies of both physical disease and psychological health we need to integrate the growing knowledge of genetic influences with our understanding of early vulnerability. Studies are needed to explore how these early risk factors shape exposure and sensitivity to later risk, and conversely how early risk may be moderated by later experiences. A common framework is also needed to combine the life course perspective with its emphasis on long-term temporal processes and the eco-social perspective which draws attention to the hierarchy of factors operating at any one time at different levels, from the macroeconomic to the molecular. Both acknowledge the need to study biological and social processes in integrated rather than competing models. The growing evidence that experiences earlier in life affect later life health informs the debate about whether the increase in life expectancy is associated with a compression or extension of morbidity. It draws attention to the possible health implications of the changing life experiences of women born in the second half of the twentieth century in developed and less developed countries. A life course perspective also provides promising explanations for social inequalities in women's health and possibilities for effective action.

18.1 Introduction

The aim of this book has been to review the factors at each stage of a women's life that contribute first to her reproductive health and then to her burden of morbidity and mortality in middle-age. In this concluding chapter we highlight some of the key findings, common themes, and gaps in knowledge raised by contributors to this book. Elucidating the complex pathways between childhood and adult life presents theoretical and methodological challenges for life course epidemiology and some of these are discussed briefly. We conclude by commenting on the relevance of our findings for policy and for understanding the future health of women born in the post-war period who are just reaching middle-age.

18.2 Key findings and common themes: linking the past to the present

18.2.1 Adding a temporal perspective to adult health and conventional risk factors

The long-term stability of a number of individual characteristics or environmental circumstances is a relatively simple way which links the past to the present. Various contributors reported continuity in health states or risk factors across the life course although in most cases tracking was relatively moderate. Nevertheless, prior health status is often one of the more important predictors of later health status. This was specifically noted in relation to depression and psychological distress and to gynaecological health, but is also relevant after the onset of chronic physical disease. As regards reproductive health, there is a tendency to repeat pregnancy outcomes both within individual women and across generations.

Contributors acknowledged the enduring importance for adult health and disease of many aspects of adult lifestyle, including both behavioural factors such as smoking, exercise, alcohol and diet, reproductive factors, body weight and shape, and proximal risk factors like blood pressure. High blood pressure, adverse lipid profiles and obesity have been shown to persist from childhood to adulthood in women. Behavioural risk factors, particularly smoking, and to a lesser extent diet and inactivity also track into adult life. Childhood socioeconomic circumstances strongly predict adult socioeconomic circumstances. At the very least, a life course approach in epidemiology emphasizes the need to take account of how age at onset, duration of exposure and changes with age in these conventional risk factors influence adult disease risk. For example, repeat measures of proximal risk factors such as blood pressure may well give better risk assessment for cardiovascular disease than a single measure in middle life. It may be weight gain, rather than actual weight, in adult life that is important in relation to breast cancer (Chapter 3). Physical exercise in childhood may be particularly important for adult bone density (Chapter 7). There are many similar questions yet to be addressed, such as whether the effect of cigarette smoking on timing of menopause is driven by the duration or critical timing of exposure (Chapter 4, commentary). A practical problem in applying a temporal perspective to conventional risk factors is that even longitudinal studies often only have one baseline measure and one contemporary measure of a risk factor rather than repeat measures of exposure across the life course. This places restrictions on aetiological insights that can be generated, and even in cases where there are more than two measures, the conventional data analysis methods may not be able to deal with the added complexity (Section 18.4).

18.2.2 The childhood origins of adult diseases and adult risk factors

Social and economic circumstances throughout life demonstrate powerful associations with a wide range of health outcomes. Exploring how the patterns of these associations differ by childhood and adult socioeconomic status has provided clues to aetiology and the role of childhood. For example, associations between childhood socioeconomic position and adult health outcomes that are independent of adult socioeconomic position, as reported for adult cardiovascular disease (Chapter 5), obesity (Chapter 14), and health behaviours (Chapter 13) suggest causal processes operating in early life. We need to understand *how* the early social environment leaves enduring biological imprints on the body and shapes subsequent behaviour which may help to explain inequalities in adult health and disease between socioeconomic groups.

In reviewing the evidence, contributors outlined how adverse physical and psychosocial environments in early life, through mechanisms related to nutrition, infectious disease, and stress may affect biological and neurobiological processes of individuals during growth and development with long-term consequences for adult disease risk. Many of the epidemiological studies with a focus on adult chronic diseases such as cardiovascular disease and diabetes have investigated the associations between measures of early body size and later function or disease (Section 18.2.2.1). Studies with a focus on psychological and behavioural outcomes have generally investigated associations with markers of childhood adversity or measures of early behaviour and temperament (Section 18.2.2.2).

18.2.2.1 Early growth and development and adult chronic disease

Contributors found evidence from longitudinal studies that women with markers of poor growth *in utero* and/or in infancy were more at risk of adult coronary heart disease, stroke, hypertension, diabetes and other indicators of diabetes risk, and obesity. Initial criticism that observed relationships between early growth and adult disease reflected lifetime social disadvantage rather than underlying early biological risk has, so far, proved unfounded in those studies with sufficient socioeconomic information to test this adequately. The authors of the cardiovascular and diabetes chapters concurred that twin and other family studies indicate that both genetic and intrauterine factors are likely to be involved. The important factor underlying any environmental programming effect is still a matter of debate with the role of maternal nutrition remaining controversial. The relationships between maternal body composition and diet both before and during pregnancy and subsequent disease risk in offspring are less consistent across studies than the relationships between early growth and adult disease. Twin studies suggest the supply of nutrients to the fetus rather than maternal undernutrition may be the underlying cause in the developed world.[1]

The association between low birthweight and increased coronary heart disease, stroke and diabetes risk appears to be greater among those who are large in adult life. Such effects may be due to catch-up growth during infancy, weight gain during childhood or weight gain in later life and may be disease and sex-specific. The importance of the timing of growth in childhood height has been investigated by studying the differential associations between leg length and trunk length (in childhood and adulthood) on disease outcome. Leg length is the component of stature found to be inversely associated with cardiovascular disease, possibly suggesting that restricted pre-pubertal growth increases risk (Chapter 5).

The influence of poor early growth on other health outcomes that have been less studied in this respect were also reviewed. Evidence suggests that impaired growth *in utero* or in infancy may compromise adult muscle function and bone strength independently of its effect on skeletal size. Poor growth in height during puberty may be associated with an increased risk of hip fracture many years later (Chapter 7). *In utero* and early postnatal effects on pregnancy outcome and reproductive ageing are also plausible but remain largely untested and are areas ripe for future research (Chapters 2 and 4).

Contributors found evidence that heavy birthweight and rapid childhood growth can also carry long-term health risks. The risk of breast cancer, particularly premenopausal disease, is highest in those of high birthweight and the risk seems to be exacerbated by rapid postnatal height growth. Leg length was found to be positively associated with breast cancer risk thus highlighting the importance of rapid childhood growth (Chapter 3). The offspring of mothers with diabetes tend to be heavy at birth and have a considerable increase in diabetes risk themselves (Chapter 6).

It remains unclear whether the relationships between adult disease risk and indicators of prenatal and postnatal growth reflect the same underlying growth trajectory. Recent research (discussed in Chapter 3) is exploiting the few life course studies with repeat measures of height and weight during childhood and adolescence and information on timing of menarche to model the growth trajectory and its relationship to later disease. It is important to distinguish what drives skeletal growth, weight gain, and the rate of maturation.[2]

18.2.2.2 Early psychosocial environment and adult health

Many contributors (see especially Chapters 8, 9, and 12–14) linked a number of aspects of the early psychosocial environment to adult psychological and behavioural outcomes. Evidence suggests that family factors such as adverse parenting practices, family conflict, parental divorce, and parental illness have long-term effects on adult depression and risky health behaviours such as smoking and alcohol consumption. Early relationships between young children and their parents and siblings can have lifelong effects on social support through the quantity and quality of later social relationships. Adult body image is negatively affected by parental comments and teasing received during childhood and adolescence. Role modelling may partly explain the associations between parental health behaviours and weight concerns and those of their children. Generally, however, it is not clear which transmission route—parents, peers, or genes—have the strongest influence on health behaviours. While many studies show an effect of childhood socioeconomic status on adult obesity, specific social, psychosocial (and behavioural) factors have rarely been examined although one study suggests the importance of parental neglect. Studies of childhood adversity of an extreme kind, involving physical or sexual abuse, have shown associations with a diverse range of adult health outcomes including depression and adult health behaviours, and also with physical health such as pregnancy outcome and urogenital disorders.

In a number of outcomes more detailed prospective research is needed to confirm and extend these findings and clarify the pathways that link the childhood psychosocial environment to adult health and other outcomes. Research on the childhood origins of depression (discussed in Chapter 8) has been more extensive than research on other health outcomes. It has already identified a number of chains of risk for adult depression involving extrinsic factors (such as persisting environmental adversities) and intrinsic factors (such as self image, coping skills, and cognitive schema) that may be more widely relevant. There is also growing evidence that early stress can affect neurobiological processes increasing vulnerability to depression and perhaps other disorders. As with studies of chronic physical disease we need to integrate the growing knowledge of genetic influences with our understanding of early vulnerability. Both can affect later health by shaping individual exposure and sensitivity to later environmental stressors. A particularly interesting group for further study is apparently resilient women. Research has rarely focused on the lifetime characteristics of women who have good adult outcomes despite having suffered adversity in childhood.[3] More studies that distinguish between factors affecting the onset of disorders or the initiation of behaviours and those that affect their maintenance, recurrence, or progression are required.

18.2.3 Integrating a life course perspective with the social and cultural context

In recent years, the study of the relationships between socioeconomic factors and health has been informed by the life course perspective, which emphasizes long-term temporal processes, and the ecosocial perspective, which draws attention to risk factors operating at a number of levels, from the macroeconomic to the molecular. There is a need to combine these perspectives, both of which acknowledge the need to integrate biological and social risk processes, into a unified framework (see commentaries on Chapters 11 and 13).[4,5]

In this book there are various examples of the importance of time and place on women's health and its risk factors. For example, in Western countries the uptake and maintenance of health behaviours, such as smoking and physical activity, are clearly context specific and show striking secular trends (Chapter 13). Health behaviours and other risk factors, such as parity and timing of births, or health outcomes, such as body image or obesity, vary over time in terms of their social distribution as cultural norms change. For example, childhood socioeconomic status predicts later smoking in some cohorts but not others. The social and cultural context during adolescence is particularly important since behaviours and body image may endure throughout life despite subsequent changes either by the individual in terms of class or in terms of the prevailing social context. Thus the eco-social perspective needs to incorporate a temporal dimension.

Rapid or dramatic changes in the wider environment can cut across and shift health and socioeconomic trajectories, with immediate and possible long-term effects on the health of populations. For example, an abrupt upturn in mortality among women and men was seen among the countries of Eastern Europe after the collapse of the Soviet Union (Chapter 16, commentary). A life course approach should incorporate both acute and delayed effects that may play out in a cohort fashion. The authors of Chapter 17 propose that the social opportunities, psychological experiences, and meaning of the transition during the 1990s from political apartheid to democratic government in South Africa may well have varied for women of different ages, and have differential health effects. This question is hard to address empirically, and is further complicated by the large and growing problem of human immunodeficiency virus (HIV) infection and acquired immunodeficiency syndrome (AIDS) in sub-Saharan Africa that is clearly affecting younger rather than older women. In this region, HIV infection is more common among women than men and leads to reduced fertility, transmission from mother to child, and eventually maternal death due to AIDS or opportunistic infections. A high prevalence of HIV and sexually transmitted diseases among women has also been found in a large cohort study in southwestern Uganda using newly developed minimally invasive testing methods to assess infection (Chapter 15). Their immediate and long-term sequelae on the health of women and their offspring has profound individual and public health implications. In developed[6] as well less developed countries the risk of HIV infection and AIDS is highest for women living in deprived neighbourhoods and needs to be understood within the wider social, political, and cultural context.

Change in the social context may affect the relationship between risk and outcome. This is illustrated by the results of a developmental contextual model presented in Chapter 11. The aim was to understand how the childhood acquisition of developmental resources (by which the authors meant educational achievement and psychosocial adjustment) was shaped by the immediate setting (home, family, and school) influenced, in turn, by the wider social context and cultural norms in two birth cohorts (1958 and 1970). Their results show, for example, that the effect of school composition on educational resources was much less in the later born cohort while the influence of parental aspirations was stronger. The authors suggest that this reflects the change in the educational system in Great Britain in 1965 from selective secondary education to the comprehensive system and the changes in occupational aspirations of parents particularly mothers during the 1970s.

Alternatively, cross-cohort and international comparisons that show similar relationships between risk and outcome, even though the social context influences the prevalence of the risk factor, would provide evidence of underlying biological or psychological mechanisms. For example, although divorce has become more common, a psychological effect on offspring may persist even if the stigmatizing and socioeconomic consequences are reduced.[7] Similarly, the biological effects of maternal sexually transmitted infections on mothers and their offspring are likely to be the same in any social context. However, the social context will influence exposure to infection, the extent of untreated infections in the mother and access to effective treatment of the sequelae for mother and offspring, thus altering subsequent morbidity and mortality patterns.

18.2.4 Reproduction and health

The preceding chapters make clear that the study of the relationships between reproduction and health would benefit from an integrated life course approach (Chapters 3–8 and 14). Reproductive characteristics tend to be correlated and may simply be cross-sectional markers of the same underlying process but few studies have attempted to investigate the combined effects of all such factors. Characteristics of menarche, menstrual cycles, pregnancy, and menopause show the clearest relation with breast cancer and fibroids, and relationships between parity and menopausal age, and between menopausal age and osteoporosis have been clearly demonstrated. In these examples reproductive characteristics are likely to be markers of sex hormone levels. It remains to be clarified whether it is the timing of exposure to certain sex hormones, their long-term levels, or in some cases their cyclical nature that is important for subsequent disease. Increased understanding of the life course trajectories of the hypothalamo–pituitary–gonadal axis, and other hormonal axes, provides the possibility of linking epidemiological observations with underlying hormonal mechanisms (Chapter 10).

There is also some evidence that reproductive characteristics affect obesity, cardiovascular disease, diabetes, osteoarthritis, and depression but the underlying biological processes are less clear. For example, while sex hormones may be implicated, the effect of parity on diabetes risk may be accounted for by obesity (Chapter 6). A common third factor may link reproductive outcomes to later chronic disease (Chapter 2). For example, infertility and disordered cycle length associated with the polycystic ovary syndrome are markers of insulin resistance. Intrauterine influences may operate on reproductive function as well as on chronic disease. There is also evidence suggesting that physiological and psychological stressors in adolescence or adult life can affect menstruation, fertility, pregnancy outcome, and possibly timing of the menopause by activating the hypothalamic-pituitary-adrenal (HPA) axis, which could also affect long-term disease risk. Assessing these possible common mechanisms involves a life course perspective on reproductive health, as well as on chronic disease.

The study of reproductive risk factors provides a good example of the need to consider both social and biological risk processes. For example, it may be difficult to disentangle the social effects of childbearing and child rearing from the biological effects of pregnancy, parity, and timing of births on later cardiovascular disease. Clarification will depend on longitudinal studies with better measures of stress and repeat measures of hormonal status using minimally invasive techniques (Chapter 10). Recent research using such techniques suggests that pubertal status may be more implicated in the sharp rise in depression after menarche than the accompanying social changes (Chapter 8).

18.2.5 Gender and ethnic differences

In the life course perspective time is seen as a powerful explanatory factor that locates individuals by chronological and physiological age, by period and by cohort.[8] As with socioeconomic status, gender and ethnicity are powerful explanatory factors in the ecosocial perspective and also need to be considered from a temporal perspective. Investigation of differences between men's and women's health, or between ethnic groups can shed light on long-term biological and social processes.[9,10] In turn, understanding these processes may allow us to assess the extent to which these differences are mainly social (to do with cultural norms and discrimination), bio-social (socially patterned exposures that have become 'embodied' into the biological and psychological attributes of individuals in these groups) or mainly biological. There may be differences in the prevalence of health outcomes or their natural history across the life course, and in relationships between risk factors and health outcomes. These differences must be carefully established, and caution exercised where gender, ethnic, or socially sensitive methods have been used, or where certain groups have been studied less than others. The traditional focus of cardiovascular disease epidemiology on White middle-aged men has been fairly criticized. In contrast, some disorders may be seen as being more pertinent to women (such as poor body image) simply because they have been investigated much less in men.[11] Formal tests of difference should be employed rather than simply comparing subgroups (Chapter 5). In this book, life course explanations for gender and ethnic differences in health and health behaviours were discussed but were not the focus of most chapters and these areas are ripe for future research.[12] Exceptions were the focus on gender differences for cardiovascular disease (Chapter 5) and depression (Chapter 8) and the discussion of ethnic differences in reproductive outcomes (Chapter 2).

In relation to cardiovascular disease it is the similarities between men and women in the effects of common risk factors that are perhaps as notable as any differences (Chapter 5, commentary). Although women are more obese than men they have have fat distributed differently with men having greater central obesity. The waist–hip distributions for men and women are completely distinct and so central obesity has been suggested as a prime candidate to explain the greater cardiovascular risk among men. Although a possible explanation, any other sex-specific risk factor could be implicated (Chapter 5). The authors of Chapter 6 attributed any excess diabetes risk in women to their greater levels of obesity.

Gender differences in outcomes such as depression may have different explanations at different life stages. Whereas longitudinal studies suggest that hormonal explanations are important in gender differences in depression at puberty (Chapter 8), differences (where they exist) in middle-age are more likely to be due to differential social roles and circumstances (Chapter 4). A number of gender differences in lifetime risk factors were highlighted that may account for differences in later outcome. Abusive roles, for example, may play a more significant role in gender differences for depression than previously realized (Chapter 8). The effects of parental divorce on psychological and behavioural outcomes are more delayed in girls than boys and need further exploration. Women are more prone to osteoporosis and muscle weakness than men because of their smaller skeletons and their dependence on the protective effects of oestrogen that are lost at menopause. Physical activity, one of the main protective factors for the strength of bones (as well as muscle), drops off earlier for girls than boys and will compound these differences (Chapter 7). In the social context physical activity may be seen as a masculine behaviour and thus not compatible with the image that many adolescent girls wish to portray. Smoking on the other hand is becoming an increasingly feminized activity (Chapter 13). Studying gender differences in the role of social support on health draws attention to the qualitatively different meaning of social ties and processes linking social relationships to health of women compared with men (Chapter 12).

18.3 Theoretical and methodological challenges

A life course approach considers the joint effects of risk factors at different life stages on adult health and disease and the pathways that link them together. This book has highlighted multiple risk factors relating to many women's health outcomes but the underlying biological and social pathways often remain to be elucidated. In many cases evidence has come from the piecing together the findings from disparate studies and a review of risk factors from each stage of the life course. This has meant, for example, that interactive effects of early and later life factors on later health have rarely been tested. An exception is in relation to early and later body size where such an approach is now commonly used. It is beginning to be employed to study, for example, whether early vulnerability interacts with menopause to influence psychological distress or well-being (Chapter 4) or moderates the behavioural response to new opportunities and constraints in adult life (Chapter 13).

The development of a life course approach to women's health would of course benefit from longitudinal studies with good quality data from birth to death. Contributors noted a number of new minimally invasive techniques (for measuring, for example, hormone levels, DNA, diet and exercise, and exposure to infection and stress) that allow more rigorous testing of hypotheses. To study the decline of physiological or cognitive function or the natural history of disease in its early stages is still often hindered by a lack of appropriately sensitive methods for assessing mild impairment or disease manifestation and small changes over time. Perhaps even more important than data quality is the clarification of hypotheses regarding the underlying mechanisms and the ways in which they may be operationalized so that they can be tested quantitatively using appropriate statistical methods. Contributors to this book have helped to define hypotheses that could be tested but many methodological challenges remain.

Even in longitudinal studies when data from across the life course has been collected it is rarely analysed within the concepts of a life course framework or even allowing for the temporal relationships between risk factors. The traditional use of generalized linear models in epidemiology, and their continued use for much life course epidemiology research, where the idea is to explain the variation in the outcome variable by a number of independent risk factors, does not fit easily with the life course concepts of pathways and risk accumulation.

The definition of a confounding variable states that it should not lie on the causal pathway between risk factor and outcome and must represent an independent causal effect on the outcome.[13] If the effect of a risk factor is adjusted for an intermediate variable on the pathway to disease outcome using a regression model, then the estimated direct effect of the risk factor on disease may be biased. The use of a technique called G-estimation has been proposed in epidemiology to obtain an unbiased estimate of the direct effect.[14]

The concepts used in life course epidemiology such as chains of risk, risk accumulation, critical and sensitive periods are beginning to be clarified[4] and this will encourage their operationalization for statistical analysis in a more systematic way. All these concepts raise particular methodological problems, even at the very basic level. For example, how should risk accumulation associated with poor socioeconomic status be measured and then defined in an analysis? As a summation of social class scores at different points across the life course, in which case what time points should be chosen, or as the duration of time spent in a low social class? Summation of measures may provide a stronger relationship with the outcome than a single measure but is this actually evidence of a cumulative effect? The lack of examples of interactions in the current literature may be due to the statistical problems in testing for an interaction where tests have low statistical power and are model dependent. The rationale for such tests must be provided by plausible biological and social hypotheses and the difference between epidemiological interaction and statistical interaction should be recognized.[13] With the inclusion of genetic data in life course studies, the concept of interaction is becoming more important as an environmental exposure may only increase disease risk for those with a certain genetic marker.

The prospective birth cohort study is the ideal design for studying life course hypotheses. Such studies come with their own set of methodological challenges, however. A birth cohort takes many years to get to the stage where questions regarding adult disease can begin to be answered. The use of existing birth cohort studies relies on the scientific hypotheses of the past for its data, and may not have all the relevant data to test contemporary hypotheses. Studying rare, or even relatively rare, outcomes can be difficult as the number of cases will be too few for detailed analysis (Chapter 3, commentary). Even where high response rates are maintained, inevitable losses to follow-up lead to considerable missing data which further complicates analyses. Within a longitudinal study the measurement of risk factors, intermediate markers, and disease outcomes may change as more refined measures become available and thus measurement error may vary over time. Other measures, such as measures of cognitive development, must of necessity change with age. The repeated measures may be missing vital points, such as heights and weights for each individual at the time of peak growth velocity. Hence, even where repeated measures of exposure are available, there may still be problems to contend with.

Modelling the steps along the hypothesized pathways is the next challenge. There is a large literature on methods for the analysis of longitudinal data and statistical computer packages with routines to analyse repeated measures adequately are now widely available. It is possible to consider the life course trajectory of a health outcome, such as blood pressure, or the developmental growth trajectory using repeat measures of height and weight in childhood and adolescence. Fitting the trajectory into a model relating to later disease outcome is more problematic. For some hypotheses one possibility may be to use parameters from such models (for example a slope representing rate of change between two time points) in a regression model (Chapter 3).[15] Alternative statistical techniques may be required. Path analysis and structural equation modelling (SEM)[16,17] have been used more extensively in the social science and psychological literature and SEM is indeed used in Chapter 11. Other useful tools include the related graphical models.[18,19] In all such methods a diagram indicating the pathways between variables is employed and a diagram indicating the proposed temporal pathway is an obvious way to develop a life course hypothesis. The interpretation of the findings and the assessment of causality may still be difficult and the flexibility of such techniques means that an appropriate degree of caution should be exercised with models being based on sound theoretical hypotheses. Further research is still needed to determine the advantages and disadvantages of these analytical strategies over the traditional regression approaches. In summary, a life course approach adds complexity to study design and analysis and the challenge is to find ways to model this complexity which can be readily interpreted.

18.4 Relevance of our findings for women today and implications for policy

18.4.1 Promoting maternal and child health

An obvious, but controversial, question raised by life course research is whether intervention during pregnancy should be investigated to ensure good fetal growth. While there is general agreement that 'victim blaming' of mothers must be avoided, opinions differ on the immediate policy relevance of the research. This is highlighted in the cardiovascular disease chapter (Chapter 5) where the authors suggested that it is too early to make policy recommendations whereas the discussant would like to see the evidence used to promote good maternal and child health. In Chapter 6 it is argued that the effect of maternal diabetes has potentially enormous implications for accelerating the incidence of diabetes worldwide and poses a greater future public health challenge than the effects of maternal under-nutrition in pregnancy. The increasing obesity of women both in the developed and developing countries also has enormous implications on future diabetes and other chronic disease risk for mothers and offspring (Chapter 14). In Chapter 2 the author suggests that pregnancy complications and birth outcomes may unmask chronic disease processes in their early stages. This offers the opportunity of earlier and therefore possibly more effective intervention but any strategy must be carefully considered so as not to cause undue worry and stress for women.

18.4.2 Control of infectious diseases

Our book raised concerns that were especially relevant for women's health policy in developing countries. Infectious diseases are prevalent, often go untreated and represent important public health problems. The impact of sexually transmitted disease control in pregnancy could have potentially large effects on the health and survival of women and their infants (Chapter 15). HIV infection and AIDS present an enormous problem for women worldwide but particularly in sub-Saharan Africa. Depression of immunocompetence by HIV also raises the risk of other infections and lies behind the resurgent trends in tuberculosis. While government strategies to reduce the price of medications are important to contain this epidemic, policies that encourage safe sexual practices, protect women against sexual coercion and rape and promote a more settled rather than migrant labour force are also needed (Chapter 17).

18.4.3 Policies that take account of social context

The argument that women's health has to be studied within its social and cultural context has implications for policy. This context exerts differential effects on women compared with men and suggests that gender sensitive interventions may be required.[20] The difference in exercise habits between men and women is one example. In relation to health behaviours and body image any policy must take into account the prevailing fashion or 'norm' of the time and place rather than just targeting the individual, since such strategies have generally been of limited success in the past. Similarly, in the commentary for the diabetes chapter (Chapter 6) Rich-Edwards argues that interventions in relation to this disease should take into account the enormous corporate and social pressure on the lives of girls and women and focus on institutional change.

18.4.4 Cohort changes in disease experience, survival, and function

The links observed between risks at different life stages and health in later life will have important policy implications if the health effects are large enough to affect temporal disease trends in the population, or between social groups within a population, and if effective and practical interventions exist. Many of the early life effects are small and the amount of variation in health outcomes explained by a single risk factor is also often small. One test of their importance is whether such factors help explain variations in disease across populations in time and place or whether their effects are overwhelmed by later risk factors perhaps working in opposite direction. Examination of trends in growth tempo and final height suggest some possible link with the upward trends in breast cancer and the declining trends in stroke over the twentieth century (Chapter 16). If, as we suspect, it is a combination of factors that is important, extension of the simple ecological correlation analysis is necessary. Modelling of more than one factor in ecological models or comparisons of cohort studies across time or place are needed to develop aetiologically informed analyses of population differences (Chapter 16, commentary). The former requires time series of all the relevant factors while the latter requires all cohorts to have the relevant measures on its individuals.

The evidence of earlier life influences on later health and disease found by contributors to this book feeds into the debate about whether the recent rapid decline in all-cause mortality at older ages has been accompanied by a compression or extension of morbidity.[21–24] Since the 1970s the decline in adult mortality has accelerated in most established market economies; improvements have been more rapid for men in middle and early old age (Chapter 16) and for women at older ages.[25] Mortality and morbidity do not necessarily have parallel trends in a population.[26] Increases in disability prevalence in the 1960s and 1970s raised concern that disability free life expectancy at age 65 years was at best stagnating and might be getting worse.[27–29] Little evidence of an extension of morbidity was found if only severe disability states were included, and recent research suggests that disability may now be falling at all levels in developed countries.[30] While current conditions, including earlier diagnosis and improved treatment and management of chronic disease,[31] may play a part in these recent favourable trends, they may also be driven by cohort improvements in physiological functioning.[32,33] Genetic factors may play some role in the survival and maintenance of function of individuals[34] but are unlikely to be important in the short-term improvements observed.

A life course perspective prompts us to consider the balance of contributions from factors at different life stages on the cohort survival and maintenance of function in old age, and to ask if the balance differs by cohort and by place. The evidence for older cohorts is inconsistent. For example, simple examination of the changes in age-specific mortality rates amongst the oldest old (aged 80 or over and born between 1870 and 1910) in a number of countries shows that the timing of onset of the rapid mortality decline has been simultaneous in different age groups. This suggests that period rather than cohort effects have dominated the decline at these ages.[25] If true, and given it was these birth cohorts where cohort effects on survival at younger ages was observed in some European countries (see Chapter 16), it would be an interesting example of how the balance between the effects of current and past conditions may change within a cohort's lifetime. More complex analysis on US cohorts born at around the same time (between 1887 and 1917)[35] does show cohort effects in survival and maintenance of function. This may reflect differential experiences in the middle years[35] or even earlier in life.

It is particularly important to consider how the life experiences of cohorts born since the 1930s differ from the experiences of earlier born cohorts in ways that may have a differential impact on their maintenance of health and function and disease risk in middle and old age. This is because it is the cohorts born between the 1930s and 1960s who will fuel the increase in the percentage of the population aged 60 years and over (anticipated to reach 30% of women in established market economies by 2020)[36] and their health will have profound implications for health and welfare services. In comparison with earlier cohorts they experienced rapid improvements in the risk of falling ill and made quicker recoveries from their illnesses,[37] benefiting from the introduction of antibiotic treatment for infectious diseases in the 1930s. These cohorts were either affected least by the Second World War or not at all and have spent the first half of their lives in the relatively prosperous post-war period. Thus they are likely to have accumulated a 'stock' of good health before they entered middle-age and we would predict that they will show considerable improvements in survival and functioning in later life in comparison with the preceding cohorts. Evidence from the UK suggests that these cohorts already have had better than average improvements in mortality compared with earlier *and later* birth cohorts (Chapter 16). This reminds us that health conditions do not necessarily improve over successive cohorts. Adverse trends in risk factors such as child obesity (see Chapter 14), adolescent smoking,[38] poverty, and socioeconomic inequality (see below) may inhibit further improvements in functioning as these later cohorts reach middle age. To establish changes in cohort functioning, and the reasons for any change, will require cohort comparisons at all stages of life using comparable measures of exposures and outcomes. The data for this research will come not only from better long-term monitoring of the health of populations, but also from life course studies which allow lifetime exposures to be examined in relation to changes in individual functioning. The setting up of new birth cohorts in countries such as Australia, the US, and the UK explicitly acknowledge the importance of this approach.

18.4.5 Social inequalities in health

A life course perspective contributes to the current and increasingly dynamic debate on social inequalities in women's and men's health. Social inequalities have been widening in women's mortality and life expectancy[39–41] as well as in markers of health such as height.[42] Explaining social inequalities in health and the reasons for the widening gap could make an important impact on public health if followed by appropriate interventions.[43,44] Explanations for social inequalities in cause-specific adult mortality[45] and other health outcomes may lie in socially patterned exposures at different stages of the life course. We have shown that they may operate through physiological and psychosocial processes, particularly developmental mechanisms. They also operate through the strong continuities in social advantage and disadvantage across the life course which are becoming more and more the result of a woman's own progress through the employment structure rather than a result of marriage (see Chapter 11).

The economic recession of the late 1970s and early 1980s and the restructuring of the economies of many industrialized nations in the last quarter of the twentieth century led to an increase in poverty and income inequality in industrial nations.[46–48] These increases, coupled with changes in family formation and disruption affected cohorts in different ways and were socially patterned by class, education, and gender. Graham[44] has succinctly highlighted the effect of these changes in the UK:

> Putting together the evidence, it is clear that shifts in employment, family formation and government policy have combined to reconfigure the lifecourse pathways along which individual socioeconomic position is determined. The unequal but relatively predictable lifecourse pathways of the 1950s and 1960s are giving way to a polarization of life chances and living standards. Those from privileged backgrounds and with education are gaining most from the changes in the labour market, and can anticipate high and sustained lifetime earnings. Conversely, those from poorer backgrounds are both losing out in the labour market and are more likely to face additional disadvantages associated with early cohabitation and early parenthood. These processes of social polarization have important lifecourse dimensions, impacting disproportionately on children and young people at life stages identified as influencing adult health.

Children, especially children living with single parents or whose parents have divorced, have been particularly affected by the increase in poverty.[47,49–51] The increased polarization in the transition from school to adulthood was evident from a comparison of two British birth cohorts (born in 1958 and 1970).[52] This study also showed more diverse patterns of transition for women than for men, and more fluid transition patterns for the later cohort, including growing unemployment, shrinking labour force participation, and more time in education. Social class differences persisted but gender differences altered as more opportunities for post school training and education became available to young women.[53] Recent evidence from Sweden[54] and Denmark[55] suggests that younger women's relations with the labour market can be an important contributing factor to their ill-health, as well as bringing positive benefits.

Adverse social and economic experiences in younger life have worrying implications for the development of lifetime health, social and personal resources in these younger birth cohorts, including the resources to parent the next generation. There is concern that what has been described as the 'growing chaos' in the lives of young people today strengthens the social gradients in all kinds of aspects of human development with long-term effects on human capital and hence the wealth of nations.[56] Fiscal and social security policies can have an important impact on reducing or increasing inequalities in living standards across social groups and across the life course and these vary considerably among industrial nations.[44] A mix of universal, targeted, and health interventions, discussed elsewhere,[56] is needed to improve the developmental health of children and young people. These policies will draw on the scientific evidence reviewed here and elsewhere which links childhood health, education, and social circumstances to health and inequalities in health in later life. The transition from research to policy would be aided by the development of an interdisciplinary science of health inequalities which is informed by a life course perspective.[44]

18.5 Conclusions: integrating life course epidemiology and women's health research

A life course approach offers a conceptual framework for organizing the study of women's health. It represents a synthesis of earlier aetiological models, such as biological programming, adult lifestyle and the social model of disease causation. Its long-term temporal perspective makes it scientifically interesting, conceptually and methodologically challenging, inherently interdisciplinary, and policy relevant. The future value of a life course approach to women's health will depend on its success in meeting four challenges. One is identifying risk and protective factors at each stage of a woman's life that influence independently, cumulatively, or interactively her chance of health and the risk of disease in later life. The second challenge is to shed light on the underlying biological, behavioural, and psychosocial pathways that operate across a woman's life and across generations. The third challenge is its ability to explain social, geographical, and temporal patterns of disease distribution in women. Its fourth challenge is the recommendation of policy interventions that are effective and sensitive to women's needs at each life stage. This book goes a long way towards meeting the first challenge. It has taken the first steps towards the second and third and the fourth remains relatively untouched. These areas are ripe for future research. We hope that this book will encourage other researchers interested in women's health to take up these challenges.

References

1 **Leon D**. Twins and fetal programming of blood pressure. *Br Med J* 1999;**319**:1313–4.

2 **Cole TJ**. Secular trends in growth. *Proc Nutr Soc* 2000;**59**:317–24.

3 **Singer B, Ryff CD, Carr D, Magee WJ**. Linking life histories and mental health: a person-centered strategy. In Raftery A, ed. *Sociological methodology*. Washington, D.C.: American Sociological Association, 1998, pp. 1–51.

4 **Ben-Shlomo Y, Kuh D**. A life course approach to chronic disease epidemiology: conceptual models, empirical challenges, and interdisciplinary perspectives. *Int J Epidemiol* 2002;**31**:285–93.

5 **Hertzman C, Power C, Matthews S, Manor O**. Using an interactive framework of society and lifecourse to explain self-rated health in early adulthood. *Soc Sci Med* 2001;**53**:1575–85.

6 **Zierler S, Kreiger N**. Reframing women's risk: social inequalities and HIV infection. *Annu Rev Public Health* 1997;**18**:401–36.

7 **Ely M, Richards MPM, Wadsworth MEJ, Elliot BJ**. Secular changes in the association of parental divorce and children's educational attainment—evidence from three British birth cohorts. *J Soc Pol* 1999;**28**:437–55.

8 **Wadsworth MEJ**. *The imprint of time: childhood, history and adult life*. Oxford: Oxford University Press, 1991.

9 **Worthman CM**. Hormones, sex, and gender. *Annu Rev Anthropol* 1995;**24**:593–616.

10 **Ness RB, Kuller LH**. Women's health as a paradigm for understanding factors that mediate disease. *J Women's Health* 1997;**6**:329–36.

11 **Phillips KA, Castle DJ**. Body dysmorphic disorder in men. *Br Med J* 2001;**323**:1015–6.

12 **Kreiger N**. Refiguring 'race': epidemiology, racialized biology, and biological expressions of race relations. *Int J Health Serv* 2000;**30**:211–6.

13 **Rothman KJ**. *Modern epidemiology*. Boston: Little, Brown and Company, 1986.

14 **Robins JM, Greenland S**. Identifiability and exchangeability for direct and indirect effects. *Epidemiology* 1992;**3**:143–55.

15 **dos Santos Silva I, De Stavola BL, Mann V, Kuh D, Hardy R, Wadsworth MEJ**. Prenatal factors, childhood growth trajectories and age at menarche. *Int J Epidemiol* 2002;**31**:405–12.

16 **Mullen B**. A general structural equation model with dichotomous, ordered categorical, and continuous latent variable indicators. *Psychometrika* 1984;**49**:115–32.

17 **Bollen KA**. *Structural equations with latent variables*. New York: John Wiley, 1989.

18 **Cox DR, Wermuth N**. Multivariate dependencies—models, analysis and interpretation. *Monographs on statistics and applied probability*. London: Chapman & Hall, 1996.

19 **Pearl J**. *Causality: models, reasoning, and inference*. New York: Cambridge University Press, 2000.

20 **Doyal L**. Sex, gender, and health: the need for a new approach. *Br Med J* 2001;**323**:1061–3.

21 **Fries JF**. Aging, natural death, and the compression of morbidity. *N Engl J Med* 1980;**303**:130–5.

22 **Fries JF**. The compression of morbidity: near or far? *Milbank Memorial Fund Q* 1989;**607**:208–32.

23 **Gruenberg EM**. The failures of success. *Milbank Memorial Fund Q* 1977;**55**:3–24.

24 **Barrett-Connor E**. Are we living longer or dying longer? In Poulter N, Thom S, eds. *Cardiovascular Disease: Risk Factors and Intervention*. Oxford: Radcliffe Medical Press, 1993:89–99.

25 **Kannisto V**. *Development of oldest-old mortality, 1950–1990: evidence from 29 developed countries*. Odense: Monographs on Population Aging, 1. Odense University Press, 1994.

26 **Riley JC**. Mortality and morbidity: trends and determinants. *World Health Stat Q* 1998;**53**:177–90.

27 **Bebbington AC**. The expectation of life without disability in England and Wales. *Soc Sci Med* 1988;**27**:321–6.

28 **Robine JM, Ritchie K**. Healthy life expectancy: evaluation of global indicator of change in population health. *Br Med J* 1991;**302**:457–60.

29 **Bebbington AC**. The expectation of life without disability in England and Wales. *Popul Trends* 1991;**66**:26–9.

30 **Mathers CD, Robine JM**. International Trends in Health Expectancies: a Review. *Aust J Aging* 1998;**17**(Suppls):51–5.

31 **Freedman VA, Martin LG**. Contribution of chronic conditions to aggregate changes in old-age functioning. *Am J Public Health* 2000;**90**:1759–60.

32 **Freedman VA, Martin LG**. Understanding trends in functional limitations among older Americans. *Am J Public Health* 1998;**88**:1457–62.

33 **Vaupel JW, Carey JR, Christensen K, Thomas E, Yashin AI, Holm NV** *et al*. Biodemographic trajectories of longevity. *Science* 2001;**280**:855.

34 **Finch CE, Tanzi RE**. Genetics of Aging. *Science* 1997;**278**:407–11.

35 **Manton KG, Stallard E, Corder L**. Changes in the age dependence of mortality and disability: cohort and other determinants. *Demography* 1997;**34**:135–57.

36 **Murray CJL, Lopez AD**. *The global burden of disease: a comprehensive assessment of mortality and disability from diseases, injuries and risk factors in 1990 and projected to 2020*. WHO & World Bank. Cambridge, Mass.: Harvard University Press, 1996.

37 **Riley JC**. *Sickness, Recovery and Death*. Hampshire: MacMillan Press, 1989.

38 **World Health Organization Regional Office for Europe**. *Smoking, drinking and drug taking in the European Region*. Copenhagen: World Health Organisation, 1997.

39 Harding S, Bethune A, Maxwell R, Brown J. Mortality trends using the Longitudinal Study. In Drever F, Whitehead M, eds. *Health inequalities. Decennial supplement.Series DS No. 15* London: The Stationery Office, 1997, pp. 143–55.

40 Whitehead M, Diderichsen F. International evidence on social inequalities in health. In Drever F, Whitehead M, eds. *Health inequalities.Decennial supplement. Series DS–o. 15.* London: The Stationery Office. 1997, pp. 44–69.

41 Hattersley L. Trends in life expectancy by social class—an update. *Health Stat Q* 1999;**2**:16–25

42 Kuh DL, Power C, Rodgers B. Secular trends in social class and sex differences in adult height. *Int J Epidemiol* 1991;**20**:1001–9.

43 Independent Inquiry into Inequalities in Health. *Report of the Independent Inquiry into Inequalities in Health.* London: The Stationery Office, 1998.

44 Graham H. Building an inter-disciplinary science of health inequalities: the example of lifecourse research. *Soc Sci Med,* in press.

45 Davey Smith G, Gunnell D, Ben-Shlomo Y. Life-course approaches to socioeconomic differentials in cause specific adult mortality. In Leon D, Walt G, eds. *Poverty, inequality and health: an international perspective.* Oxford: Oxford University Press, 2000, pp. 88–124.

46 Smith DJ. Living conditions in the twentieth century. In: Rutter M, Smith DJ, eds. *Psychosocial Disorders in Young People: Time Trends and Their Causes.* Chichester: John Wiley & Sons Ltd, 1995.

47 Bradbury B, Jenkins SP, Micklewright J. *The dynamics of child poverty in industrialised countries.* Cambridge: Cambridge University Press, 2001.

48 Freeman RB. *When earnings diverge: causes, consequences and cures for the new inequality in the US.* Washington, D.C.: National Policy Association, 1997.

49 Cornia GA. *Child poverty and deprivation in industrialised countries: recent trends and policy options.* Florence: UNICEF International Child Development Centre: Innocenti Occasional Papers, No.2., 1990.

50 Corcoran ME, Chaudry A. The dynamics of child poverty. *Future Child* 1997;**7**:40–54.

51 DiLiberti JH. The relationship between social stratification and all-cause mortality among children in the United States: 1968–1992. *Pediatr* 2000, pp. 105.

52 Schoon I, McCulloch A, Joshi H, Wiggins R, Bynner J. Transitions from school to work in a changing social context. *YOUNG: Nordic J Youth Res* 2001;**9**:4–22.

53 Bynner J, Parsons S. Getting on with qualifications. In Aldershot, ed. *Getting on, getting by, getting nowhere. Twenty-something in the 1990's.* Ashgate: 1997, pp. 11–29.

54 Novo M, Hammarstrom A, Janlert U. Do high levels of unemployment influence the health of those who are not employed? A gendered comparison of young men and women during boom and recession. *Soc Sci Med* 2001;**53**:293–303.

55 Helweg-Larsen K, Knudsen LB, Petersson B. Women in Denmark—why do they die so young? Risk factors for premature death. *Scand J Soc Welfare* 1998;**7**:266–76.

56 Keating D, Hertzman C. *Developmental health and the wealth of nations: Social, biological and educational dynamics.* New York: The Guilford Press, 1999.

Index

Entries in **bold** refer to figures, those in *italics* refer to tables